Practical Endodontics
♦ *A Clinical Atlas* ♦

Practical Endodontics
◆ *A Clinical Atlas* ◆

Edward Besner, BS, DDS
Former Associate Clinical Professor, Department of Endodontics,
Georgetown University School of Dentistry, Washington, D.C.; Lecturer in
Endodontics, Institute for Graduate Dentists, New York; Consultant in Endodontics,
Veterans Administration Dental Training Center, Washington, D.C.;
Founder and Past President, Virginia State Academy of Endodontics;
Diplomate of the American Board of Endodontics

Andrew E. Michanowicz, BS, DDS
Former Clinical Professor and Chairman, Graduate Section of Endodontics,
Department of Restorative Dentistry, University of Pittsburgh, Pittsburgh,
Pennsylvania; Consultant in Endodontics, Allegheny General Hospital,
Division of Dental Medicine, Pittsburgh, Pennsylvania; Consultant in Endodontics,
Montefiore Hospital, Department of Dental Medicine, Pittsburgh, Pennsylvania;
Lecturer in Endodontics, Veterans Administration Hospital, Pittsburgh, Pennsylvania;
Diplomate of the American Board of Endodontics

John P. Michanowicz, BS, DDS
Former Associate Clinical Professor, Graduate Section of Endodontics,
Department of Restorative Dentistry, University of Pittsburgh, Pittsburgh, Pennsylvania;
Associate Professor, Medical College of Pennsylvania; Consultant in Endodontics, Department of
Dentistry, Allegheny General Hospital, Pittsburgh, Pennsylvania;
Consultant in Endodontics, Department of Dentistry, Montefiore Hospital,
Pittsburgh, Pennsylvania; Lecturer in Endodontics,
Veterans Administration Hospital, Pittsburgh, Pennsylvania;
Fellow of the American Association of Endodontics

With 923 illustrations

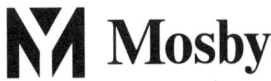

St. Louis Baltimore Boston Chicago London Madrid Philadelphia Sydney Toronto

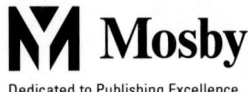
Dedicated to Publishing Excellence

Publisher: George Stamathis
Editor-in-Chief: Don Ladig
Executive Editor: Linda L. Duncan
Assistant Editor: Melba Steube
Project Manager: Carol Sullivan Wiseman
Senior Production Editor: David S. Brown
Senior Designer: Jeanne Wolfgeher
Manufacturing Supervisor: Betty Richmond
Illustrator: Jane Kobukata Gordon

Copyright © 1994 by Mosby-Year Book, Inc.

All rights reserved. No part of this publication may be reproduced, stored in a retrieval system, or transmitted, in any form or by any means, electronic, mechanical, photocopying, recording, or otherwise, without prior written permission from the publisher.

Permission to photocopy or reproduce solely for internal or personal use is permitted for libraries or other users registered with the Copyright Clearance Center, provided that the base fee of $4.00 per chapter plus $.10 per page is paid directly to the Copyright Clearance Center, 27 Congress Street, Salem, MA 01970. This consent does not extend to other kinds of copying, such as copying for general distribution, for advertising or promotional purposes, for creating new collected works, or for resale.

Printed in the United States of America

Mosby-Year Book, Inc.
11830 Westline Industrial Drive
St. Louis, Missouri 63146

Library of Congress Cataloging in Publication Data

Besner, Edward.
    Practical endodontics : a clinical atlas / Edward Besner, Andrew
  E. Michanowicz, John P. Michanowicz. — 1st ed.
      p.   cm.
    Includes index.
    ISBN 0-8016-7798-X
    1. Endodontics—Atlases. I. Michanowicz, Andrew E.
  II. Michanowicz, John P. III. Title.
    [DNLM: 1. Endodontics—atlases. WU 17 B555p 1994]
RK351.B469 1994
617.6'342—dc20
DNLM/DLC
for Library of Congress   93-7003
                                                               CIP

94 95 96 97 CA/MY 9 8 7 6 5 4 3 2

Dedicated to my wife, *Marlynne,* for her
support and sacrifices, and my daughters,
Robin, Tara, and *Allison.*
Edward Besner

Dedicated to my wife, *Louise,* for her loving
support, and my children, *Lou Ann* and
Andrew Michael and *their families.*
Andrew E. Michanowicz

Dedicated to *my children* and *my parents* for
their support, love, and sacrifices.
John P. Michanowicz

In Memory

◆

Louis I. Grossman
"The Father of Endodontics"

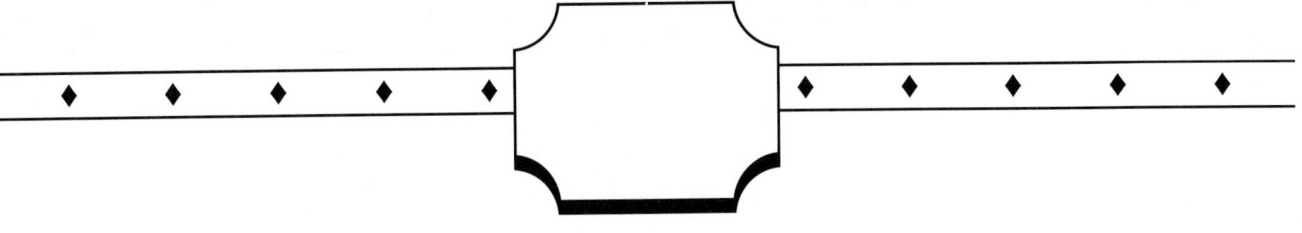

Preface

Endodontics has evolved from "root canal treatment" and from being taught as part of subjects such as Oral Medicine to a full-fledged specialty. However, endodontics continues to be a viable part of general practice.

There has been a constant inundation of new techniques and materials that make it difficult for the practitioner to choose one or more techniques for his or her treatment plan. To compound the problem each specialty has moved further in its own direction in teaching and practice, thereby making each specialist removed from the other specialties and general practice.

A lack of consistency has resulted. This book is a summation of all the authors' experiences in clinical practice so that the outcomes of the techniques and treatment outlined are reliable and predictable.

The text was written to be a guideline for the general practitioner and as a chairside manual during the treatment of endodontics. For additional information relating to the biological basis of endodontic therapy, one should refer to other textbooks and current literature.

This edition will be an invaluable aid to the student to help select a specific technique for treatment and to be aware of the alternatives.

The book will also serve as a reference and guide to other specialties in selecting the optimal course of treatment when combined therapy with other specialties requires a multidisciplined approach.

Thanks and appreciation are extended to our former residents and students from the University of Pittsburgh and Georgetown University who are now our colleagues. During their training they nurtured the desire for us to continue teaching and fostered the challenge for the future that culminated in the writing of this book.

Finally our thanks are given to our referring colleagues whose confidence in us helped us enjoy our clinical success, which is manifested in this book.

Edward Besner
Andrew E. Michanowicz
John P. Michanowicz

Acknowledgments

We would like to extend our gratitude and deepest appreciation to Toni Ewing, Nancy Gran, and Kathy Rak for their invaluable efforts in compiling, recording, and typing of the data and text. Their countless hours in recalling patients and retrieving information, combined with their photographic skills, have helped to bring the text to fruition. The hours resulted in time away from their families and our thanks is extended to them.

Our appreciation is also extended to the numerous manufacturers of endodontic products who were more than willing to offer assistance with their products.

Special Acknowledgment

We would like to thank our endodontic colleague Dr. Albert (Ace) Goerig for his valuable contribution to the chapters on Radiographic Interpretation and Restoration of the Endodontically Treated Tooth. Dr. Goerig is a Diplomate of the American Board of Endodontics and lectures internationally on endodontics. Dr. Goerig maintains a private practice limited to endodontics in Olympia, Washington.

Also, many thanks to June Buck for her essential contributions to the above chapters.

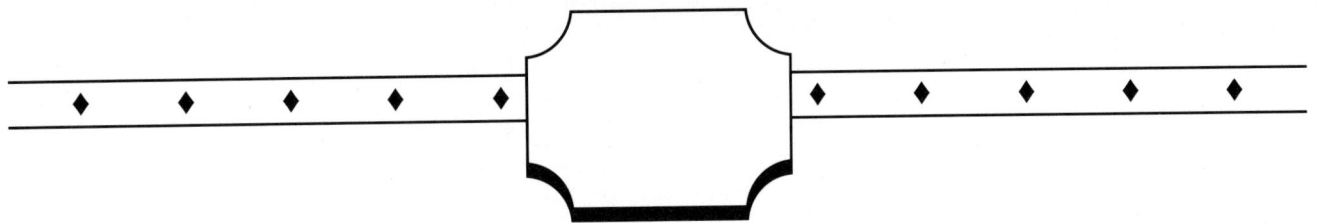

Contents

1 Introduction, 1

2 Diagnosis, 21

3 Radiographic interpretation, 41
Albert Goerig

4 Sterilization procedures and endodontic armamentarium, 63

5 Anatomical variations, 95

6 Routine endodontic therapy, 105

7 Low temperature thermoplasticized gutta percha (Ultrafil), 141

8 Comparison of other filling techniques, 159

9 Restoration of the endodontically treated tooth, 171
Albert Goerig

10 Endodontic complications and emergencies, 185

11 Nonsurgical retreatment, 197

12 Surgical endodontics, 227

13 Traumatic injuries, 243

Practical Endodontics
♦ *A Clinical Atlas* ♦

Introduction

In recent years, dentistry has changed its orientation more toward the prevention of dental disease. It stresses the replacement of affected dental structures resulting from disease or traumatic injury. Part of this success has been brought about by the dentist's ability to understand and respond to the need for the protection of the dental pulp and the supporting periodontium.

Endodontics is that discipline responsible for the diagnosis and treatment of the dental pulp and surrounding periodontal tissue. To appreciate the full scope of endodontics, an understanding of pulpal and periodontal pathology and treatments is necessary.

SCOPE OF ENDODONTICS

I. Pulpal and Periodontal Pathology
   A. Dentin exposure
   B. Pulp exposure
   C. Pulp pathology
   D. Pulp calcification
   E. Internal resorption
   F. External resorption
   G. Periapical and lateral pathology
   H. Periodontal-endodontic lesions
II. Endodontic Therapy
   A. Dentin protection
   B. Pulp capping
   C. Pulpotomy or apexification
   D. Pulpectomy and root canal therapy
   E. Endodontic surgery
      1. Amalgam resection or apicoectomy
      2. Amalgam repair
      3. Radisectomy (root amputation)
      4. Hemisectomy
   F. Endodontic implant
   G. Replantation and splinting
   H. Bleaching
   I. Retreatment of endodontically treated teeth
      1. Iatrogenic perforations
      2. Removal of separated instruments
      3. Removal of silver cones
      4. Removal of posts
      5. Removal of gutta percha
      6. Removal of root canal cements

Pulpal and Periodontal Pathology

DENTIN EXPOSURE ♦ Caries, either coronal or radicular, is the most common cause of pulpal irritation. This stimulation to the protoplasmic extensions of the dentinoblasts produces inflammation of the pulp. Attrition by abrasion, fractures of the dentin, dental preparations, and gingival recession are other prime examples of causes of pulp irritation due to dentin exposure. Bacterial toxins may penetrate toward the pulp along the dentinal tubules.

PULP EXPOSURE ♦ Caries is the most common cause of pulp exposure. Even before the actual pulpal exposure, bacterial toxins have set up pulpal inflammation. With the exposure, more toxins and bacteria penetrate into the pulpal tissues. Iatrogenic causes and coronal and radicular fractures are responsible for pulp exposures, resulting in injury or death of the pulp (Fig. 1-1).

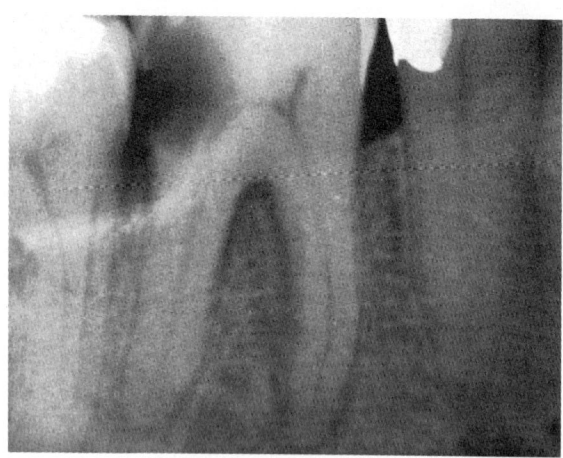

Figure 1-1 Pulpal pathology. Radiograph of a mandibular first molar with a carious exposure on the distal surface of the tooth. Root canal therapy is indicated for this tooth.

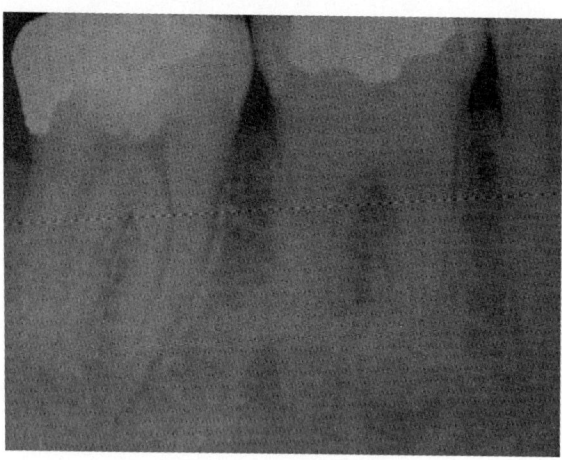

Figure 1-2 Pulp calcification. Radiograph of a mandibular first molar with calcification of canals and an area of radiolucency periapically. Root canal therapy is indicated. An attempt should always be made to treat an endodontic problem by a non-surgical approach. If the canals cannot be negotiated, then a surgical approach should be considered.

PULP PATHOLOGY ♦ Pulpal inflammation, abscesses, and pulpal necrosis are the most common types of diseases seen in the pulp. Chronic inflammation usually precedes any acute reaction. Bacteria may establish entry into the pulp through vascular means. With this anachoretic action, bacteria may originate from any part of the body, pass through the blood stream, and settle in an area of pulpal inflammation (Fig. 1-1).

PULP CALCIFICATION ♦ All pulps of vital teeth are stimulated to slow calcification. Traumatic injuries have broght about very rapid and almost complete calcifications. If no pulpal or apical pathology occurs, the tooth needs only watching. Other causes for rapid calcification are deep caries, deep irritating fillings, and trauma of occlusion (Fig. 1-2).

INTERNAL RESORPTION ♦ It is interesting that at times a traumatic injury that may cause calcification of the pulp is also capable of producing internal resorption. The dental destruction by resorption results from a metaplastic pulpal condition. Perforations of the coronal or radicular portion of the tooth most often result in pulpal contamination and thereby pulpal necrosis. Internal resorption is evident because the pulp canal wall is not visible in the resorbed dentin (Figs. 1-3,*A*, and 1-4).

EXTERNAL RESORPTION ♦ Unlike internal resorption, external root resorption is not caused by pulp dystrophy. It is the result of some chronic periodontal alteration that causes a resorption of the cemental and dentinal wall. Progression of this process may penetrate the pulp, setting up some pathology. Pulp necrosis does not produce a halt to this active process. Apical resorption with or without pulpal involvement may be a result of traumatic injury, trauma of occlusion, or orthodontic procedures (Figs. 1-3,*B*, 1-5, and 1-6).

PERIAPICAL AND LATERAL PATHOLOGY ♦ These pathologies are produced by extension of noxious pulpal stimuli and bacterial by-products into the tissues beyond the root. There are a number of pathologies, some acute and others chronic in nature. Suppurative by-products resulting from a low-grade inflammation may drain into a variety of anatomical structures, including mucosal or cutaneous surfaces, as a draining fistual (Fig. 1-7).

PERIODONTAL-ENDODONTIC LESIONS ♦ The extension of periodontal disease into the pulp has not been documented as pulpal disease on the periodontium. A sinus tract extending along the periodontal ligament may open into the gingival sulcus. This extension may pass through lateral canals in the area of the furcation of multirooted teeth, resembling a periodontal lesion. A successful endodontic treatment produces a termination of this sinus tract. At times a combination of endodontic and periodontal therapy is needed to correct the lesion (Fig. 1-8).

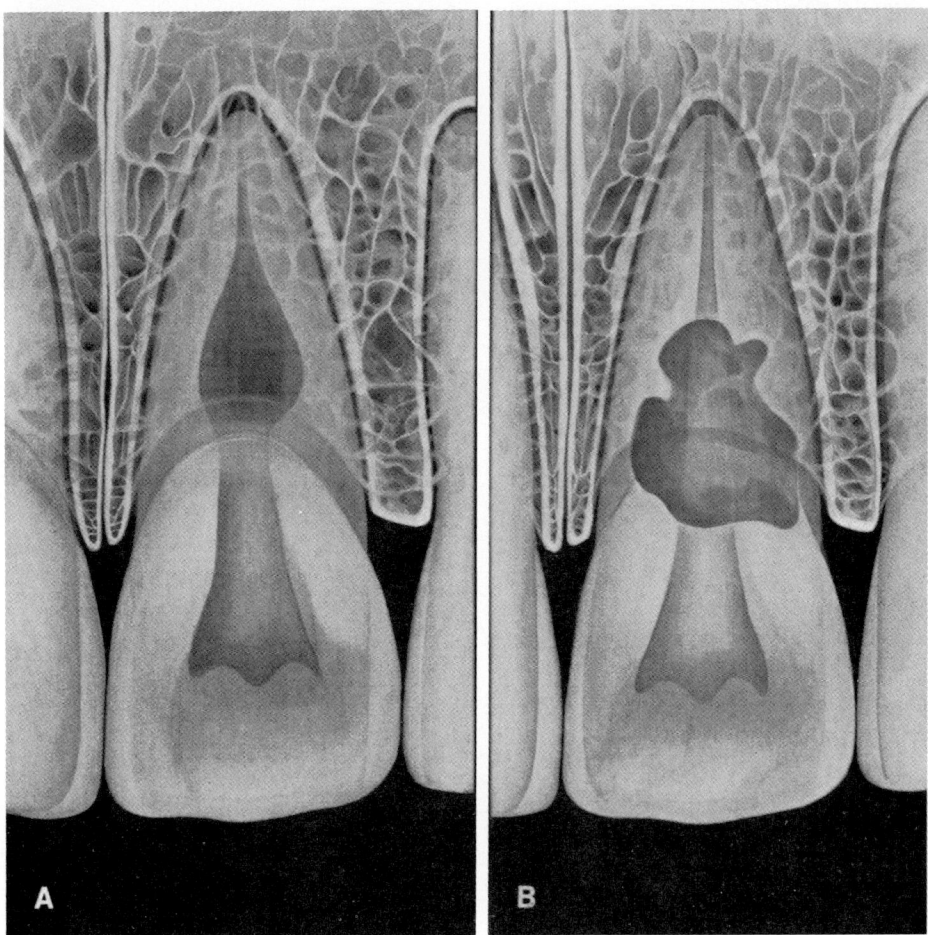

Figure 1-3 Drawing showing resorption. Internal and external root resorption show different characteristics radiographically and the treatment of each of these conditions differs. **A,** Internal root resorption is usually seen radiographically by following the outline of the canal. There is no disruption of the canal wall. Treatment involves removing the pulp. **B,** External root resorption is usually seen radiographically with the canal running right through the area of the resorption. There is disruption of the canal wall. Treatment involves sealing the resorbed area. If the resorption has perforated into the root canal, then endodontic therapy also becomes necessary.

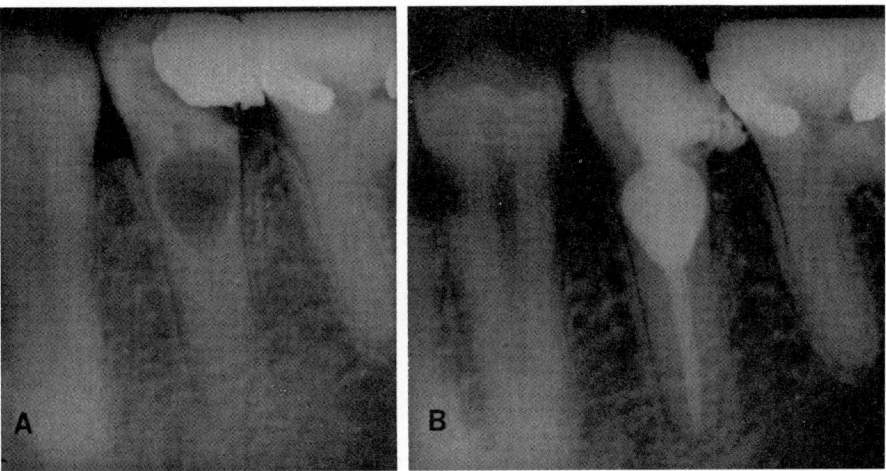

Figure 1-4 A, Preoperative radiograph of a mandibular second premolar depicting an extensive internal resorption. **B,** Postoperative radiograph of obturated canal and internally resorbed area after using the vertical condensation technique.

4   PRACTICAL ENDODONTICS

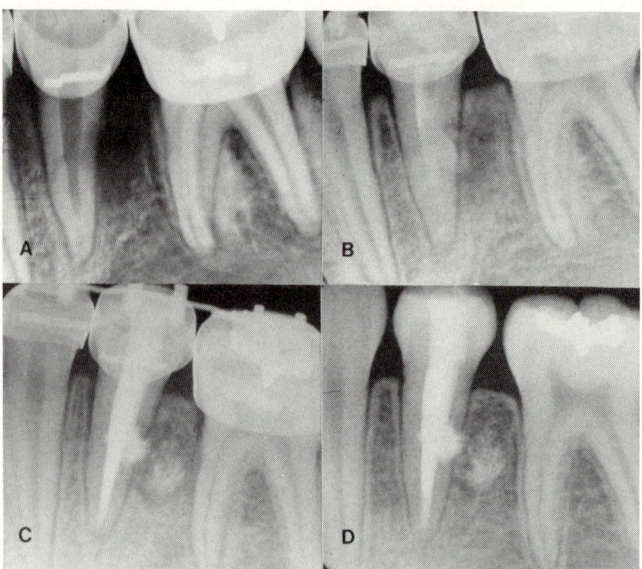

Figure 1-5 Non-surgical treatment for external root resorption. **A,** Preoperative radiograph of a mandibular second premolar demonstrating external root resorption. The resorption has perforated into the canal midway along the root on the distal side. **B,** The canal has been cleansed and shaped, and calcium hydroxide paste has been placed in the canal. The paste was changed every 4 weeks over a six-month period. **C,** Postoperative radiograph showing the obturation of the canal with gutta percha and sealer and the sealing off of the perforated defect. Note some of the sealant expressed into the adjacent osseous tissue. **D,** Six-month postoperative radiograph showing healing has taken place. (Courtesy of Dr. Martin Levin.)

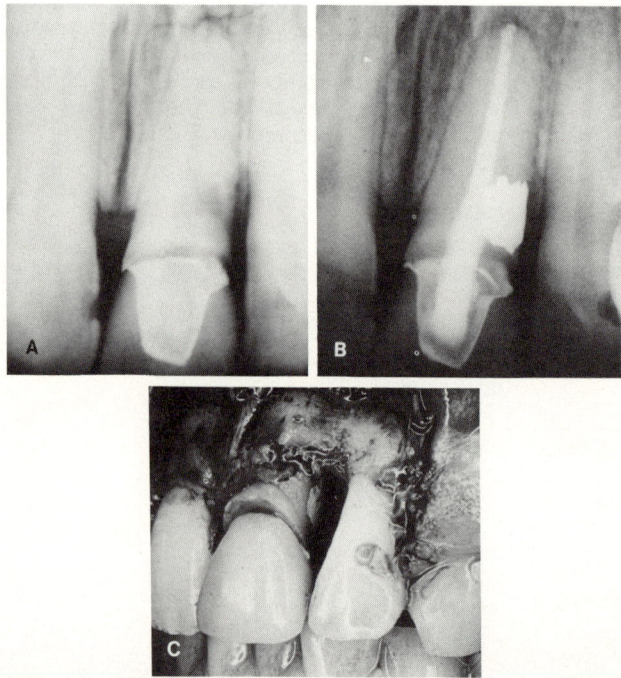

Figure 1-6 Surgical treatment for external root resorption. **A,** Preoperative radiograph of a maxillary central incisor with external root resorption on the distal surface of the root. **B,** Postoperative radiograph showing complete obturation of the canal and a surgical amalgam repair. **C,** View of surgical area with amalgam repair.

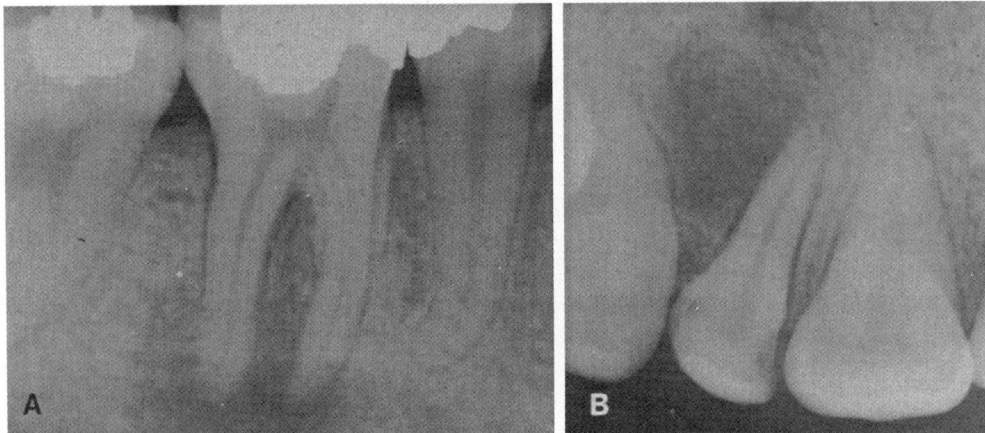

Figure 1-7 Periapical and lateral pathology. **A,** Radiograph of a large periapical lesion around the mandibular first molar. **B,** Radiograph of lesion laterally around the maxillary lateral. In both cases, the area of radiolucency was attributed to a necrotic pulp.

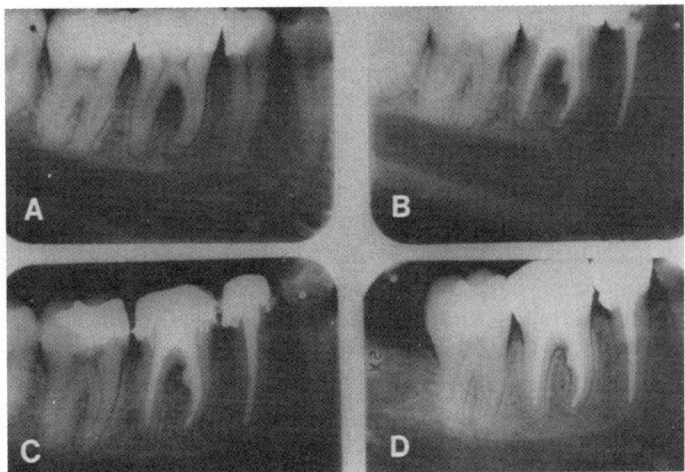

Figure 1-8 Periodontal-endodontic lesion. **A,** Radiograph of pulpally involved mandibular first molar showing severe furcation involvement. **B,** Treatment of tooth demonstrating lateral canal in the furcation. **C,** Six-month postoperative radiograph showing filling in the furca bone. **D,** Complete repair of the bone in the furca 1 year after root canal therapy. (Courtesy of Dr. Thomas Mullaney.)

Endodontic Therapy

DENTIN PROTECTION ♦ All exposed dentin should be covered before any irreversible pulp changes can result. It is important to seal these dentinal tubules; where applicable, a base should be placed under the restoration.

PULP CAPPING ♦ Pulp capping is the protection of a small pulp exposure by stimulating secondary dentin with a sedative dressing. Calcium hydroxide paste is placed in direct contact with the exposed pulp. Even after the formation of secondary dentin, pulpal pathology and necrosis may develop.

PULPOTOMY OR APEXIFICATION ♦ A pulpotomy is the removal of the coronal portion of the pulp and the placement of calcium hydroxide over the assumed healthy pulp. Apexification is the removal of a non-vital pulp and the placement of calcium hydroxide in the total canal. Both procedures are considered only tentative and both are to induce apical closure and the continued development of an immature tooth (Fig. 1-9).

PULPECTOMY AND ROOT CANAL THERAPY ♦ Pulpectomy consists of complete debridement of the pulp tissue and shaping of the entire root canal system, then obturated three dimensionally. This endodontic therapy is the most predictable (Fig. 1-10).

ENDODONTIC SURGERY ♦ Periapical surgery is indicated only when a routine endodontic procedure cannot be performed, such as a broken instrument in the canal and an area of radiolucency at the apex; a calcified canal with an area of radiolucency at the apex; or a perforated canal near the apex. In these cases, where there is good access, the retrograde amalgam can be performed. This procedure is used only to improve on the apical seal (Fig. 1-11).

A radisectomy or root amputation is the removal of one or more roots of a multirooted tooth. This procedure is most frequently used where there is extensive root caries or a root perforation that cannot be treated by routine endodontic therapy. Periodontal involvement of a root of a multirooted tooth can be treated with root canal therapy in the retained roots and root amputation of the periodontally involved root (Fig. 1-14).

Hemisectomy is the sectioning of a crown of a multirooted tooth. This may be followed with retaining both roots and constructing premolar crowns (premolarization or twinning) or with the removal of one of its roots and the attached portion of the crown (Fig. 1-15). This treatment is frequently used when one root is perforated beyond repair or calcified where an

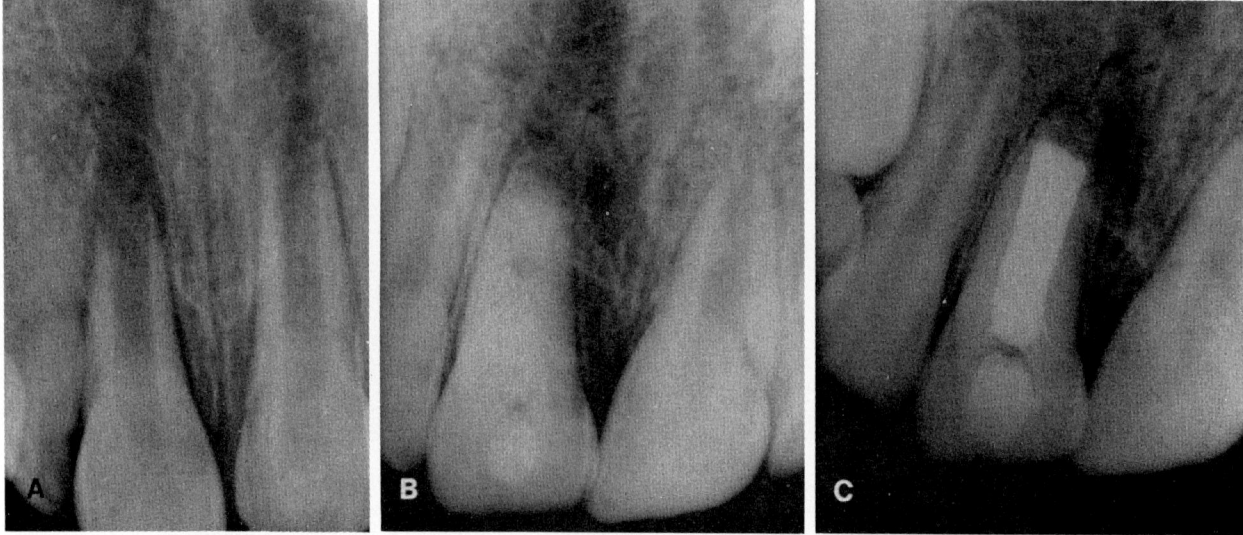

Figure 1-9 Series of radiographs demonstrating the apexification procedure. **A,** Preoperative radiograph showing open apex. The maxillary left central presented with pressure symptoms, and vitality tests gave a nonvital response. **B,** Radiograph showing the canal cleansed and shaped and obturated with calcium hydroxide. The calcium hydroxide dressing does not have to be changed unless leakage of the coronal seal is observed or absorption of the calcium hydroxide is observed radiographically. The tooth is examined clinically and radiographically in 3 months and then at 6-month intervals until apexification is complete. **C,** Postoperative radiograph showing a dentinal stop formation and the canal completely obturated with gutta percha.

amalgam resection is not possible. This therapy may also be indicated when one of the roots is periodontally involved and will not respond to any routine treatment.

ENDODONTIC IMPLANT ♦ This is an endodontic therapy in which the pulpal tissue has been debrided and the canal prepared and obturated with a titanium pin that is extended beyond the apex and into the alveolar bone. It is used to give greater stability to the tooth by producing a more favorable crown-root ratio (Fig. 1-16). It may also be used to splint two fractured segments or to increase the length of the root in root resorption cases.

REPLANTATION ♦ This is the replacement of a tooth that has been avulsed by some traumatic injury. If the tooth can be returned to its socket within a short period of time, the prognosis is most favorable (Fig. 1-18). Intentional replantation is the removal of a tooth from its socket, sealing the apices, and replanting the tooth to its socket. This procedure is indicated when a routine root canal therapy or apical surgery cannot be performed (Fig. 1-17).

BLEACHING ♦ Vital bleaching is the lightening of a tooth that has usually been stained by tetracycline therapy during the development of the tooth (Fig. 1-23). Non-vital bleaching is the lightening of a tooth that has been endodontically treated. The dentinal tubules have been stained by pulpal hemorrhage or dental products. Superoxol (30 or 35 percent hydrogen peroxide) is used as the oxygenating bleaching agent (Fig. 1-22).

RETREATMENT ♦ Retreatment is the undoing of the root canal fill and often the restorative part of the tooth. Basic endodontic principles are then followed to change the success of treatment (Fig. 1-24).

Text continued on p. 17.

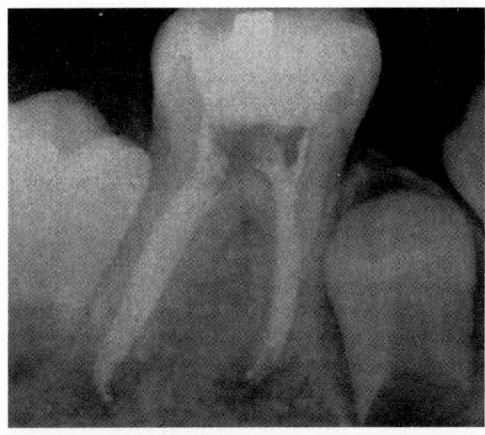

Figure 1-10 Pulpectomy and root canal therapy. Radiograph of a mandibular first molar with completed root canal therapy. Notice the shaping of each canal with the obliteration of the root canal system.

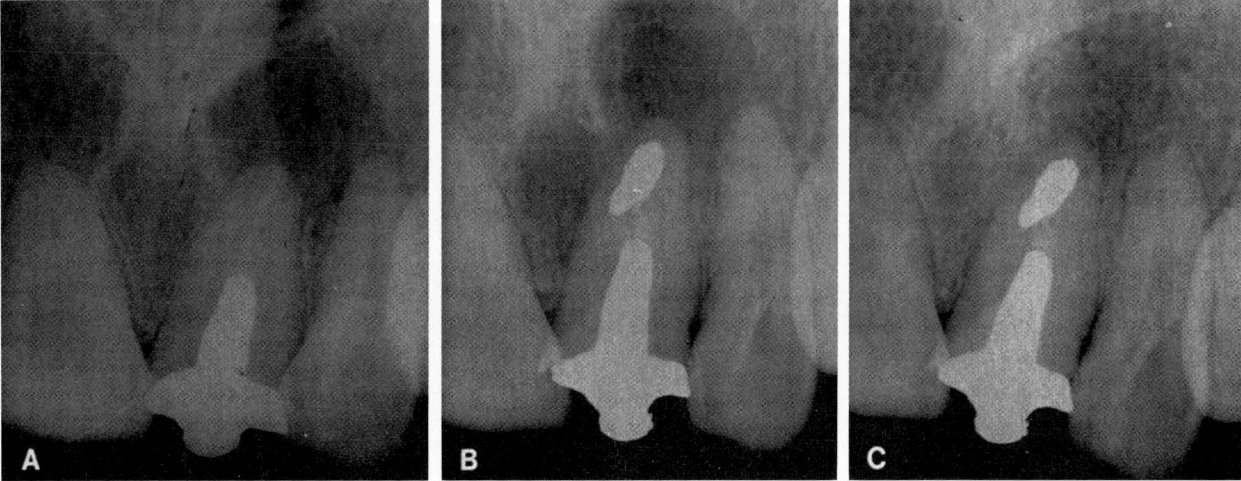

Figure 1-11 A, A failure of root canal due to improperly treated canal before placement of post and core. **B,** An amalgam retrofill placed apically to seal off the canal. **C,** Six-month postoperative radiograph showing healing taking place.

8 PRACTICAL ENDODONTICS

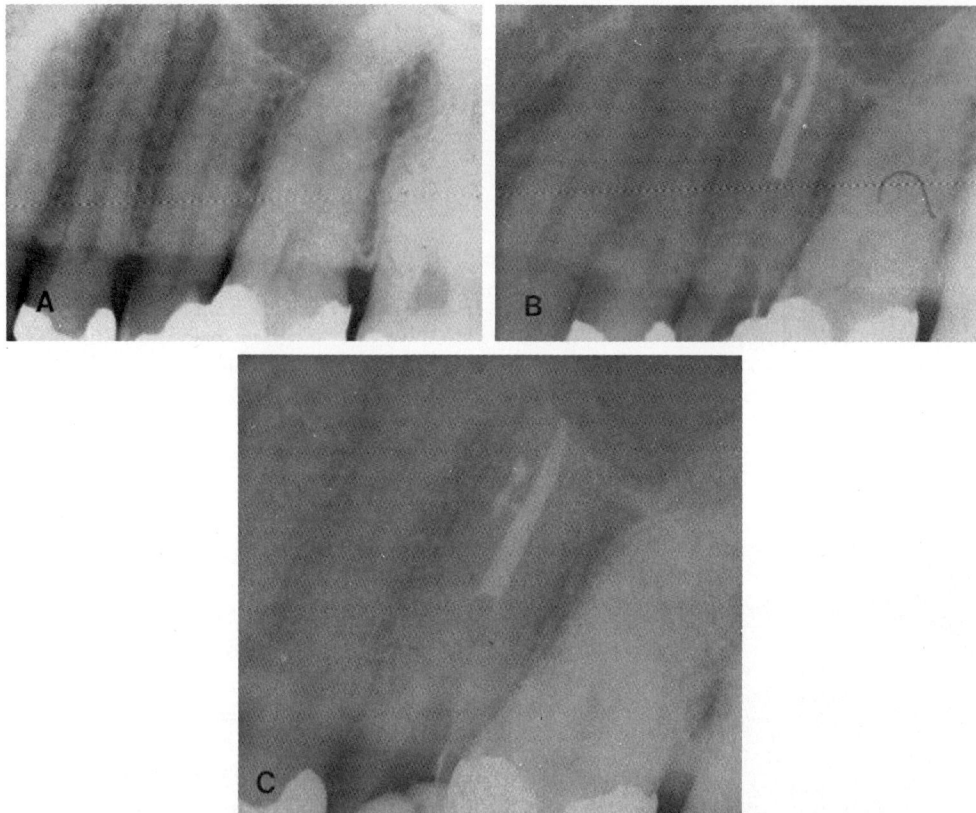

Figure 1-12 Series of radiographs demonstrating an apicoectomy procedure. **A,** Preoperative radiograph showing curved root in the apical area of the maxillary second premolar. **B,** Radiograph showing well condensed gutta percha in canal with lateral canal on mesial aspect. However, the integrity of the apical canal had not been maintained. Patient continued to have symptoms. **C,** Apicoectomy had to be performed to eliminate the ledge and to achieve a complete apical seal. After this procedure was performed, the tooth became asymptomatic.

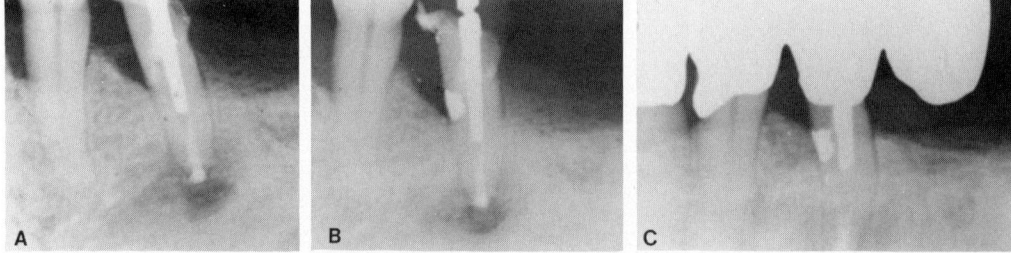

Figure 1-13 Series of radiographs demonstrating treatment of a perforation with an amalgam repair. **A,** Radiograph of a perforation at the level of crestal bone created by a bur. **B,** Amalgam repair by a surgical approach. A cavity preparation was made at the point of the perforation, and amalgam was condensed into the preparation. A recontouring of the bone was done to correct the periodontal defect. **C,** One-year postoperative radiograph showing healing taking place. Note that the level of bone on the buccal surface does not go above the amalgam as appears from the radiograph. No pocket depth could be demonstrated.

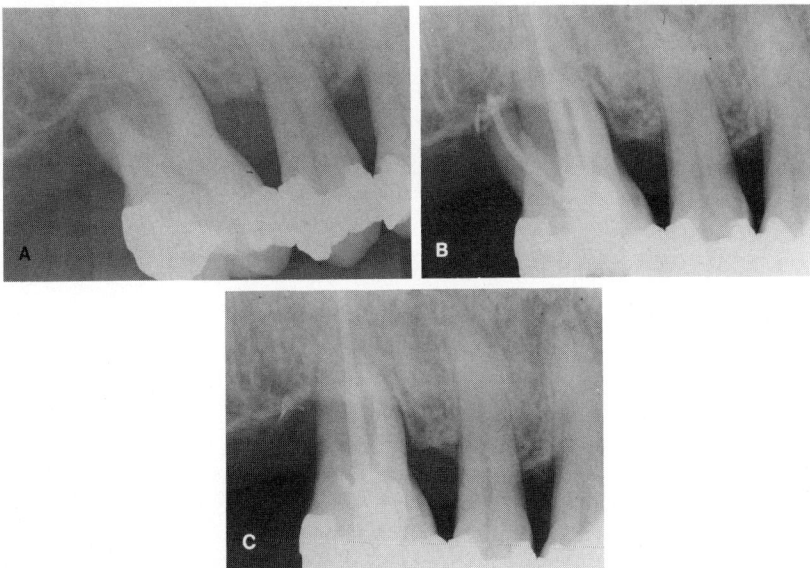

Figure 1-14 Series of radiographs demonstrating a radisectomy. **A,** Preoperative radiograph showing osseous defect around the distal root. **B,** Radiograph after root canal therapy. Distal root had been filled due to the length of time before patient could have distal root amputated. **C,** Postoperative radiograph showing distal root removed.

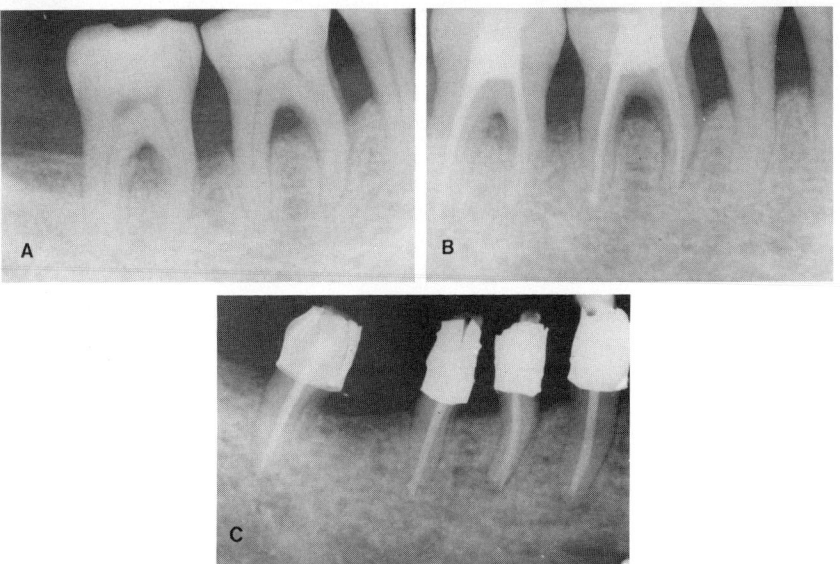

Figure 1-15 Series of radiographs demonstrating hemisections. **A,** Preoperative radiograph showing severe defect of the supporting apparatus in the area of the furca of the first and second molars. **B,** Root canal therapy performed on the mesial and distal roots of both teeth. **C,** Both molars were sectioned in two. The mesial root of the second molar was removed. The distal root of the second molar, both roots of the first molar, and the second premolar were prepared for crowns.

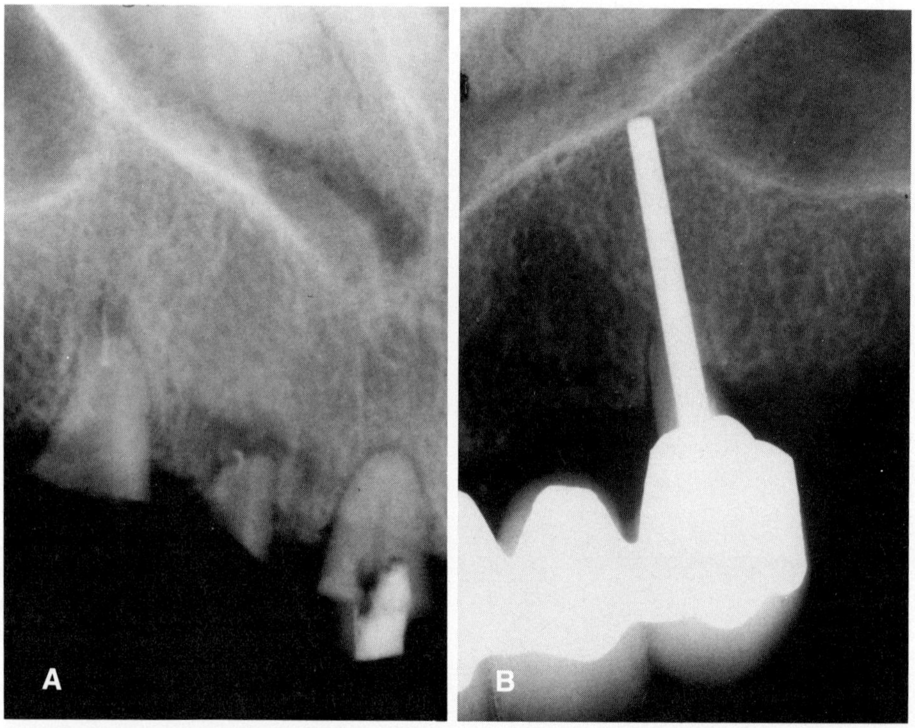

Figure 1-16 The use of an endodontic implant for internal stability and increasing the crown to root ratio. **A,** Radiograph of a short root in the maxillary cuspid. **B,** Radiograph after tooth is restored with an endodontic implant.

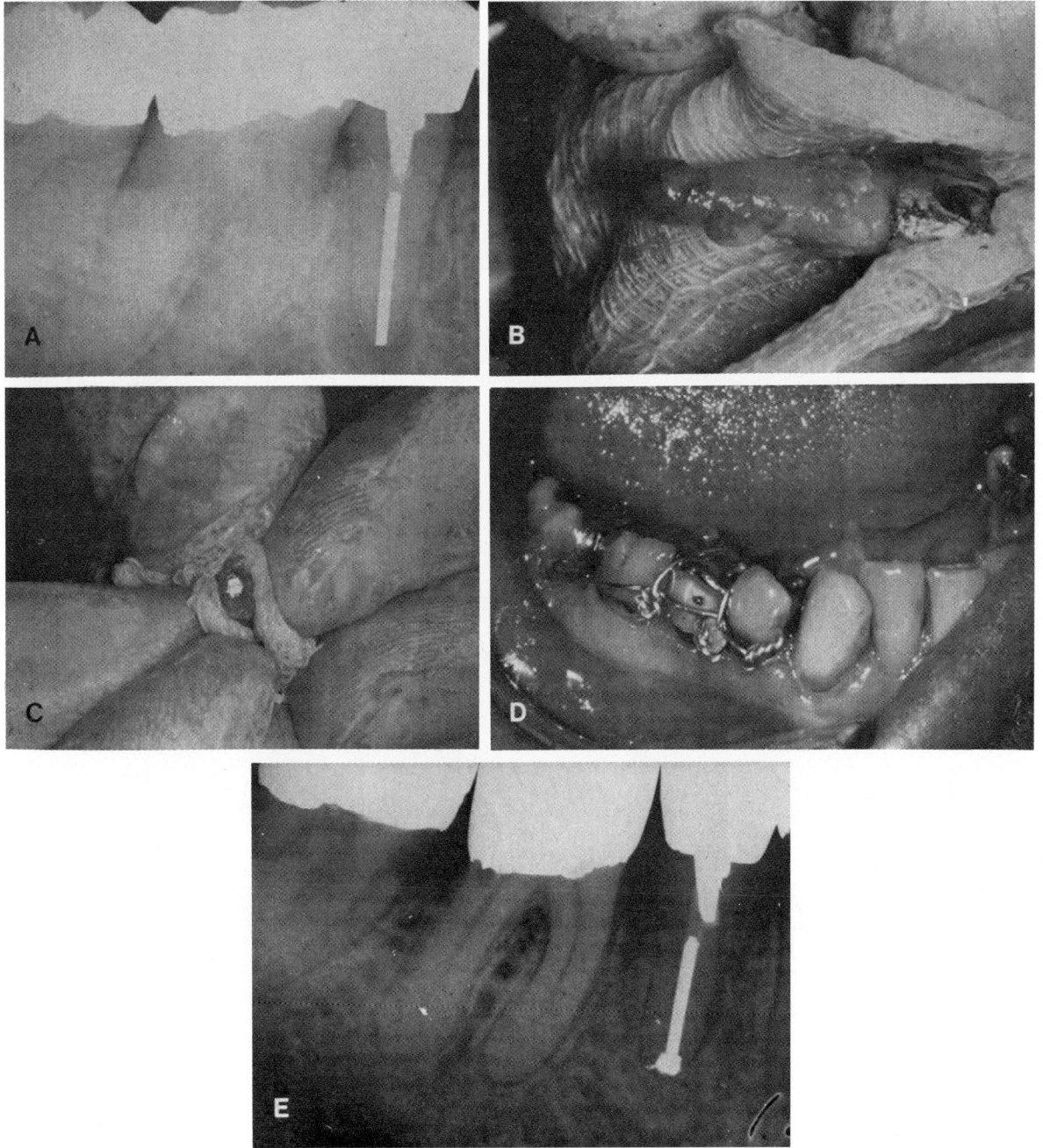

Figure 1-17 Series of radiographs and photographs showing an intentional replantation procedure. **A,** Preoperative radiograph of the mandibular second premolar showing a silver point in the canal with a post crown. An area of radiolucency can be seen. The tooth could not be retreated due to the position of the silver point in the canal. A retrograde amalgam would have been difficult because of the location of the mental foramen. **B,** The tooth was removed and held in a wet gauze sponge saturated with saline solution. **C,** A retrograde amalgam was placed at the apex. **D,** Tooth was placed back into the socket and stabilized with a wire splint. **E,** A 1-year postoperative recall showing healing taking place.

12 PRACTICAL ENDODONTICS

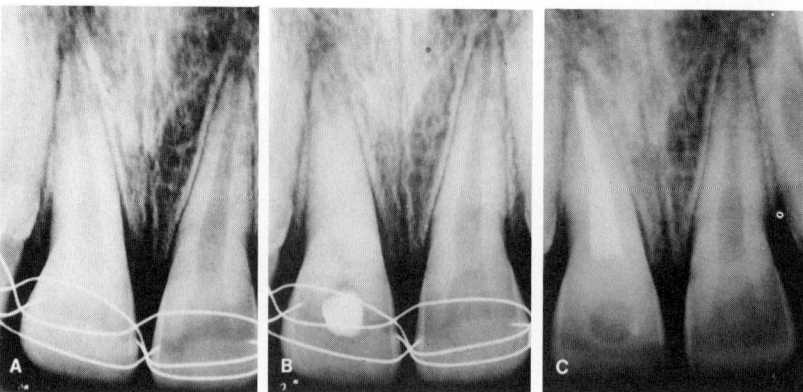

Figure 1-18 Treatment of an avulsed tooth. **A,** Maxillary central replanted and stabilized with a wire splint. **B,** Root canal therapy started two weeks after the accident. The canal had been cleansed and shaped and calcium hydroxide placed in the canal. This material was changed every 4 weeks for a period of 6 months. After no evidence of root resorption could be seen for a 6-month period, the root canal was sealed with gutta percha. **C,** Radiograph of completed root canal therapy.

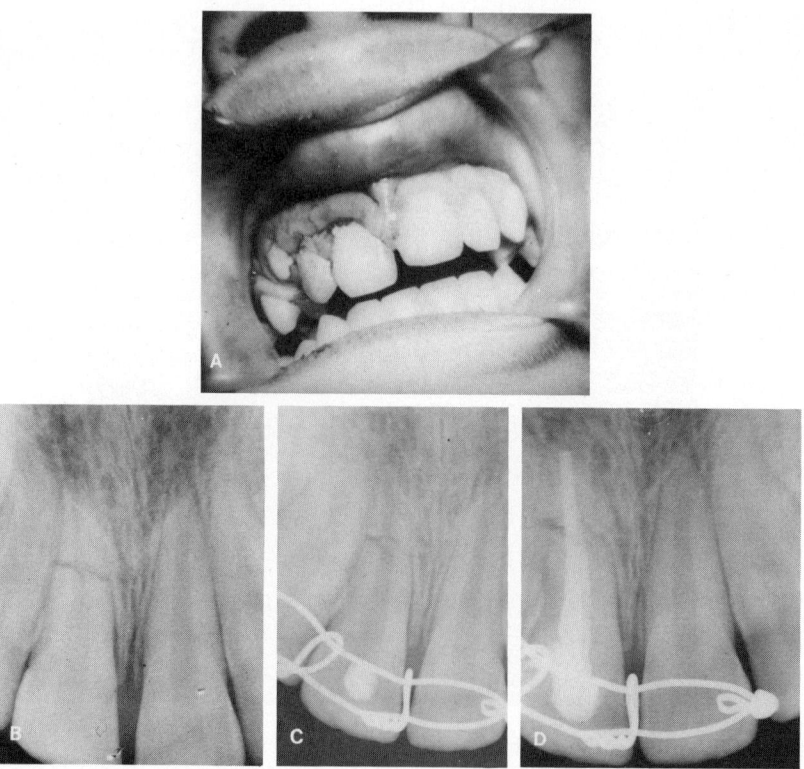

Figure 1-19 Series of photographs and radiographs demonstrating splinting technique using wire ligature splint. **A,** Patient fell, forcing the center incisor lingually. **B,** Radiograph showing horizontal root fracture in same tooth. **C,** Wire splint in place. The wire is looped around the involved tooth and one adjacent tooth on one side and two on the other side. A wire is placed interproximally, one leg above and one leg below the contact point. Each interproximal wire is twisted, and the ends are cut and tucked interproximally. **D,** Radiograph showing endodontically treated tooth and wire splint in place. In most cases of horizontal root fractures, the pulp will remain vital. An accurate response to vitalilty tests cannot be obtained until a few months after the accident. In this case, endodontic symptoms developed.

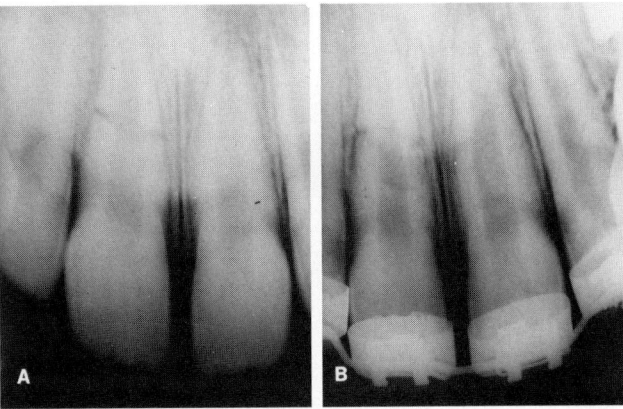

Figure 1-20 Splinting using orthodontic bands and arch wire. **A,** Horizontal root fracture in the mid-root of a maxillary central. **B,** Splinting using orthodontic bands and wire. In this case, the pulp maintained its vitality.

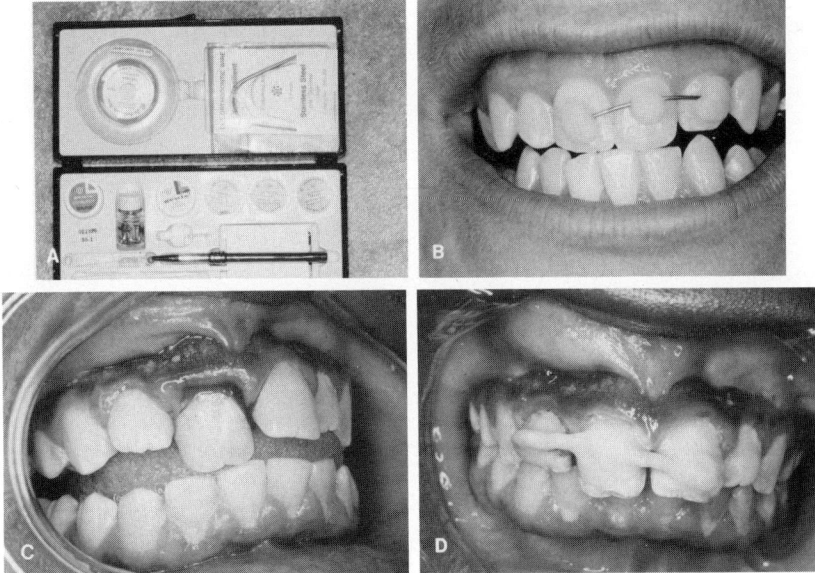

Figure 1-21 Splinting using acid etching technique. **A,** Kit with acid etching material, wire, and composite material. **B,** A wire is adapted to the involved tooth and one adjacent tooth on each side. The teeth are acid etched, a composite material is placed on the teeth, and the wire is then embedded in the material. **C,** A traumatic injury causing the maxillary right central to be displaced lingually. **D,** The tooth was repositioned into proper occlusion and the acid etching technique used. The composite material was applied to the involved tooth and one adjacent tooth on each side, and the wire was embedded in the material. The wire was then coated with the composite for aesthetics. (Courtesy of Dr. Robert Sears.)

14 PRACTICAL ENDODONTICS

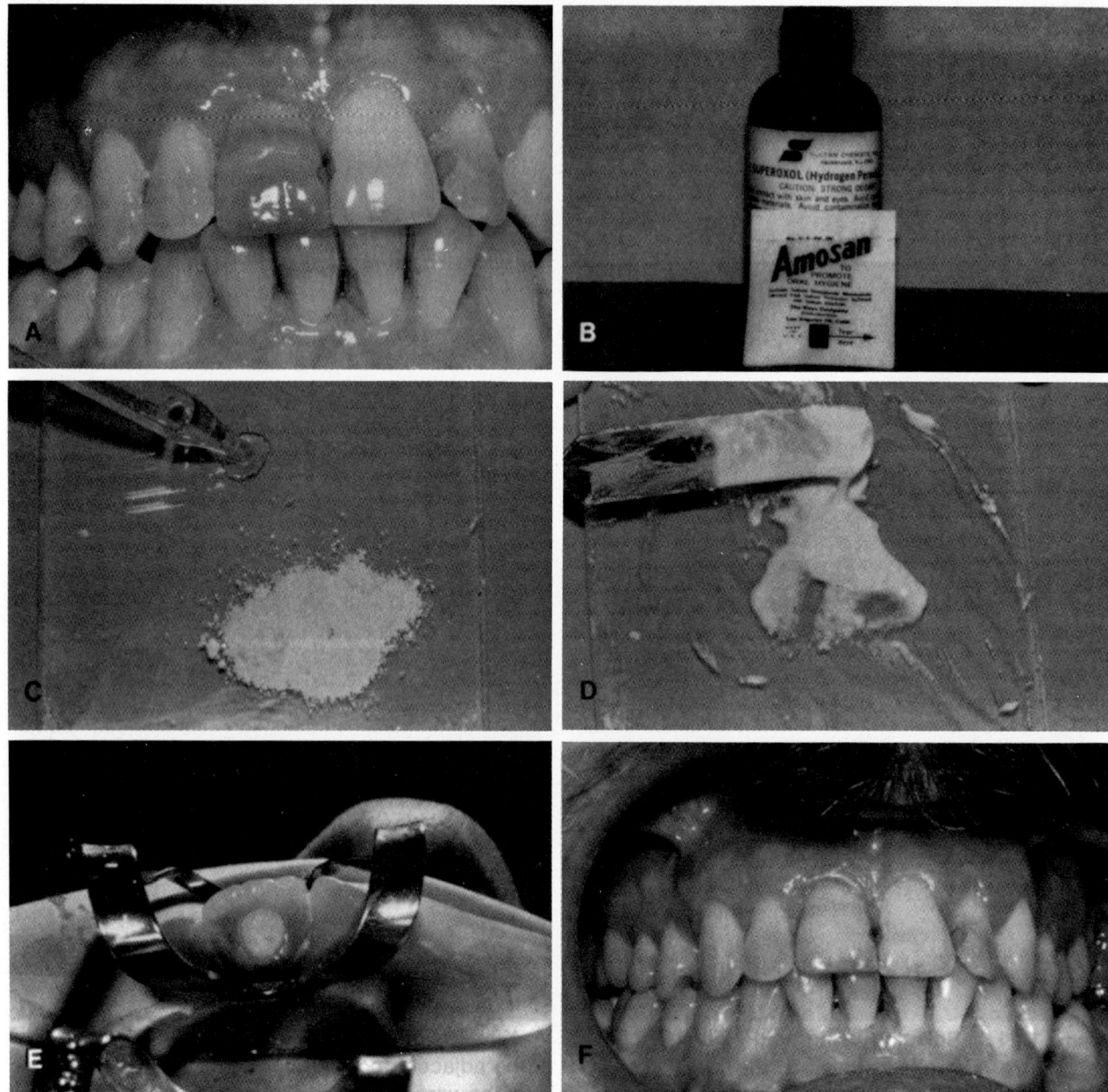

Figure 1-22 Series of photographs demonstrating a technique for bleaching the non-vital tooth. **A,** Discoloration of maxillary central incisor. **B,** Bleaching material (Superoxol and Amosan). Amosan contains sodium perborate, which is the bleaching agent. This mixed with Superoxol bleaches the crown. **C,** Placing one drop of Superoxol with Amosan Powder. **D,** Mixing Superoxol and Amosan. **E,** Placing the paste in the chamber after the chamber had been cleaned out to the cervical line. A layer of cement should be placed on the floor of the pulp chamber above the gutta percha before starting the bleaching process. A cotton pellet is placed over the paste, and a seal is placed on top. This is known as the "Walking Bleach." **F,** Bleaching result after 4 days. In some cases, the paste has to be changed every 5 to 7 days if discoloration persists. Studies have shown that Superoxol (30% hydrogen peroxide) may cause cervical resorption. Superoxol may be substituted with water and sodium perborate.

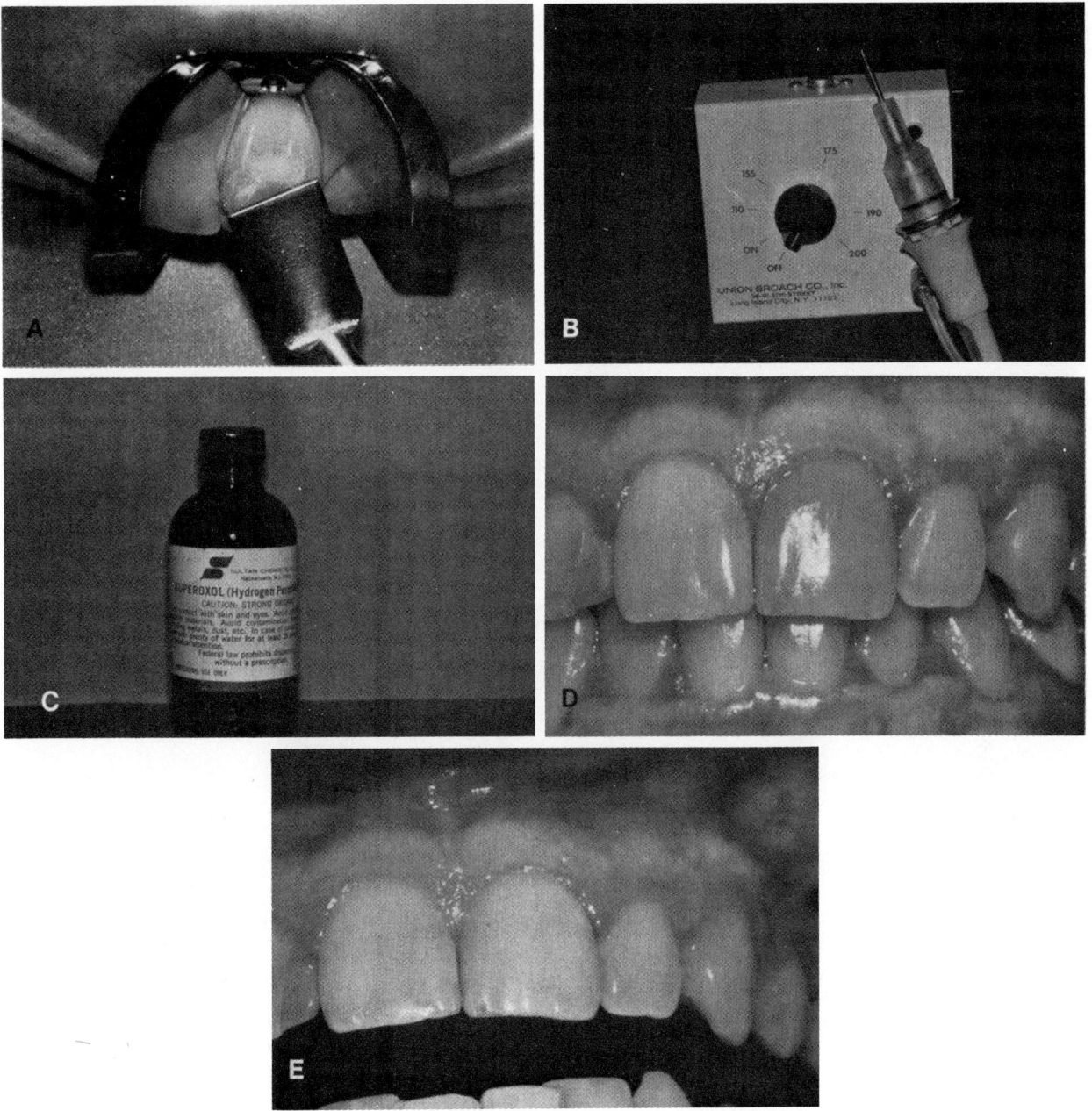

Figure 1-23 Series of photographs demonstrating bleaching of the vital tooth. **A,** Cotton pellet saturated with Superoxol placed on the stained tooth. A heating device is placed on the cotton. **B,** The heating instrument used is the Indiana heating instrument, which can regulate the amount of heat. **C,** Superoxol. **D,** Preoperative photograph of stained maxillary central. **E,** Postoperative photograph showing removal of stain.

16 PRACTICAL ENDODONTICS

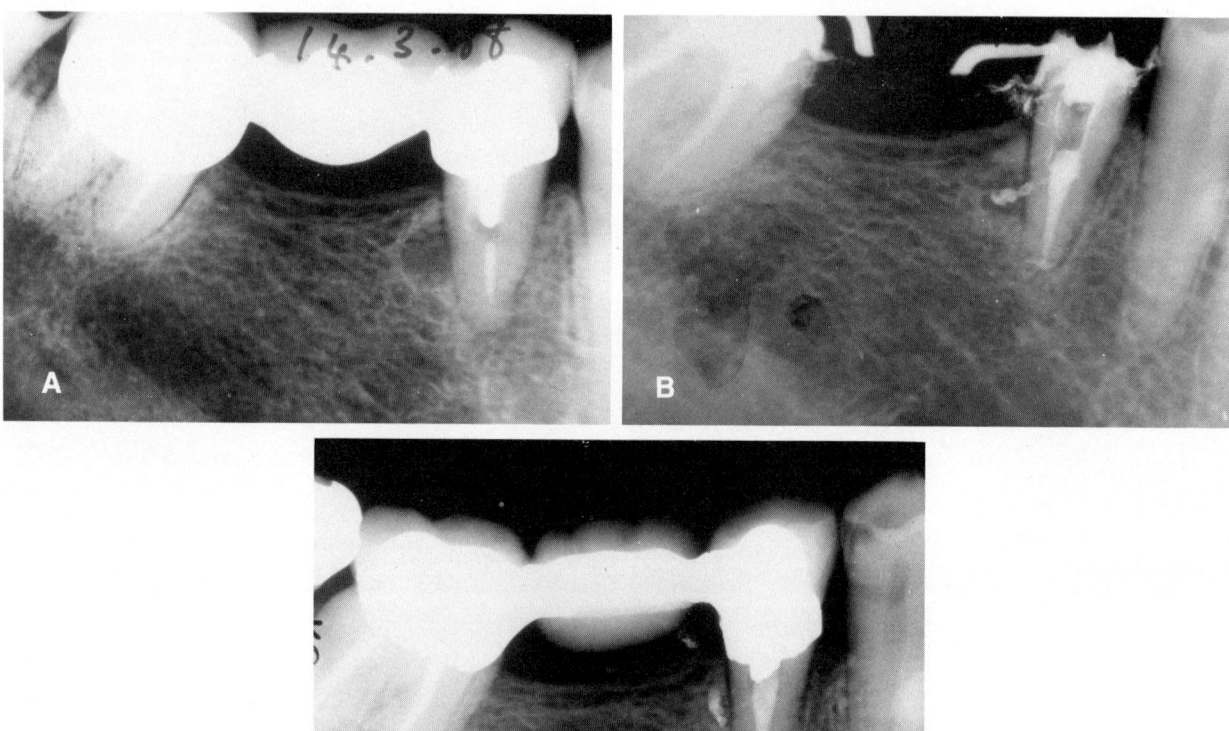

Figure 1-24 Series of radiographs demonstrating nonsurgical retreatment. **A,** Radiograph showing lateral radiolucency in midroot of an endodontically treated tooth. **B,** Post, bridge, and gutta percha removing and retreatment of root canal system demonstrating lateral canal at level of lateral radiolucency. **C,** Year recall demonstrating healing. (Courtesy of Dr. Pierre Machtou.)

BASIC ENDODONTIC CONCEPTS

It is the intent of the authors to limit the scope of this text to the treatment of the endodontically involved pulp and extended periapical lesion by a non-surgical approach. More than 90 percent of all endodontic problems can be treated by this one therapy. For a predictable and reproducible success in endodontic therapy, these important factors are necessary:

1. A careful and complete diagnosis must be made on each and every suspected tooth.
2. Careful interpretation of the radiograph should be made:
   - Outside of root:
     1. length of root
     2. curvature of root
     3. root formation
   - Inside of root:
     1. internal anatomy
     2. calcifications
     3. branching of canal
     4. resorptions
     5. pulp stones
     6. foreign bodies
     7. previous root canal
3. Emphasis should be placed on cleansing and shaping of canals rather than relying on intracanal medicaments (Figs. 1-25 and 1-26).
4. The internal anatomy of the root canal should be followed, and the integrity of the apex should be maintained (Figs. 1-27, 1-28, and 1-29).
5. Extra canals should be sought (Fig. 1-30).
6. Complete obturation of the entire root canal system both apically and laterally is our treatment objective (Figs. 1-31 and 1-32).
7. Gutta percha should be the filling material of choice (Fig. 1-33).
8. Surgery should be performed only to improve on the apical seal, not to remove pathosis (Fig. 1-33).

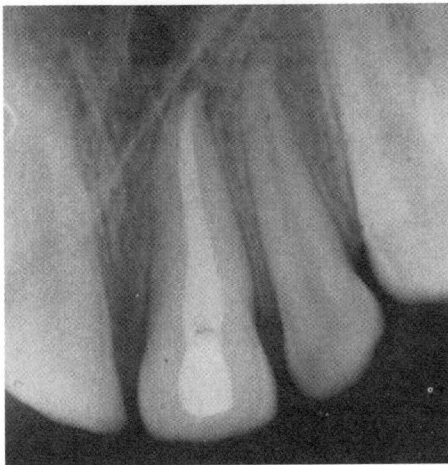

Figure 1-25 Radiograph of an endodontically treated maxillary central incisor. The canal has been properly cleansed and shaped to allow for complete obturation. Note the taper of the apical third of the canal and the body (middle third) of the canal. There is a gradual conical shape to the gutta percha.

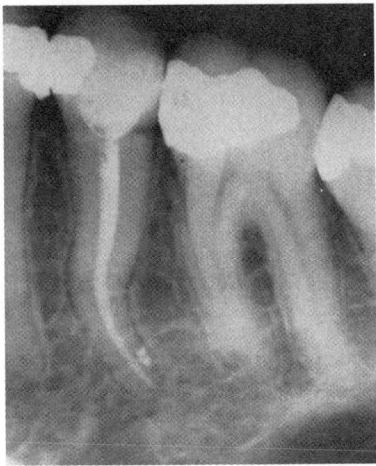

Figure 1-26 Radiograph of an endodontically treated mandibular right second premolar. With proper cleansing and shaping even for a curved canal, proper obturation has been made possible.

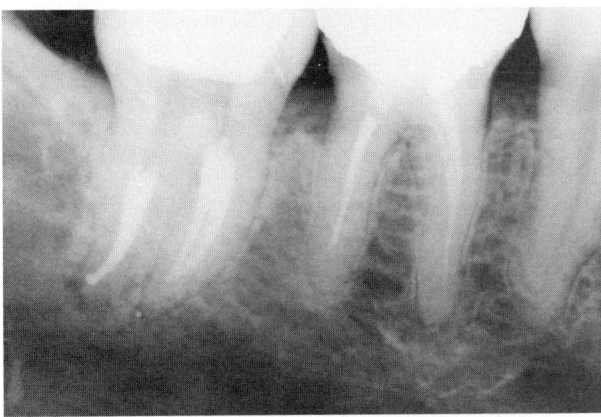

Figure 1-27 Radiograph of two endodontically treated teeth. Note the difference in treatment of the first and second molar. The integrity of the internal anatomy of the first molar was not followed.

18   PRACTICAL ENDODONTICS

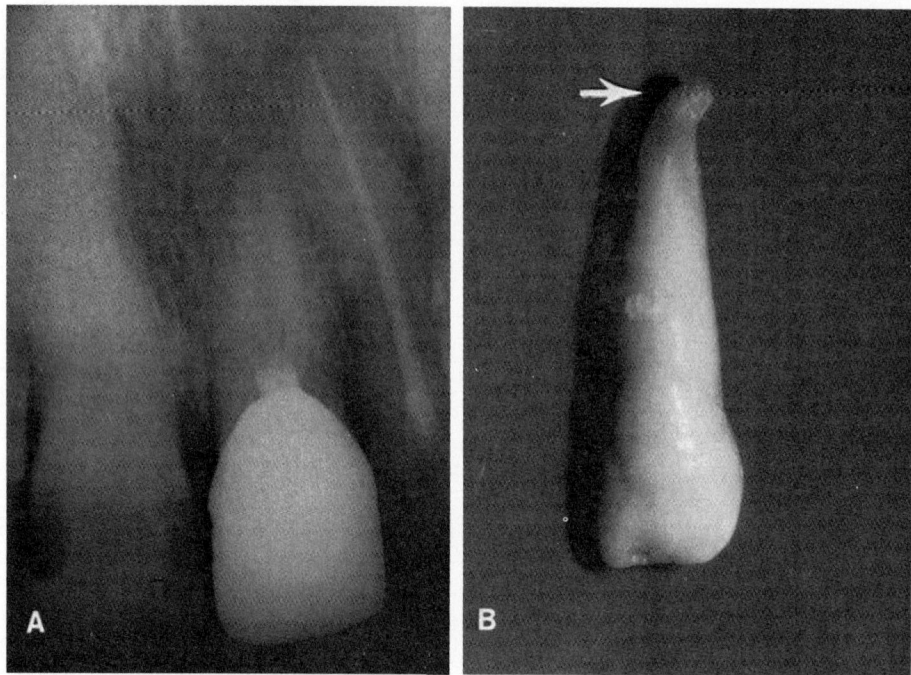

Figure 1-28 **A,** Radiograph of an endodontically treated lateral incisor. Note how the internal anatomy of the canal has been violated by perforation in the apical area. **B,** Examination of the tooth following extraction reveals that the integrity of the apex was not maintained. *Arrow* shows area of perforation.

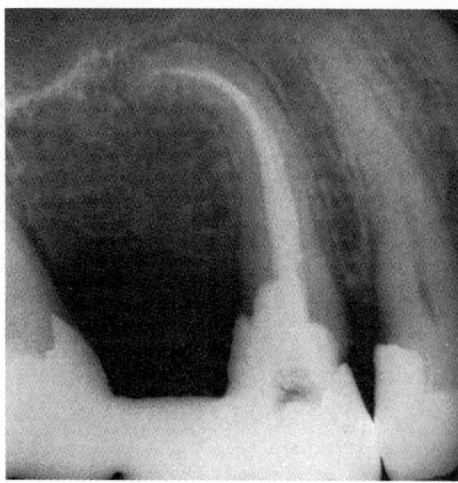

Figure 1-29 Even with a severe curvature of the canal, the internal anatomy and the integrity of the apex have been maintained.

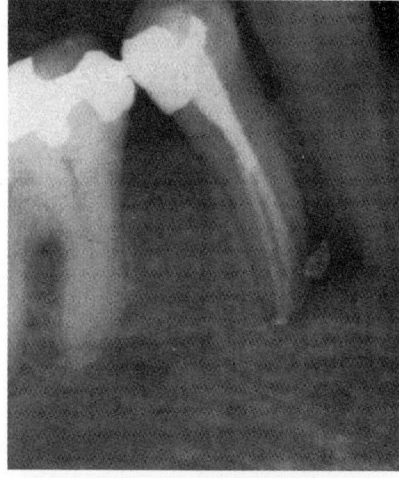

Figure 1-30 Radiograph of a mandibular premolar with a complex canal system. When treating a tooth endodontically, one is treating a root canal system. It is necessary to examine for extra canals. Sealant has been expressed.

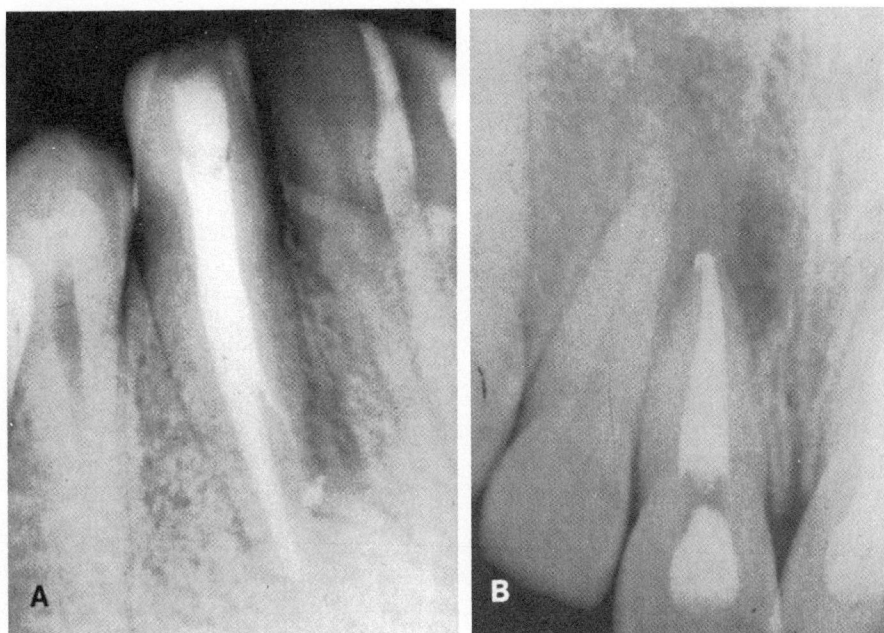

Figure 1-31 Complete obturation of the root canal system. **A,** Radiograph of accessory canal in the mandibular cuspid. Notice the density of the gutta percha in the root canal. **B,** Radiograph of maxillary central incisor. Notice the density and shape of the apical, middle, and coronal third of the root canal.

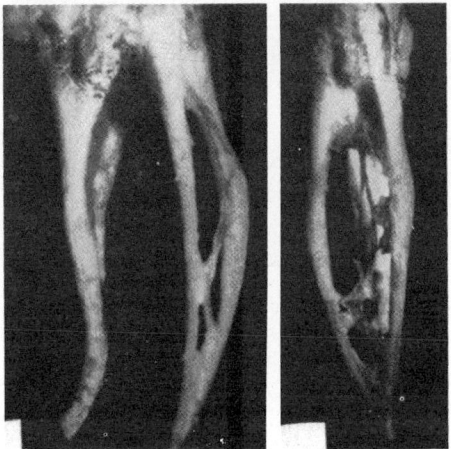

Figure 1-32 The photographs are of a lower molar that had root canal therapy completed; the tooth structure had been dissolved away, leaving the gutta percha intact. Notice the network of canals and the one homogeneous material that totally obliterates the root canal system. (From Davis SK, Brayton SM, and Goldman M: The morphology of the prepared root canal: a study utilizing injectable silicone, *Oral Surg* 34: 642-648, 1972.)

20   PRACTICAL ENDODONTICS

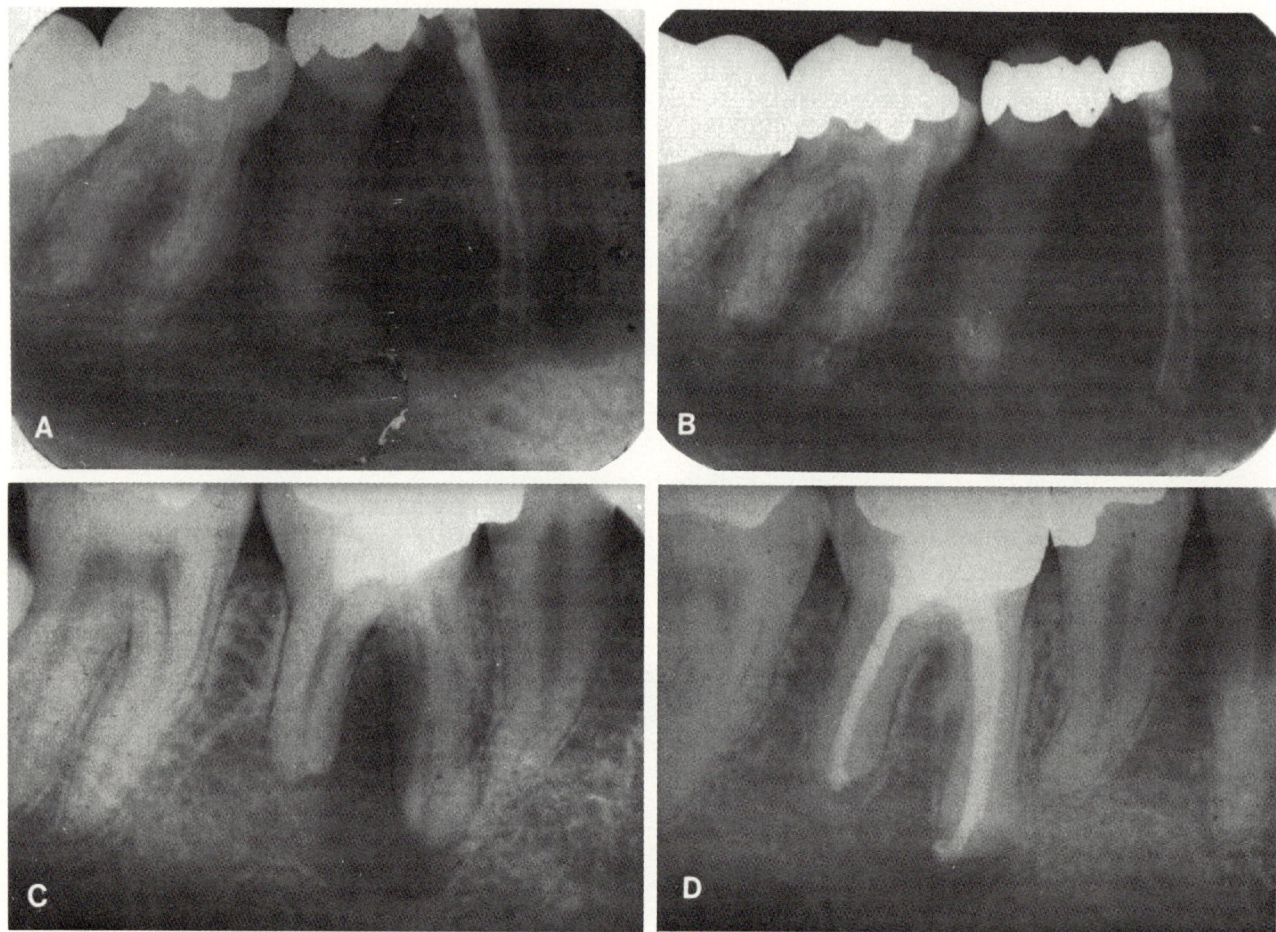

Figure 1-33 Surgery should be performed only to improve on the apical seal. **A,** Radiograph of an endodontically treated lesion. **B,** One-year postoperative radiograph of the previous tooth indicating a filling in of the previous lesion with bone. **C,** Radiograph of a pretreated endodontically involved molar with a rather large apical and interradicular lesion. **D,** Postoperative 6-month radiograph of the previous tooth demonstrating the ability of total healing by a nonsurgcial endodontic approach.

2

Diagnosis

The diagnostic approach to endodontic problems must be organized; it cannot be hit or miss. Although a tentative diagnosis can often be made with a single test, other diagnostic aids must be used for confirmation. No one test is that reliable.

The sequence of the diagnostic process is as follows:

I. Medical history
II. Dental history
III. Subjective symptoms
IV. Clinical observations
V. Clinical tests

STEP I: MEDICAL HISTORY

The medical history should include a record of sensitivities or reactions to any drug or antibiotic, the presence of cardiovascular disease (especially valvular disease with a history of rheumatic fever), blood dyscrasias, hormonal disease, and so forth.

Purpose: Knowledge of these medical factors might modify subsequent local treatment.

Table 2.1 is a medical history form that can be used to receive useful information concerning the overall medical status of the patient.

The box on p. 23 lists systemic conditions a patient may have or drugs he or she may be taking and the limitations these place on treatment.

Premedication of patients with a history of rheumatic fever, heart murmurs, or congenital heart disease is mandatory.

The box on p. 24 is adapted from a chart by the American Heart Association for the prevention of bacterial endocarditis.

Individuals with artificial pacemakers present a special type of problem in patient management. Because they rely on artificial cardiac stimulation for pacing the heart, it is extremely important that the dentist refrain from performing any procedure that would interfere with pacemaker function. Procedures such as pulp testing, sonic devices for determining root length, or electrosurgery are contraindicated. In any medically compromised patient the attending physician should be consulted before dental treatment.

STEP II: DENTAL HISTORY

The dental history should include the following questions:
1. What is the patient's past total dental treatment?
2. What is the chief complaint?
3. What is the history of the chief complaint?
4. Has the patient had any recent fillings?
5. Were there any unusual problems concerning the tooth, such as pulp capping or pulpotomy procedure, or a large restoration performed?
6. Has the tooth ever been subjected to a sharp blow in an accident of some kind?
7. Has a swelling or a gum boil around the tooth ever been noticed? If yes, what did the patient do?
8. Has there been any drainage from the tooth or gum?

Purpose: Often the problem tooth can be localized by taking the dental history.

TABLE 2-1 ♦ *Medical History*

Questions	Yes	No	Comments
1. Are you in good health?			
2. Have you had any change in health since last year?			
3. Have you had major or minor surgery in the past 5 years?			
4. Are you now being treated by a physician? If so, for what condition?			
5. Are you now taking any drugs or medication? If so, what medication?			
6. Are you pregnant? If so, approximate date of delivery?			
7. Have you ever fainted?			

8. Have you ever had any of the following?
    High blood pressure
    Low blood pressure
    Rheumatic fever
    Heart murmur
    Kidney disease
    Hepatitis
    Asthma
    AIDS
    Cancer
    Sinusitis
    Heart condition
    Diabetes
    Liver disease
    Nervous disorders
    Hay fever
    Anemia
    Abnormal bleeding
    Alcoholism
    Drug addiction
    Epilepsy			

9. Have you ever undergone psychiatric therapy?			
10. Do you have any allergies? If so, to what are you allergic?			
11. Are you allergic to local anesthetic? If so, what anesthetic?			

12. Have you ever had any ill effects from the following?
    Novocaine
    Penicillin or other antibiotics
    Aspirin
    Codeine
    Any other drugs			

13. Do you wear a pacemaker?			
14. Do you presently or have you had any other medical problems?			

The Medically Compromised Patient

Patient having *hyperthyroidism*:
1. No epinephrine in the anesthetic (use Carbocaine or Citanest).
2. Increase the amount of sedative if patient requires it.

Patient having *ulcers*:
1. No aspirin can be used.
2. If using penicillin, must use Penicillin V rather than Penicillin G (In all situations Penicillin V is preferable when administered orally).
3. No tetracycline can be used if patient is taking antacids.

Patient having *gout*:
No aspirin can be used.

Patient on *CNS stimulants* such as *amphetamine*:
Increase the sedative if the patient requires it.

Patient is an *alcoholic*:
1. Aspirin must not be used before or after the consumption of alcohol.
2. Sedatives must be used cautiously.

Patient taking *antidepressant drugs (MAO inhibitor)*:
1. General anesthesia must be used cautiously.
2. Narcotic analgesics must be used cautiously.
3. Antisialagogue such as atropine or banthine should be used in decreased dosage if patient requires it.

Patient taking *antihypertensive drugs,* such as *reserpine*:
1. General anesthesia must be used cautiously.
2. Sedatives must be used cautiously (the dosage may have to be reduced).

Patient taking *sulfonamides*:
No procaine anesthetic or procaine penicillin can be used.

Patient on oral *antidiabetic* agents, such as *Phenoformin* or *Diabinese*:
1. Barbiturates must be used cautiously.
2. Aspirin must be used cautiously.

Patient having *convulsive* disorders:
No Darvon can be used.

Patient having *liver* damage:
Use acetaminophen (Tylenol) cautiously when patient requires it.

Patient having *head injuries*:
No narcotics can be used.

Patient must not take *aspirin* when:
1. Patient is taking an anticoagulant.
2. Patient has blood dyscrasia.
3. Patient has had a kidney transplant.

Must be cautious when taking *aspirin*:
1. When patient has asthma.
2. When patient is a diabetic.
3. When patient is in her last month of pregnancy.

Patient must not take *tetracycline* when:
1. Patient has been taking penicillin.
2. Patient has been taking antacid.

Patient must use *barbiturates* cautiously when:
1. Patient is taking griseofulvin (antifungal drug).
2. Patient is taking Dilantin.
3. Patient is taking steroids.

When *prophylactic antibiotics* must be used:
1. Penicillin is preferable with patients who have a history of rheumatic fever, a heart prosthesis, or diabetes.
2. Erythromycin is preferable with patients who have kidney disorders.

For the Prevention of Bacterial Endocarditis: Recommendations by the American Heart Association.

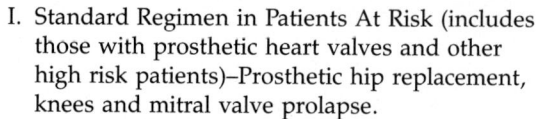

I. Standard Regimen in Patients At Risk (includes those with prosthetic heart valves and other high risk patients)–Prosthetic hip replacement, knees and mitral valve prolapse.
   Amoxicillin 3.0 g orally 1 hour before procedure, then 1.5 g 6 hours after initial dose. (See pediatric dosages below.)
For amoxicillin/penicillin-allergic patients:
   Erythromycin ethylsuccinate 800 mg or erythromycin stearate 1.0 g orally 2 hours before a procedure, then one-half the dose 6 hours after the initial administration. (See pediatric dosages below.)
   -OR-
Clindamycin 300 mg orally 1 hour before a procedure and 150 mg 6 hours after initial dose.*

II. Alternate Prophylactic Regimens For Dental/Oral/Upper Respiratory Tract Procedures in Patients At Risk:
   A. For patients unable to take oral medications:
      Ampicillin 2.0 g IV (or IM) 30 minutes before procedure, then ampicillin 1.0 g IV (or IM) OR amoxicillin 1.5 g orally 6 hours after initial dose. (See pediatric dosages below.)
      -OR-
      For ampicillin/amoxicillin/penicillin-allergic patients unable to take oral medications:
      Clindamycin 300 mg IV 30 minutes before a procedure and 150 mg IV (or orally) 6 hours after initial dose. (See pediatric dosages below.)
   B. For patients considered to be at high risk who are not candidates for the standard regimen:
      Ampicillin 2.0 g IV (or IM) plus gentamicin 1.5 mg/kg IV (or IM) (not to exceed 80 mg) 30 minutes before procedure, followed by amoxicillin 1.5 g orally 6 hours after the initial dose. Alternatively, the parenteral regimen may be repeated 8 hours after the initial dose. (See pediatric dosages below.)
For amoxicillin/ampicillin/penicillin-allergic patients considered to be at high risk:
   Vancomycin 1.0 g IV administered over 1 hour, starting 1 hour before the procedure. No repeat dose is necessary. (See pediatric dosages below.)

Note: Initial pediatric dosages are listed below. Follow-up oral dose should be one-half the initial dose. Total pediatric dose should not exceed total adult dose.

Amoxicillin*:	50 mg	Vancomycin:	20 mg
Clindamycin:	10 mg	Ampicillin:	50 mg
Erythromycin ethylsuccinate or stearate	20 mg	Gentamicin:	2.0 mg

For Genitourinary/Gastrointestinal Procedures

I. Standard regimen:
   Ampicillin 2.0 g IV (or IM) plus gentamicin 1.5 mg/kg IV (or IM) (not to exceed 80 mg) 30 minutes before procedure, followed by amoxicillin 1.5 g orally 6 hours after the initial dose. Alternatively, the parenteral regimen may be repeated once 8 hours after the initial dose.*
For amoxicillin/ampicillin/penicillin-allergic patients:
   Vancomycin 1.0 g IV administered over 1 hour plus gentamicin 1.5 mg IV (or IM) (not to exceed 80 mg) 1 hour before the procedure. May be repeated once 8 hours after initial dose. (See pediatric dosages below.)

II. Alternate oral regimen for low-risk patients:
   Amoxicillin 3.0 g orally 1 hour before the procedure, then 1.5 g 6 hours after the initial dose. (See pediatric dosages below.)

Note: Initial pediatric dosages are listed below. Follow-up oral dose should be one-half the initial dose. Total pediatric dose should not exceed total adult dose.

Ampicillin:	50 mg	Gentamicin:	2.0 mg
Amoxicillin:	50 mg	Vancomycin:	20 mg

Note: Antibiotic regimens used to prevent recurrence of acute rheumatic fever are inadequate for the prevention of bacterial endocarditis. In patients with markedly compromised renal function, it may be necessary to modify or omit the second dose of gentamicin or vancomycin. IM injections may be contraindicated in patients receiving anticoagulants.

---

*The following weight ranges may also be used for the initial pediatric dose of amoxicillin:
33 lbs: 750 mg
33 to 66 lbs: 1500 mg
66 lbs: 3000 mg (full adult dose)

STEP III: SUBJECTIVE SYMPTOMS

Careful questioning of the patient must be conducted to evaluate the patient's problem completely. The following are typical questions that may be asked:
1. Is the pain present now?
2. What type of pain is it (sharp, dull)?
3. Is the pain localized or diffuse?
4. Is there throbbing?
5. Is the pain intermittent or continuous?
6. Is the pain increased by cold, heat, pressure, mastication, lying down, sweet, or sour?
7. Do you have to take anything hot or cold to bring on the pain?
8. Is the pain spontaneous?
9. Does it go away by itself or do you have to take medication?
10. Does hot or cold make it feel better?
11. Does the tooth feel loose? If yes, when did you first notice it?
12. How long does the pain last?

Purpose: A tentative diagnosis can often be made from the subjective symptoms.

STEP IV: CLINICAL OBSERVATIONS

These are the objective signs observed by the clinician in and around the mouth. It is important to note the following:
1. Extraoral swelling (Fig. 2-1)
2. Lymph node involvement
3. Intraoral swelling (Fig. 2-2)
4. Fistula (sinus tract)-intraoral, extraoral

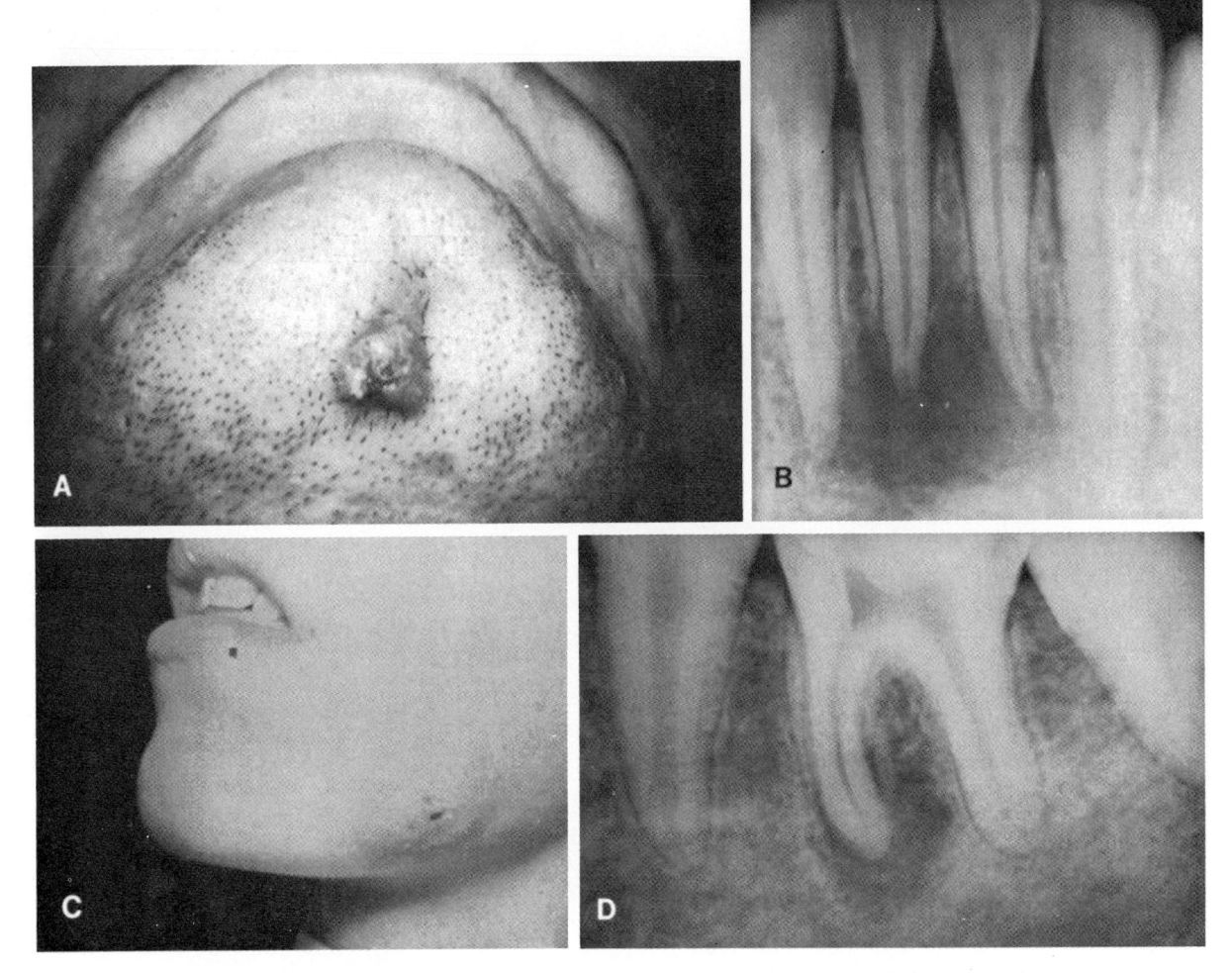

Figure 2-1 Part of the clinical observation is to note any abnormalities not only intraorally, but extraorally as well. **A,** Photograph of drainage to the surface of the chin from a fistula of a suppurative apical periodontitis. Case was misdiagnosed by patient's physician and treated with antibiotics over a 10-year period. **B,** Radiograph of involved tooth enabled proper diagnosis and proper therapy. **C,** Extraoral draining fistula. Patient sought treatment of a plastic surgeon to remove lesion near the angle of the mandible. **D,** A radiograph was taken demonstrating a periapical radiolucent area around the mesial root of the mandibular first molar.

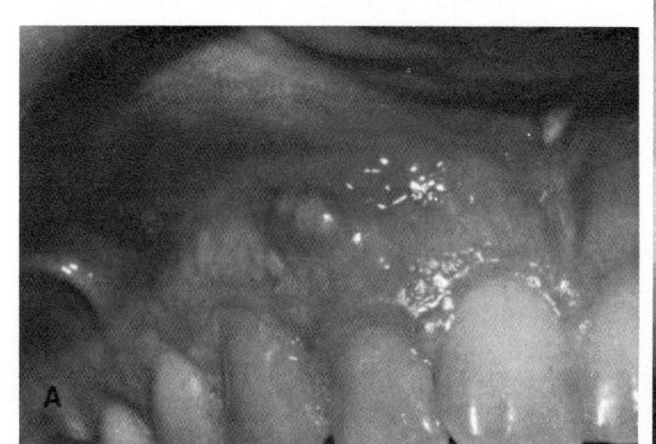

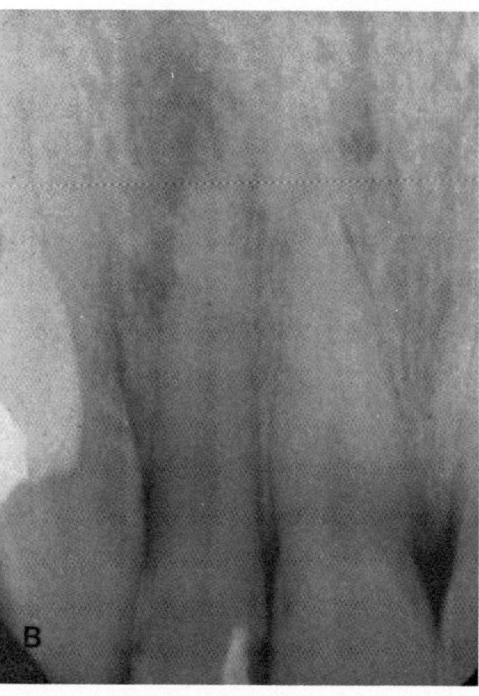

Figure 2-2 After noting any abnormalities extraorally, the focus of attention is then intraoral. **A,** Photograph of a chronic draining fistula over lateral incisor giving rise to a parulus (gumboil). **B,** Radiograph shows a periapical lesion of the lateral draining into the parulus seen in the previous picture.

5. Tooth discoloration
6. Traumatic injuries such as crown and root fractures
7. Presence of a deep carious lesion
8. Recurrent caries beneath a restoration
9. Type and extent of restoration
10. Developmental defects of teeth
11. Gingival recession
12. Color of gingival tissue
13. Temperature elevation
14. Traumatic occlusion
15. Loose, leaking, or fractured restorations
16. Mobility

Purpose: Often the problem tooth can be localized, and the dentist may see other contributing factors involved. A judgment on whether the involved tooth is worth salvaging can also be made.

STEP V: CLINICAL TESTS

These tests are mandatory to confirm any tentative diagnosis that has been made so far. All eight of these tests must be used, and in certain cases the selective tests must be used in addition.

Diagnostic Tests (Fig. 2-3) (Table 2-2)

1. Electric pulp test (Fig. 2-5)
2. Thermal tests
   Cold—Ethyl chloride or ice (Fig. 2-6)
   Hot—Gutta percha heated (Fig. 2-7)
3. Percussion (Fig. 2-8)
4. Palpation (Fig. 2-9)
5. Mobility (Fig. 2-10)
6. Periodontal evaluation (Fig. 2-11)
7. Occlusal evaluation (Fig. 2-12)
8. Radiograph (Fig. 2-13)

Selective Tests for Difficult Diagnostic Situations (Fig. 2-4)

9. Test cavity preparation (Fig. 2-14)
10. Anesthetic test (Fig. 2-15)
11. Transillumination (Fig. 2-16)
12. Biting (Fig. 2-16, *D*)
13. Staining (Fig. 2-16, *E,* 2-17)
14. Gutta percha point tracing with radiograph (Fig. 2-19)

Purpose: The status of pulp and periapical tissue can be evaluated, and a diagnosis can be confirmed.

TABLE 2-2 ♦ *Diagnosis*

	Vital Pulp		Non-vital Pulp	
	Reversible Pulpitis	Irreversible Pulpitis	Chronic	Acute
1. History	Slight sensitivity	Constant or intermittent pain	May have had pain at some time	Usually have no severe pain
2. Electric pulp test	Response	Response	No response	No response
3. Thermal test				
Cold	Response	Marked prolonged response	No response	No response
Hot	Response	Marked prolonged response	No response	May or may not have response
4. Percussion	No sensitivity	Usually no sensitivity	No sensitivity	Sensitivity
5. Palpation	Not palpable	Not palpable	Not palpable	May be palpable
6. Radiograph	No periapical radiolucency, but deep restoration or caries	May or may not show periapical changes at apex	Periapical radiolucency	May or may not have periapical radiolucency

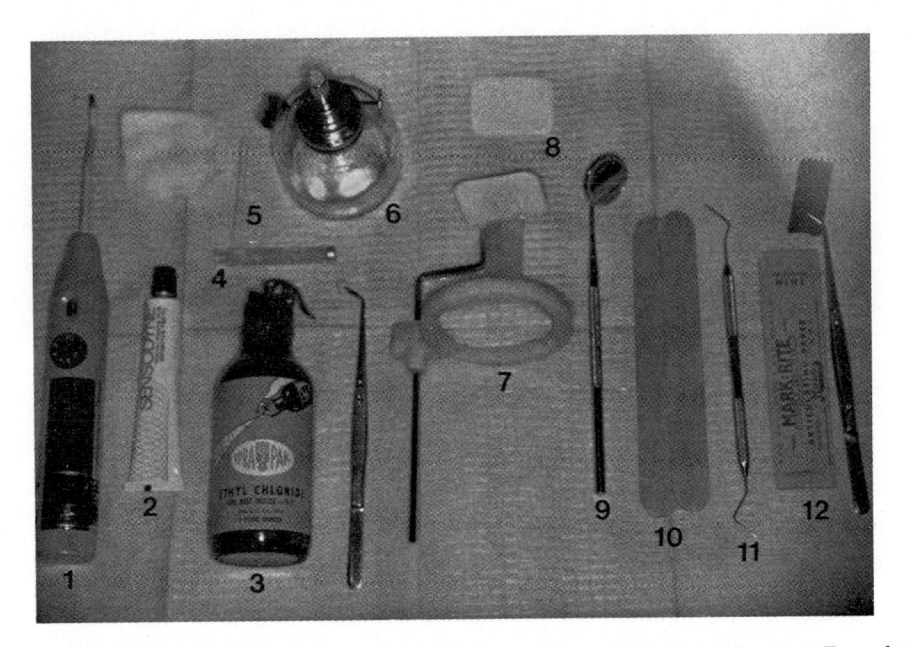

Figure 2-3 Diagnostic testing equipment useful for an endodontic evaluation. From left to right: *1*, battery pulp tester; *2*, tooth paste used as an electrolyte for the pulp tester; *3*, ethyl chloride spray bottle, cotton pellet held in cotton pliers used with ethyl chloride (cold test); *4*, anesthetic carpule filled with water and frozen (cold test); *5*, stick of gutta percha and *6*, alcohol lamp (heat test); *7*, XCP film holder and *8*, x-ray film; *9*, mirror (percussion test); *10*, tongue blades (mobility test); *11*, periodontal probe; *12*, articulating paper and cotton pliers used as holder (to check occlusion).

28 PRACTICAL ENDODONTICS

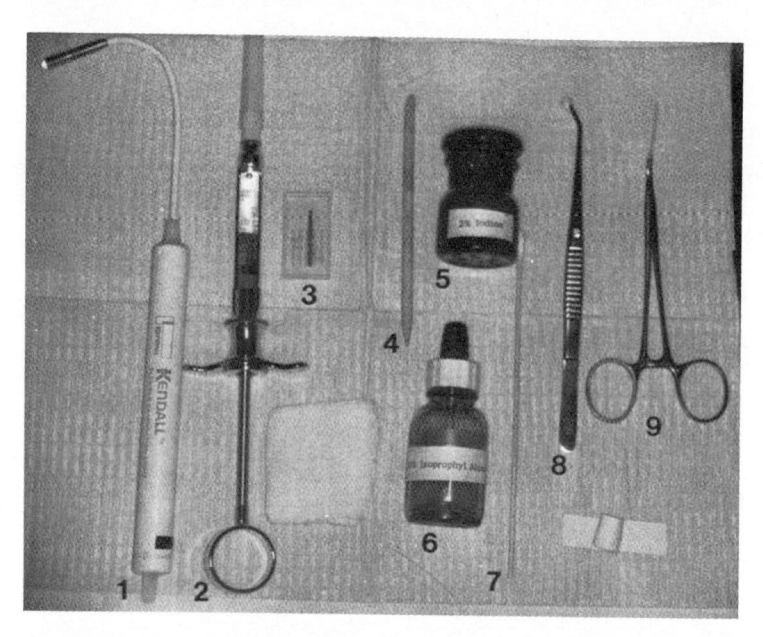

Figure 2-4 Diagnostic testing equipment for more difficult diagnostic situations. From left to right: *1*, fiber optic (transillumination); *2*, anesthetic syringe with carpules (selective anesthetic); *3*, bur (test cavity to determine pulp vitality); *4*, orangewood stick (check for fractured tooth); *5*, iodine (staining for fractured tooth); *6*, isopropyl alcohol (to wash stain off the tooth); *7*, cotton swab and *8*, cotton pellet held in cotton pliers (to dry tooth); *9*, gutta percha point held in hemostat (tracer for sinus tract).

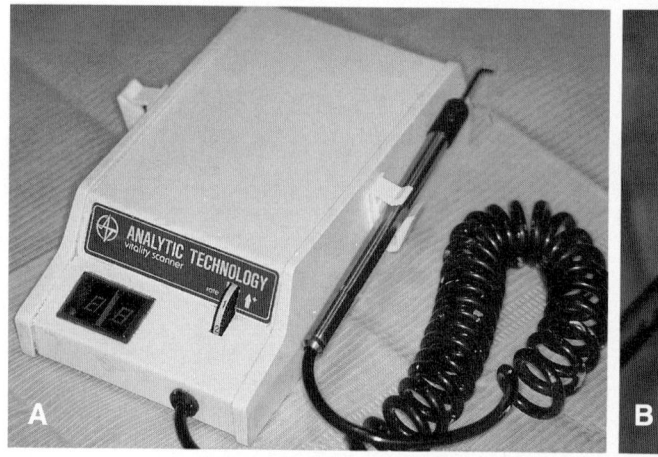

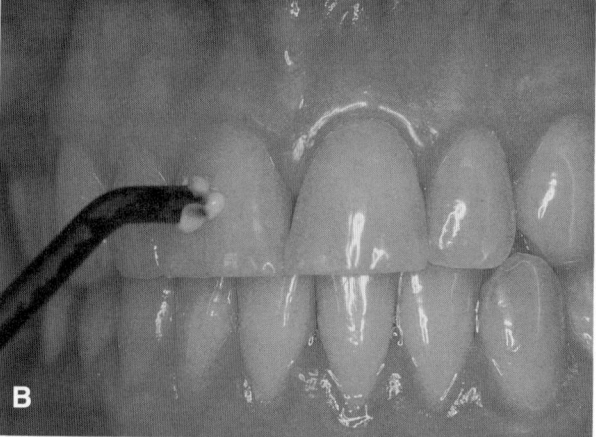

Figure 2-5 Electric pulp tester used to produce a stimulus to excite a response. **A,** Pulp tester, (Analytic Technology), is battery operated. **B,** Application of pulp tester. Tip of pulp tester is applied to cervical-middle third of tooth. Small amount of toothpaste on tip ensures better conduction of current to dry surface of tooth.

Clinical Tests: Diagnostic Armamentarium

1. Electric Pulp Test
    Technique: The electrode coated with an electrolyte is placed on sound tooth structure. The current is increased slowly until the patient signals a response (Fig. 2-5).
    Purpose: Gives an indication of pulp vitality when compared to the control tooth.

2. Thermal Test—Cold
    Technique: Ice (in an anesthetic Carpule) or ethyl chloride spray (sprayed on a cotton pellet) is applied to the tooth (Fig. 2-6).
    Purpose: A response and immediate remission is normal. An increase in intensity that lingers is abnormal. No response may be normal or abnormal.

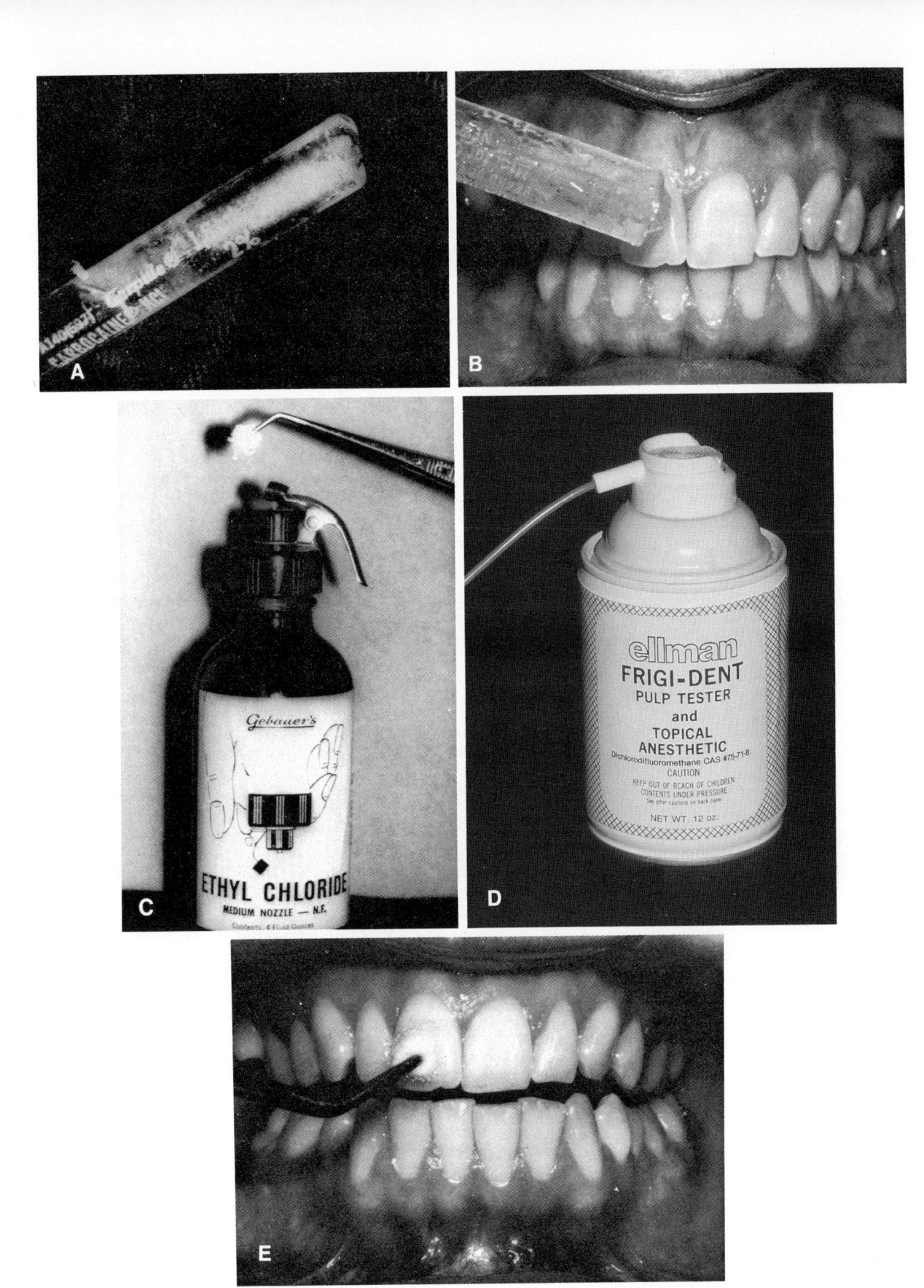

Figure 2-6 Cold test may be performed with ice, ethyl chloride spray, or Freon. **A,** Small cylinder of ice (frozen water in anesthetic carpule) is an easy source. **B,** Ice cylinder is placed on the tooth surface to produce a response. **C,** If refrigeration is not available, ethyl chloride may be sprayed on a cotton pellet held in a cotton plier. **D,** Freon, which is sprayed directly on the tooth, can also be used (Ellman International, Inc., Hewlett, NY). **E,** Frosting has been produced on cotton pellet with the ethyl chloride spray, and the cold surface is placed on the tooth.

30 PRACTICAL ENDODONTICS

Thermal Test—Hot

Technique: Gutta percha temporary stopping is heated and applied to the tooth (Fig. 2-7).

Purpose: A response and immediate remission is normal. An increase in intensity that lingers is abnormal. No response may be normal or abnormal.

3. Percussion

    Technique: The incisal edge or occlusal surface of the tooth is tapped with the end of a mirror (Fig. 2-8).

    Purpose: Suggest inflammation of the periodontal ligament.

4. Palpation

    Technique: Pressure is applied to the soft tissue over the root of the tooth (Fig. 2-9).

    Purpose: Location of an intraoral swelling.

5. Mobility

    Technique: Apply pressure with two tongue blades, one placed on lingual and one on buccal, after drying the tooth with 2 × 2 gauze sponge (Fig. 2-10).

    Purpose: Determines the degree of alveolar attachment and gives some idea of the periodontal status around the tooth. It also determines if the crown is loose or the entire tooth is loose. Look for fluid seepage under crown or in the sulcus.

6. Periodontal Evaluation (Periodontal Probe)

    Technique: The periodontal sulcus is probed all around the tooth (Fig. 2-11).

    Purpose: Differential diagnosis can be made between a periodontal and endodontic lesion.

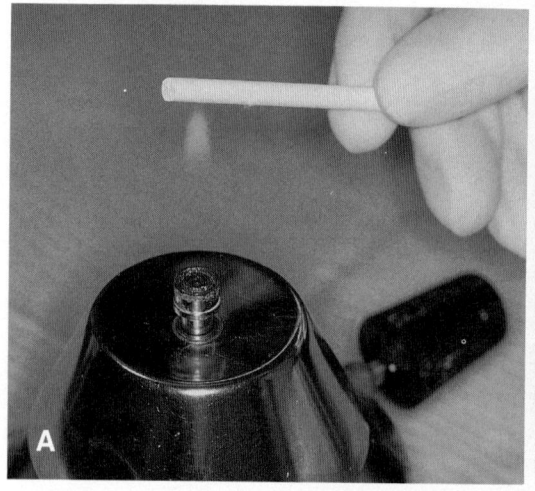

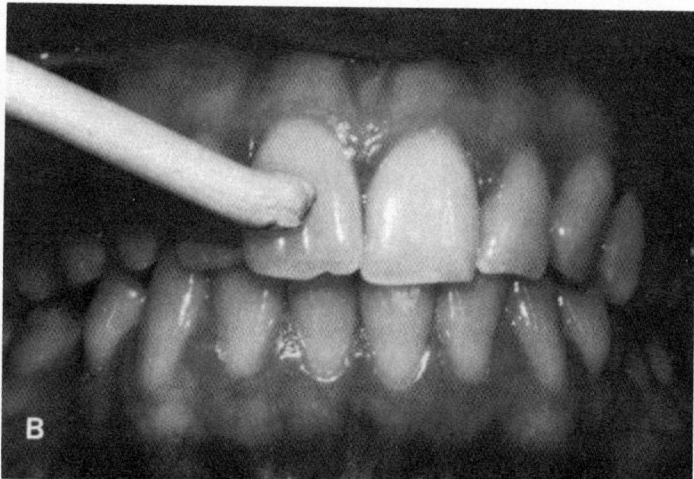

Figure 2-7 Hot test. **A,** A stick of gutta percha is heated over a flame. **B,** The gutta percha is then applied to the cervical-middle third of the tooth. Care should be taken not to overheat the gutta percha and allow the melted material to adhere to the tooth. This could overheat the tooth, producing permanent damage.

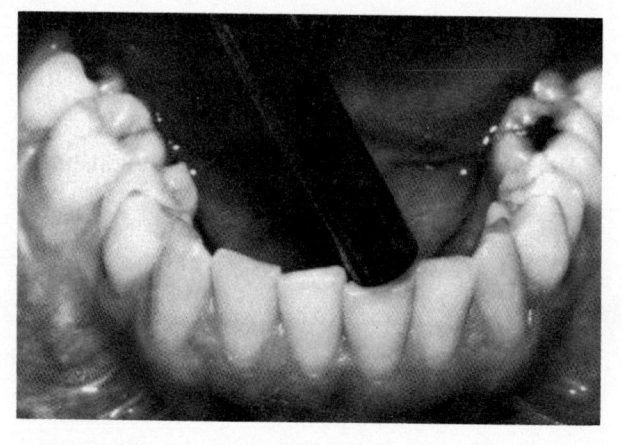

Figure 2-8 Percussion test. Using the butt end of a mirror handle to tap against a tooth to elicit sensitivity of an acute apical periodontal tissue.

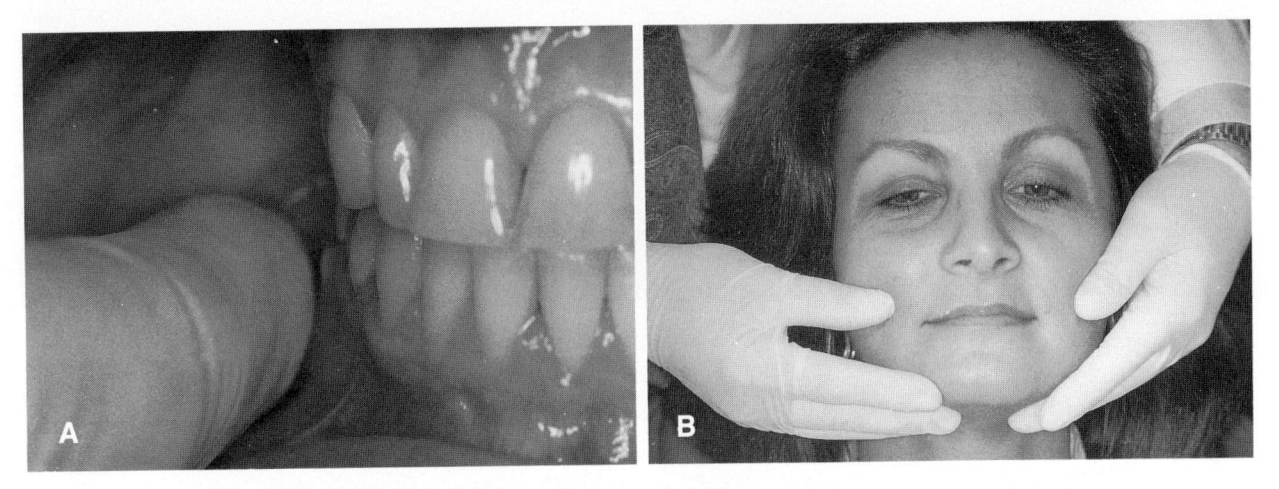

Figure 2-9 Palpation. **A,** Application of finger pressure over apices of suspected teeth to determine tenderness or intraoral swelling. **B,** Palpation need not be limited intraorally but may extend to lower border of the jaw and neck to locate tender or swollen lymph nodes.

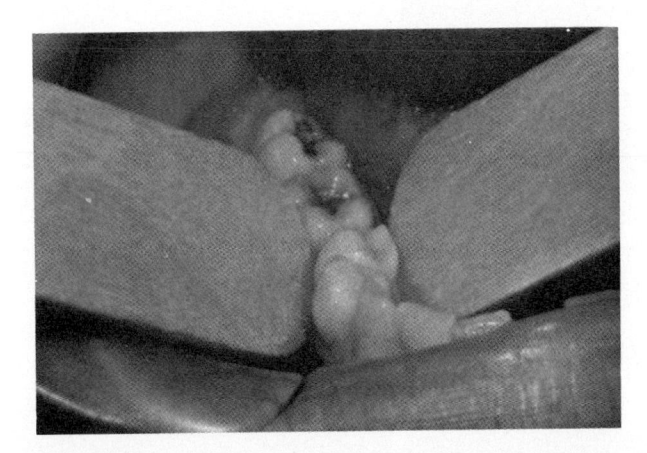

Figure 2-10 Mobility. With two tongue blades or instrument handles (placed on buccal and lingual surfaces), pressure is applied in both directions to establish movement and degree of mobility.

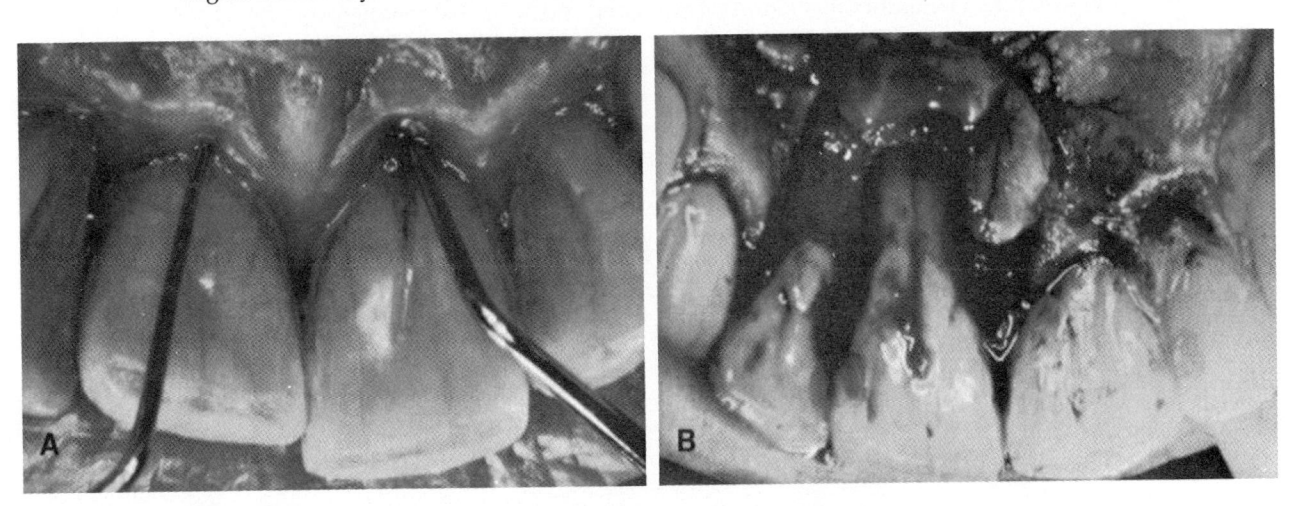

Figure 2-11 Periodontal evaluations are necessary to establish alveolar bone support. A draining fistula may be establishing access along the periodontal ligament, or a combined lesion (periodontal-endodontic) may be present. No tooth that is periodontally poor should be treated endodontically. **A,** Palatal groove on maxillary central incisor with periodontal probe in place showing the depth of the pocket. **B,** Palatal tissue is flapped back to expose the root surface. The periodontal defect can be seen, as can the anatomical palatal groove running along the root surface. This tooth has a guarded prognosis from a periodontal standpoint. (From Seibert JS: In Goldman HM and Cohen W: *Periodontal Therapy*, ed 5, St Louis, 1973, Mosby. Courtesy of Major W Thomas, Frankfurt, Germany.)

7. Occlusal Evaluation (Articulating Paper)

Technique: Place articulating paper in the mouth and have the patient go into all the occlusal movements (Fig. 2-12).

Purpose: Aids in differential diagnosis between an endodontic lesion and occlusal problem. Can also see a contributing factor to the endodontic problem.

8. Radiograph

Technique: Exposure of periapical radiographs from the long cone technique (Fig. 2-13).

Purpose: Shows periapical pathosis and factors that predispose to pulpal involvement.

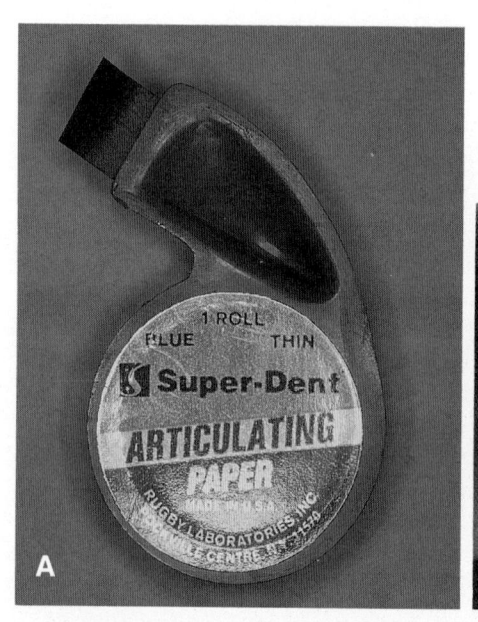

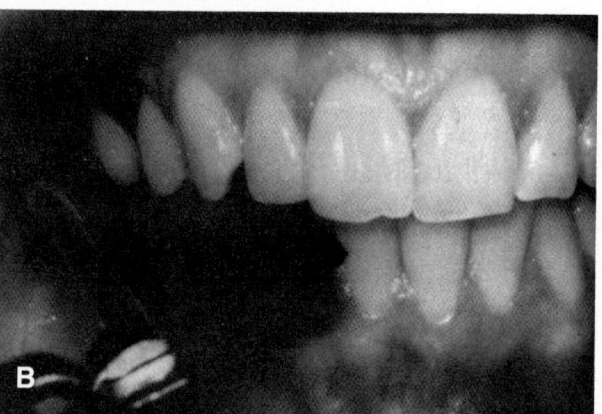

Figure 2-12 Occlusal evaluation. **A,** Articulating paper. **B,** Articulating paper held by a Miller forcep allows access to all teeth. It is necessary to have patient demonstrate contacts in eccentric and centric occlusal relations. Too frequently the cause of trouble is occlusal rather than endodontic in origin.

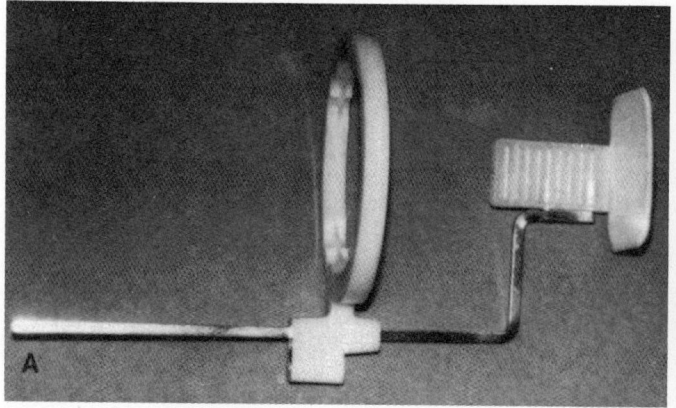

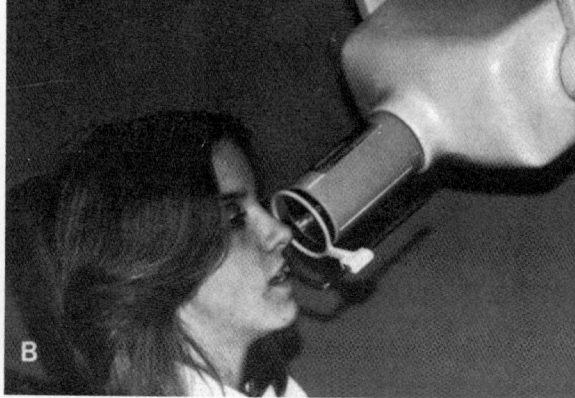

Figure 2-13 Radiographic evaluation. **A,** XCP holder for x-ray film. **B,** Application of the XCP holder; the long cone is lined up with the ring.

Selective Tests for Difficult Diagnostic Situations (Fig. 2-4)

9. Test Cavity Preparation
   Technique: A small Class I cavity preparation is made through the crown down to the dentin with a round bur. When the bur touches the dentin, a response should be elicited on a vital tooth (Fig. 2-14).
   Purpose: Used when the suspected tooth has a full crown or extensive restoration and all other tests are negative.

10. Anesthetic Test
    Technique: Infiltration anesthesia of the maxilla (moving from an anterior direction) and block anesthesia of the mandible (Fig. 2-15).
    Purpose: Aids in locating which arch the pain is coming from or used in differential diagnosis to rule out a dental problem.

11. Transillumination
    Technique: Light from a fiber optic is applied from the buccal or lingual to illuminate the tooth (Fig. 2-16, *A-C*).
    Purpose: Can be used as an aid in diagnosing a fracture.

12. Biting
    Technique: Place an orangewood stick on each cusp of the tooth and have the patient bite down (Fig. 2-16, *D*).
    Purpose: Identification of a fractured tooth.

13. Staining
    Technique: First method: Remove filling from suspected tooth and place 2% iodine in the cavity preparation. The iodine will stain the fracture line dark (Fig. 2-16, *E*).
    Second method: Mix a dye in zinc oxide and eugenol and place it in the cavity preparation after the filling has been removed. The dye will seep out and line the fracture.
    Third method: Have the patient chew a disclosing tablet after taking out the filling of the suspected fractured tooth. The fracture line will be stained.
    Purpose: Isolation of a cracked tooth.

14. Gutta Percha Point Tracing with Radiograph
    Technique: Place a gutta percha point through the fistulous tract and take a radiograph (see Fig. 2-19).
    Purpose: Can localize the endodontic lesion to the specific tooth. Aids in differential diagnosis between a periodontal and an endodontic lesion.

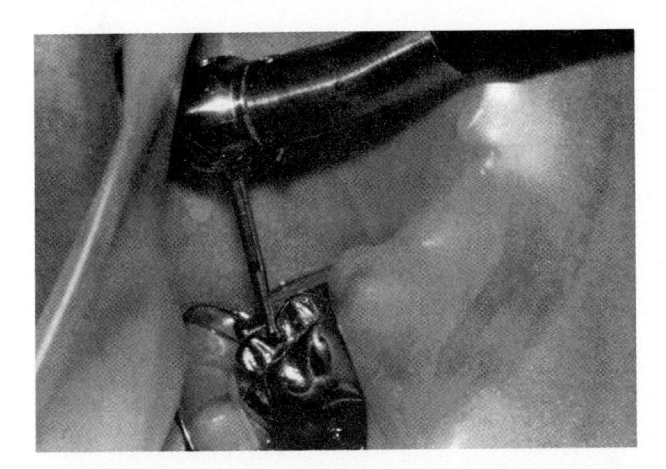

Figure 2-14 Test cavity. A small Class I opening is made through the crown and into dentin. If pain is elicited the pulp is vital.

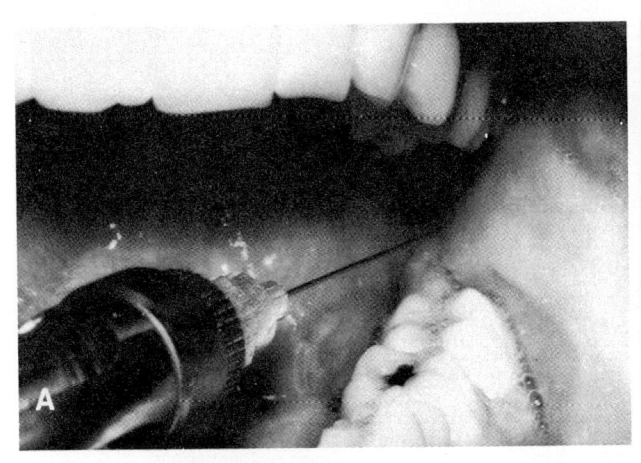

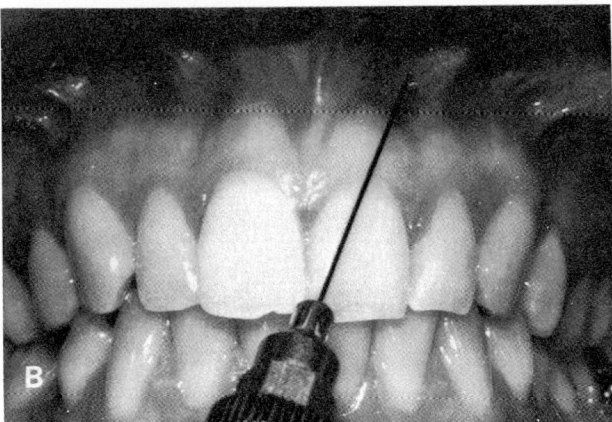

Figure 2-15 Anesthetic test. **A,** Mandibular block is administered to determine whether the source of pain is in the maxillary quadrant or mandibular quadrant. If pain disappears following the block, the origin may be established. **B,** Infiltration of a tooth may establish whether the source of pain is in that tooth.

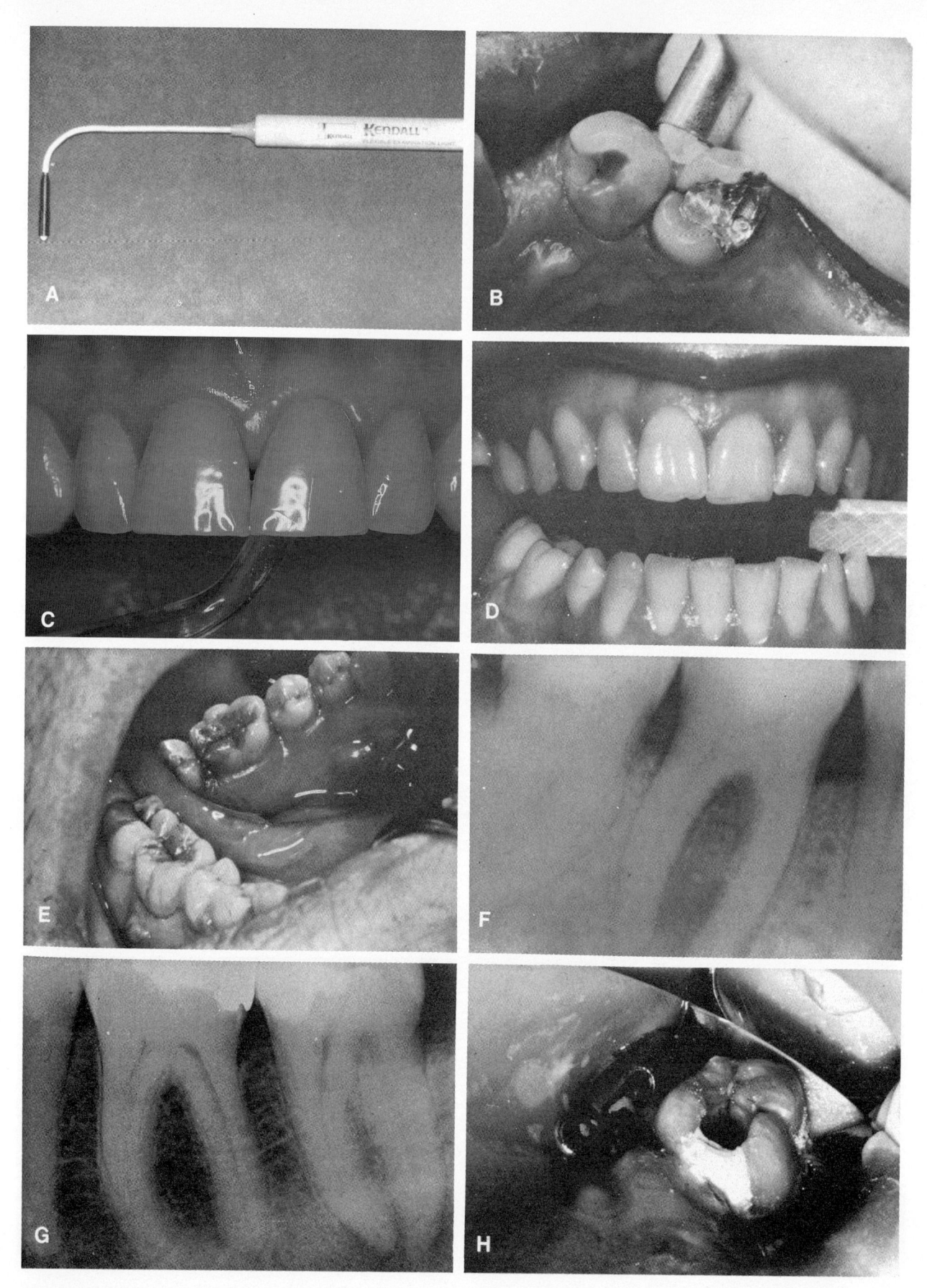

Figure 2-16 For legend, see opposite page.

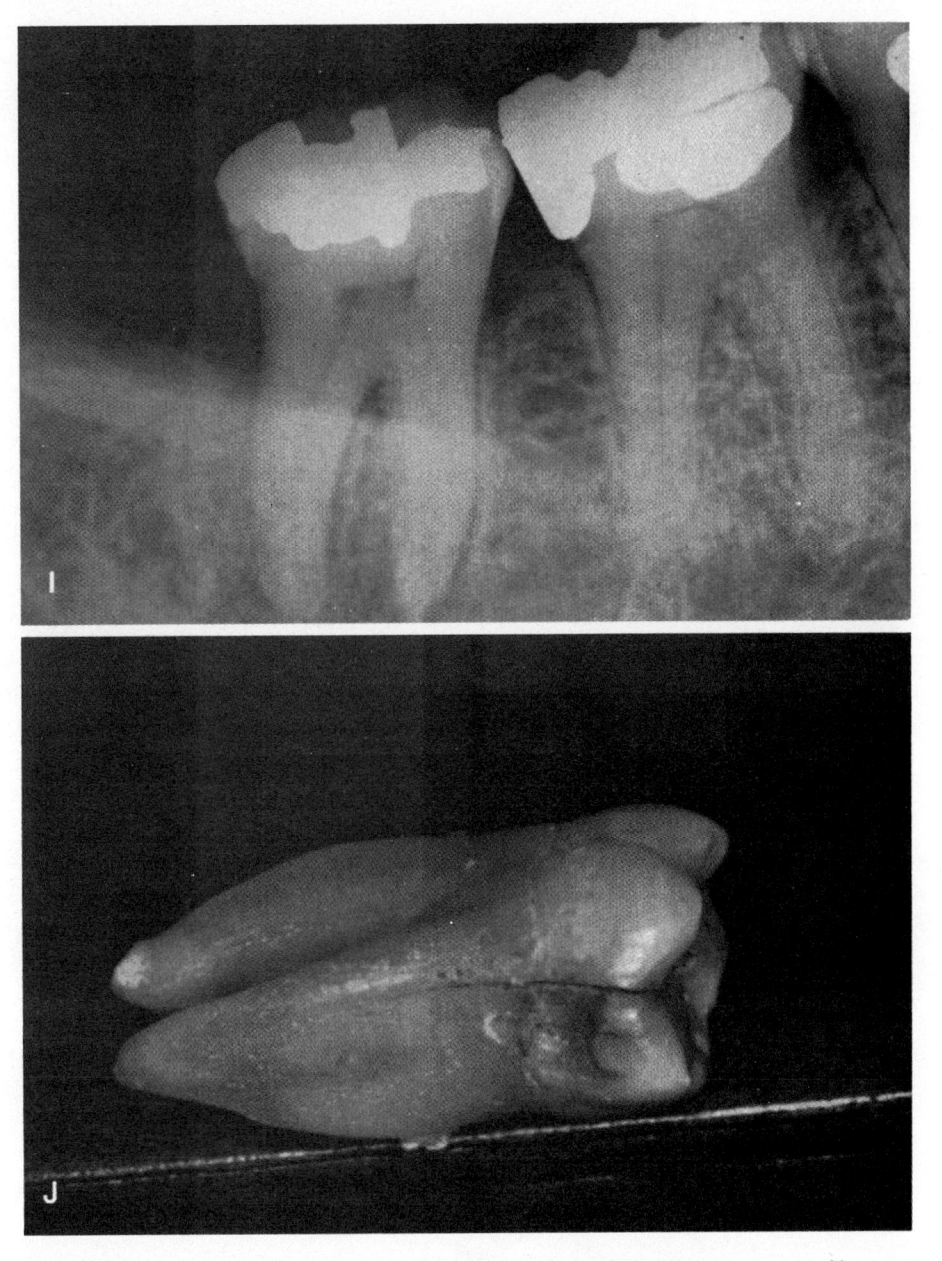

Figure 2-16 Tests for the "cracked tooth syndrome." **A,** Transillumination. A fiber optic device has made this method very easy. **B,** Fiber optic has been placed in the interproximal area in an effort to search for dental fractures. **C,** Transillumination is produced by placing the fiber optic on the palatal surface of the tooth. **D,** Bite test. Wooden stick is placed between opposing teeth, and the patient is asked to bite down. A fractured tooth would have pain elicited upon its release. **E,** Application of 2% iodine solution placed on the occlusal surface of suspected tooth. **F,** Radiograph of the tooth showing a periapical lesion on a tooth with no evidence of caries or causative influence. **G,** Patient presents with symptoms of a cracked tooth. Radiograph of symptomatic mandibular second molar. **H,** After filling is removed, fracture line can be seen. **I,** A mandibular second molar that presented with symptoms of severe pain upon mastication. **J,** Extracted tooth showing an incompleted fracture line running on the distal surface of the crown extending below the cervical line.

Occasionally the results of diagnostic tests will be inconclusive. The patient must be given analgesics until the diseased tooth reveals itself. A tooth must not be treated without a definite diagnosis. When doubt exists, it is best to do nothing at that point; the patient should be kept under observation and brought back for further testing at a later date.

Tests for the Cracked Tooth Syndrome

1. Transillumination (Fig. 2-16, *A-C*)
2. Bite test (Fig. 2-16, *D*)
3. Staining (Fig. 2-16, *E* and 2-17)

The cracked tooth syndrome refers to a crack within the crown of the tooth without any pulpal involvement. It usually manifests itself as sensitivity to certain biting pressures. It becomes very painful when biting in one direction. Also, extreme reaction to cold sets it off. A differential diagnosis must be made between centric prematurities, sinusitis, posterior teeth that give inconclusive pulp tests, and cracked tooth syndrome. Any tooth with a large amalgam filling or a gold filling that does not onlay or protect the cusps should be suspected. The older the patient or the greater the intercuspation and wear, the greater the possibility of cracks. One should always think in terms of a cracked tooth when all other tests prove negative.

DIFFERENTIAL DIAGNOSIS

I. DIFFERENTIAL DIAGNOSIS OF ANATOMICAL LANDMARKS AND PATHOLOGICAL LESIONS FROM ENDODONTIC LESIONS

To avoid mistakes in diagnosis it is necessary to have a full knowledge of the most common radiolucent areas around the apices, whether they represent normal anatomical areas or radiolucent areas caused by other diseases.

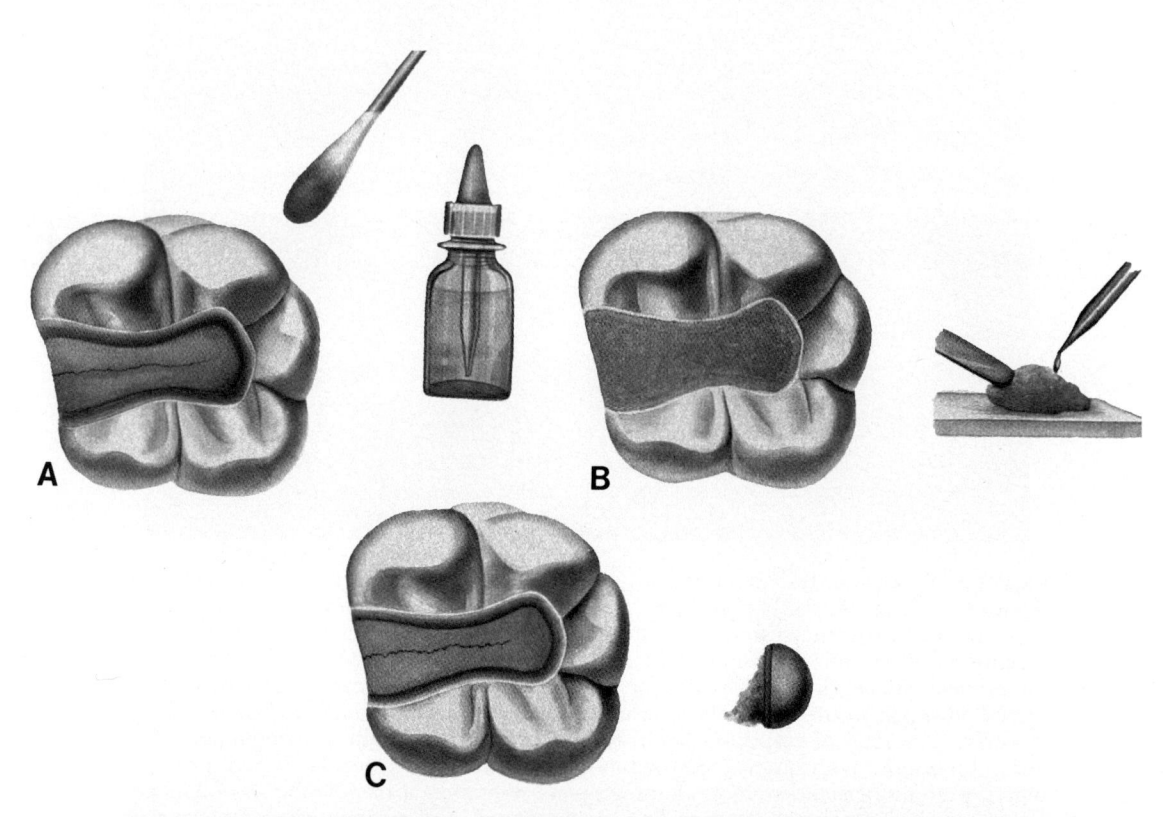

Figure 2-17 Application of stain for suspected tooth fracture. **A,** *Method I:* After removing filling, iodine or methylene blue dye is applied to cavity preparation to disclose fracture. **B,** *Method II:* After removing filling, a dye is incorporated into a mixture of zinc oxide and eugenol, placed into cavity preparation. This is then checked for fracture. **C,** *Method III:* After filling is removed, patient is instructed to chew on a disclosing tablet and then the tooth is checked for a fracture. If a fracture is present, a dark stain can be seen on the fracture line.

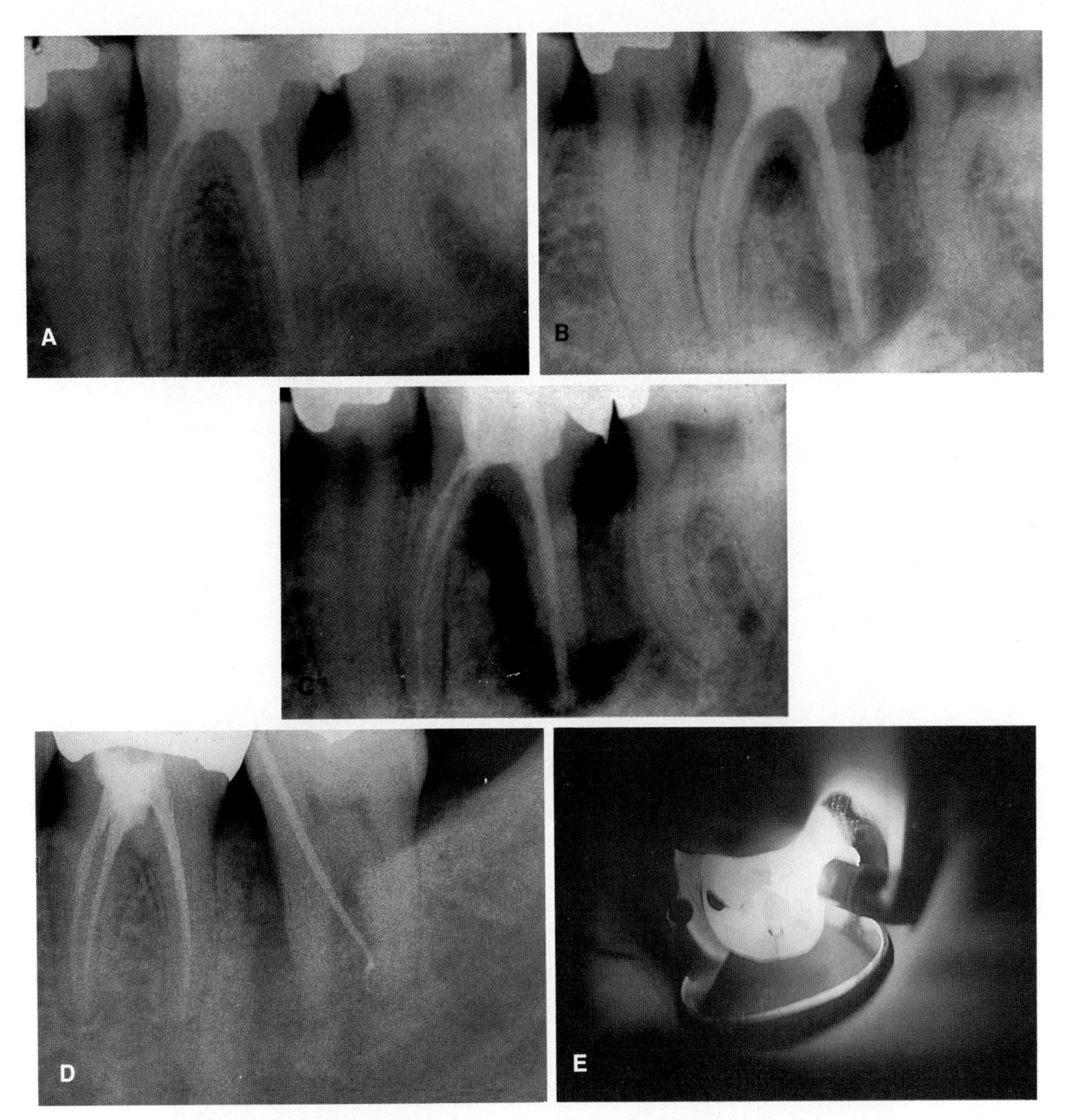

Figure 2-18 Diagnosis of root fracture. **A,** Radiograph of a mandibular first molar right after root canal therapy was completed. **B,** One-year recall of same tooth. Notice radiographic changes around the distal root and in the furcation. **C,** Fifteen-month recall showing progressive destruction of bone around the distal root. Notice that the radiographic changes are not just in the periapical area but are creeping along the surface of the distal root. It is a halo type lesion that typically envelops the root in the advanced stages. Radiographic changes are only seen in these advanced stages when complete root fractures are present. **D,** Preoperative radiograph of mandibular right second molar with gutta percha point through fistulous tract. **E,** Fiber optic showing vertical fracture mesial to distal on same tooth.

38 PRACTICAL ENDODONTICS

A. Anatomical Landmarks That May Be Superimposed over Root Apices
   1. Anterior palatine foramen
   2. Nostril spots
   3. Mental foramen
   4. Inferior alveolar canal
   5. Maxillary sinus
   6. Prominent nutrient canals

B. Pathological Lesions That Might Be Mistaken for an Endodontic Lesion
   1. Median maxillary cyst
   2. Globulomaxillary cyst (Fig. 2-20, B and C)
   3. Hemorrhagic traumatic bone cyst
   4. Lateral periodontal cyst
   5. Neoplasm
   6. Periapical fibroosteoma (cementoma) (Fig. 2-20, A)

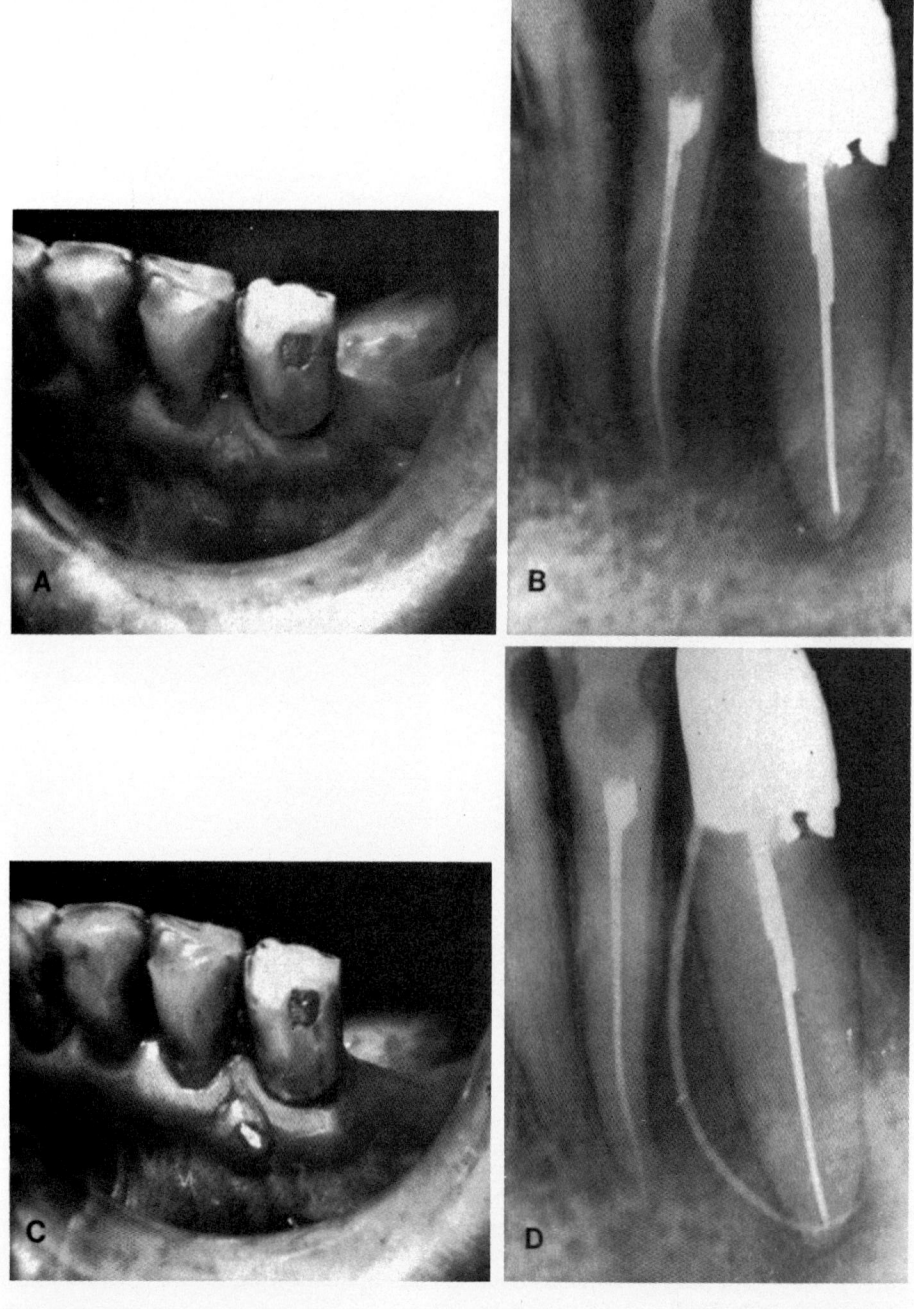

Figure 2-19 Intraoral fistula tracing. **A,** Photograph of an intraoral fistula between the lateral and cuspid. **B,** Radiograph of periapical rarefaction between lateral and cuspid. **C,** A gutta percha point is placed through the fistulous tract. **D,** A radiograph is then taken that points to the apex of the cuspid. This demonstrates that the cuspid is causing the fistulous tract.

To establish a differential diagnosis and to eliminate the possibility of confusing any anatomical or pathological areas with areas of periapical pathosis, several procedures may be used:

1. Take several roentgenograms at various angles. Anatomical areas will shift from the apex with the change of angulation. A radiolucent area caused by pulpal pathosis will not move.
2. Study the roentgenograms carefully. The presence of an unbroken lamina dura is a strong indication that no periapical pathosis is present.
3. Take electric pulp tests. If a response is elicited, this may establish the vitality of the tooth and prevent error in recognition of lesions (such as cementoma) that bear a strong roentgenographic resemblence to a granuloma or a cyst. If no response is elicited, the lesion may be presumed to be a sequela of pulpal pathosis.

II. REFERRED PAIN

The most common examples of pain referral in the oral cavity are:

1. Pain referred to the maxillary molars and bicuspids from the maxillary sinus
2. Pain from the maxillary molars referred to the mandibular molars
3. Pain from the mandibular molars referred to the ear
4. Pain referred from a dysfunction of a temporomandibular joint
5. Pain referred from trifacial neuralgia
6. Pain of psychosomatic origin

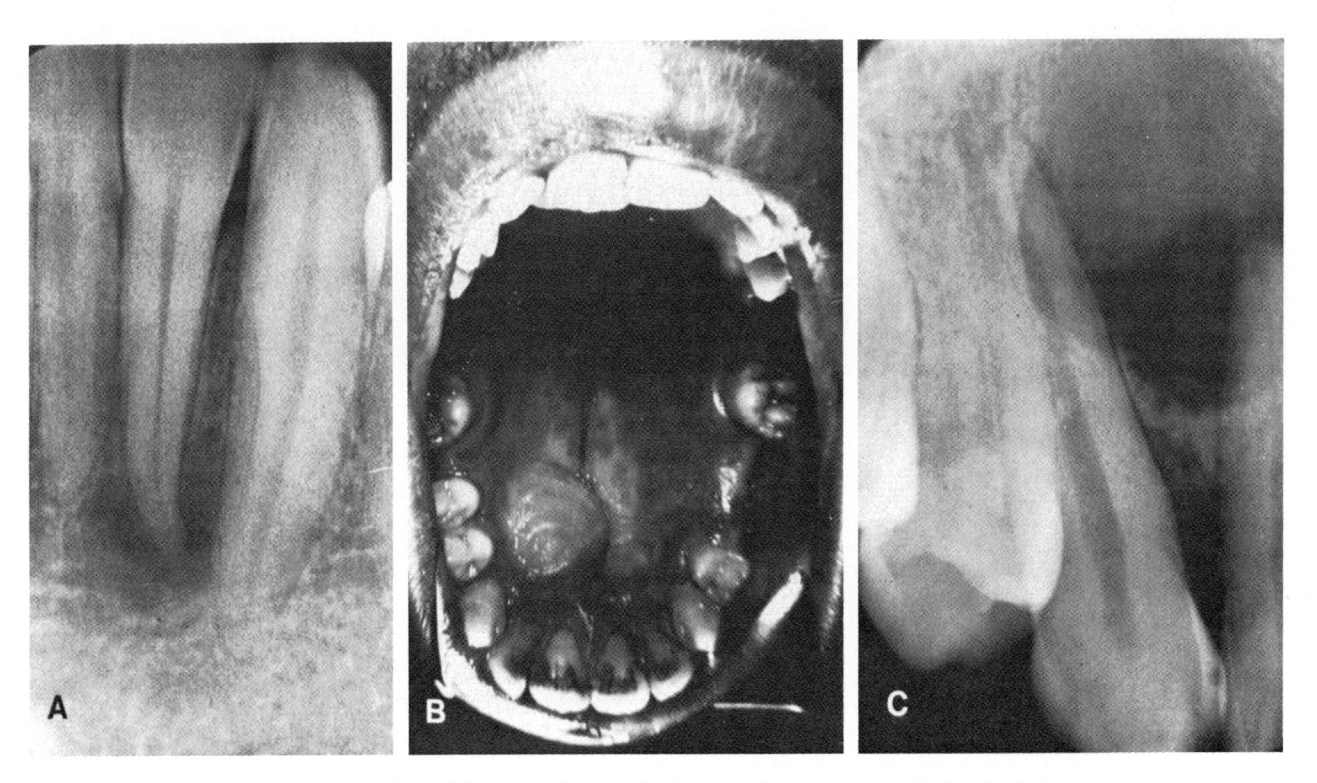

Figure 2-20 Pathological lesions that might be mistaken for an endodontic lesion. **A,** Radiolucent lesion around the lateral incisor. This tooth tested vital. A diagnosis of a cementoma was made. **B,** Photograph of an intraoral swelling. A radiograph of this area was taken. **C,** Radiograph of swelling in *B*. All maxillary anterior teeth gave vital response. A diagnosis of a globulomaxillary cyst was made.

3

Radiographic Interpretation

Knowledge of endodontic radiography is essential for proper diagnosis, instrumentation, and obturation, but the radiograph has limitations. It is a two-dimensional picture of a three-dimensional object and cannot distinguish between healthy and unhealthy pulp tissue or the various stages of pulpal degeneration. In many situations, especially in the mandible, pulpal infection can spread to the periapical area, but go undetected on the radiograph.

The radiograph still offers the single most pertinent piece of diagnostic information. As the dentist comes to understand the limitations of the radiograph and strives to improve his or her radiographic technique and interpretation, endodontic treatment will become easier and more successful. The techniques outlined in the following sections have proven to be successful and predictable.

NORMAL ANATOMIC LANDMARKS

In diagnosis, the clinician must first be able to distinguish abnormal findings from normal landmarks. Normal anatomic landmarks of the mandibular (Fig. 3-1) and maxillary (Fig. 3-2) jaw are shown. Many times these structures can imitate or hide lesions of endodontic or nonendodontic origin. Also encroachment on or damage to these areas during endodontic instrumentation, obturation, and apical surgery have led to numerous litigation cases against dentists. In particular, overextension of instruments or obturation materials into the mandibular canal can cause temporary or permanent paresthesia of the patient's lip. The mandibular canal generally follows a path that passes near the apices of the mandibular second molars and then drops down away from the roots near the border of the mandible and then exits at the mental foramen near the apices of the first or second premolars (Fig. 3-1, *A*).

If the roots of the maxillary molars and bicuspids are adjacent to the maxillary sinus, any instrumentation beyond the apical foramen can irritate the schneiderian membrane, lining the maxillary sinus (Fig. 3-3). Overextension of filling material in these cases can result in a constant low grade postoperative discomfort associated with the treated tooth and the sinus.

ENDODONTIC RADIOGRAPHIC LANDMARKS AND TERMINOLOGY

To accurately cleanse, shape, and obturate the root canal space, a knowledge of the apical root canal anatomy is essential. Often the term *apex* is mistakenly used to denote the location where the canal exits the root. The apex is the anatomic end of the root, while the apical foramen is the correct term used to denote the terminus of the canal where it exits onto the root surface (Fig. 3-4). Occasionally, the apical foramen opens at the anatomic root apex, but in the majority of cases the apical foramen exits on the root surface between 0.5 to 1.0 mm from the root apex (Fig. 3-5).

At this canal terminus, there is usually a natural constriction (minor diameter), which often coincides with the cementodentinal junction (CDJ) (Fig. 3-5). If

Text continued on pg. 46.

42 PRACTICAL ENDODONTICS

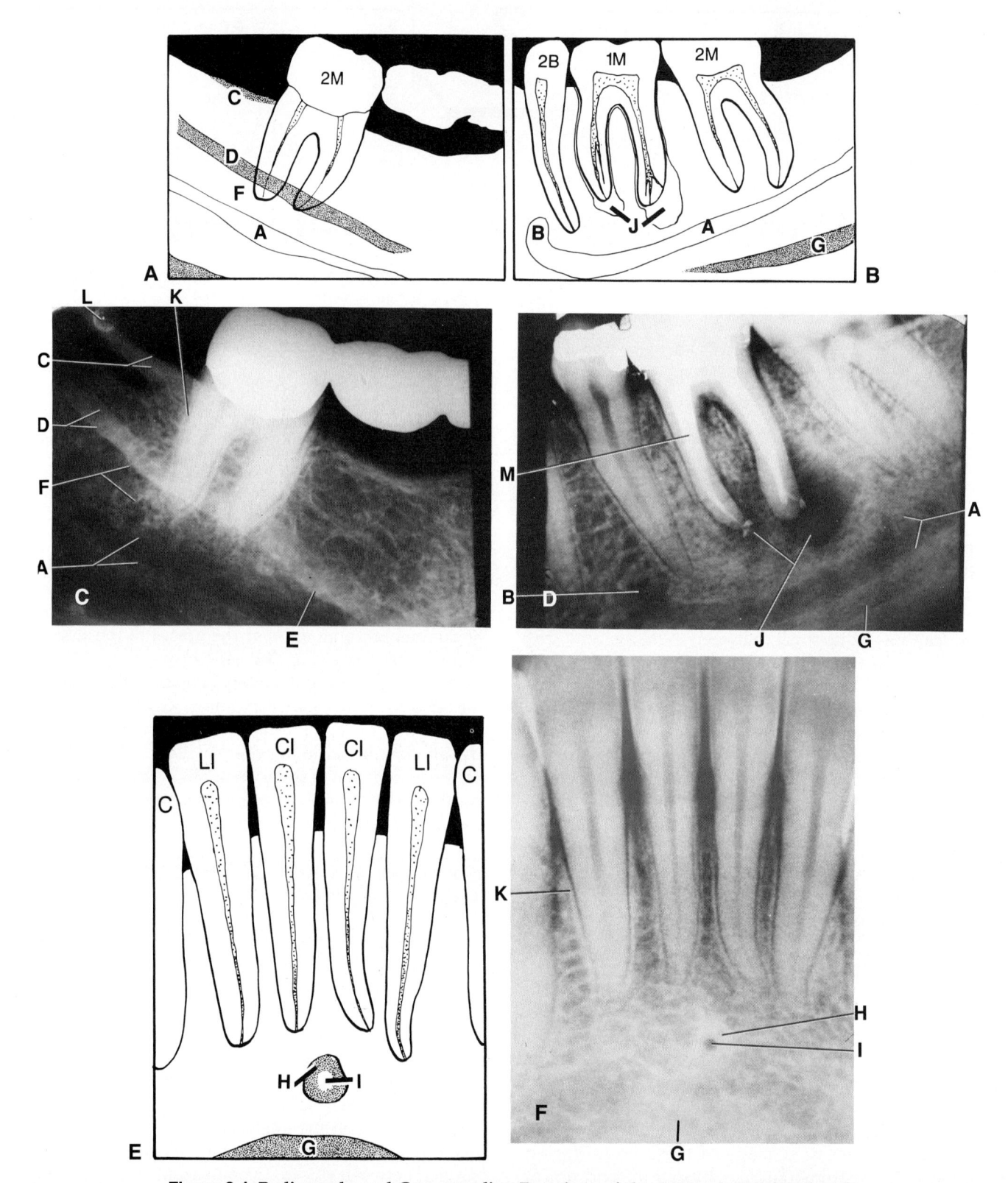

Figure 3-1 Radiographs and Corresponding Drawings of the Anatomic Landmarks of the Mandibular Arch. A, Mandibular canal. **B,** Mental foramen. **C,** External oblique ridge. **D,** Internal oblique ridge. **E,** Submaxillary fossa. **F,** Mylohyoid line. **G,** Cortical bone of the inferior border of the mandible. **H,** Genial tubercle. **I,** Lingual foramen. **J,** Periapical radiolucency. **K,** Lamina dura. **L,** Identification dot. **M,** Root canal filling.

Chapter 3 ♦ Radiographic Interpretation 43

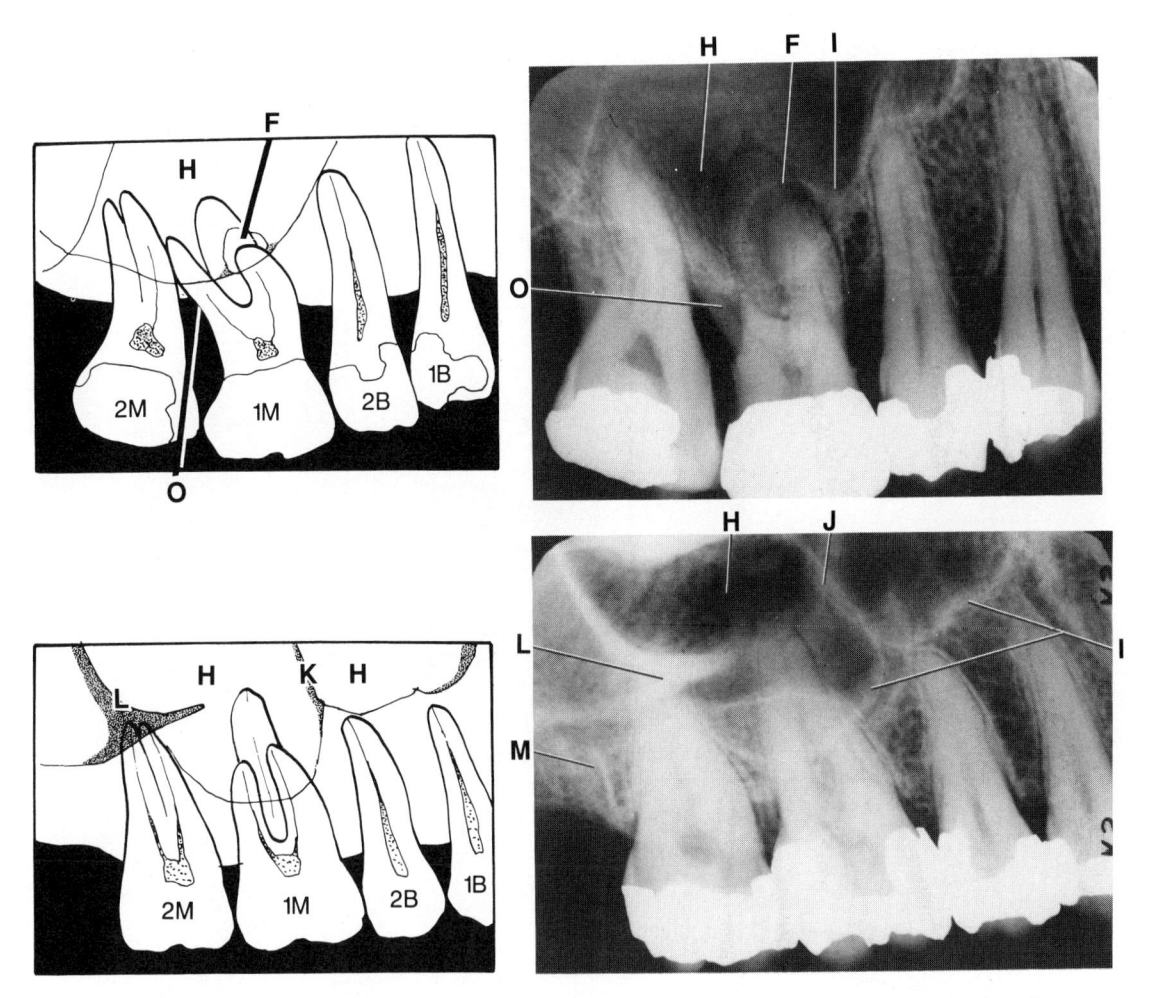

Figure 3-2 Radiographs and Corresponding Drawings of the Anatomic Landmarks of the Maxillary Arch. **A**, Nasal fossa. **B**, Anterior nasal spine. **C**, Nasal septum. **D**, Median palatine suture. **E**, Incisive foramen. **F**, Periapical lesion. **G**, Root canal filling. **H**, Maxillary sinus. **I**, Floor of the maxillary sinus. **J**, Bone septum between nasal fossa and maxillary sinus. **K**, Maxillary sinus septum. **L**, Zygomatic process. **M**, Maxillary tuberosity. **N**, Lamina dura. **O**, Periodontal bone loss.

44 PRACTICAL ENDODONTICS

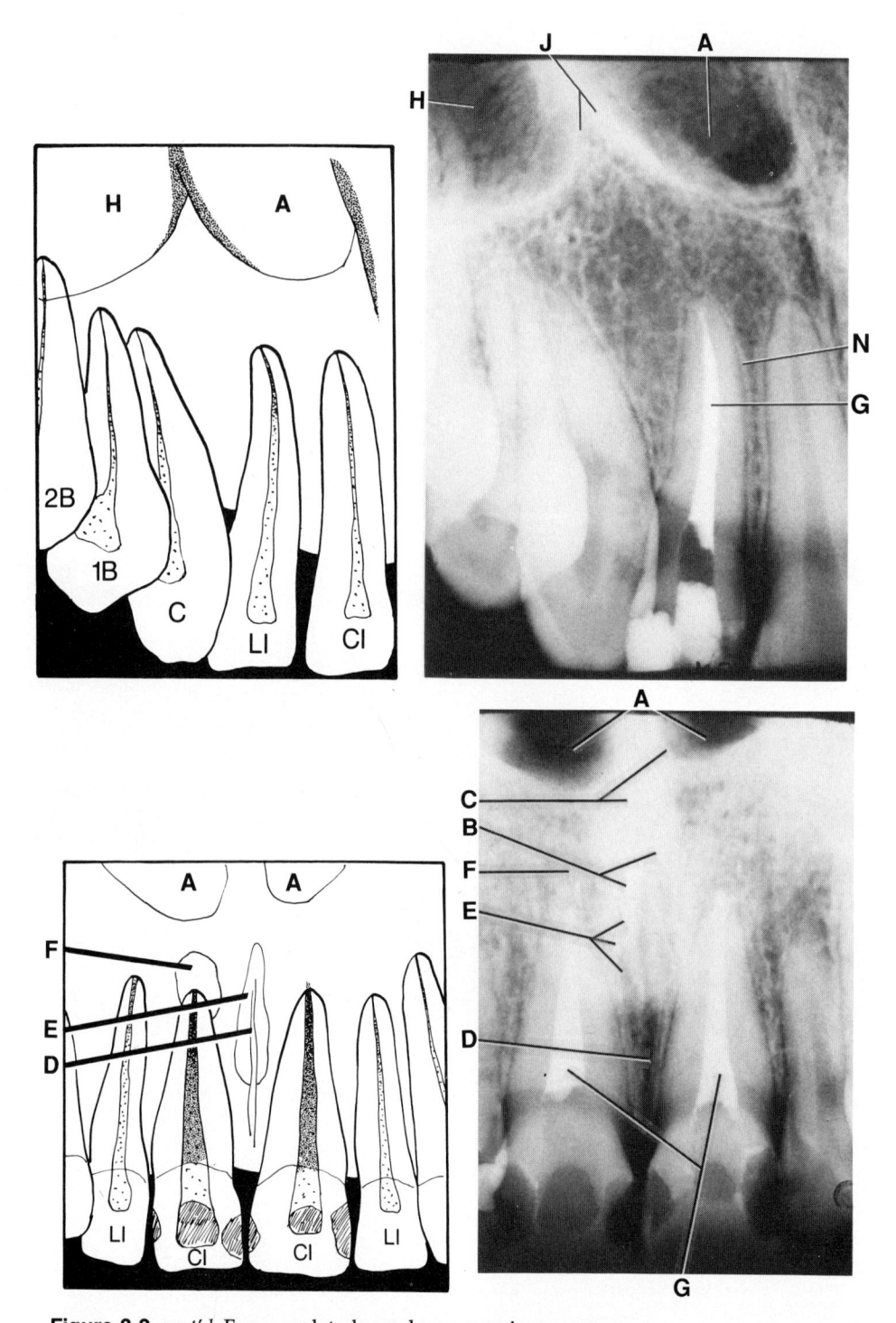

Figure 3-2 *cont'd* For complete legend, see previous page.

Chapter 3 ♦ Radiographic Interpretation 45

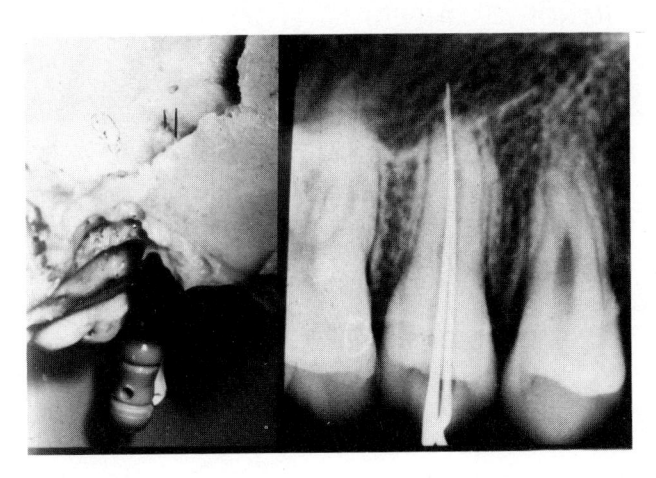

Figure 3-3

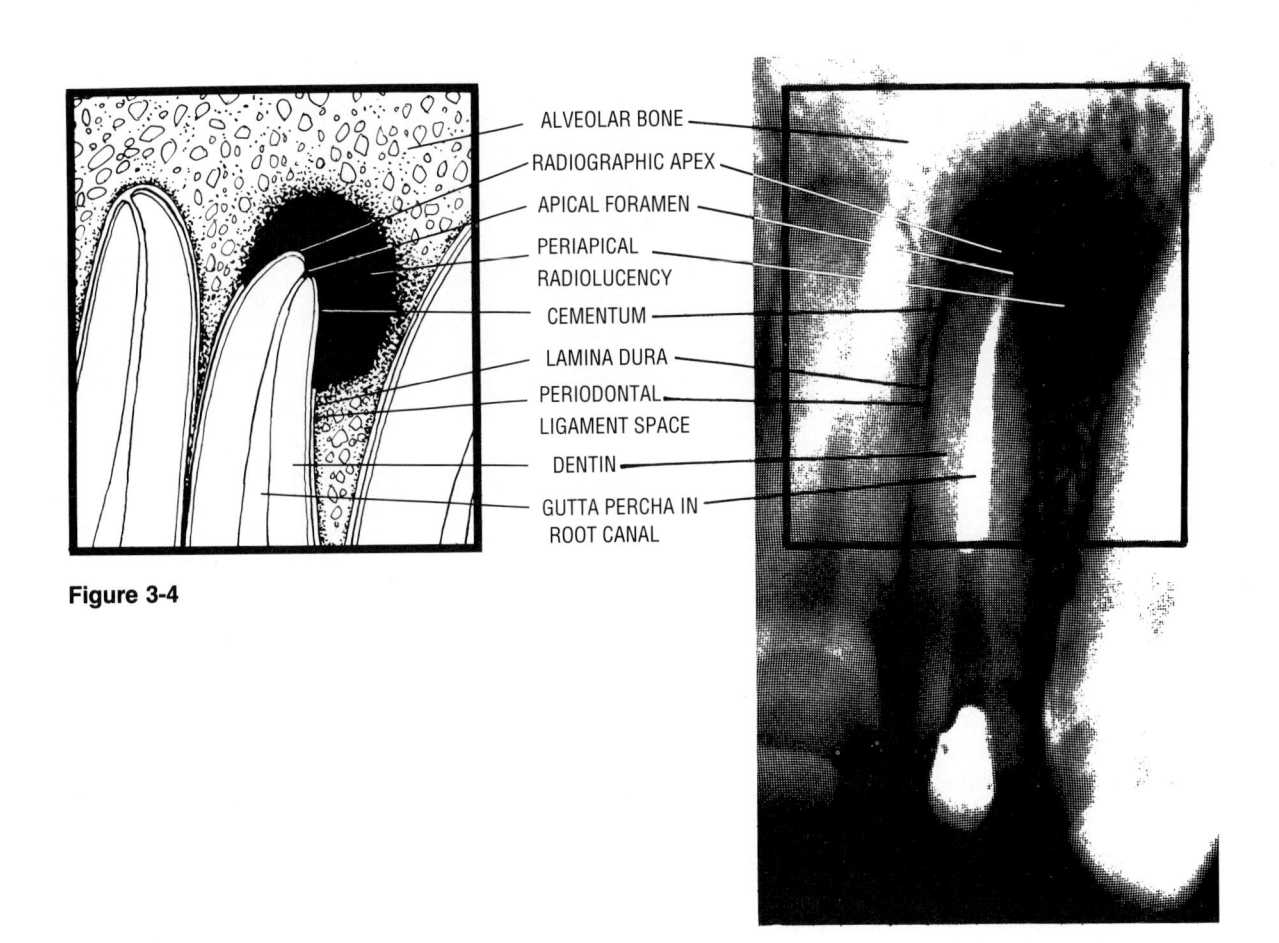

- ALVEOLAR BONE
- RADIOGRAPHIC APEX
- APICAL FORAMEN
- PERIAPICAL RADIOLUCENCY
- CEMENTUM
- LAMINA DURA
- PERIODONTAL LIGAMENT SPACE
- DENTIN
- GUTTA PERCHA IN ROOT CANAL

Figure 3-4

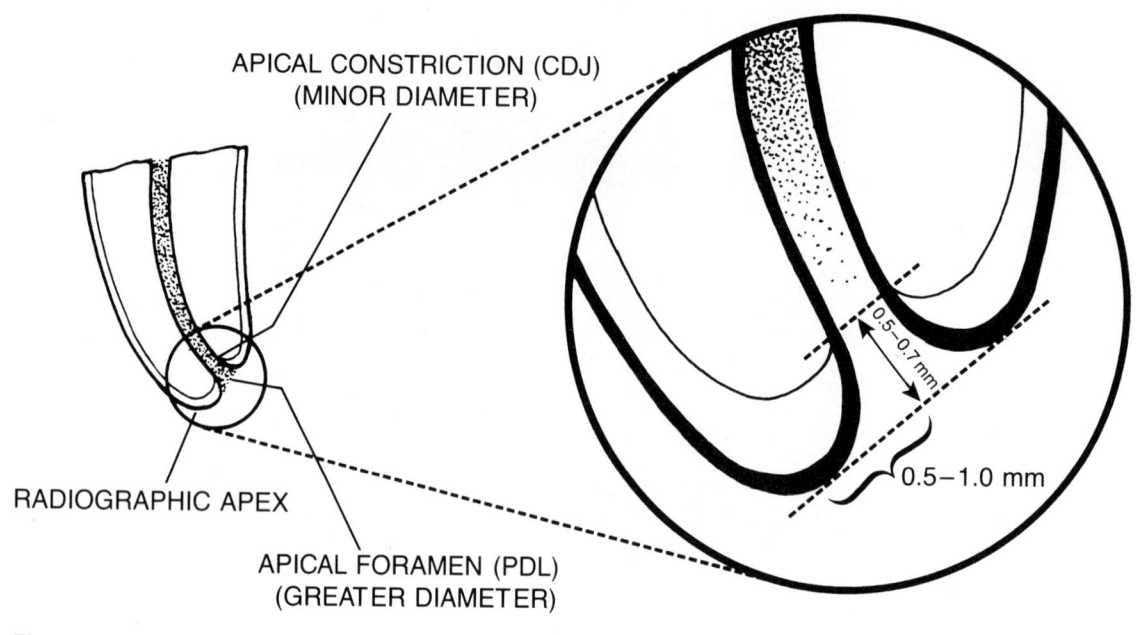

Figure 3-5

this natural constriction is maintained during cleansing and shaping, it will serve as the apical seat and dentin matrix to contain the filling material within the canal. The distance from the apical constriction (CDJ) to the apical foramen (PDL) is approximately 0.5 mm to 0.7 mm. The apical seat for the root canal filling is developed at this point.

In a healthy tooth, there is an intact narrow periodontal ligament space surrounded by a compact layer of bone called the lamina dura. As pulpal infection spreads to the periapical tissues, bone is resorbed and the periodontal ligament space appears wider or the lamina dura loses its continuity (Fig. 3-6).

About 20% of the time the apical foramen, where the root canal exits, lies on the buccal or lingual surface of the root and cannot be accurately seen on the radiograph (Fig. 3-7, A and B). This can lead to instrumentation beyond the foramen and an irritation to the periapical tissues. By changing the horizontal angulation 10 to 20 degrees, the foramen may move to the edge of the root where it can be better visualized, thus avoiding this complication (Fig. 3-7, C and D). In deciding between the two radiographs, the one that shows the file closest to the PDL is the most accurate representation of the apical anatomy.

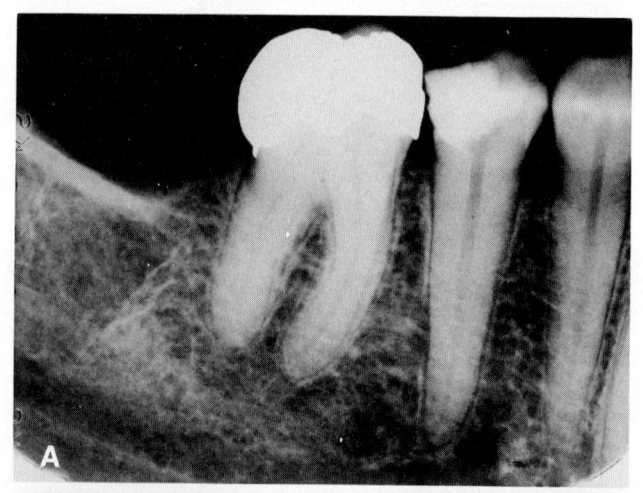

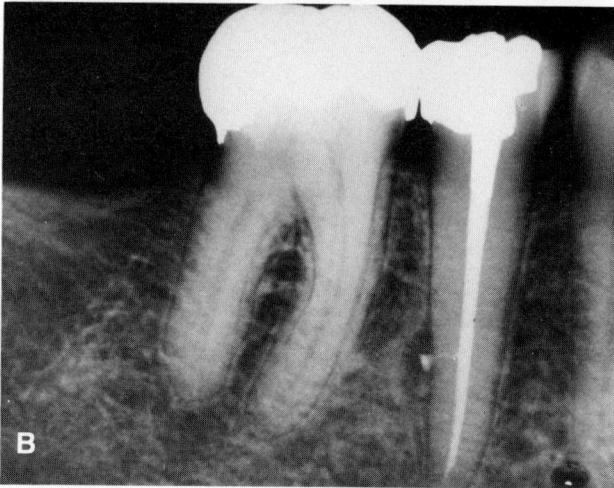

Figure 3-6

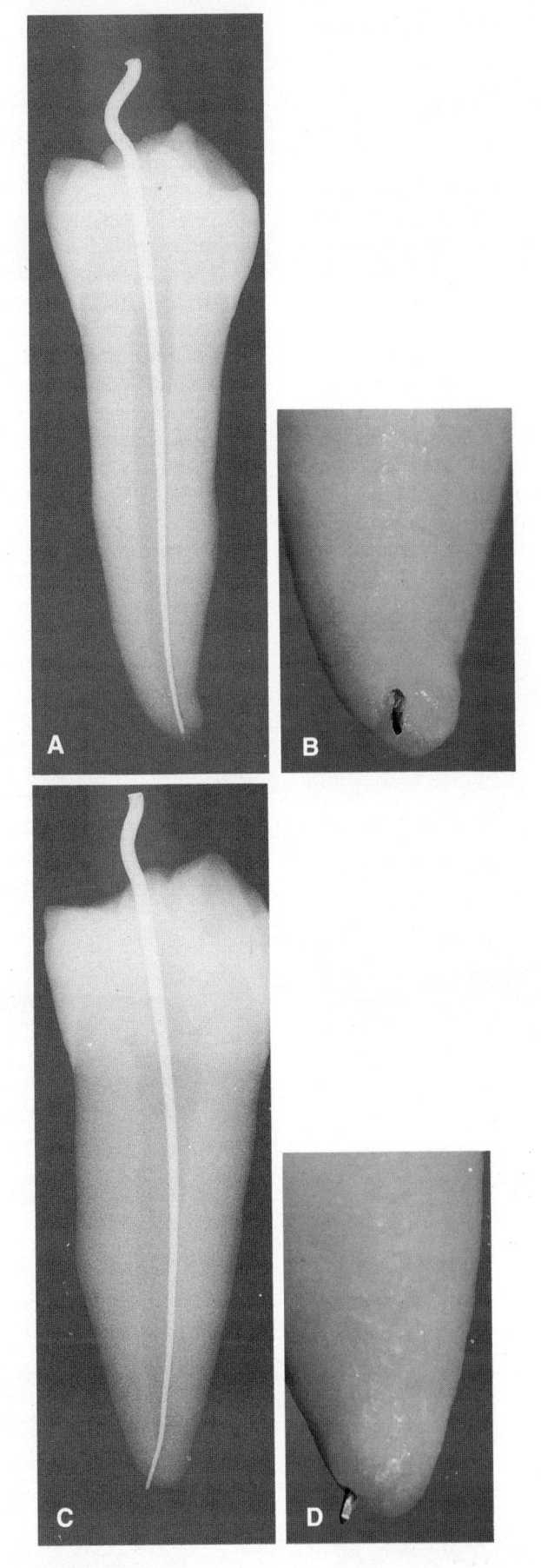

Figure 3-7

HELPFUL HINTS IN RADIOGRAPHIC DIAGNOSIS

Pulpal degeneration begins coronally and moves apically, which is why a radiolucent lesion can be seen on the lateral aspect of the root before one appears at the apex. When lateral lesions are seen, suspect a necrotic pulp and a lateral canal (Fig. 3-6). Periradicular lesions normally surround the portals of exit. The canal exit usually points to the center of the lesion (Fig. 3-8). Once the position and location of apical foramen is known, the correct direction and degree of bend can be placed on the instrument. This can also be verified by observing the direction of instrument curve as it is removed from the canal.

Root outline reflects the shape of the canal. Cone-shaped roots as seen on an angled view usually indicate a single canal or that the two canals in the same root come together and exit at one foramen (Fig. 3-9, *left*). Short, wide (blunt) roots indicate that each of two canals may have its own separate foramen (Fig. 3-9, *right*). Number of canals is best determined from an angled-view radiograph.

The clinician should routinely view the radiograph from the outside toward the center. Look for periapical lesions, caries, periodontal disease, defective fillings, superimposed normal anatomic structures, etc., that could account for the patient's discomfort. Many dentists focus on the obvious, which lies in the center of the radiograph and may fail to see the real cause of the patient's problem on the edge of the radiograph (Fig. 3-10). Note periradicular lesion on the first premolar.

Sharp changes in the radiographic density of the canal shadow (sometimes called the *fast break*) usually indicates either bifurcation (or trifurcation) into smaller diameter canals (Fig. 3-11, *A*) or a wide buccolingual canal width that becomes narrower apically such as seen in many cuspids (Fig. 3-11, *B*). Unclear or double root images may indicate ribbon-shaped roots or possibly two separate roots. Vertical radiolucent lines on the root are either root canals or lines representing the outline of the root. Canals are lines that funnel into the pulp chamber while the lines that go into the periodontal ligament are outlines of the root as seen in the first molar (Fig. 3-12). Nature is

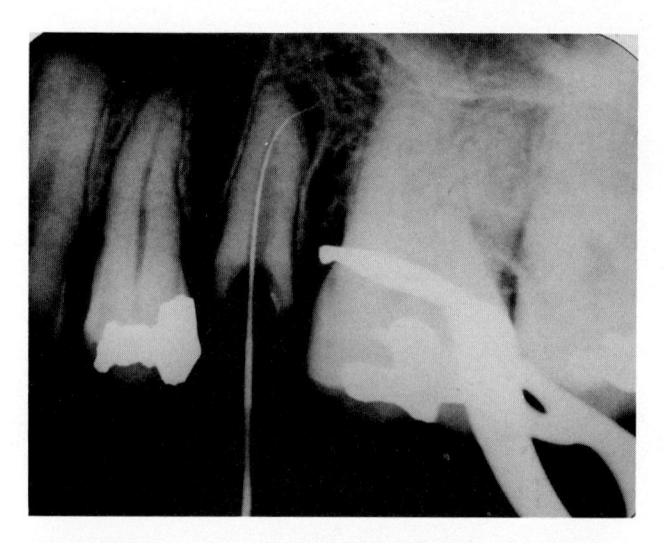

Figure 3-8

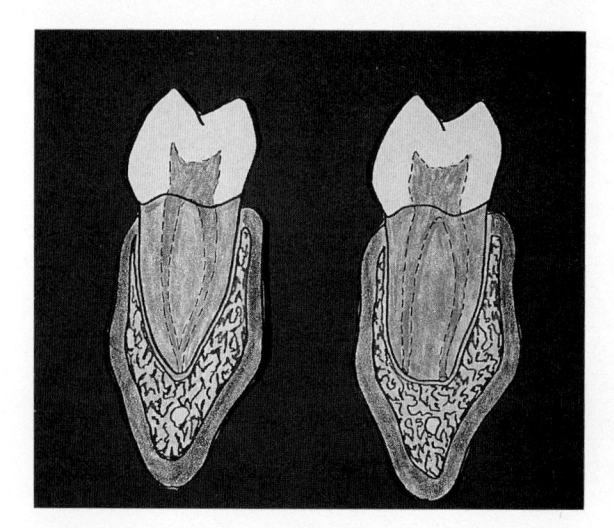

Figure 3-9

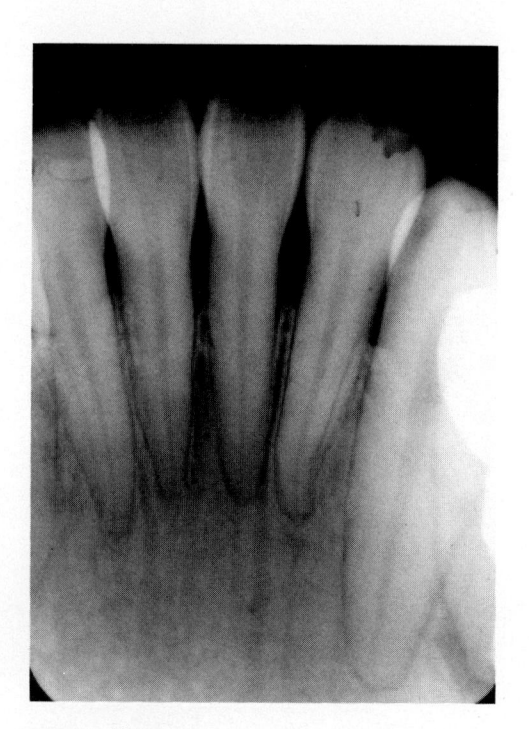

Figure 3-10

Chapter 3 ♦ Radiographic Interpretation 49

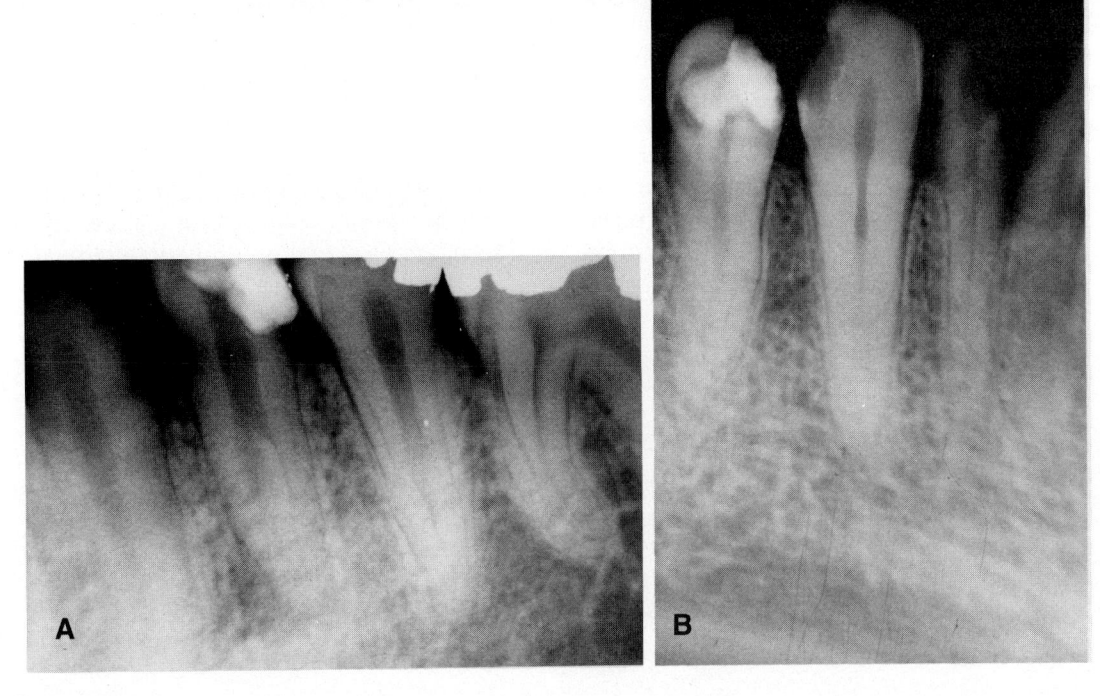

Figure 3-11

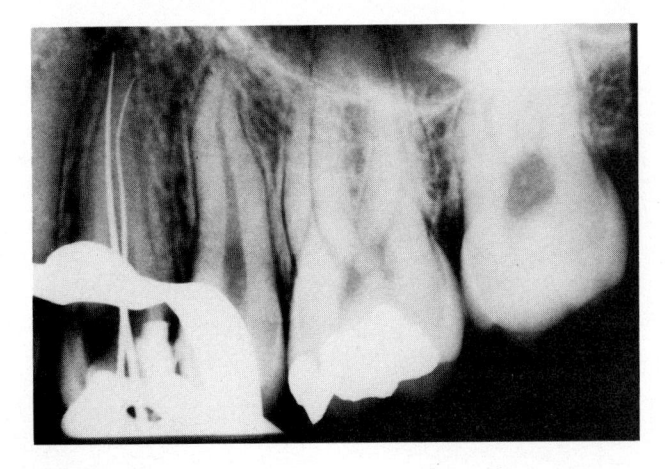

Figure 3-12

50   PRACTICAL ENDODONTICS

usually symmetrical in development, so if canals are not centrally placed, especially on a horizontal angle shot, suspect more than one canal in the root. Root canal failure of the lower molar is shown in Fig. 3-13, A. Note that at a distal angled x-ray shows the missed canal off to one side of the root (Fig. 3-13, B). As a general rule, more distinct (sharply defined edge) objects are usually on the lingual side closest to the radiographic film.

A sinus tract is a channel from a chronic apical abscess to an epithelial surface. All sinus tracts should be traced to help determine the source of the infection (Fig. 3-14, A-B). To trace these tracts, place a fresh gutta percha point (size 25 or 30) in the sinus tract until it stops. Now take a radiograph of the area. The tip of the gutta percha will point to the infected area, which could be two or three teeth away from the exit of the sinus tract. Sinus tracts can even cross the midline.

Radiopaque lesions such as condensing osteitis may indicate a sick pulp or even mask periapical infections (Fig. 3-15). A pulp chamber that is reduced in size or calcifying, or a tooth with a full crown, deep restoration, or pulp capping should be prime suspects in difficult diagnostic cases.

Radiolucent lesions associated with a vital tooth are usually not of endodontic origin (Fig. 3-16). These lesions may represent anatomic landmarks, pe-

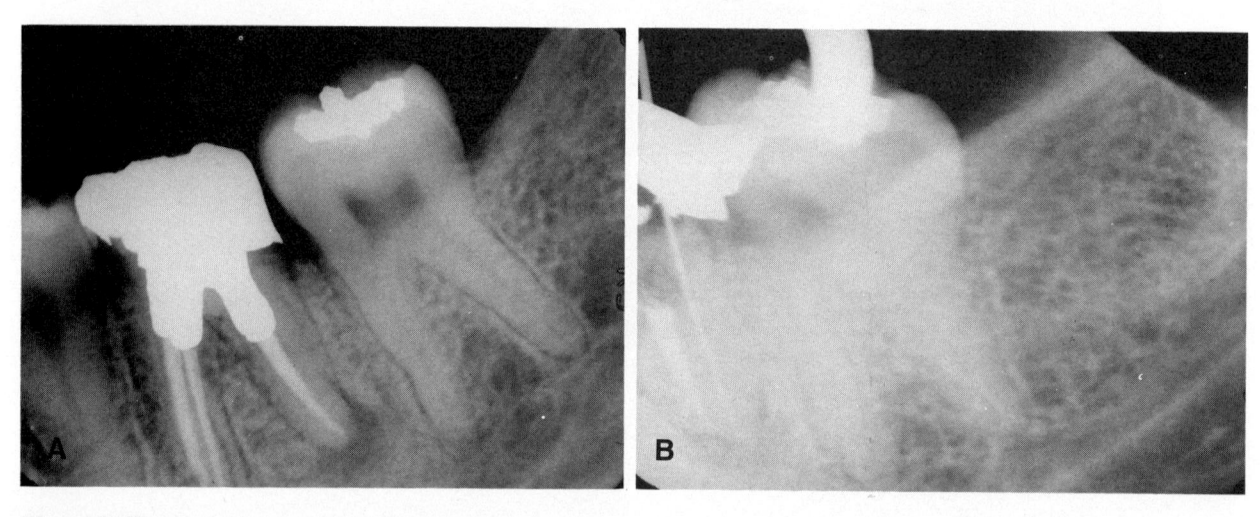

Figure 3-13

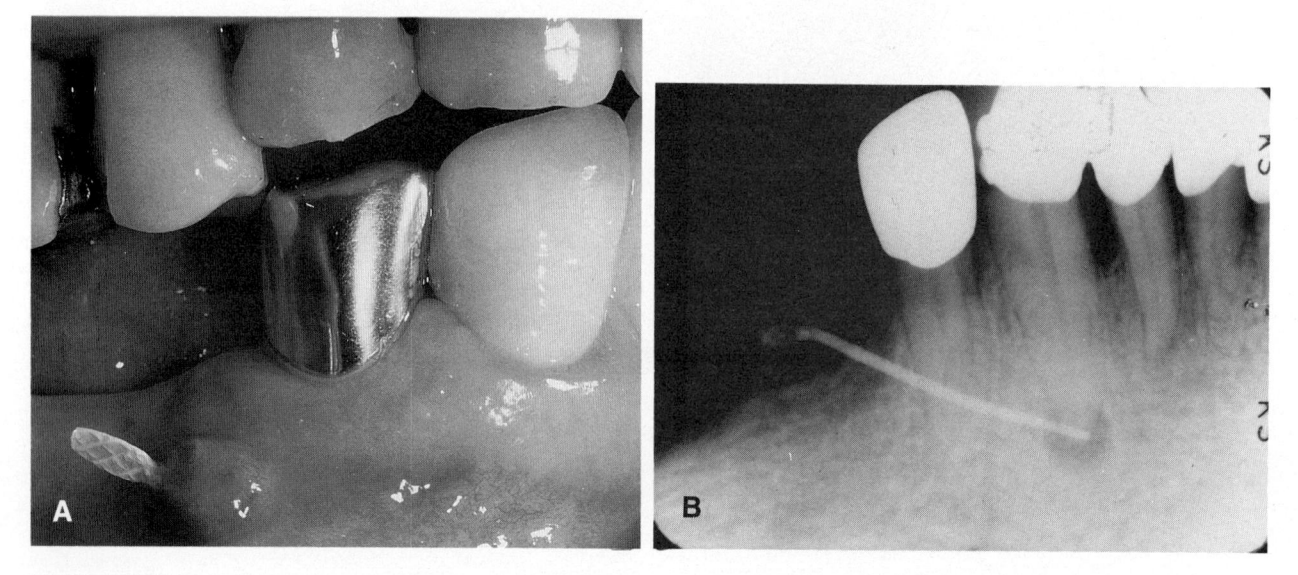

Figure 3-14

riodontal disease, or a lesion of nonendodontic origin, e.g., periapical fibrous dysplasia (cementoma), odontogenic keratocyst, traumatic bone cysts. The mental foramen many times is interpreted as a periapical lesion at the apex of the mandibular second premolar (Fig. 3-17, *left*). If it is the mental foramen, a change in the horizontal radiographic angulation will move the radiolucency away from the root apex (Fig. 3-17, *right*). A true periapical lesion will always stay at the apex.

Variations in angulation will alter the radiographic image of a lesion with regard to size, shape, and positional relationship to other structures. A lesion can easily be missed if only one preoperative radiograph is made (Fig. 3-18, *A*). Clinician must remember that the radiograph is a two-dimensional picture of a three-dimensional subject. If the diagnosis cannot be made with one radiograph, then another radiograph from a different angle should be taken. Here the second radiograph shows a periapical radiolucency of the second premolar (Fig. 3-18, *B*). A more accurate diagnosis or canal measurement can result when two radiographs from different angles are taken and compared. The first radiograph should be made straight on (at right angle to the buccal or labial surface of the tooth) and the second radiograph is made from a mesial or distal horizontal angle depending on the location of the tooth in the arch (Fig. 3-19). By comparing the two radiographs, the clinician can more readily see the third dimensional of the object viewed. The best measurement radiographs of premolars are usually taken from the mesial angle, while the best angle for molars is from the distal.

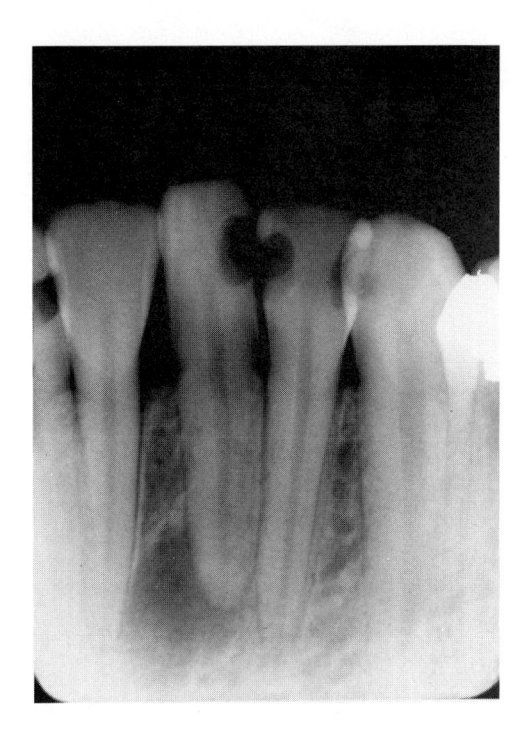

Figure 3-16

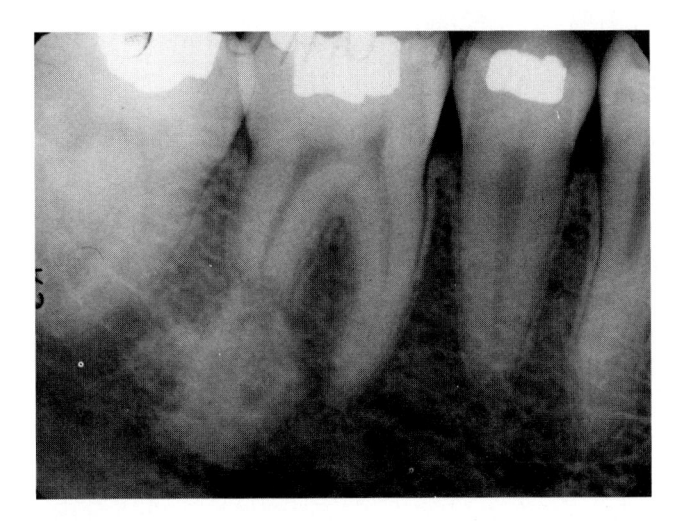

Figure 3-15

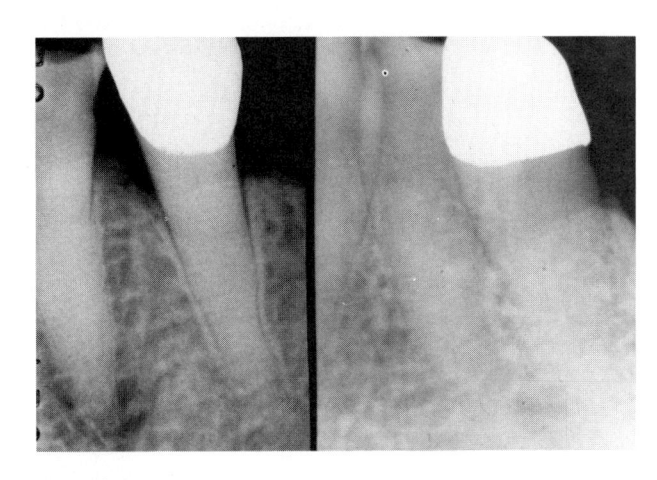

Figure 3-17

52 PRACTICAL ENDODONTICS

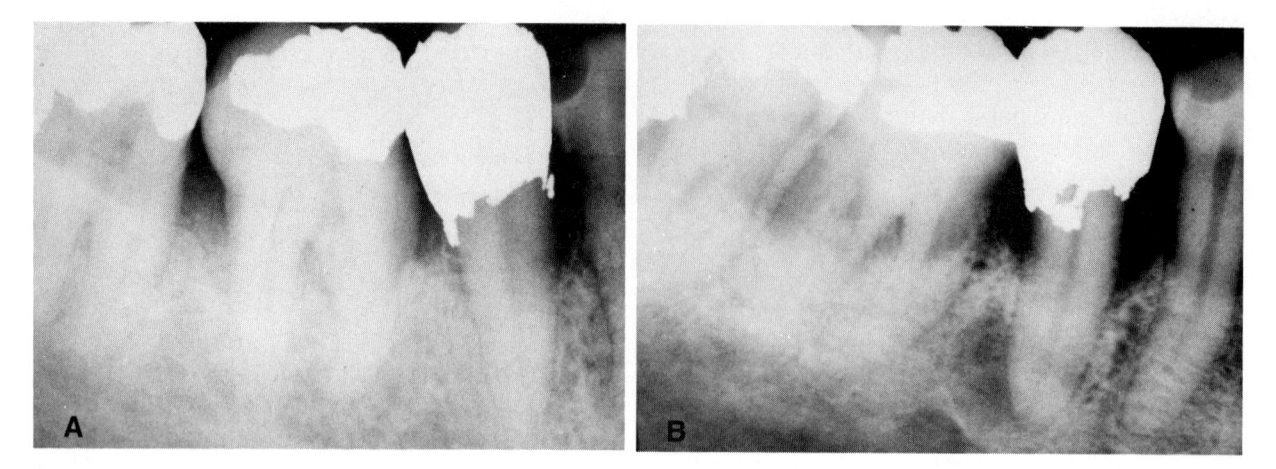

Figure 3-18

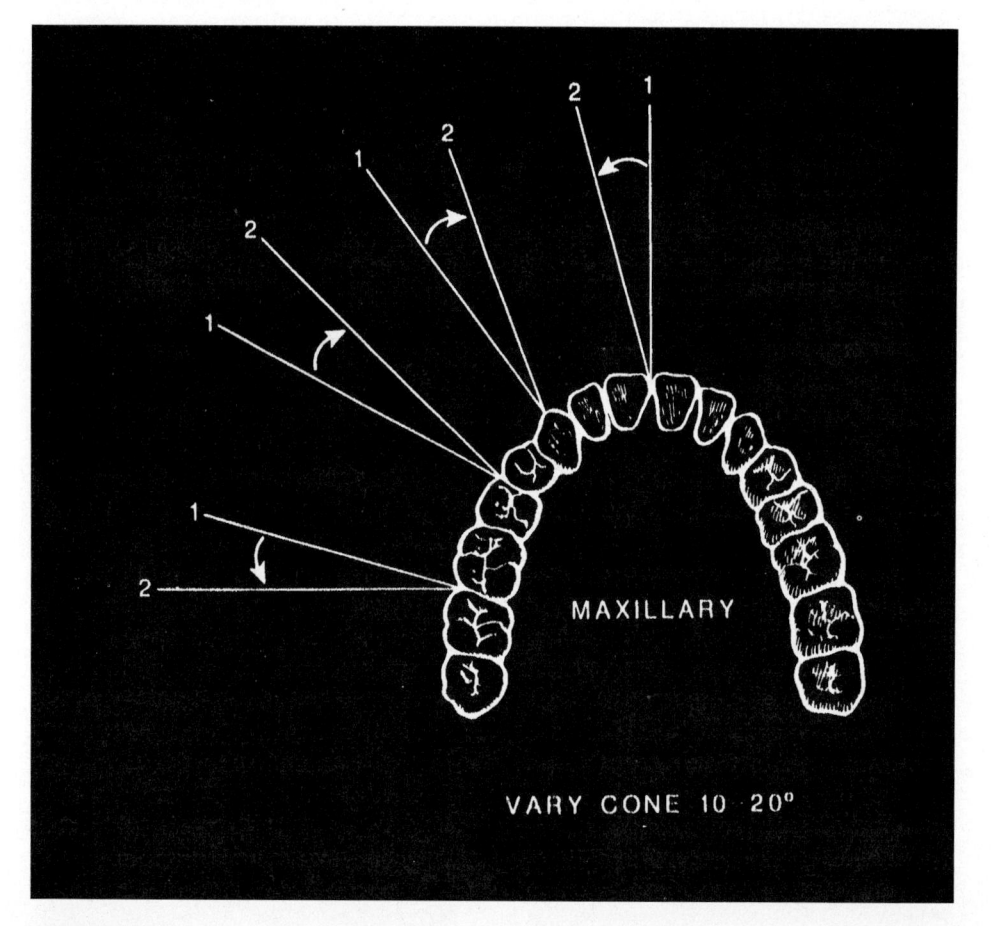

Figure 3-19

BUCCAL OBJECT/SLOB RULE

The buccal object rule (BOR) is used to determine the relative buccal lingual location of objects in the oral cavity. Although sometimes confusing, the use of a simple mnemonic can make it easier to understand. This mnemonic is the word SLOB (same lingual, opposite buccal). Simply stated, the lingual object will always follow the x-ray tube head. For example, if the radiograph of the maxillary premolar is taken from the mesial then you will see the lingual canal and root on the mesial. If the x-ray cone is moved to the distal, the lingual canal/root on the radiograph will appear to move to the distal, while the buccal root or object will appear to have moved in the opposite direction to the mesial.

The buccal object rule is very helpful in endodontic radiography and is used to:
1. Determine number, location, shape, size, and direction of various roots and root canals during cleansing, shaping, and obturation.
2. Move anatomic landmarks, such as the zygomatic process, thereby improving radiographic visualization of obscured objects.
3. Distinguish between normal anatomic landmarks and the radiolucent shadows associated with pathosis of the roots of teeth.
4. Determine the buccal or lingual position of perforations, and resorptive processes.
5. Distinguish between internal and external root resorption.
6. Locate radiopaque foreign bodies in trauma cases.
7. Locate anatomic landmarks (i.e., mandibular canal, maxillary sinus) in relation to the root apex during root canal therapy and periapical surgery.

In the past, two known radiographs with different horizontal angulation have been used to determine the position of the lingual or buccal object. This usually requires the making of additional radiographs from known positions. However, by using certain clues, the clinician can determine with the use of only one radiograph from which horizontal angulation (mesial or distal) the radiograph was made. Once this is known, the SLOB rule is used to determine if the object lies on the buccal or lingual. Six clues can be used to determine whether the radiograph was taken from the mesial or distal.
1. In the MAXILLARY ARCH, the most important clue is the position of the palatal root of the maxillary molars (Fig. 3-20). Normally, radiographs are taken at a straight right angle to the tooth, and the palatal root is visualized as lying between the two buccal roots. If the palatal root lies behind the mesiobuccal root, the x-ray beam came from mesial direction (Fig. 3-20, *A* and *B*). Now by looking at the maxillary premolars on the same radiograph, the SLOB rule can be used to determine that the root appearing to the mesial is the lingual root. Conversely, if the radiograph was taken from the distal, the palatal root of the maxillary first molar will lie behind the distobuccal root. Again by using the SLOB rule, we can predict that the lingual canal of the maxillary premolars will appear distal to the buccal canal (Fig. 3-20, *C* and *D*).

Other direction indicators of horizontal angulation in the maxillary arch are:
2. If the cuspid is seen in the radiograph, the radiograph was probably made from a mesial angle.
3. When contacts overlap, the radiograph was made from either the mesial or distal but not straight on.
4. The lingual roots or cusps lie closest to the film and appear more distinct than the buccal roots and cusps.
5. Maxillary radiographs are usually made from a positive vertical angle (+10 to +45 degrees), and thus the palatal roots appear to be longer than the buccal roots.
6. The lingual cusp and the lingual portion of the rubber dam clamp will appear higher (more radicular), having moved in the direction of the x-ray cone.

The most important clue in the MANDIBULAR ARCH is seeing the cuspid or molars in the radiograph (Fig. 3-21). If the cuspid is seen, the radiograph was probably taken from the mesial (Fig. 3-21, *A-B*) but if the radiograph was shot from the distal horizontal angle (Fig. 3-21, *C-D*), then the second and third molars and not the cuspid will be seen in the film.

Other important clues in the mandibular arch are the movement of the rubber dam clamp arms and the cusps of the premolar teeth. Most mandibular radiographs are taken at a negative vertical angulation (0 to −10 degrees). The buccal cusp is the highest (most coronal) cusp and moves in the opposite direction of the x-ray cone. The lingual (most radicular) cusp moves in the direction of the x-ray cone. This same rationale is used for the lingual arm (most radicular) of the rubber dam clamp. The contacts overlap when the radiograph is made from a mesial or distal horizontal angulation.

54 PRACTICAL ENDODONTICS

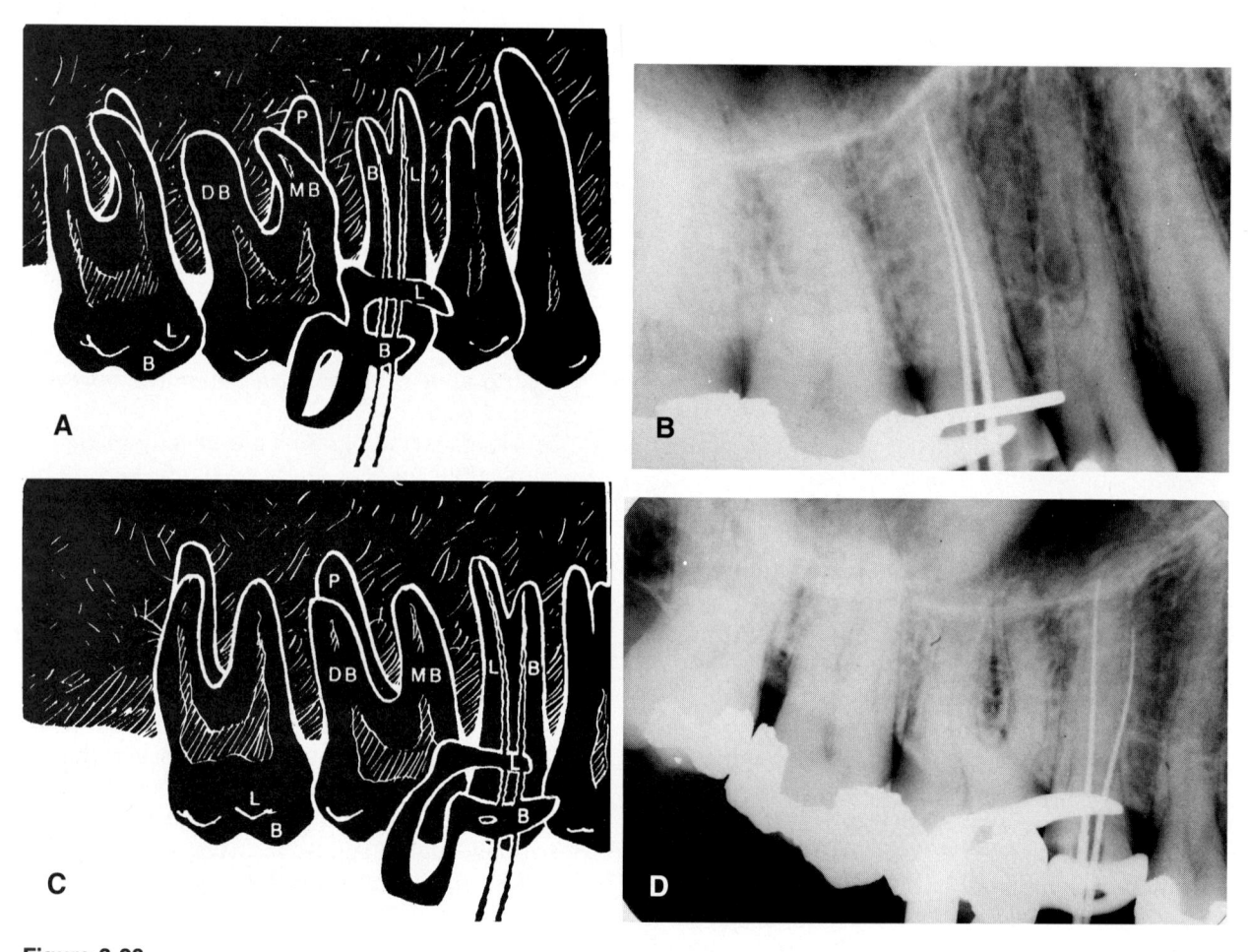

Figure 3-20

Chapter 3 ♦ Radiographic Interpretation 55

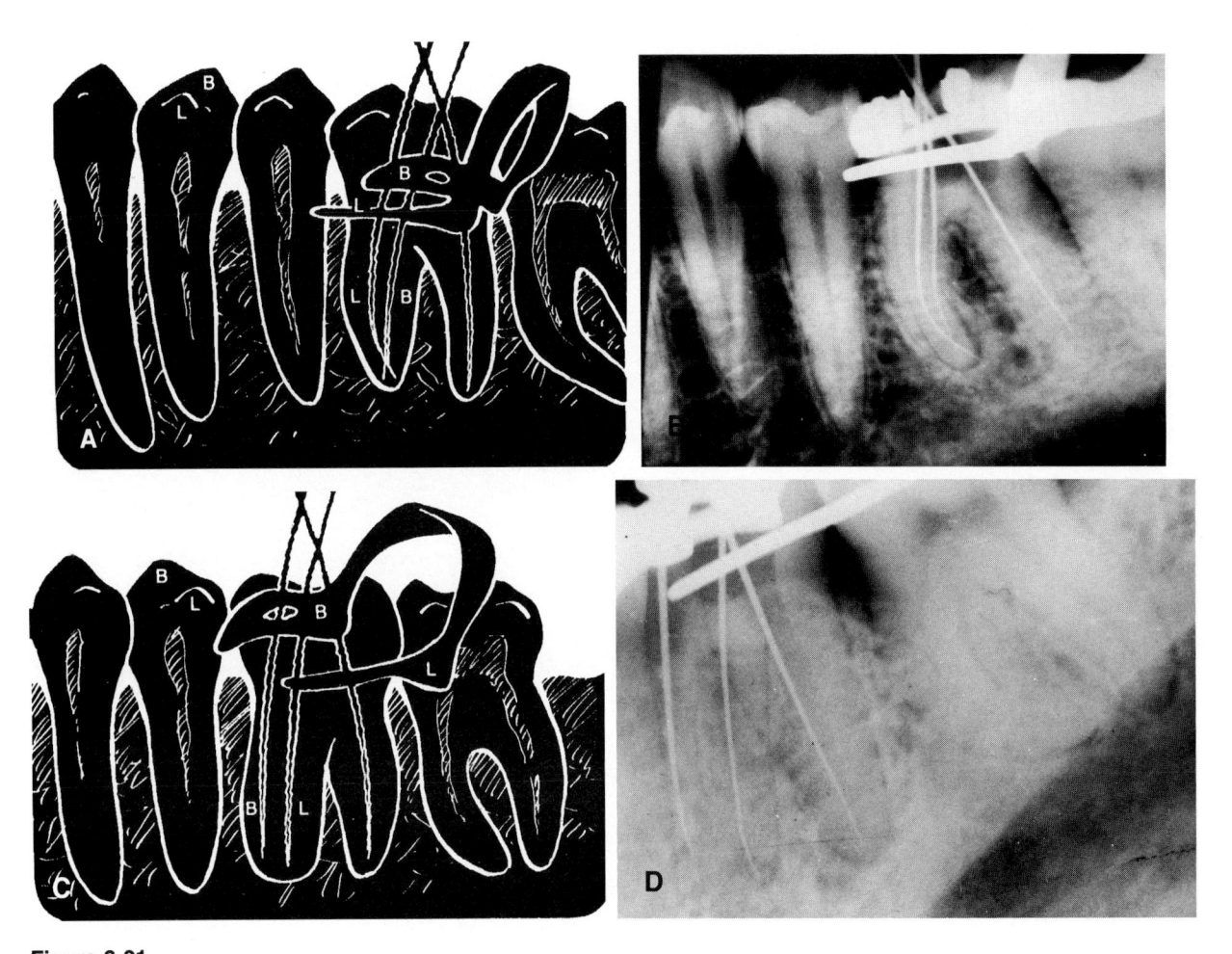

Figure 3-21

HELPFUL HINTS IN RADIOGRAPHIC TECHNIQUE

Paralleling (right-angle) radiograph technique is recommended over the bisecting angle technique. Parallel radiographs show less distortion and minimal enlargement, are more accurate, and reduce the chance of the zygomatic process overlapping the roots in maxillary molar teeth. A parallel radiograph can provide a picture of near true dimensions of the real tooth within the dental arch. Initial canal measurements and other cleansing, shaping, and obturation measurements of the canal can then be reliably made from these radiographs (Fig. 3-22).

To obtain a parallel radiograph, the tooth should be parallel to the radiographic film and outside edge of the cone head (perpendicular to radiographic beam) (Fig. 3-23, A-B). In multirooted teeth, the film should be parallel to an imaginary line that bisects the roots (Fig. 3-24, A-B). Many devices are available to help the assistant align the cone head parallel with the radiograph (Fig. 3-25). Paralleling devices to hold all films are highly recommended. This is particularly true with elderly patients or young children who do not have the manual dexterity to hold the film. Having the patient hold the film with his or her finger may cause bending of the film. Some dentists remove the rubber dam frame for ease in film placement, resulting in saliva contaminating the operating field.

This can be prevented by sliding the film holder under the rubber dam (Fig. 3-23, B) or by partially removing the rubber dam when making the radiograph (Fig. 3-24, B). The upper corner is released when making radiographs of maxillary teeth and the lower corner when making radiographs of the mandibular teeth. The use of plastic rubber dam frames will also ensure that the apices are not obscured by the frame.

When first learning, the Rinn XCP, the Crawford

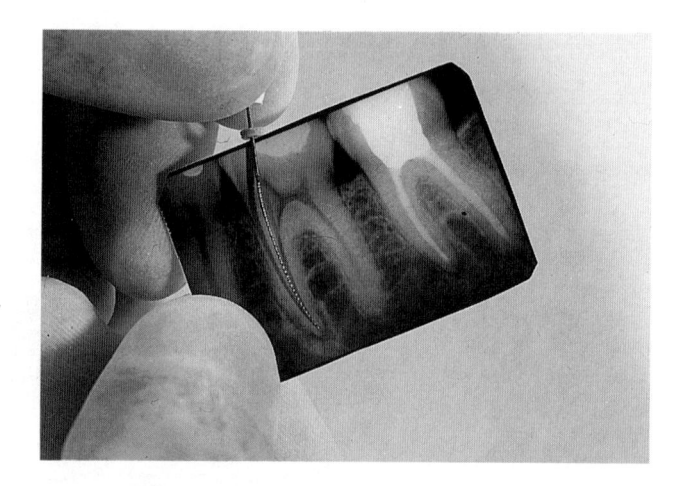

Figure 3-22

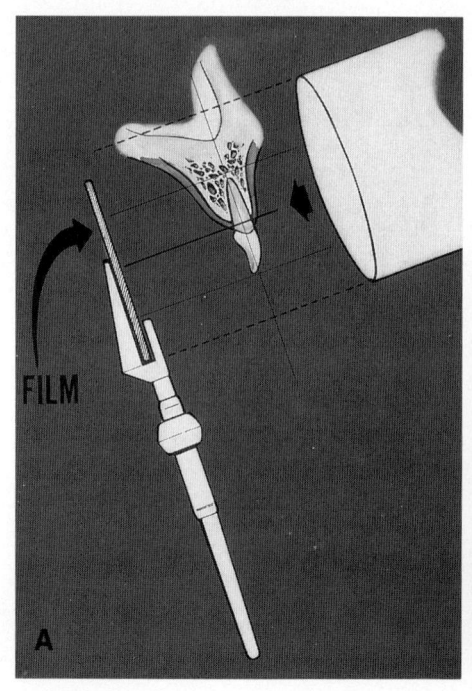

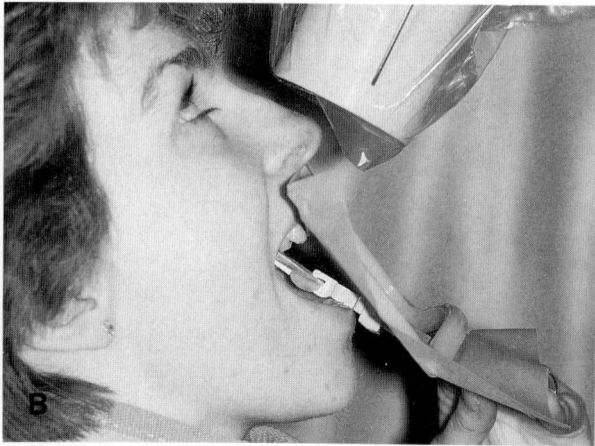

Figure 3-23

hemostat, or Rinn Snap-A-Ray with the paralleling ring is best used to teach the novice parallel relationships. With more experience, less complicated devices such as the plain Snap-A-Ray, hemostat, or Endo-Ray can be used. These products require less set-up and sterilization time. An inexpensive disposable film holder can be made by taping the radiograph to a tongue blade (Fig. 3-26). After being used on a patient, it is discarded. The use of disposable items are encouraged in this era of infection control. The Endo-Ray (Fig. 3-27) is highly recommended for endodontic measurement films of posterior teeth, while the Snap-A-Ray is used for anterior endodontic measurements.

Incorrect film placement is the most common error in radiography and can lead to an improper diagnosis and missed endodontic measurements. This is followed in order of occurrence by cone cutting, processing errors, and incorrect vertical and/or horizontal angulation. These errors can usually be avoided by following a few simple procedures. Place the dot on the film toward the incisal edge so that it does not overlap the root apices in the radiograph. To ensure the periapical area is not missed, line up the film as closely as possible with the incisal or occlusal surface of the teeth. In patients with shallow palatal vaults, line the edge of the film on the occlusal surface and use a bisecting angle technique. Place the tooth to be radiographed in the center of the film. When the slope of the palate is narrow and interferes with anterior film placement, use smaller size film or use the Snap-A-Ray and place the film parallel to the tooth but further back in the mouth.

Continue to improve each new radiograph by looking at the previous radiographs of that tooth and make any new changes in exposure, film placement, and angulation. To obtain the perfect angled radiograph, leave the cone head in the same position next

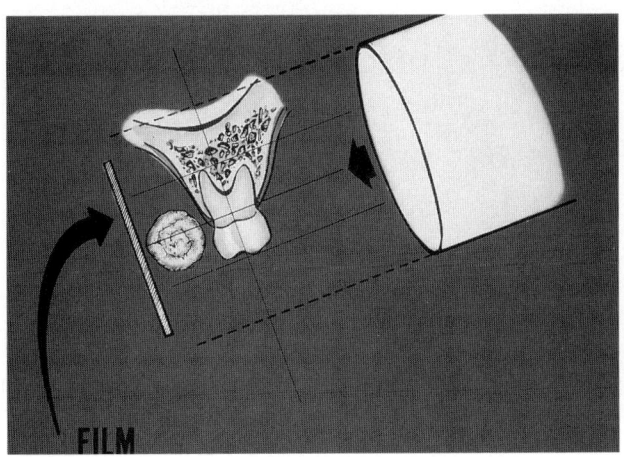

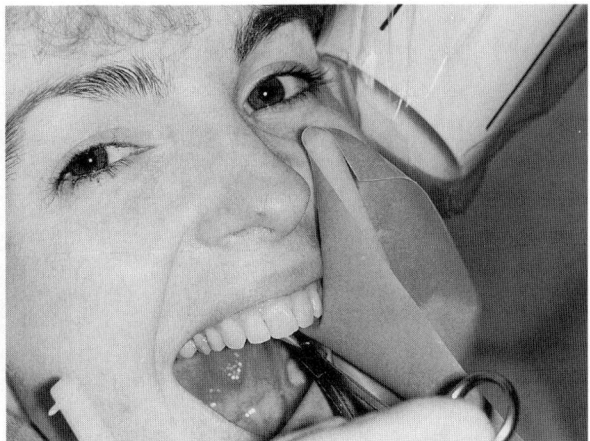

Figure 3-24

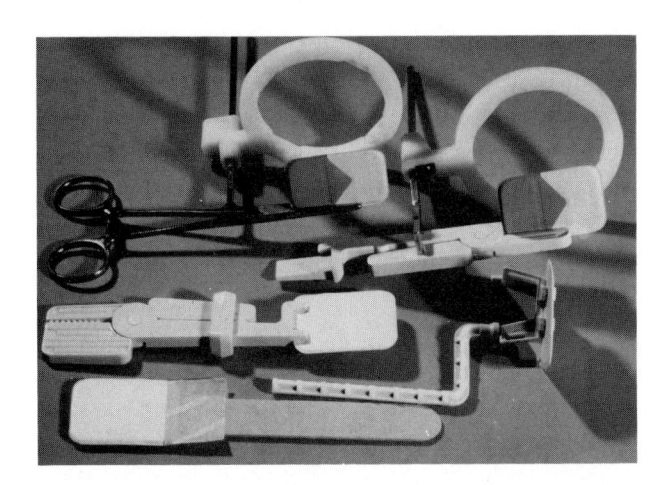

Figure 3-25

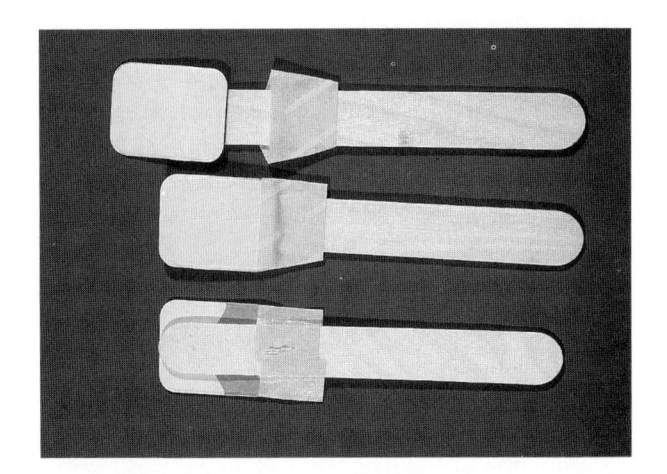

Figure 3-26

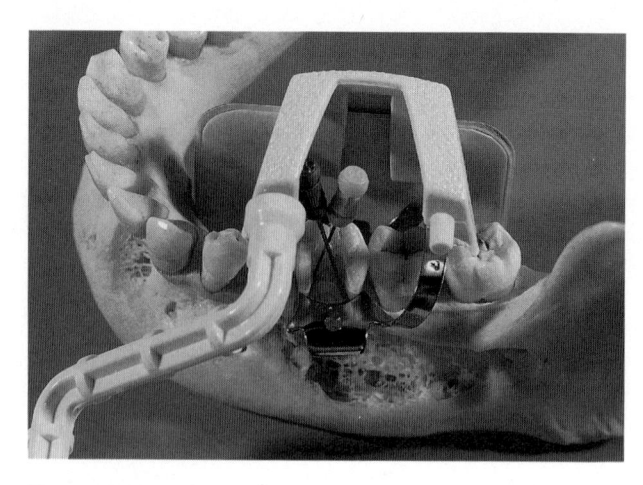

Figure 3-27

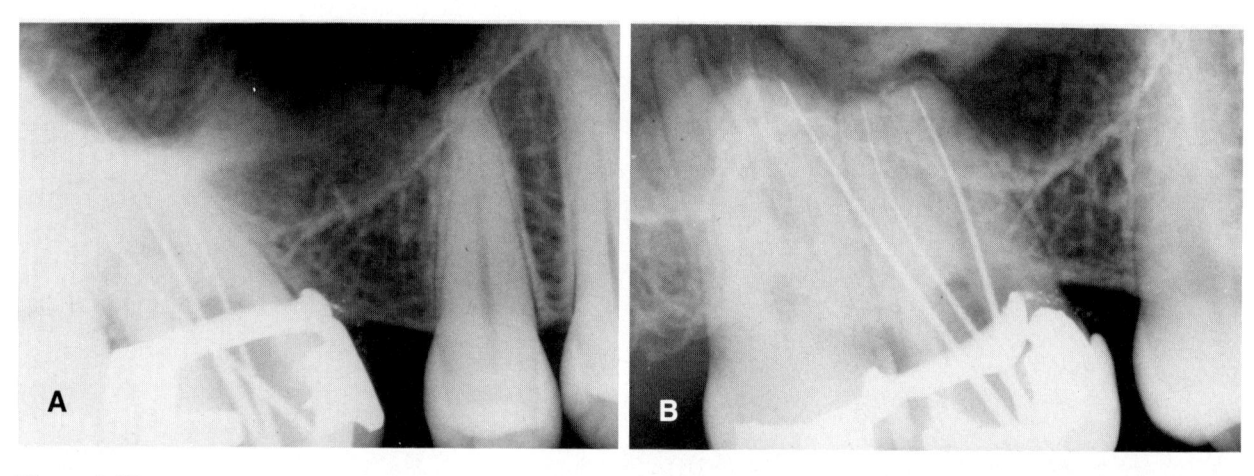

Figure 3-28

to the patient while you develop the first film. If a second picture is needed, only minor alterations of the cone head position is made to obtain the desired picture.

Make the radiograph at the proper vertical and horizontal angulation. The correct vertical angulation is obtained when the cone is at a right angle to the tooth and the tooth and film are parallel. In the maxillary posterior teeth, the vertical angulation should be less than 30 degrees to reduce the possibility of the zygomatic process overlapping the roots (Fig. 3-28, A). Shooting from the distal and at a lower angle can greatly enhance your success (Fig. 3-28, B).

To ensure proper deep placement of the film in the lingual vestibule, use your index finger to gently push down the floor of the mouth and slide the film packet next to your finger. Not only will you get the film deep enough but you reduce patient discomfort and induction of the gag reflex (Fig. 3-29).

Many mandibular posterior teeth tilt lingually. To obtain an accurate parallel radiograph, a positive 5-degree vertical angle must be used (Fig. 3-30). If the mandible is very narrow, a small or narrow film is best for making radiographs of the anterior teeth.

Increase the time setting to obtain darker endodontic radiographs. This burns out the trabeculation and improves visualization of the tooth and instruments. When working on calcified canals, place the rubber dam clamp on another tooth back so the view of the pulpal floor is not blocked by the clamp wings.

For insurance claims or for dentists with a referred endodontic practice, double film packs are recommended for the diagnostic, final treatment, and follow-up radiographs. One set is for permanent office records and the other for the referring dentist and insurance claims. Insurance companies may not accept information obtained from apex locators, so record all necessary steps on film. Rinn also makes a Mini-Ray duplicator (Model 72-1220) (Fig. 3-31) to make quick copies of radiographs for insurance companies.

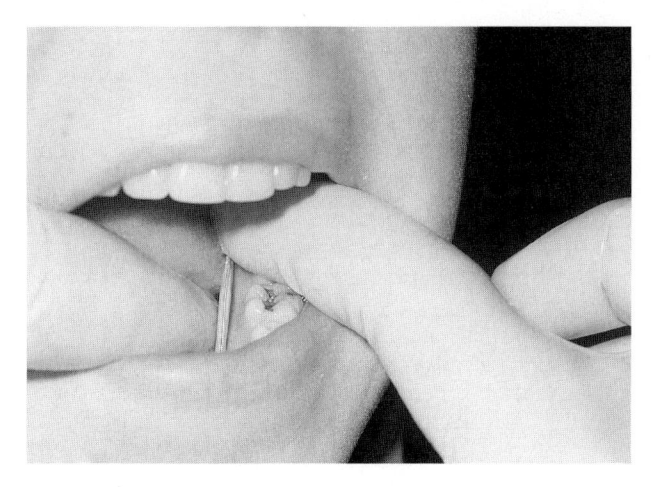

Figure 3-29

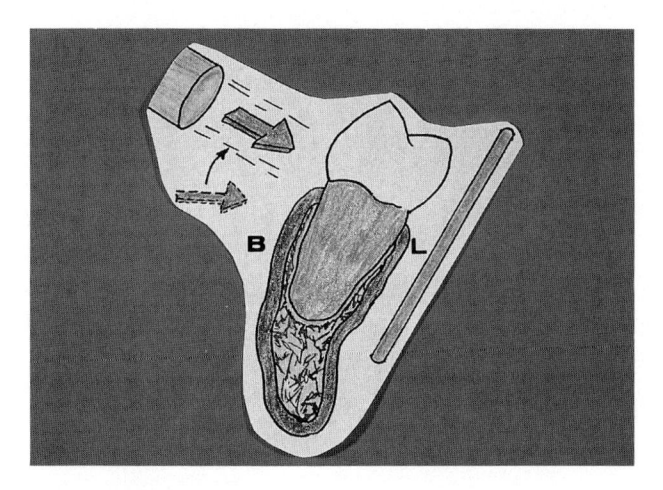

Figure 3-30

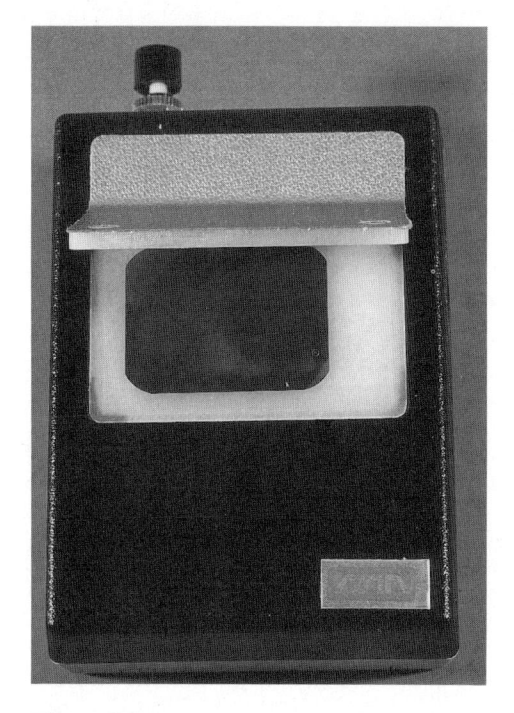

Figure 3-31

PROCESSING THE RADIOGRAPH

Each dentist must demand and maintain archivable quality radiographs. This begins with dental school training as to what is acceptable. Once clinicians have mastered the technique they can train their staff in proper radiographic techniques and film processing procedures. The clinician cannot expect the staff to learn on their own nor set their own standard of acceptability. Poorly processed radiographs have often led to a wrong diagnosis (Fig. 3-32, *A* and *B*). When improperly fixed or washed, many radiographs deteriorate over time thus destroying an important part of the dental record. Routine cleaning and maintenance of the automatic film processor and changing of chemicals is a must. The use of daylight quick processing tanks (Fig. 3-33) and high speed chemicals (Fig. 3-34) is highly recommended in every dental office, and is especially useful when performing endodontics. The table top processing box is used right in the operatory, which eliminates the trip down the hall to the darkroom. Not only can the film be read wet within 30 seconds, but high quality radiographs are obtained. It is important to wash these quick processed radiographs for 30 minutes after fixing to prevent deterioration with time. Clothing stains from

60 PRACTICAL ENDODONTICS

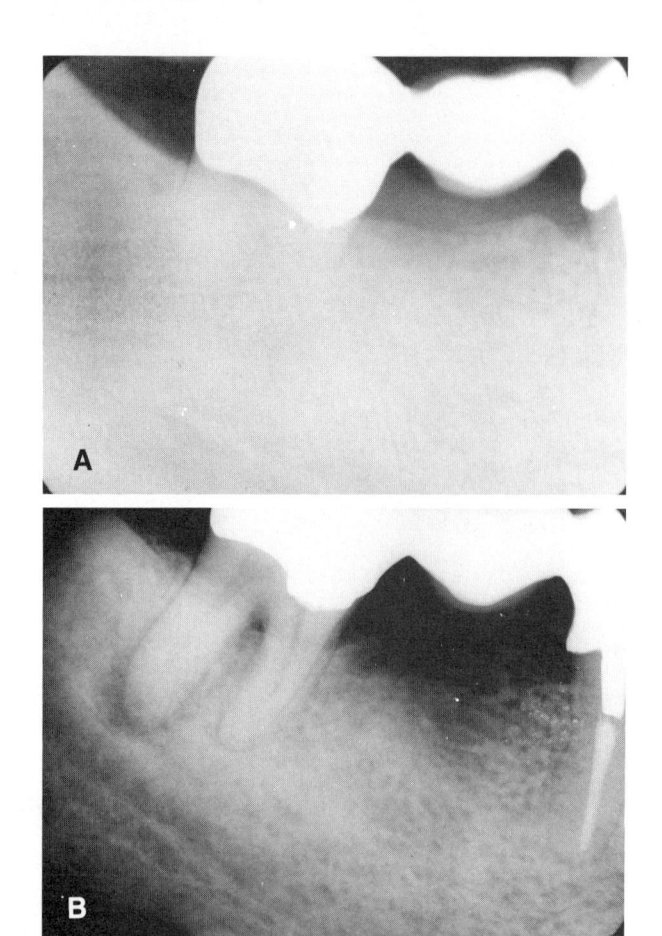

Figure 3-32

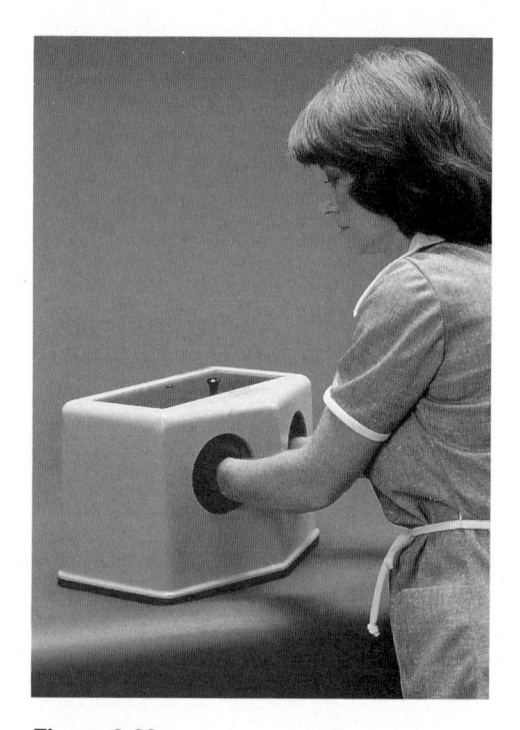

Figure 3-33

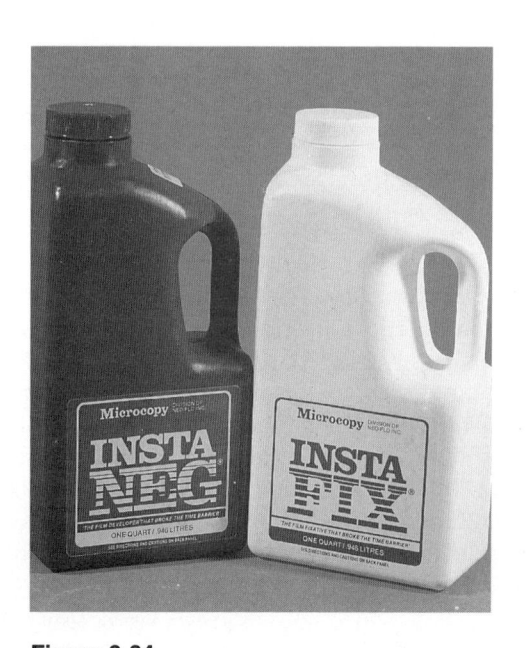

Figure 3-34

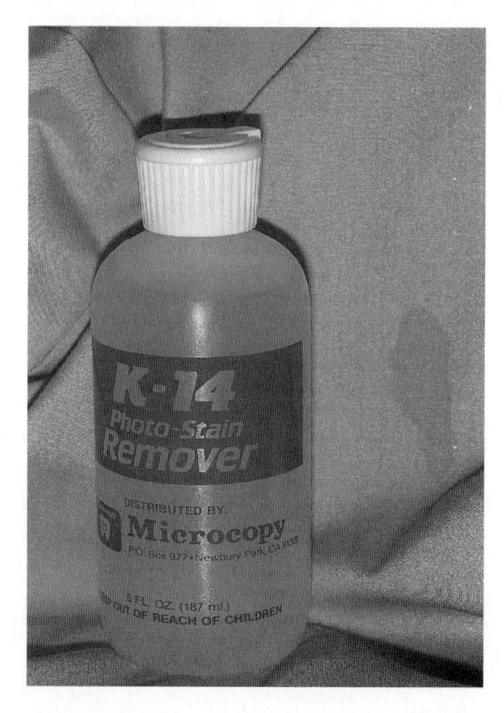

Figure 3-35

processing chemicals can be easily and quickly removed with stain removers such as Microcopy Fix-Off (Fig. 3-35). Note fixer stain on clinic smock.

RADIOGRAPHIC SAFETY

Radiographic safety is a major concern of many patients. As clinicians we are obligated to do everything we can to protect the patient, our staff, and ourselves against unnecessary radiation, and to educate patients about the minimal risk vs maximum benefits of dental radiographs. When talking with patients, instead of using the word *x-ray*, use the words *necessary x-rays* to emphasize the importance of each film.

The dentist has control over many factors that can greatly reduce radiation to patient and staff. Some of these factors are as follows: Proper x-ray equipment adjustment, filtration and collimation, the use of the lead aprons, thyroid collar, and lead film holders (Fig. 3-36). Open-end x-ray cones lined with lead or steel are recommended over short pointed cones, which produce larger amounts of scatter radiation. When more than one film is required per area, a double film pack is used with the same amount of radiation expended for a one film pack. If only one film has been made, it can be duplicated and the patient need not be radiated again. Through proper training and use of proper radiographic techniques, the need for additional retake pictures is almost completely eliminated. Electronic apex locators are also available and are reasonably accurate in verification measurement, thus reducing patient exposure. The use of radiovisiography in the office can reduce radiation by one fifth.

Operator protection is equally important. The operator should stand at least 6 feet away from the patient when taking the radiograph or be protected by a 1-mm thick lead shield. A radiation survey should be routinely conducted of the x-ray room and equipment. A film badge is also recommended to monitor radiation exposure to operator.

Radiation has two biological effects on tissues: somatic (the effect on all tissues of the body except sperm and ovum) and gonadal (genetic—the effect on the reproductive cells that is passed on to future generations). The taking of a complete mouth radiographic survey the maximum somatic dose to the face could range between 0.6 rad to 4 rad. Yet the risk of skin cancer cannot be statistically demonstrated at dose levels below 25 rad and an erythematic dose is in the range of 400 rad. The risk of harmful effects would therefore be very small. With good technique, the male genetic exposure for a complete set of in-

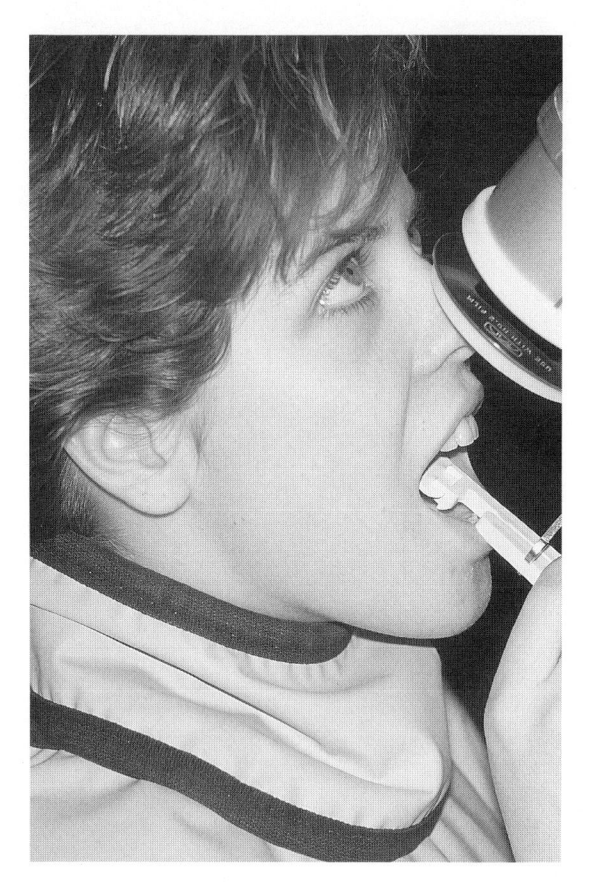

Figure 3-36

traoral radiographs is approximately 0.3 mR (which is about the same exposure each person gets from background radiation every day). The possible hazard for female ovum is only one fifth of the male. When a lead apron and D film is used, the dose to gonadal tissues with a full mouth dental series (18 intraoral films) would be .01 mR.

LEGAL CONSIDERATION IN DENTAL RADIOGRAPHY

It can be generally said that you will not be faulted for taking additional radiographs to make the right diagnosis, but will be liable if the wrong diagnosis is made because not enough radiographs were taken. This is also true with errors in cleansing, shaping, and obturation. It is important that the radiograph is of an archivable quality and does not deteriorate over the years. Besides dating the film holder, use a pencil to date the radiograph in a noncritical part of the radiograph.

4

Sterilization Procedures and Endodontic Armamentarium

"Every patient must be considered infectious and the same infection control procedure must be applied for all patients."

The ability of the dentist to practice endodontics free from diseased germs is a challenge. As early as 1978 the American Dental Association made recommendations for controlling infection in dentistry.

The Occupational Safety and Health Agency (OSHA) has now become involved in the safety regulations of the employee and dentist. They have issued guidelines that we must conform to, thus reducing risks of contracting a bloodborne disease (human immune deficiency virus [HIV] or Hepatitis B).

Bloodborne organisms can penetrate the body through various ways. The most common cause is needle sticks or contaminated surface tops. Pathogenic organisms have been known to live at least 1 week outside the body at room temperature.

Surface areas that are not disinfected preoperatively and postoperatively could pose a problem. Should one touch the contaminated surface area and place his or her hand on the mucous membrane of the mouth or eye he or she could become infected. This also poses a problem with those who have open wounds and are not properly protected.

The Council on Dental Material, Instruments, and Equipment has stated there are four basic types of sterilization practical for use in dentistry (Tables 4-1 and 4-2):

1. Steam autoclave (Fig 4-1, *A, B,* and *C*)
2. Dry heat
3. Chemical vapor (Fig 4-2)
4. Ethylene oxide chamber

TABLE 4-1 ♦ *Summary of Sterilization Conditions*

Sterilizer	Temperature	Pressure	Time
Steam Autoclave	121°C (250°F)	15 psi	15 min
unwrapped items	132°C (270°F)	30 psi	3 min
Steam autoclave	121°C (250°F)	15 psi	20 min
lightly wrapped items	132°C (270°F)	30 psi	8 min
heavily wrapped items	132°C (270°F)	30 psi	10 min
Dry heat	170°C (340°F)		60 min
	160°C (320°F)		120 min
	150°C (300°F)		150 min
	140°C (285°F)		180 min
	121°C (250°F)		12 hrs
Dry heat (rapid flow)			
unwrapped items	190°C (375°F)		6 min
packaged items	190°C (375°F)		12 min
Chemical vapor	132°C (270°F)	20-40 psi	20 min
Ethylene oxide	Ambient		8-10 hrs

From Council on Dental Materials, Instruments, and Equipment: *JADA*, 122:80, 1991.

TABLE 4-2 ♦ Sterilization and Disinfection of Dental Instruments, Materials, and Some Commonly Used Items

	Steam Autoclave	Dry Heat Oven	Chemical Vapor	Ethylene Oxide	Chemical Agents	Other Methods & Comments
Angle attachments*	+	+	+	++	+	
Burs						
Carbon steel	−	++	++	++	−	Discard
Steel	+	++	++	++	−	Discard
Tungston-carbide	+	++	+	++	−	Discard
Condensers	+	++	++	++	+	
Dapen dishes	++	+	+	++	+	
Endodontic instruments (broaches, files, reamers)	++	++	++	++		
Stainless steel handles	+	++	++	++	+	
Stainless w/plastic handles	++	++	−	++	−	
Glass slabs	++	++	++	++	+	
Hand instruments						
Carbon steel	−	++	++	++	−	
	(Steam autoclave with chemical protection [2% sodium nitrite])					
Stainless steel	++	++	++	++		
Handpieces*	(++)*	−	(+)*	++		
Contra-angles	++	−	++	++		
Instruments in packs	++	+ / Small packs	++	++ / Small packs	=	
Instrument tray setups						
Restorative or Surgical	+ / Size limit	+	+ / Size limit	++ / Size limit	=	
Mirrors	−	++	++	++	+	
Needles						
Disposable	=	=	=	=	=	Discard (++) Do not reuse
Pluggers and condensers	++	++	++	++	+	
Polishing wheels & disks						
Garnet and cuttle	=	−	−	++	=	
Rag	++	−	+	++	=	
Rubber	+	−	−	++	−	
Rubber dam equipment						
Carbon steel clamps	−	++	++	++	−	
Metal frames	++	++	++	++	+	
Plastic frames	−	−	−	++	+	
Punches	−	++	++	++	+	
Stainless steel clamps	++	++	++	++	+	
Saliva evacuators, ejectors (plastic)	−	−	−	−		Discard (++) (single use/disposable)
Stones						
Diamond	+	++	++	++	−	
Polishing	++	+	++	++	−	
Sharpening	++	++	++	−	−	
Surgical instruments						
Stainless steel	++	++	++	++	−	
Ultrasonic scaling tips	+	=	=	++	+	
Water-air syringe tips	++	++	++	++	−	Discard (++)
X-ray equipment						
Plastic film holders	(++)*	=	(+)*	++	+	
Collimating devices	−	=	=	++	+	

Infection control recommendations, *JADA* (suppl) 123:4, 1992.
*Since manufacturers use a variety of alloys and materials in these products, confirmation with the equipment manufacturers is recommended, especially for handpieces and their attachments.
++Effective and preferred method.
+Effective and acceptable method.
−Effective method, but risk of damage to materials.
=Ineffective method with risk of damage to materials.

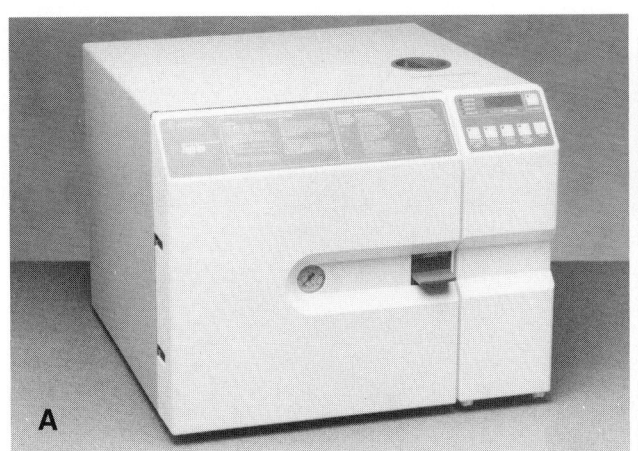

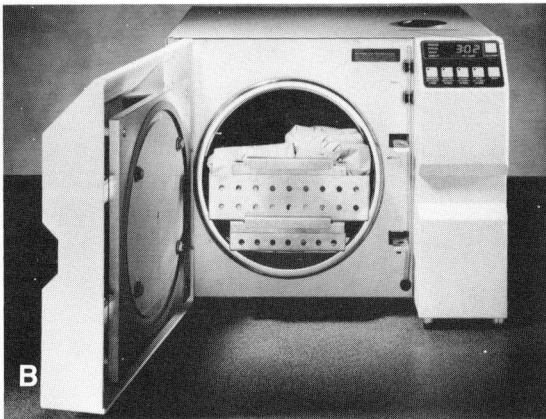

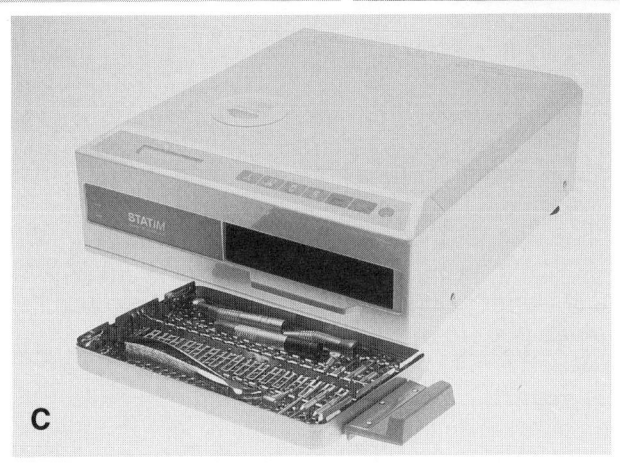

Chapter 4 ♦ Sterilization Procedures and Endodontic Armamentarium 65

Figure 4-1 The autoclave is the most effective method of sterilizing dental instruments with the least amount of expense. (*A* and *B*, American Sterilizer Co., 2424 West 23rd Street, PO Box 620, Erie, PA 16514); *C*, STATIM Cassette Autoclave 6 minute Sterilizing Cycle. (SciCan Division, Toronto, Canada.)

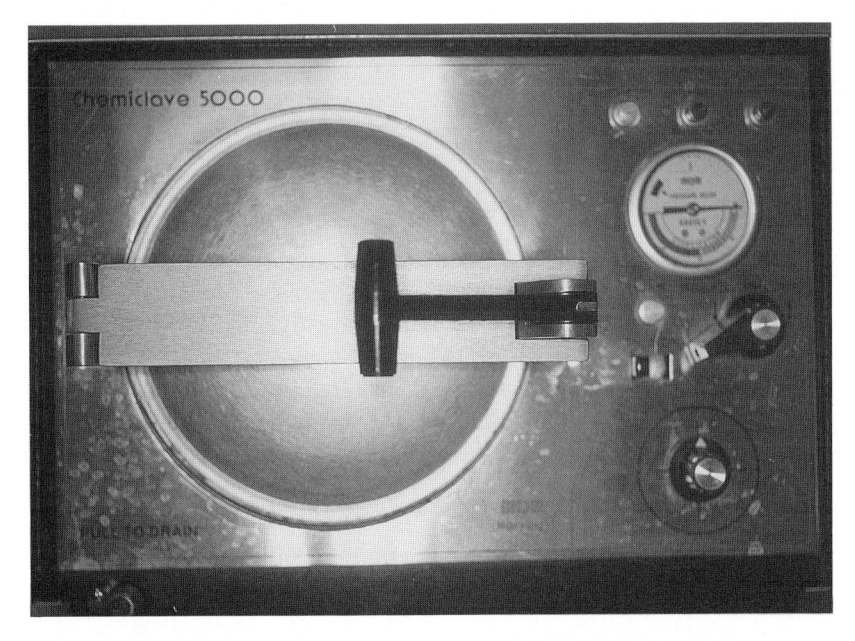

Figure 4-2 Chemical vapor used to sterilize carbon steel burs and carbon steel hand instruments. (Courtesy of Dr. CJ Miller, Dr. S Rand Werrin, and Dr. J Gruendel.)

Blood, breast milk, vaginal secretions, semen, or cerebrospinal, synovial, pleural, peritoneal, pericardial, and amniotic fluids, or body fluids containing visible blood such as saliva in dental procedures are to be considered infectious at all times.

It is important that all employees and dentists use protective barriers to prevent exposure to blood and other body fluids to which universal precautions apply (see Figs. 4-6, *A, B,* and *C;* 4-9, and 4-10).

A rubber dam should be used whenever possible to reduce and contain the spray from high speed handpieces during endodontic procedures (Fig. 4-11).

SURFACE DISINFECTANTS

Disinfectants are less effective than sterilization against pathogenic organisms. Instruments and equipment that come in contact with skin that may be exposed to spatter or spray of body fluids or those that may have been touched by contaminated hands should be disinfected.

The instruments to be sterilized with disinfectant should be placed in the ultrasonic bath before hand scrubbing. It is reported that ultrasonic cleaning of the instruments is 16 times more efficient than hand scrubbing. Ultrasound also reduces the potential for instrument sticks or punctures from the contaminated instruments. If the instruments are still visibly dirty they can then be hand scrubbed before sterilization. The dental assistant should use utility gloves while scrubbing the instruments.

There are six chemical groups the Environmental Protection Agency (EPA) recognizes as effective for surface disinfection in the dental environment. The first five also are accepted by the American Dental Association (ADA).

1. *Household bleach:* The active chemical is sodium hypochlorite and it can be diluted 1:5 to 1:100. It has an application time of 10 to 30 minutes. Gutta percha cones are disinfected using full strength household bleach for 1 minute (Fig. 4-3).
2. *Iodophors:* Active chemical is 1% available iodine. Dilution is according to manufacturers' instruction. Application time is 10 minutes. This product also has residual activity.
3. *Phenol-alcohol sprays:* Active chemicals .176% to 1.65% combined phenols with 18% to 54% ethanol, also 0.1% phenol and 79% ethyl alcohol. Application time per manufacturers' instructions.
4. *Synthetic phenol combinations:* Active chemicals 9% phenyl phenol and 1% 0-benzyle-p-chlorophenol. Dilution 1:32 and application time 10 minutes.
5. *Phenol water sprays:* Active chemicals 1.41% phenol, 0.47% sodium tetraborate, and 0.24% sodium phenate. Application time 10 minutes.

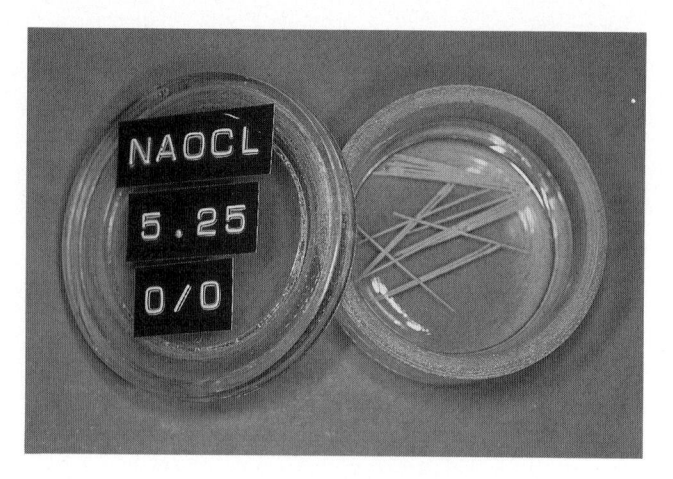

Figure 4-3 Disinfecting gutta percha cones in 5.25% household bleach for 1 minute before obturating root canal.

6. *Glutaraldehyde,* or .50% glutaraldehyde, .025% phenylphenoe, and .005 p-tertiary amylphenol. Application time 30 and 10 minutes respectively.

SPRAY - WIPE - SPRAY

This is an acceptable method of cleaning and disinfecting. No agent is available or registered with the EPA and ADA of acceptance that cleans and disinfects in one step. Therefore the importance of cleaning as a separate step from disinfection and sterilization cannot be overemphasized. All operatories and work areas should be disinfected before treating a patient.

MINIMUM DENTAL OFFICE INFECTION CONTROL PROGRAM

1. Comprehensive Medical History (Fig. 4-4)
2. Written Exposure Control Plan (Fig. 4-5)
3. Universal Precautions (Fig. 4-6)
4. Hepatitis B Vaccine
5. Postexposure Evaluation, Follow-up
6. Antiseptic Mouthrinse (Fig. 4-7)
7. Antiseptic Handwash (Fig. 4-8)
8. Disposable Face Mask (Fig. 4-9)
9. Disposable Gloves (Fig. 4-9)
10. Protective Eyewear (Fig. 4-9)
11. Protective Gowns, Laundry (Fig. 4-10)
12. Rubber Dam (Fig. 4-11)
13. Resheathing Devices (Fig. 4-12)
14. Sharps Containers (Fig. 4-13)
15. Regulated Waste Disposal (Fig. 4-14)
16. Sterilizable Handpieces (Fig. 4-15)
17. Ultrasonic Cleaner (Fig. 4-16)

Text continued on pg. 75.

Mr. Mrs. Miss .... Name of Spouse ....
Residence Address ....
City .... State .... Zip Code ....
Residence Phone .... Birth Date ....
Employment .... Spouse's Employment ....
Business Phone .... Business Phone ....
Referred by .... Family Dentist ....
Physician ....

The following medical information is necessary to carry out a correct and comprehensive dental examination and treatment planning. Any one of these items could have bearing on how we would examine you or what treatment we would recommend. This information will be kept confidential.

MEDICAL HISTORY YES NO

1. How is your general health? ....
   ....
2. Are you allergic to any medication? ....
   If yes, please name. ....
3. Do you smoke? ....
   If so, how much? ....
4. Do you take any medication, pills or tablets on a routine or daily basis? ....
   If yes, please name. ....
5. (Women) Are you pregnant? ....
6. Have you recently been under the care of a physician? ....
   If yes, why? ....
7. Do you suffer from shortness of breath or stress as you go about your daily activities? ....
   If yes, explain. ....
8. Have you had chest pains or swelling of the legs? ....
   If yes, give circumstances. ....
9. Are you a diabetic or does diabetes run in your family? ....
10. Do you have a history of any heart disease, rheumatic fever, high blood pressure or anemia? ....
11. Do you have bleeding tendencies? ....
12. Have you had any previous unpleasant local or general anesthetic experiences? ....
    If yes, give circumstances. ....
13. Have you ever had any liver disease, hepatitis, or jaundice? ....
14. Do you have any disease of the thyroid gland? ....
    If yes, please explain. ....
15. Have you had any kidney diseases or infections? ....
16. Have you had any major health problem, extensive illnesses, hospitalization or surgery that was not already covered in the above questions? ....
    If yes, please explain. ....
17. Do you have any transmissible, communicable or reportable diseases? ....
    If yes, please explain. ....

DENTAL HISTORY

1. How recently was your abscess detected or suspected? ....
   ....
2. Have you had previous root canal therapy? ....
   If yes, how long ago was it carried out? ....
3. What is the purpose of this visit? ....
   ....

Our office does not participate with dental insurance. However, we will be happy to report procedures performed by us to your insurance company so you can receive any benefits due you. We ask for your cooperation by paying any unpaid balance of your fee in full upon completion of your treatment.

I, the undersigned consent to the performing of whatever procedure may be decided upon to be necessary or advisable in the opinion of the Doctor(s).

I also understand that only the Root Canal Treatment will be done in this office. The permanent (outside) restoration (filling, inlay, crown, etc.) will be done by my regular dentist.

Signed _____

Figure 4-4 Comprehensive medical history obtained and reviewed. Not all patients can be identified as carriers of infectious diseases by their medical history. Each patient must be considered potentially infectious.

68   PRACTICAL ENDODONTICS

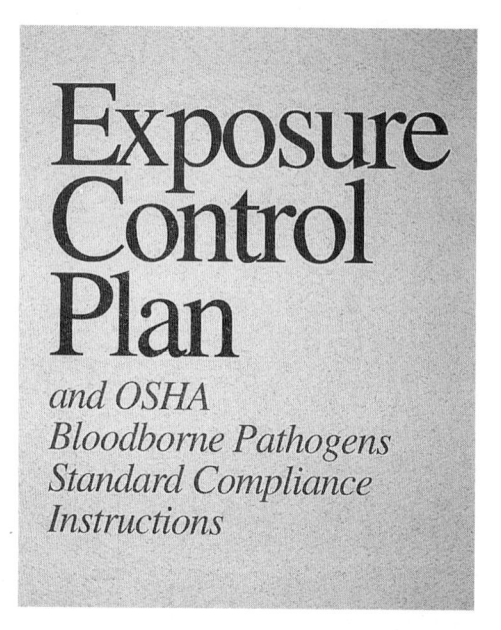

Figure 4-5 OSHA requires an Exposure Control Plan in each office that is easily accessible to the employees.

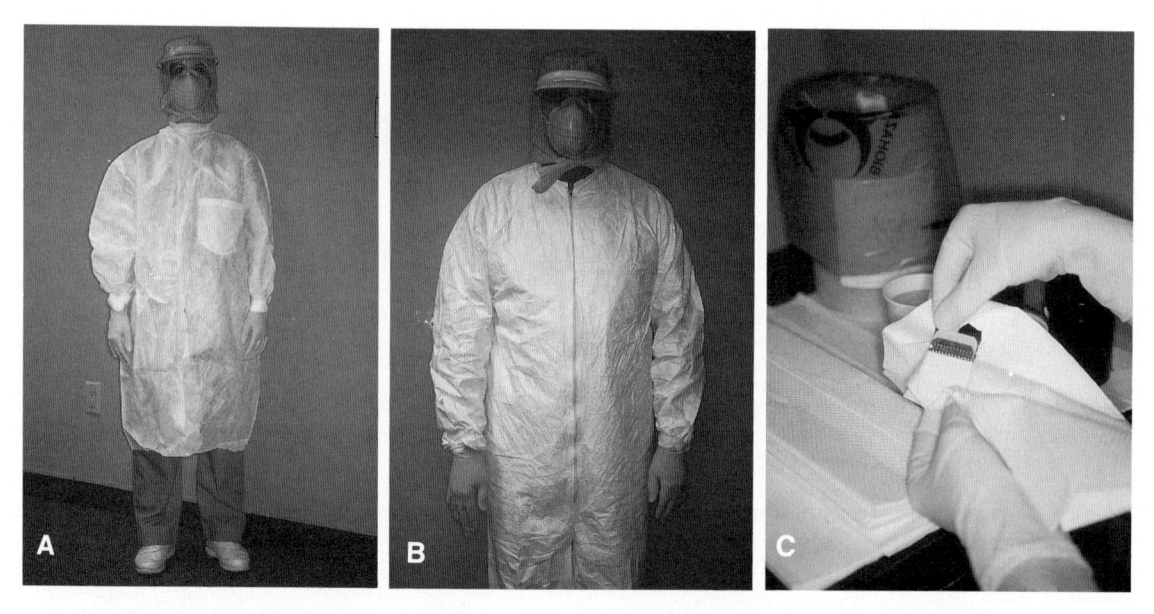

Figure 4-6 A, Protective clothing for doctor and dental assistant. **B,** Used for HIV positive and Hepatitis B patients. This is a disposable garment. **C,** Remove film from packet wearing gloves and properly dispose of outer covering. **D** and **E,** American Dental Association (ADA) infection control recommendations and procedures (ASAP).

ADA INFECTION CONTROL RECOMMENDATIONS

BEFORE PATIENT TREATMENT

IMMUNIZATION
The ADA's Council on Dental Therapeutics recommends that all dental personnel having patient contact, including dentist, dental students, and dental auxilliary personnel, receive the hepatitis B vaccine.

RECORD KEEPING
- Establish standard operating procedures.
- Classify all job tasks (see OSHA Guidelines.)
- Institute Employee Training Program.
- Maintain Infection Control Records.
- Obtain thorough Medical History.

DURING PATIENT TREATMENT

BARRIER PROTECTION
Gloves — *Latex gloves* must be worn for all procedures. Wash hands before/after gloving with *antimicrobial soap*. Change *gloves* between each patient. Discard *gloves* that are torn, cut or punctured.

Masks — *Masks* must be worn to protect the face, mouth and nose. Change masks between patients.

Eyewear — *Protective eyewear* must be worn. *Face shields* may be worn instead of glasses. Clean and disinfect between each patient.

Clothing — Wear *gowns*, *labcoats* or *protective clothing*. Change clothing prior to leaving office. Launder separately.

INFECTION CONTROL
Personal Protection — Vaccines, gloves, masks, eyewear.

Patient Screening — Identify high risk patients.

Equipment Asepsis — Clean equipment between patients. Buy equipment that is easy to clean.

Aseptic Techniques — Maintain a sterile treatment area.

Surface Disinfection — Use ADA approved disinfectant on operatory surfaces.

Instrument Sterilization — Sterilize all instruments between patients.

AFTER PATIENT TREATMENT

- Wear heavy-duty rubber *gloves*.
- Sterilize instruments.
  —Sterilize instruments that penetrate soft tissue or bone.
    — Sterilize, whenever possible, all instruments that come in contact with oral mucous membranes, body fluids, or those that have been contaminated with secretions of patients. Otherwise, use appropriate disinfection.
    — Monitor the sterilizer with biological monitors.
- Clean *handpieces, dental units*, and *ultrasonic scalers*.
    — Flush *handpieces, dental units, ultrasonic scalers* and *air/water syringes* if possible. Otherwise, disinfect them.
    — Clean and sterilize *air/water syringes* and *ultrasonic scalers* if possible. Otherwise, disinfect them.
    — Clean and sterilize *handpieces* if possible. Otherwise, disinfect them.
- Handle sharp instruments with caution.
    — Place *disposable needles, scalpels* and other sharp items intact into puncture-resistant containers before disposal.
- Decontaminate environmental surfaces.
    — Wipe work surfaces with absorbent toweling to remove debris, and dispose of the toweling appropriately.
    — Disinfect with suitable chemical germicide.
    — Change *protective coverings* on light handles, X-ray unit heads, etc.
- Decontaminate *supplies* and *materials*.
    — Rinse and disinfect impressions, bite registrations and appliances to be sent to the laboratory.
- Dispose of all wastes according to manufacturer's instructions and adhere to all applicable waste disposal regulations.
    — Place soild waste contaminated with blood or saliva in sealed, sturdy, impervious bags; dispose according to regulations.
- Wash hands and change *gloves*.

OSHA GUIDELINES

The OSHA guidelines include the following:

- All tasks, work areas and personnel in the dental offices should be classified according to the degree of risk involved.

- Standard Operating Procedure (SOPs) regarding infection control should be defined for each of these tasks or classifications. These SOPs should include both the protective equipment and mandatory work practices necessary to prevent the transmissions of disease. If your office follows the ADA's infection control recommendations, you can use those recommendations as your office's SOPs.

- As an employer, you are responsible for monitoring the compliance of your staff with the SOPs.

- You are also responsible for maintaining records of the training, instances of non-compliance, corrective actions taken to induce compliance, and instances of parenteral exposure to body fluids.

Categories of tasks, work areas and personnel
OSHA guidelines state that tasks in the dental office be evaluated and classified into one of the following three categories.

Category I:
Tasks that involve exposure to blood, body fluids, or tissues.
"All procedures or other job-related tasks that involve an inherent potential for mucous membrane of skin contact with blood, body fluids or tissues, or a potential for spills or splashes of them, are Category I tasks. Use of appropriate protective measures should be required for every employee engaged in Category I tasks."
Most, although not necessarily all, tasks performed by the dentists, dental hygienist, dental assistant and laboratory technician would fall in this category. The ADA recommends that these office personnel and the tasks they perform be classified as Category I.

Category II:
Tasks that involve no exposure to blood, body fluids or tissues, but employment may require performing unplanned Category I tasks.
"The normal work routine involves no exposure to blood, body fluids or tissues, but exposure or potential exposure may be required as a condition of employment. Appropriate protective measures should be readily available to every employee engaged in Category II tasks."

Clerical or non professional workers who may, as part of their duties, help clean up the office, handle instruments or impressions materials, or those who sent out dental materials to laboratories, would be classified as Category II.

Category III:
Tasks that involve no exposure to blood, body fluids or tissues.
"The normal work routine involves no exposure to blood, body fluids or tissues. Persons who perform these duties are not called upon as part of their employment to perform or assist in emergency medical care or first aid or to be potentially exposed in some other way."
A front office receptionist, bookeeper, or insurance clerk who does not handle dental instruments or materials would be a Category III worker.

Note: These classifications are not rigid and there may be crossover, depending upon the job performed.

Standard Operating Procedures
It should not be necessary to develop your own Standard Operating Procedures if your office follows the infection control guidelines established by the American Dental Association or the Centers for Disease Control.

OMS inc.
ATLANTA, GEORGIA U.S.A.
3120 Crossing Park/Norcross, GA 30071 / (404) 447-6766
ATLANTA, GEORGIA U.S.A.

Orthotrac
Omnitrac
ASAP

Complete Toll Free Phone Order Service
Georgia WATS — 1-800-241-3196   Other States WATS — 1-800-358-0112

Adapted from "Dental Team Infection Control Procedures" by permission of Atlanta Dental Supply Company.

Figure 4-6, *D cont'd* For complete legend, see opposite page.

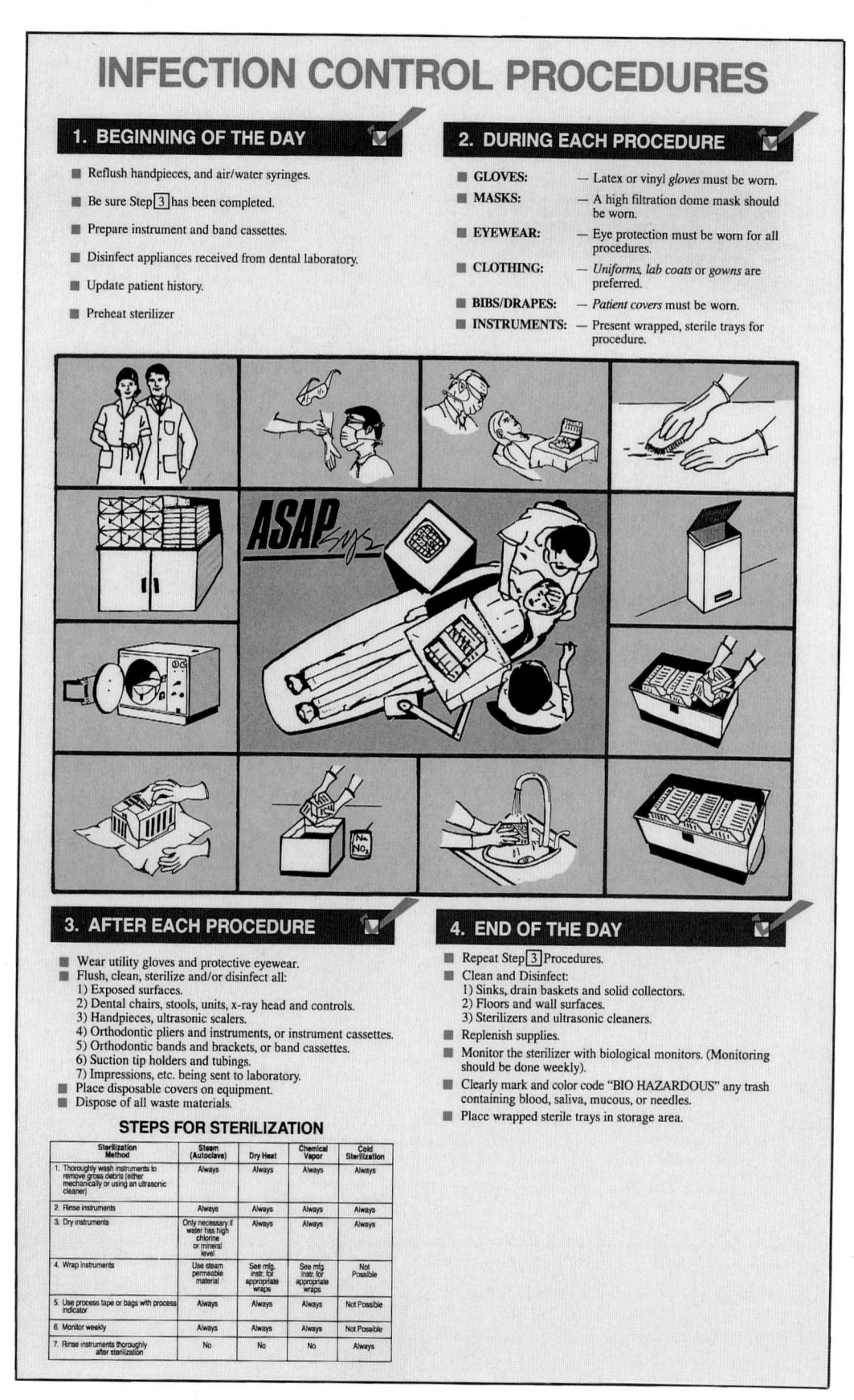

Figure 4-6, *E cont'd* For complete legend, see page 68.

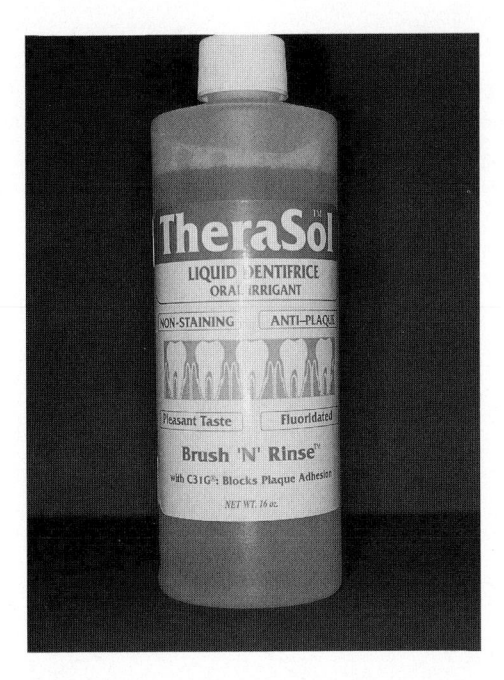

Figure 4-7 Patient rinses mouth for 30 seconds to reduce microorganisms of the oral cavity. (OraTec Corp., 285 Spring Park Place, Suite 600, Herndon, VA 22070.)

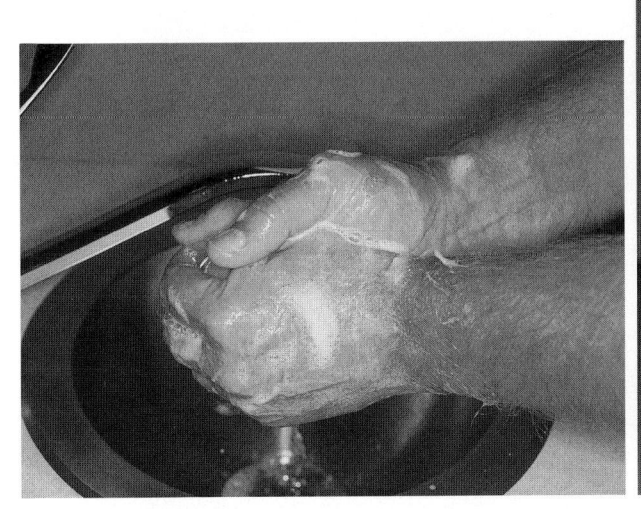

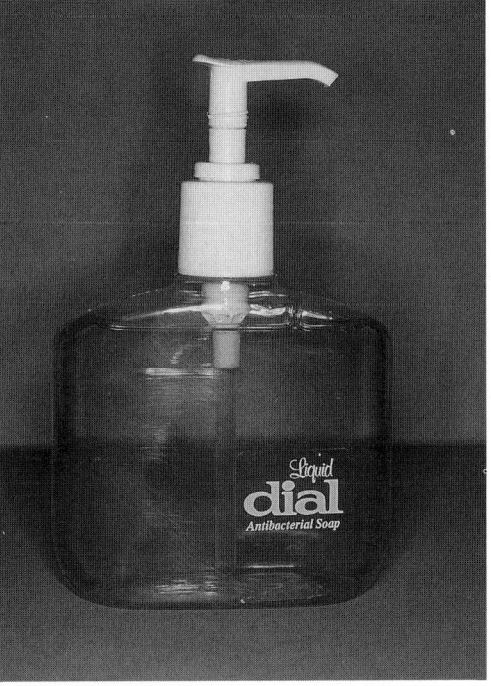

Figure 4-8 Hands must be washed before and after treatment of patient with antibacterial soap. (Dial Corp., Phoenix, AZ 85077.)

72   PRACTICAL ENDODONTICS

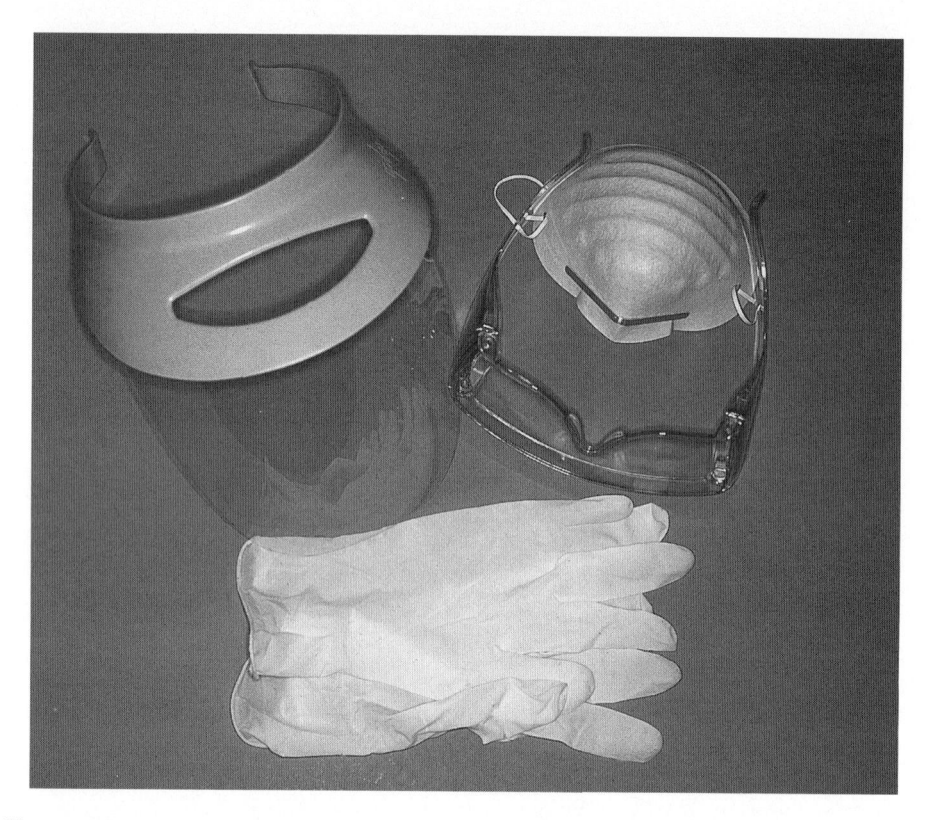

Figure 4-9 Protective coverings must be worn at all times when doctor and dental assistant come in contact with secretions, sprays, and splatters.

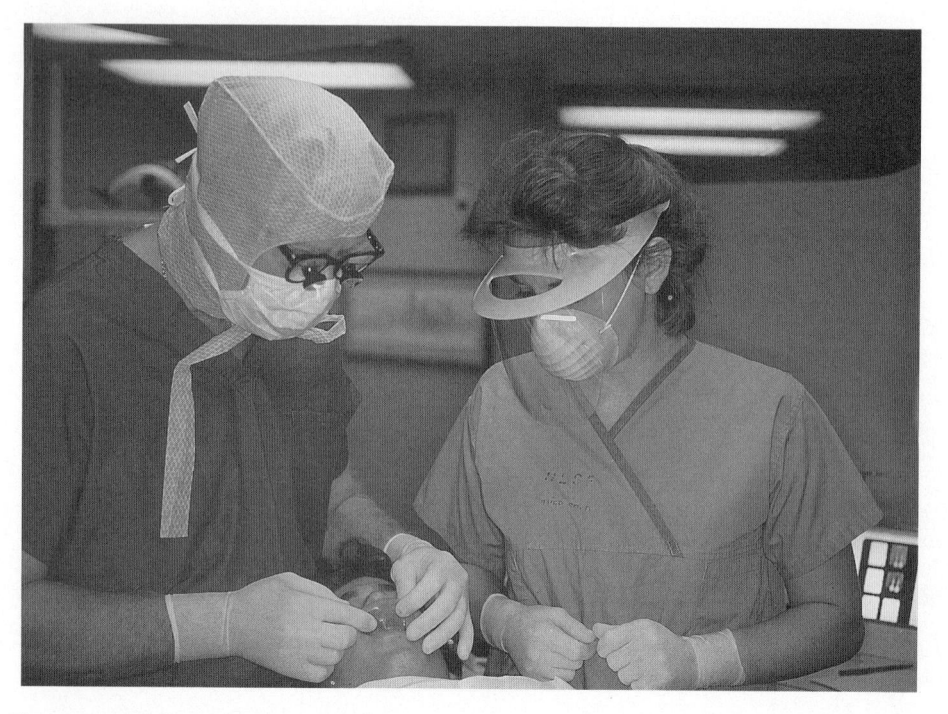

Figure 4-10 Clinical attire should be changed once a day or when it becomes visibly soiled. (See also Fig. 4-6, *A* and *B*.)

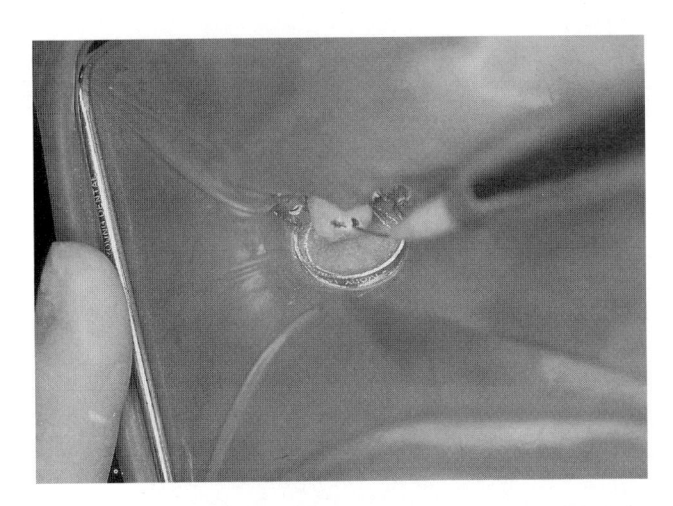

Figure 4-11 Use rubber dam to limit transmission of blood pathogens from patient's mouth. (Hygenic Corp., Akron, OH 44310.)

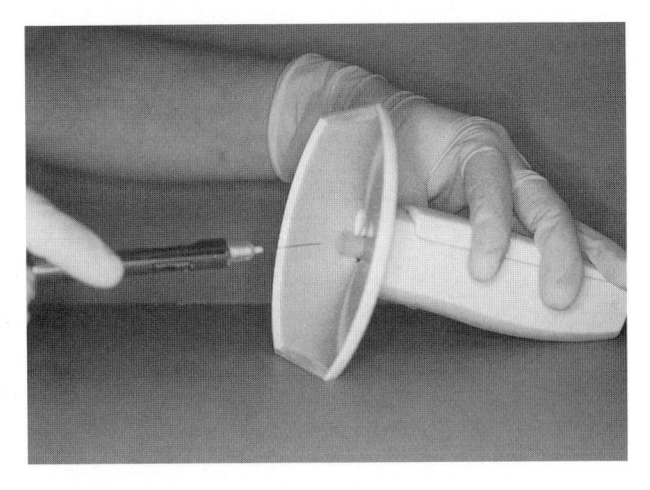

Figure 4-12 Needles are placed in resheathing devices before and after injection. (On.Gard Systems, Inc., 1900 Grant St., Suite 710, Denver, CO 80203.)

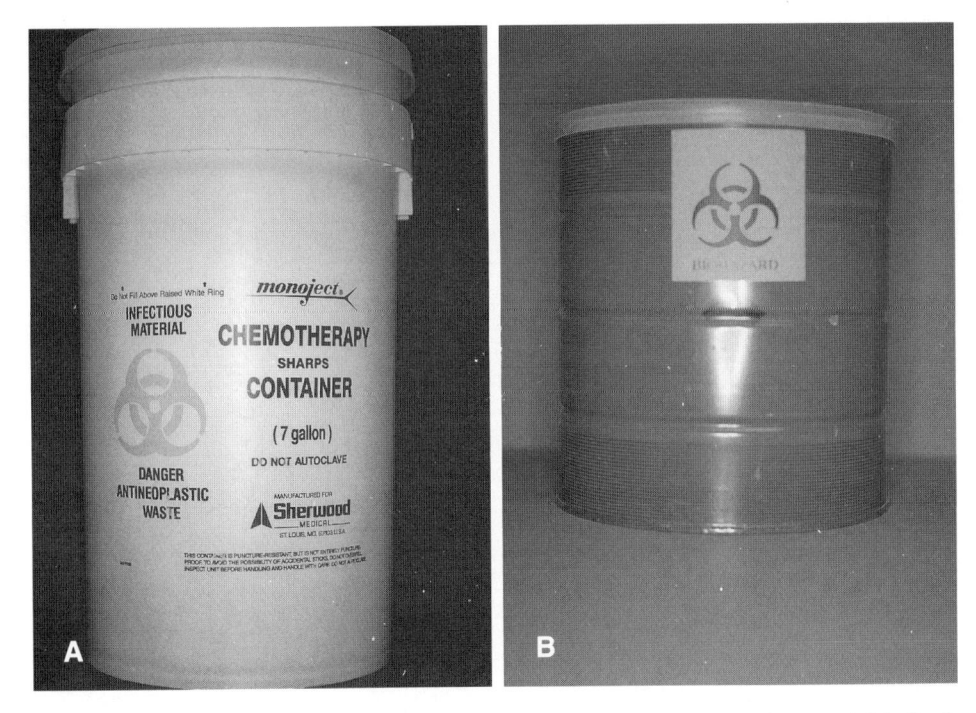

Figure 4-13 A, Must be readily available in dental operatories. (Sherwood Medical, St Louis, MO 63103.) **B,** Containers must be puncture proof.

74 PRACTICAL ENDODONTICS

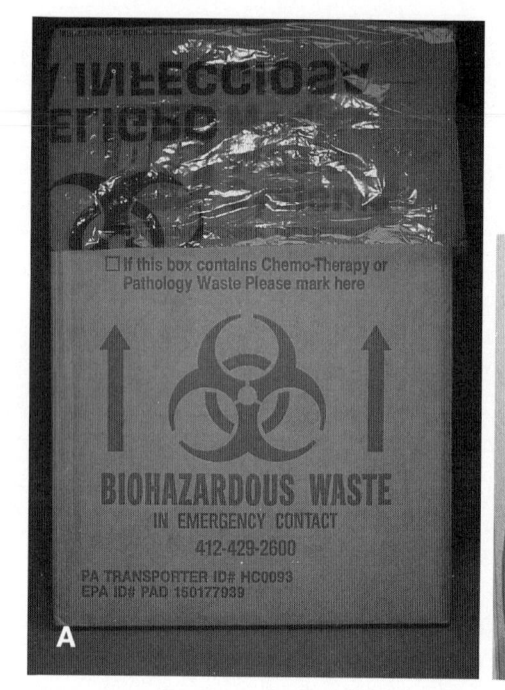

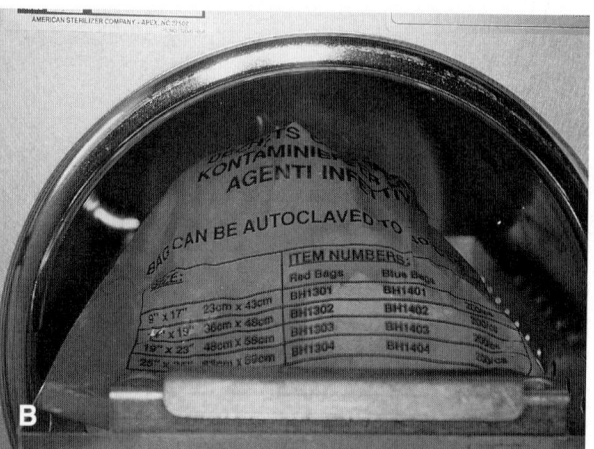

Figure 4-14 A, Container for contaminated items (e.g., gauze, gloves, rubber dams, towels, napkins, and disposable gowns). **B,** Sterilizing waste before disposal.

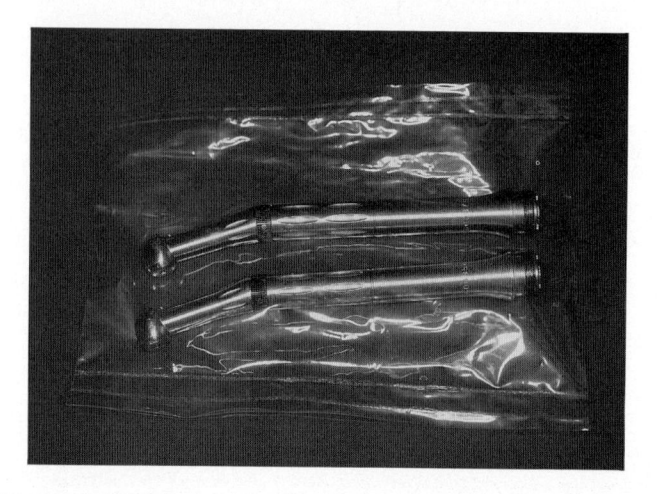

Figure 4-15 Follow manufacturer's instructions for sterilizing.

18. Instrument Packaging (Fig. 4-17)
19. Heat Sterilizer (Fig. 4-18)
20. Sterilization Monitoring (Fig. 4-19)
21. Glutaraldehyde (Fig. 4-20)
22. Surface Cleaner (Fig. 4-21)
23. Surface Disinfectant (Fig. 4-22)
24. Surface Covers (Fig. 4-23)
25. Biohazard Communication
26. Training Program
27. Recordkeeping
28. "OSHA" Poster
29. When in doubt always refer to universal precautions.

All individuals employed by a dentist should read and become aware of all safety procedures and sign on the page provided for signatures. The goal of the health professional is to eliminate the transfer of pathogenic microorganisms. This would comply with OSHA and state regulations.

ENDODONTIC ARMAMENTARIUM

The objective of this chapter is to familiarize one with the armamentaria used in endodontic therapy. The instruments listed are essential for correct endodontic treatment (Figs. 4-24 to 4-37). As always, it is the obligation of each dentist to select his or her own armamentarium and have it available in a sterile condition for the appropriate usage.

TRAY INSTRUMENTS

1. Hooked Explorer.
2. Spoon Excavator.
3. DG-16 Explorer.
4. Mosquito Hemostat.
5. Grooved Cotton Pliers.
6. Plastic Instrument.
7. Mirror.

INTRACANAL INSTRUMENTS

Root canal instruments can be divided into four general classes:

1. Exploring—locating and probing of canals (smooth broaches, path finders, and files)
2. Extirpating—debriding pulpal tissue (barbed broaches, reamers, and files)
3. Enlarging—cleansing and shaping the canal (reamers, files, and Gates Glidden drills)
4. Filling—obturating of the canal with gutta percha (spreaders and pluggers)

MATERIALS AND ARMAMENTARIUM USED FOR AN OBTURATION OF THE ROOT CANAL

1. Gutta Percha Points
2. Root Canal Sealer
3. Spreaders
4. Pluggers
5. Heat Carrier

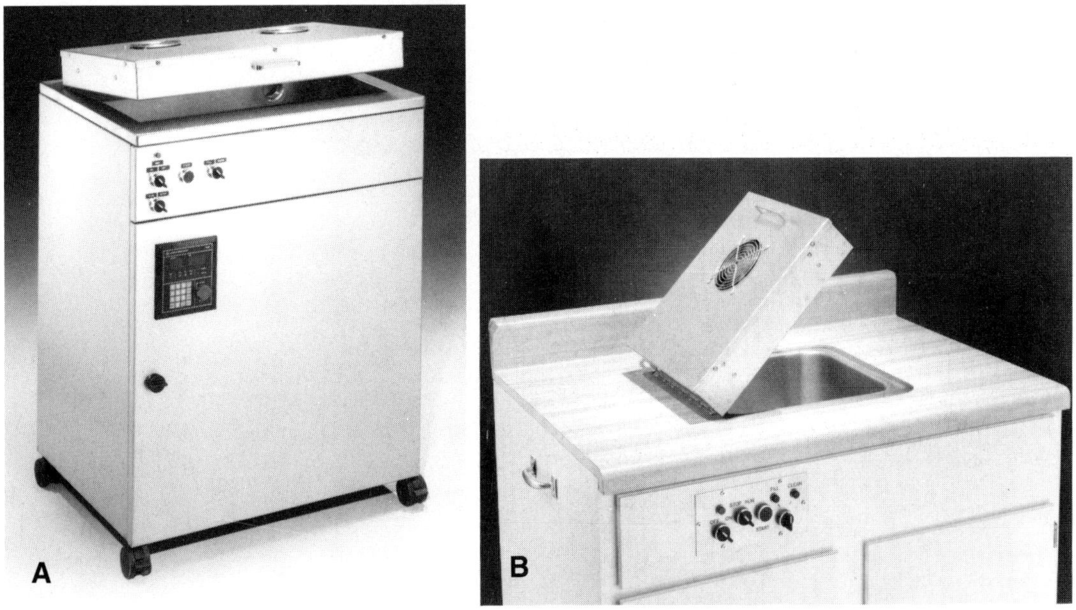

Figure 4-16 Ultrasonic cleaner is 16 times more efficient than hand scrubbing. (ESMA-DENT, PO Box 162, Highland Park, IL 60035.)

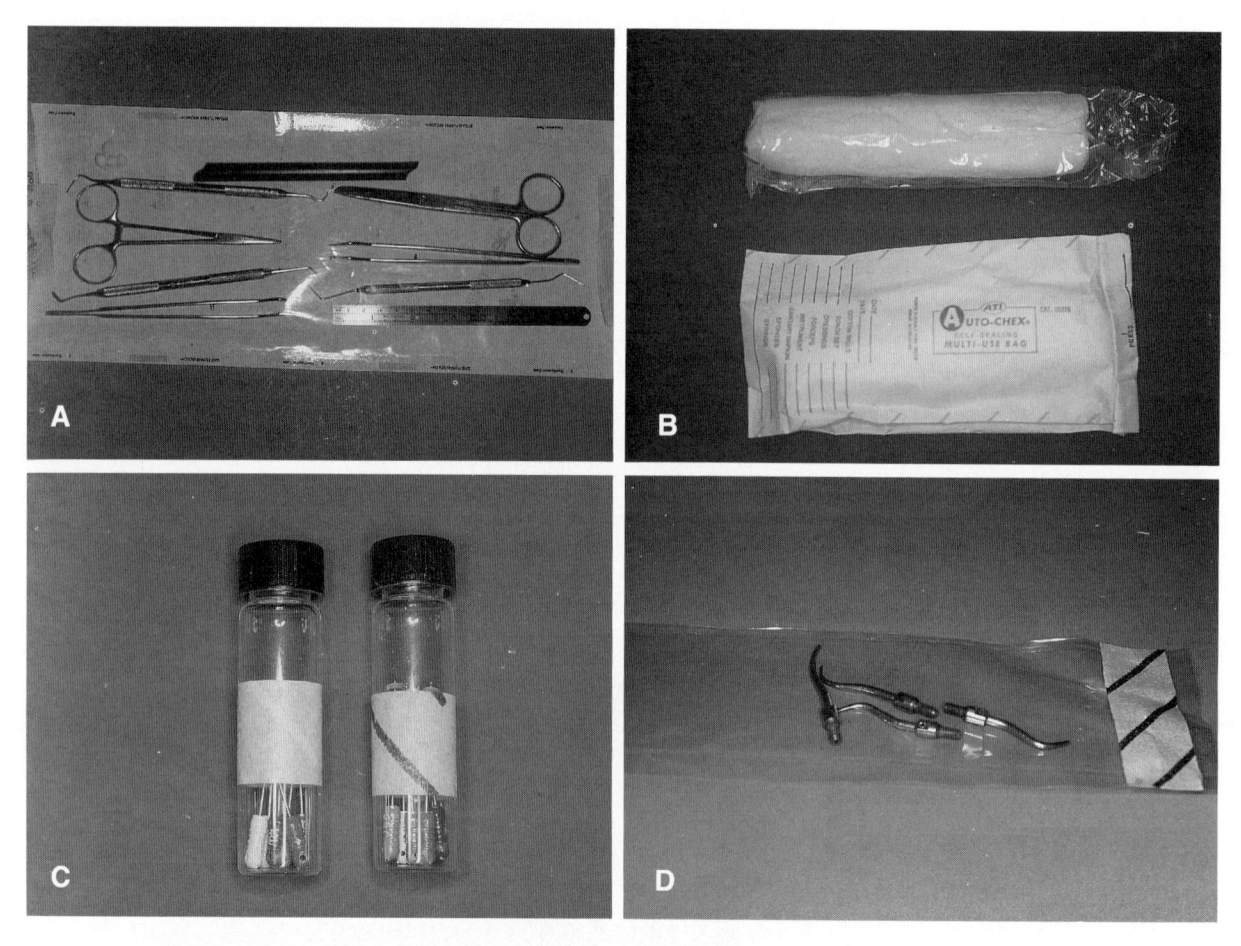

Figure 4-17 A, Instruments are placed in sleeve made of clear plastic and chemically treated indicator paper. **B,** Clear plastic bags sealed with heat and chemically treated paper bags protect instruments after sterilization. **C,** Reamers and files are placed in glass vials with chemically treated tape that indicates proper sterilization has occurred with dry heat, ethylene oxide, or steam. **D,** Sterilized air scaling tips.

Continued.

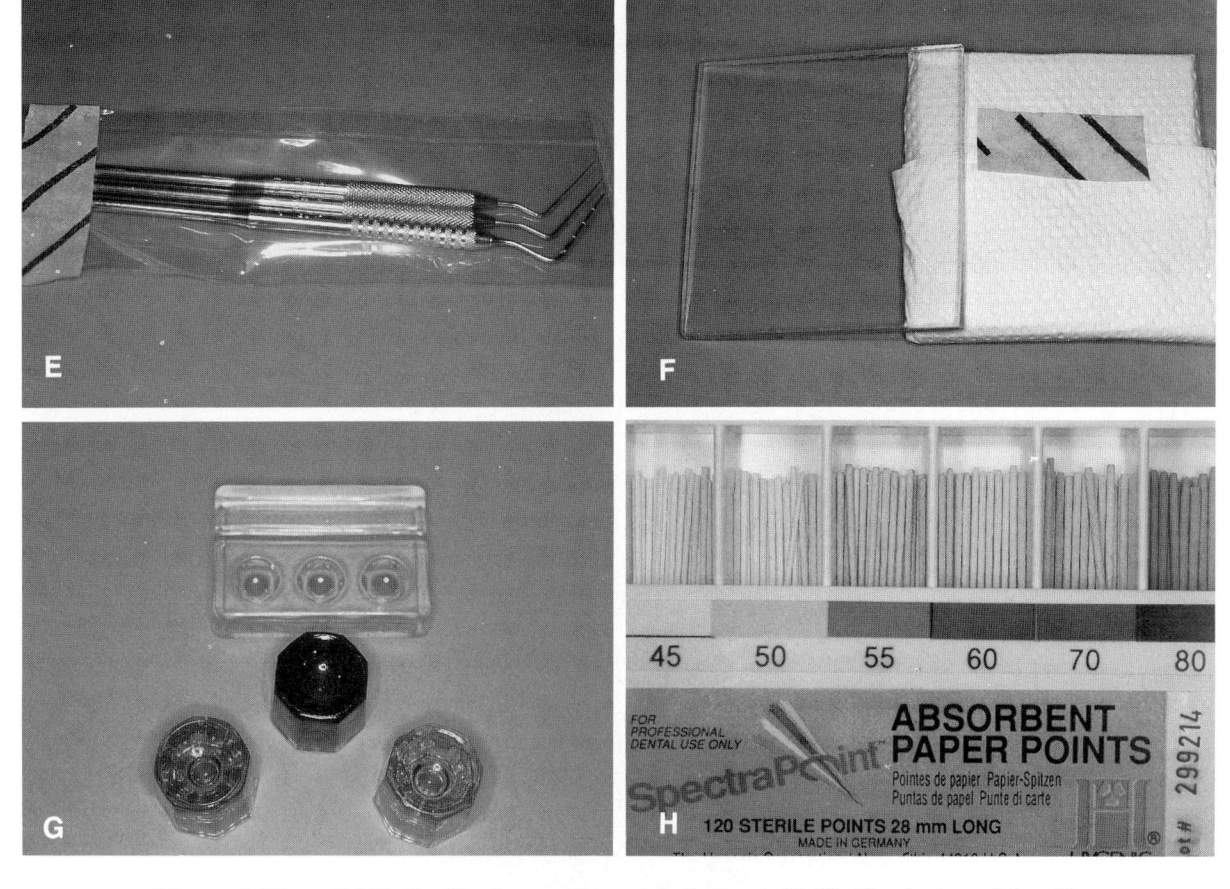

Figure 4-17, *cont'd* **E,** Sterilized spreaders and pluggers. **F,** Sterilized glass slabs. **G,** Dappen dishes and glass medicament trays can be placed in autoclave. **H,** Presterilized absorbent paper points. (Hygenic Corp., Akron, OH 44310.)

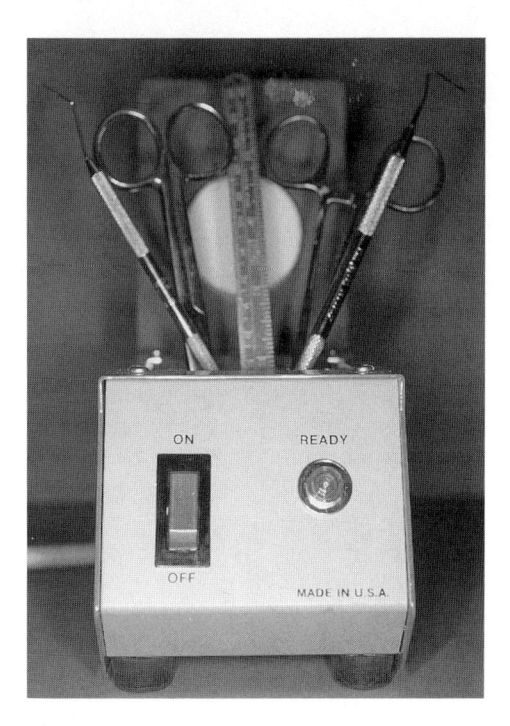

Figure 4-18 Glass bead sterilizer is an effective method for immediate sterilization. The entire instrument must be immersed in the beads for 5 seconds at a temperature of 225° to 250° C or 425° to 500° F; paper points are immersed for 10 seconds.

78 PRACTICAL ENDODONTICS

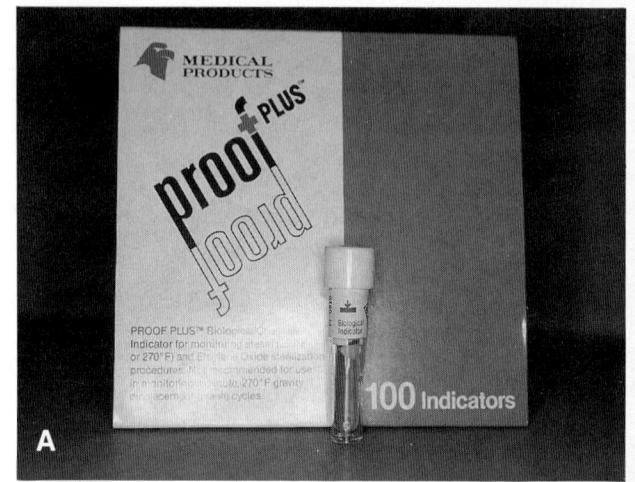

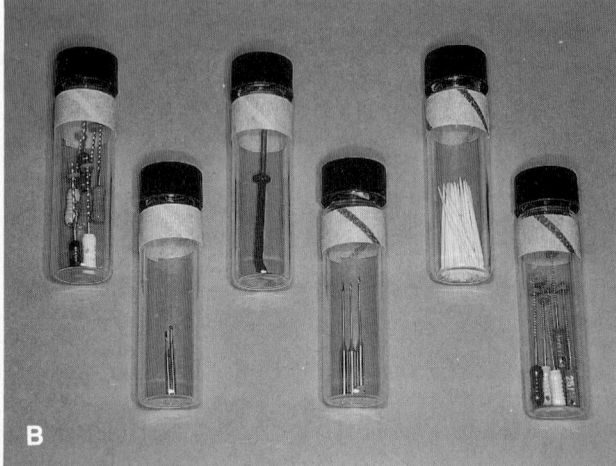

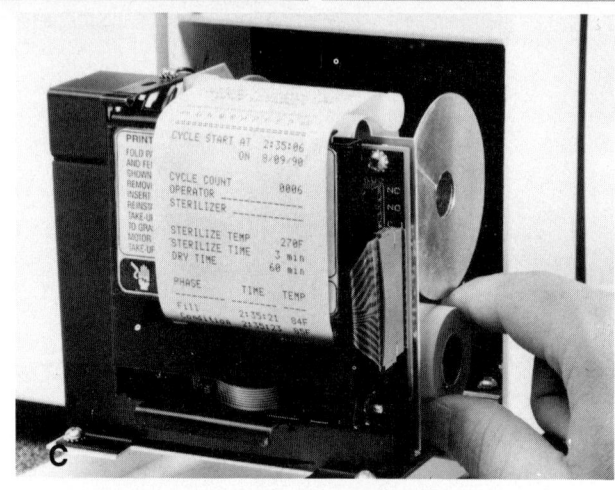

Figure 4-19 A, Biological chemical color indicator for monitoring steam and ethylene oxide sterilization. (Amsco Medical Products Div., Div. of American Sterilizer Co., Erie, PA 16514.) **B,** Chemically treated tape shows sterilization has occurred. The black marks indicate the instruments have been sterilized. **C,** The latest autoclaves have built-in monitoring devices. (American Sterilizer Co., 2424 West 23rd Street, PO Box 620, Erie, PA 16514.)

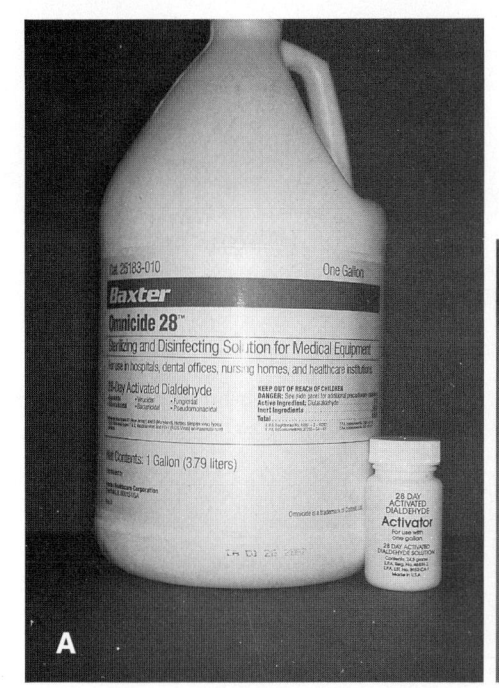

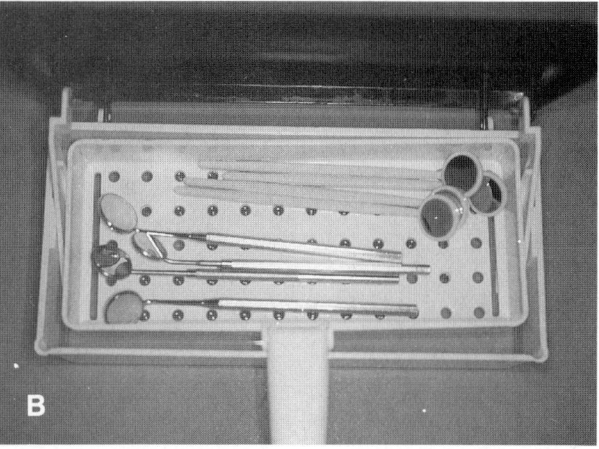

Figure 4-20 A, Glutaraldehyde is used when instruments are sensitive to heat. It should not be substituted for heat sterilization. Follow manufacturer's instructions. (Baxter Healthcare Corp., Deerfield, IL 60015.) **B,** Mirrors being disinfected in glutaraldehyde. (Baxter Healthcare Corp., Deerfield, IL 60015.)

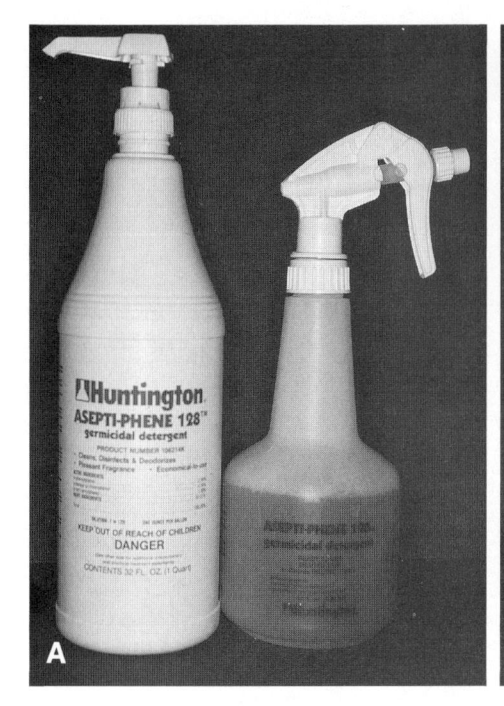

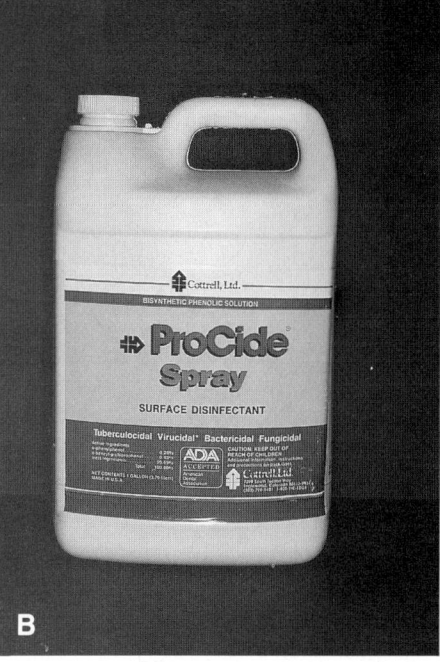

Figure 4-21 Surface cleaners and disinfectants are used with the spray-wipe-spray technique. Follow manufacturer's directions. (*A,* Huntington Lab Inc., Huntington, IN 46750; *B,* Cottrell Ltd., Englewood, CO 80112-9937.)

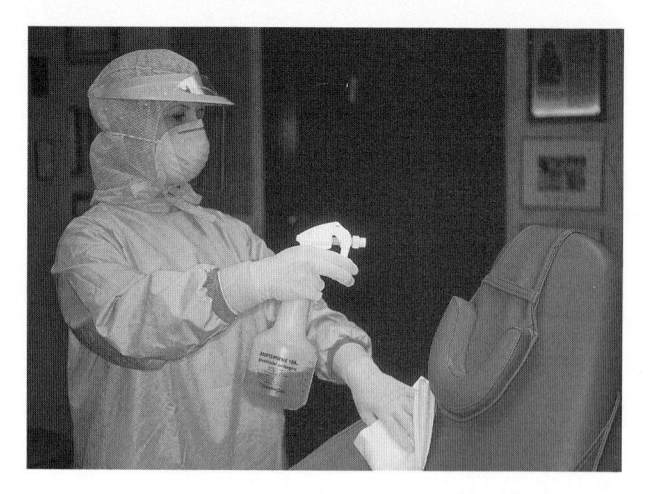

Figure 4-22 Operatory cleaned and disinfected after treating HIV positive or Hepatitis B patient. (The attire worn is not mandatory, however, gloves are to be worn.)

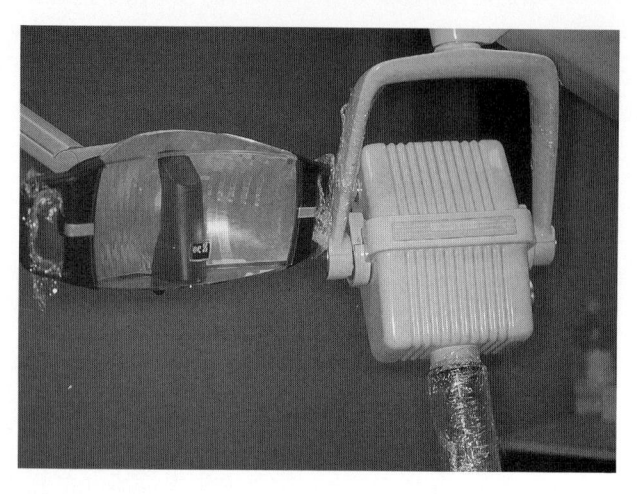

Figure 4-23 Surface covers should be changed before each appointment. Plastic wrap or aluminum foil can be used.

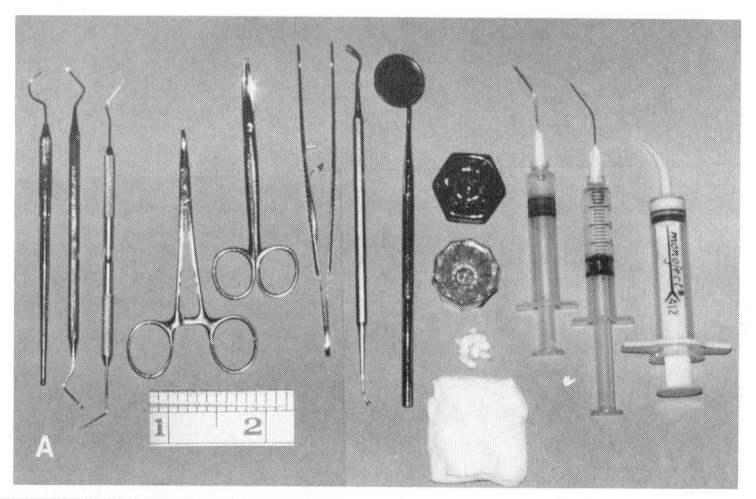

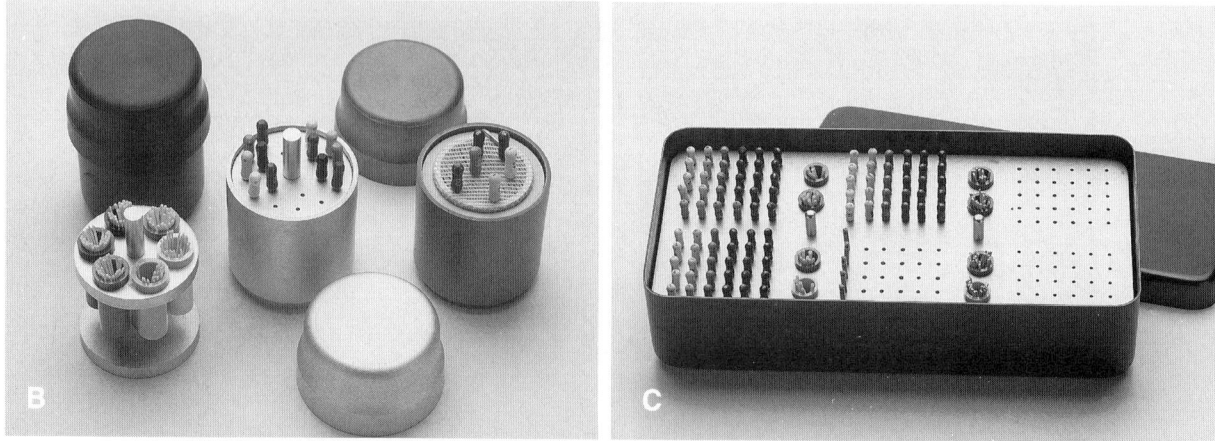

Figure 4-24 Tray Instruments. **A,** Bracket table equipment. From *left* to *right: Hooked explorer* - for cleaning pulp horn spaces in anterior teeth; *Spoon excavator* - for reaching into the pulp chamber in bicuspids and molars; *DG-16 Explorer* - for locating and exploring the root canal; *Mosquito hemostat* - for holding radiograph films; *Iris scissors* - for cutting paper points, cotton pellets, and gutta percha, *Grooved cotton pliers* - for holding paper points, cotton pellets, and gutta percha points; *Plastic instrument* - for placing cements to seal access openings in the crown; *Mirror* - for visibility; *Dappen dish* (two) - for sodium hypochlorite and hydrogen peroxide; *Cotton pellets* - for drying pulp chamber and sealing pulp chamber during visits; *2X2 gauze sponges* - for cleaning reamers and files; *Irrigating syringe* (two disposable) - sodium hypochlorite and hydrogen peroxide; *Monojet syringe* (disposable) containing RC Prep; *Ruler* - to place stops on intracanal instruments and to measure the gutta percha points. **B** and **C,** *Instrument boxes* - to store and autoclave intracanal instruments and paper points.

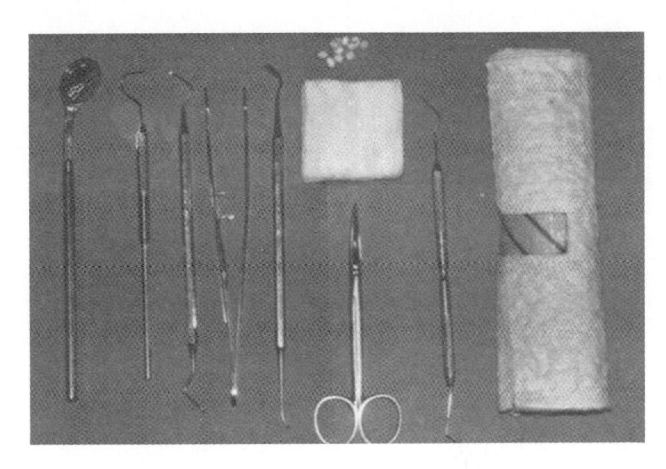

Figure 4-25 Autoclave pack. From *left* to *right:* Mirror, Hooked explorer, Spoon excavator, Cotton pliers, Plastic instrument, Scissors, 2 × 2 Cotton sponges, Cotton pellets, DG-16 explorer.

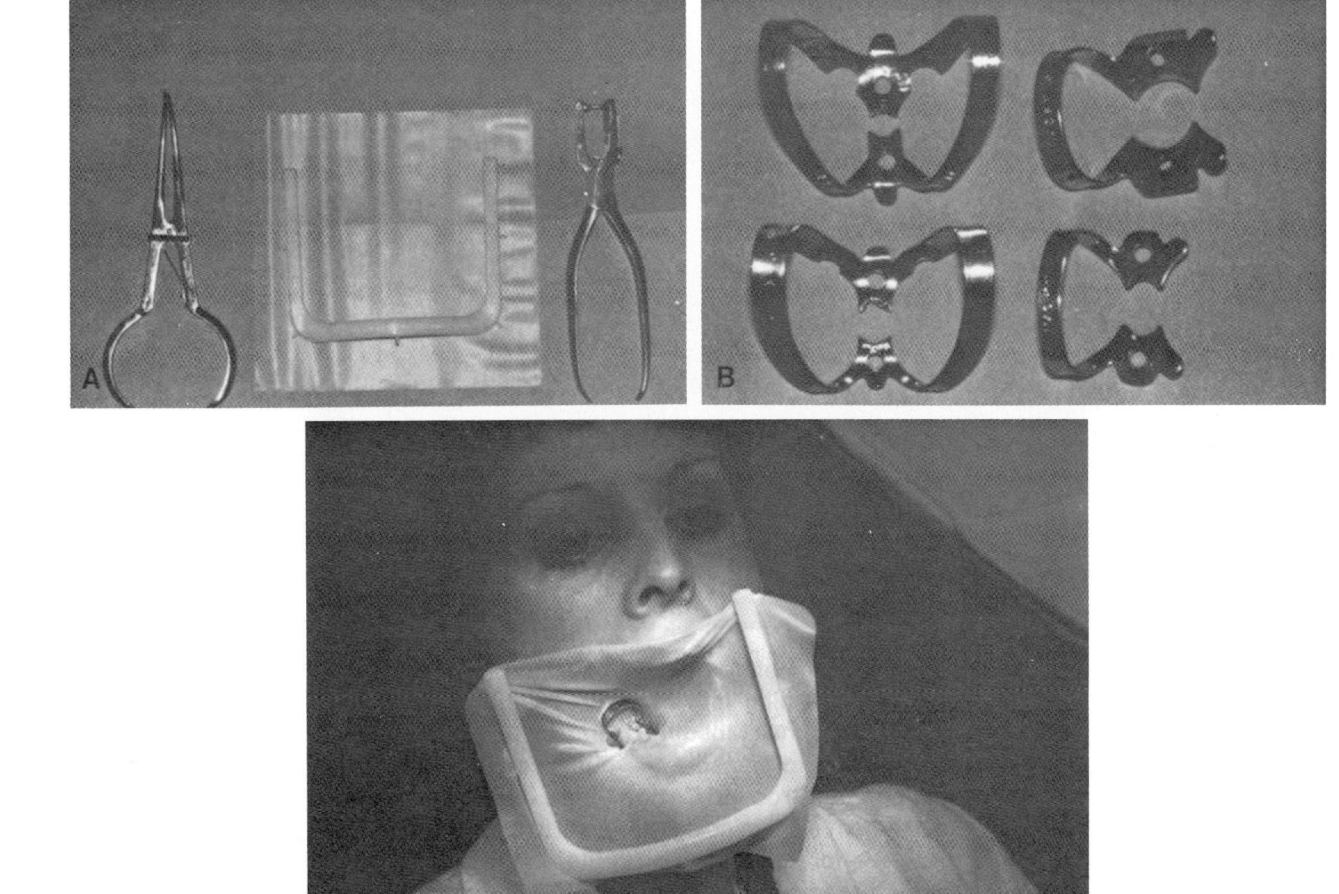

Figure 4-26 A, Rubber dam set-up. From *left* to *right:* Clamp forcep, Rubber dam and Visiframe, and Rubber dam punch. **B,** Rubber dam clamps assortment that could be adapted to most teeth. From *left* to *right:* upper row—No. 211 S. S. White, No. 5 Ivory; lower row—No. 9 Ivory, No. 2 Ivory. **C,** Application of the rubber dam.

82 PRACTICAL ENDODONTICS

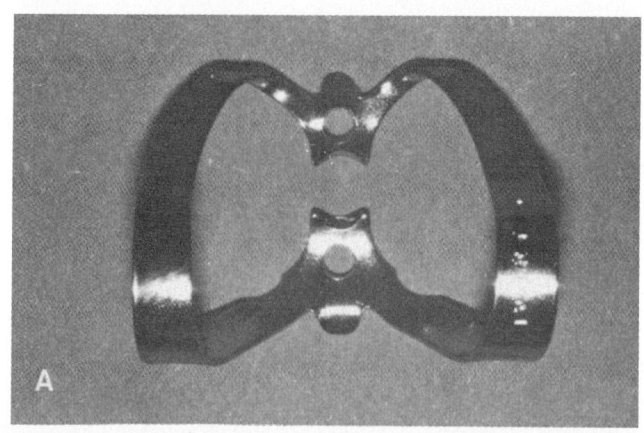

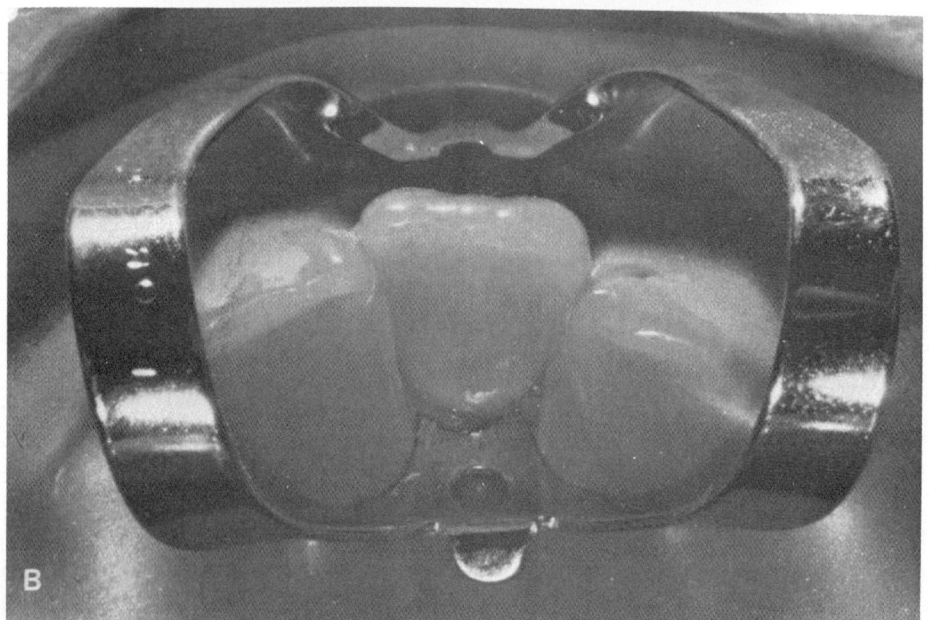

Figure 4-27 **A,** No. 9 Ivory clamp designed for the maxillary central and cuspid. **B,** No. 9 Ivory clamp in place on a maxillary central incisor.

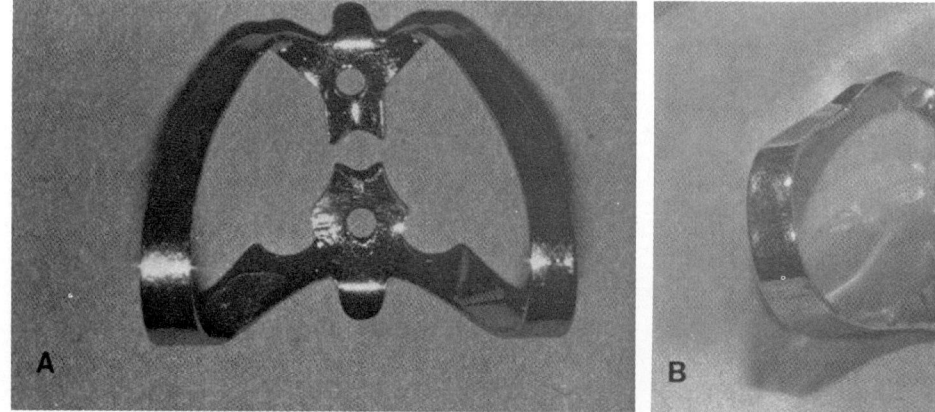

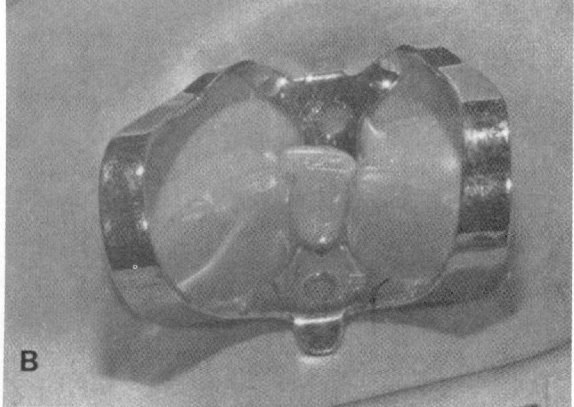

Figure 4-28 **A,** No. 211 S. S. White clamp designed for the maxillary lateral incisor and all the mandibular anterior teeth. **B,** No. 211 S. S. White clamp in place on a mandibular central incisor.

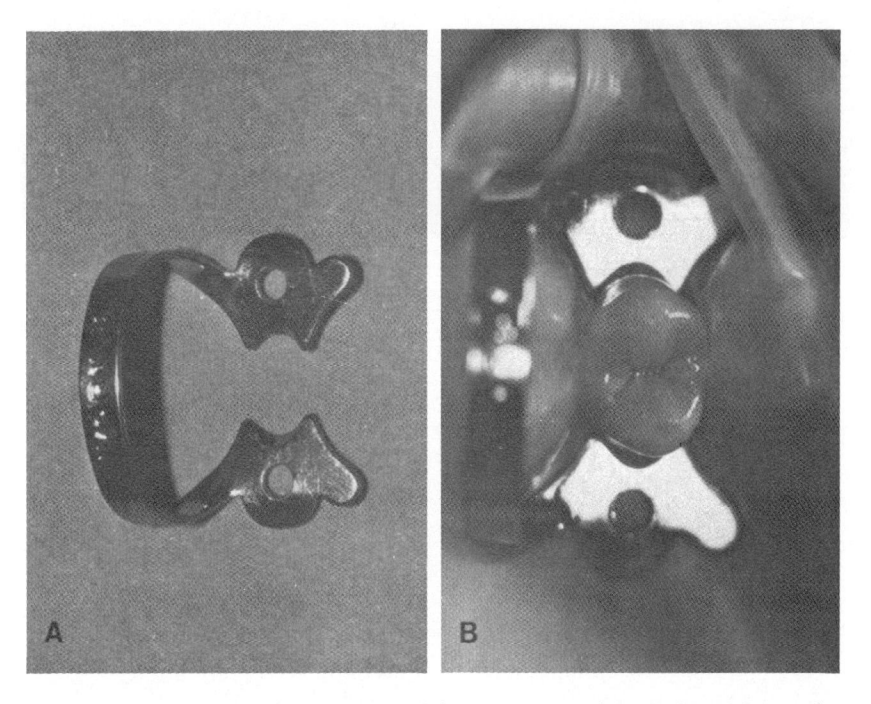

Chapter 4 ♦ Sterilization Procedures and Endodontic Armamentarium 83

Figure 4-29 **A,** No. 2 Ivory clamp designed for most premolars. **B,** No. 2 Ivory clamp in place on a maxillary premolar.

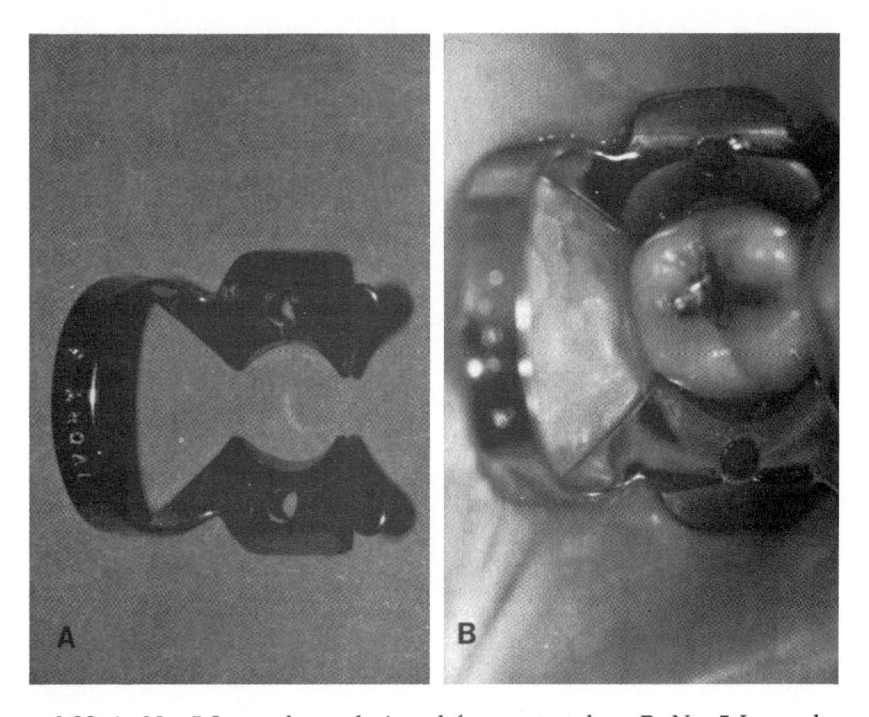

Figure 4-30 **A,** No. 5 Ivory clamp designed for most molars. **B,** No. 5 Ivory clamp in place on a mandibular molar.

84 PRACTICAL ENDODONTICS

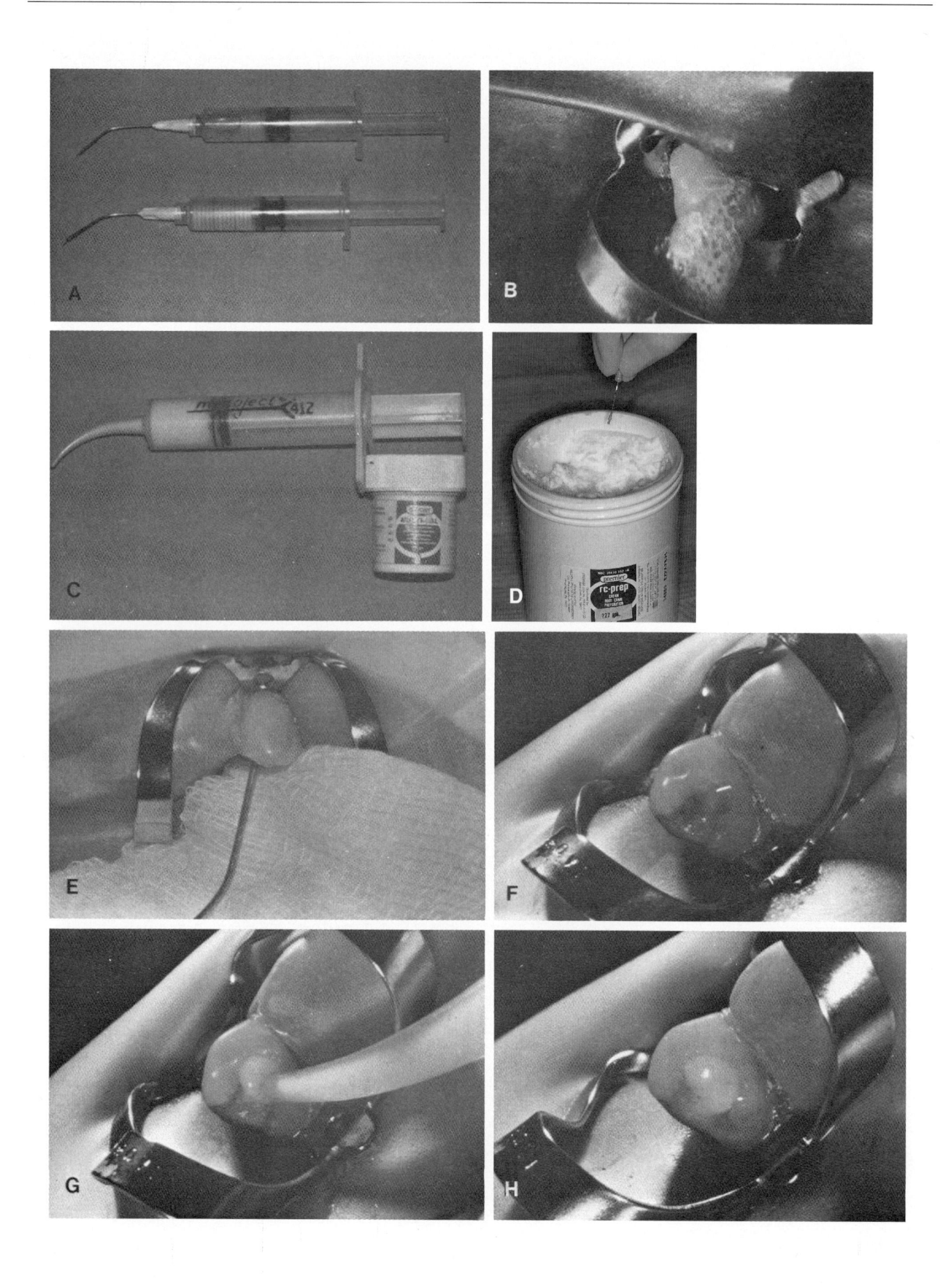

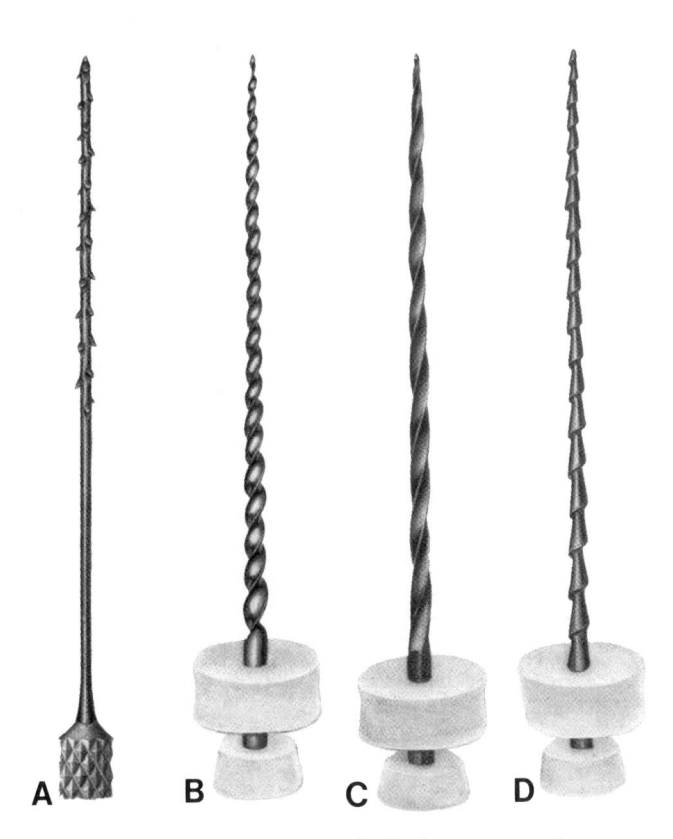

Figure 4-32 A comparison of all the intracanal instruments. **A,** Barbed broach. **B,** K-file. **C,** Reamer. **D,** Hedstrom file.

Figure 4-31 Irrigating Solutions. These solutions consist of sodium hypochlorite and hydrogen peroxide. RC Prep can also be used with sodium hypochlorite in tight canals. **A,** Photograph of two syringes, one containing 3% hydrogen peroxide and one containing 2½% sodium hypochlorite. These two solutions together liberate nascent oxygen. This effervescence brings bits of tissue debris and dentinal shavings to the surface. **B,** The effervescence from the mixture of sodium hypochlorite and hydrogen peroxide. **C,** RC Prep can be used in combination with sodium hypochlorite. It contains urea peroxide and ethylenediamine tetraacetic acid, which can be used for chelation. It may be placed in a plastic syringe to carry into the canal. **D,** RC Prep can also be used directly from the container and carried into the tooth on the flukes of a file. **E,** A disposable syringe, filled with sodium hypochlorite placed loosely into a canal. Excess is spilled onto a gauze or cotton roll. **F,** View of access with sodium hypochlorite welled up in the canal and chamber. Tooth is ready for further cleansing and shaping of the canal. **G,** Plastic syringe used to carry RC Prep into canal. **H,** View of access with RC Prep ready for cleansing and shaping.

86   PRACTICAL ENDODONTICS

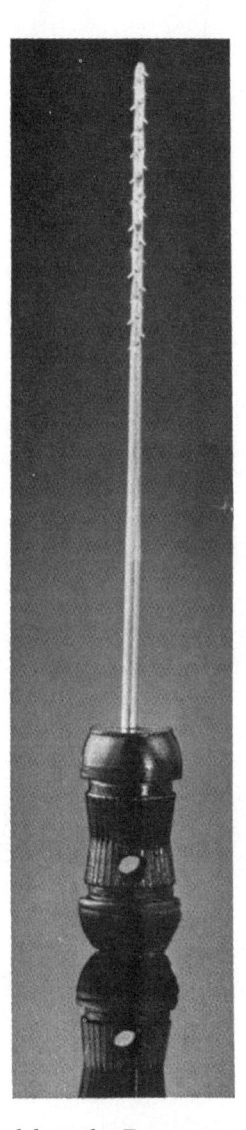

Figure 4-33 Barbed broach. For removing pulpal tissue. The barbed broach is only used in the larger canals, such as the maxillary anterior teeth and the palatal canals of the maxillary molars or the distal root of the mandibular molars. It is used only in the coronal third of the canal and should not touch the walls of the canal.

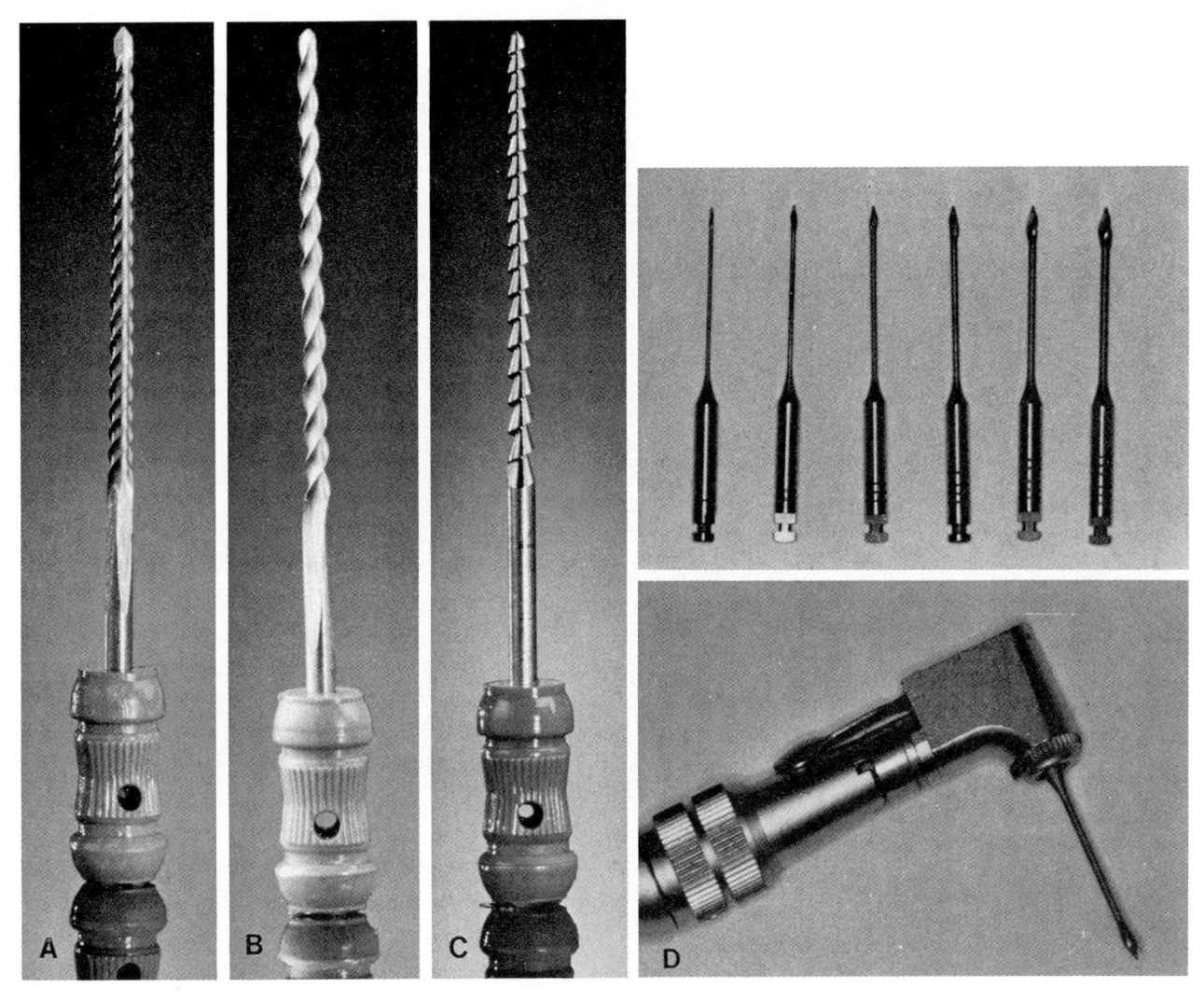

Chapter 4 ♦ Sterilization Procedures and Endodontic Armamentarium 87

Figure 4-34 K-file, reamer, Hedstrom file, and Gates Glidden drills. Used for debriding and enlarging the canal. **A,** K-files are used for the apical preparation and can also be used to prepare the body of the canal. **B,** Reamers are used only for the preparation of the body of the canal. **C,** Hedstrom files are used to widen the occlusal third of the canal and to smooth the walls of the preparation. **D,** *Top,* Gates Glidden drills come in sizes one to six. *Bottom,* They are used in a slow-speed handpiece to widen the canal orifice after the canal has been initially prepared, and they should not be inserted apically into the canal for more than a few millimeters.

88　PRACTICAL ENDODONTICS

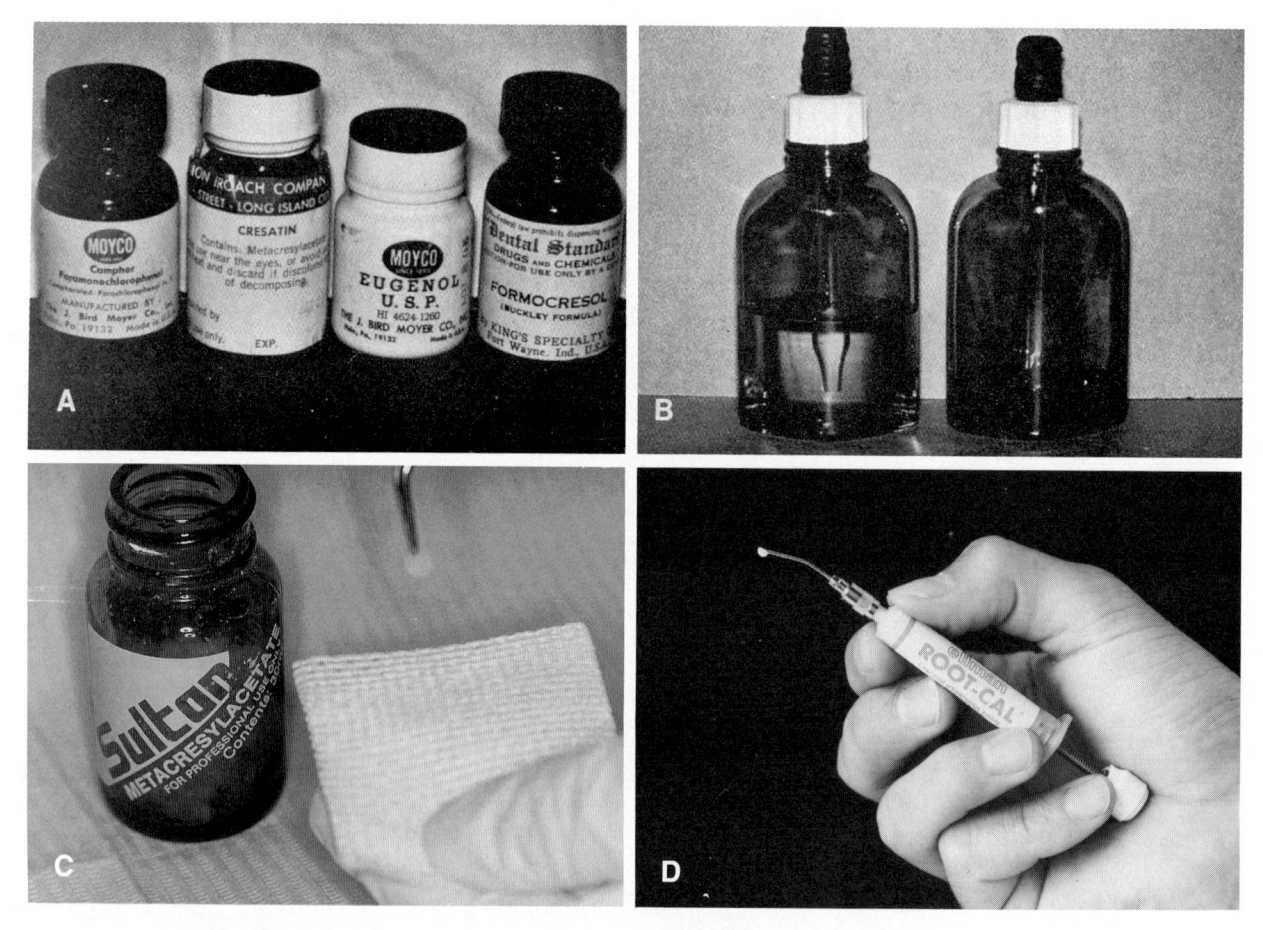

Figure 4-35 A, Intracanal medicaments. Camphorated monoparachlorophenol (CMPC) and metacresylacetate (Cresatin) are two of the most widely used medicaments. Both have a wide antibacterial spectrum. Eugenol is used for sedation where periapical irritation exists. Formocresol (formalin and cresol) is used in emergency therapy as a medicament following a pulpotomy. This latter therapy renders fixation of the remaining pulpal tissue. **B,** These medicaments are conveniently kept in eyedropper bottles. **C,** The cotton pellet is dried with a 2 × 2 gauze sponge before placing into pulp chamber. **D,** Calcium Hydroxide - between visits, this routine, intracanal medicament is placed into the root canal to reduce potential problems. It is used to dry up weeping canals, to induce apexification, to prevent root resorption, or to treat perforations.

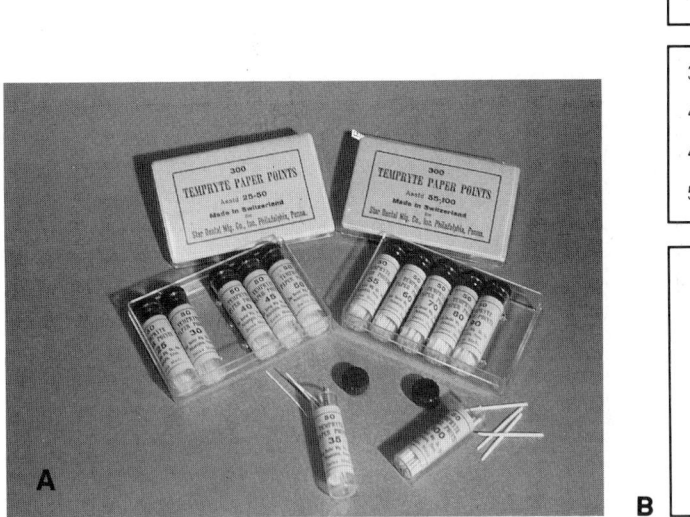

Figure 4-36 Drying of root canal is achieved by using absorbent paper points. Paper points are made to remove moisture from prepared canals. They are rigid enough to be easily inserted and withdrawn without losing shape and sized to correspond to standardized endodontic instruments (both standardized and taper). **A**, Boxes of paper points of assorted sizes. **B**, Comparison of standardized and taper paper points.

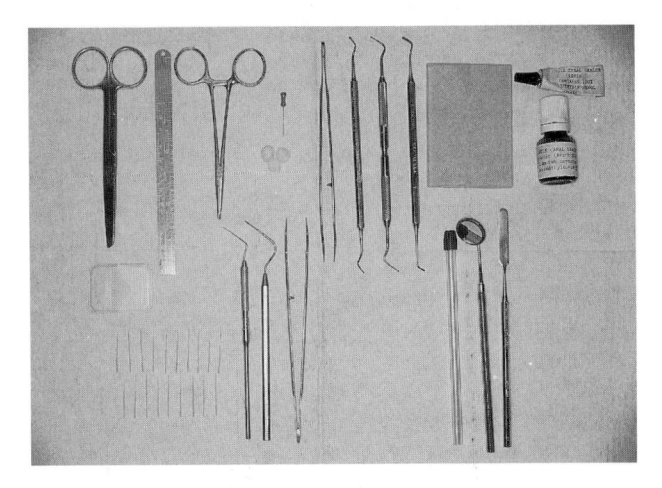

Figure 4-37 Instrument tray set-up for obturation of the root canal.

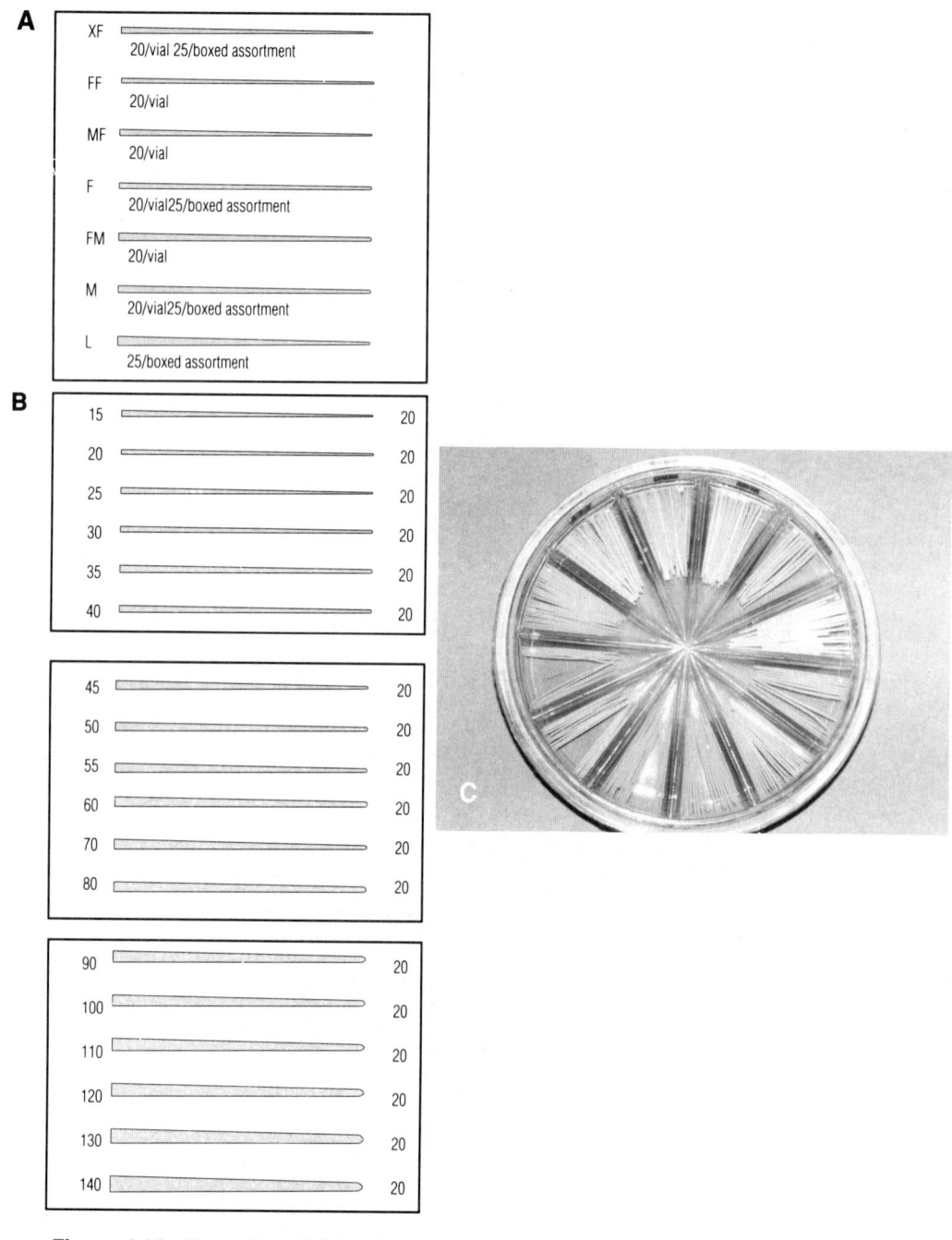

Figure 4-38 Obturation of the root canal. Materials: *Gutta percha points* - a durable, dependable radiopaque root canal filling. Since they are compressible, they can be condensed into each other and against the walls of the canal. **A**, Assortment (taper sizes) - for lateral condensation or as primary cone in the vertical condensation technique; **B**, Standardized points - sized to match corresponding size files used as primary cone. **C**, Gutta percha dish for sterilization and storage of gutta percha points.

Continued.

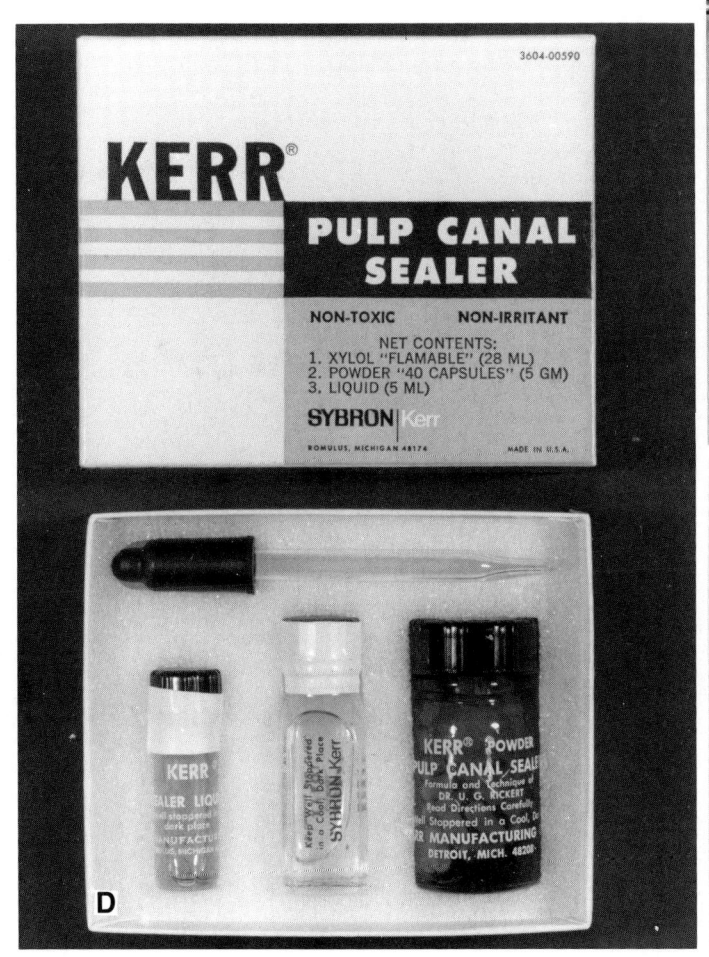

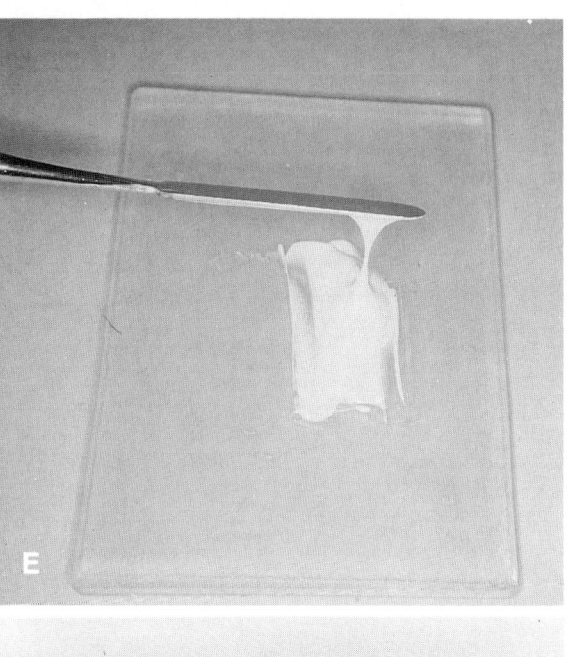

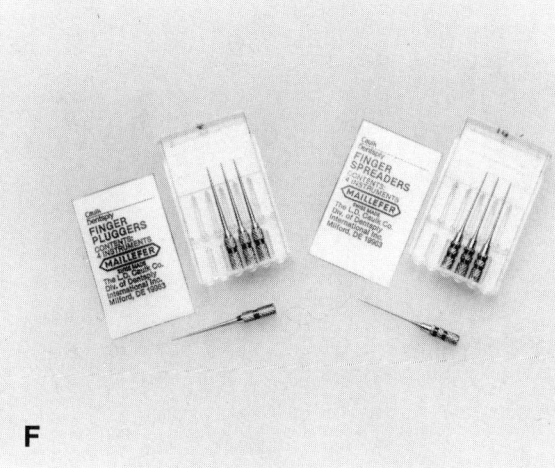

Chapter 4 ♦ Sterilization Procedures and Endodontic Armamentarium 91

Figure 4-38, *cont'd Root canal sealer* - to fill voids and discrepancies between the gutta percha and the root canal walls. **D,** Root canal cement. **E,** Consistency of cement should string out inch with spatula from glass slab. Intruments: **F,** *Spreader* - tapered instruments with spearlike point used to compress the filling material laterally against the canal walls. The spreader is placed in the canal under pressure and then withdrawn. A gutta percha point is then inserted into the space created by the spreader point. Some spreaders are long handled and some are short handled, and all come in different sizes.

92 PRACTICAL ENDODONTICS

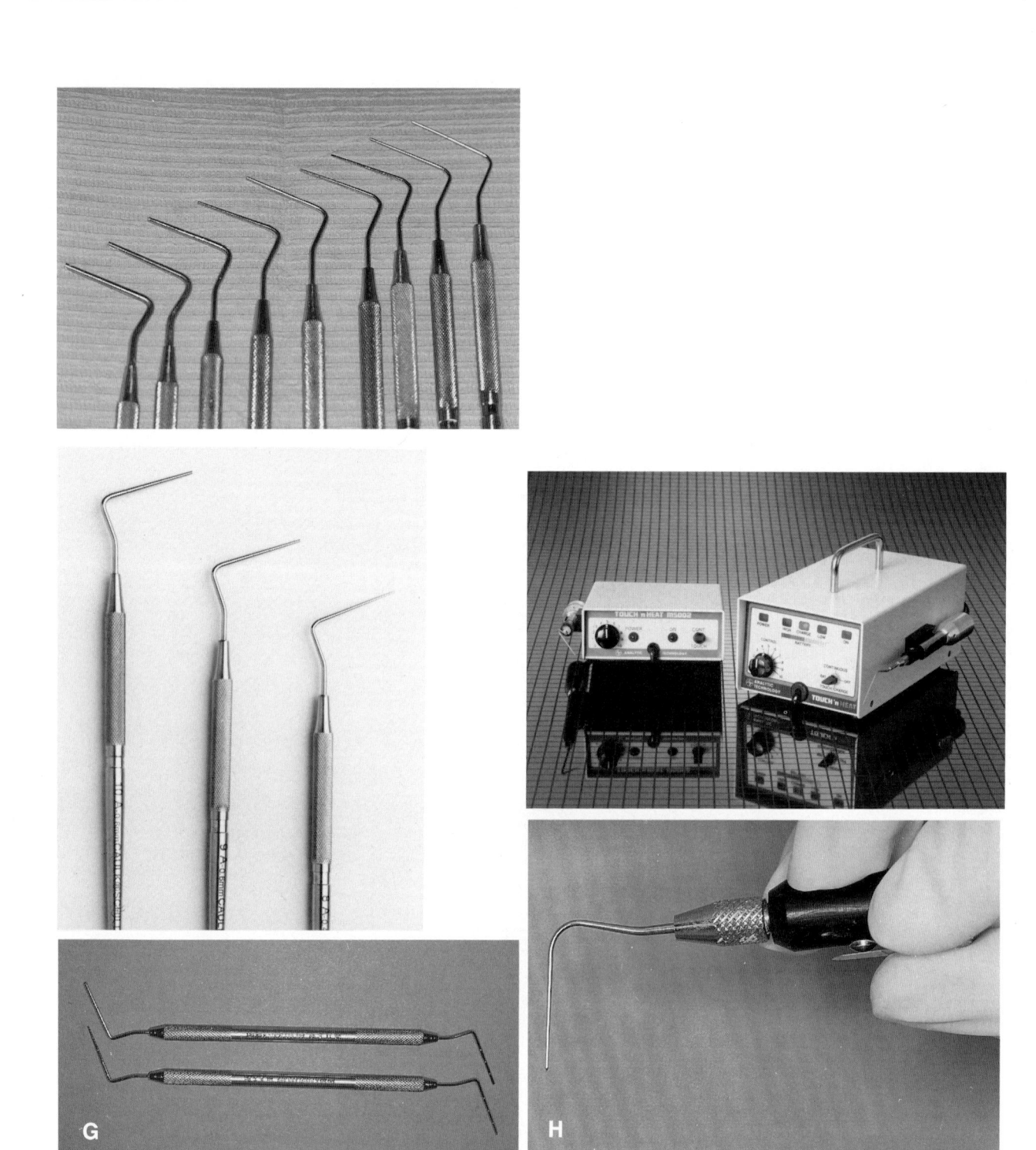

Figure 4-38, *cont'd* **G,** *Plugger* - flat-ended instrument used to compress the gutta percha mass apically. *Top,* Schlider pluggers in different sizes (nos. 8 to 12 in ½ increments). *Middle,* close-up of Schlider plugger showing 5-mm increments on plugger. This determines the depth of the plugger in the canal. *Bottom,* Double-ended pluggers. **H,** *Heat carrier. Top,* Touch 'n Heat (Analytic Technology) to warm the gutta percha. *Bottom,* Tip of heat carrier to be placed in the canal after primary gutta percha cone is cemented in place. (Analytic Technology Corp., Redmond, WA 98052.)

Continued.

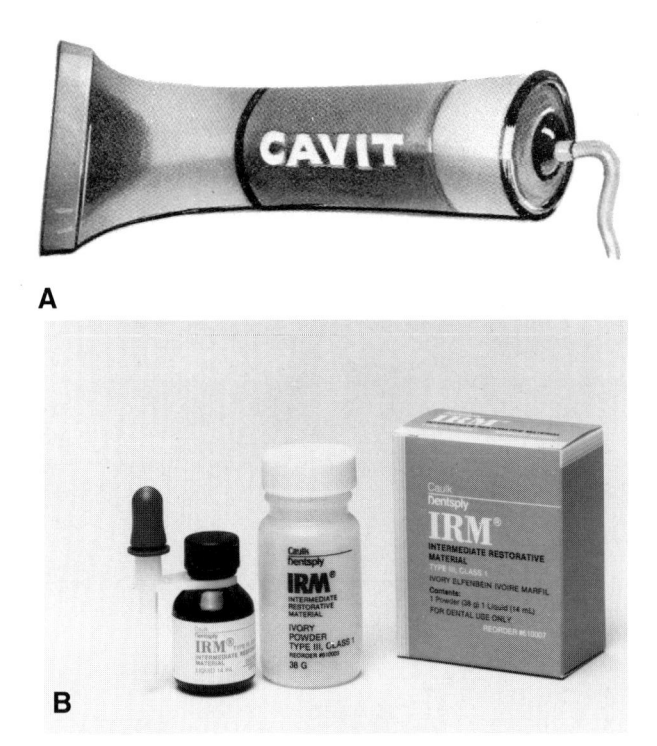

Chapter 4 ♦ Sterilization Procedures and Endodontic Armamentarium 93

Figure 4-39 Sealing agents. **A,** Cavit is an effective, convenient temporary sealing agent to close the chamber between and following endodontic therapy. **B,** IRM is an excellent seal when a harder temporary seal is needed.

5

Anatomical Variations

When practicing successful endodontics one must have a thorough knowledge of root canal morphology. Not only should one be aware of the normal anatomy of the tooth, but also the less common occurrences as well. For example, many endodontic failures could be minimized if one carefully investigates the possibility of extra root canals.

Careful study of the radiograph is the single most important approach in detecting extra root canals. Two good preoperative radiographs from different angles may show:
1. Change in radiographic density of root canal space
2. Unusual contour of roots
3. Unusual crown-root ratio—a relatively short crown to root ratio could indicate an extra canal.

The length-of-tooth radiograph is important in detecting extra canals. A dark shadow running nearly parallel to a file in a root canal space may point to an extra canal. The shadow usually runs only a short distance along the file and then becomes obscured. Also, one can suspect an extra canal when a file appears to go off to one side of the root rather than running in the center of the canal.

Clinically, one can expect extra root canals when the buccal-lingual width of the crown is wider than usual. For example, if a lower anterior tooth has a prominent cingulum and a wider than normal buccal-lingual width, chances are good that there are two canals. The extra canal is usually quite lingually. On an upper molar, a prominent mesiobuccal cusp where the width buccal-lingually on the mesial is much wider than normal would lead one to suspect an extra canal in the mesial root. Once the chamber is penetrated, an instrument such as a D-16 explorer should be used in search of extra canals. If a canal is fairly large and in a normal position in the tooth, chances are there is only one canal present in that area of the tooth. While instrumenting the canals, always be on the lookout for a possible extra canal or branching off of the main canal. Sometimes another canal is not discovered until the cleansing and shaping of the other canals are completed. This gives one better visibility for searching.

EXTRA ROOT CANALS THAT ARE OFTEN MISSED

Mandibular Incisors

The lingual canal is the canal most often missed when treating mandibular incisors. The lingual side of the access cavity should be extended so as to find the extra canal. This access opening will also make cleansing and shaping of both canals easier. Extra canals are more prevalent in short bulky roots. Two canals are found in about 40% of cases. Two canals with separate foramen occur, however, in 13% of cases (Fig. 5-1).

Maxillary Molars

The mesiolingual canal is the canal most often missed when treating maxillary molars. The extra orifice is usually found 1 to 4 mm lingual to the mesiobuccal canal orifice. The frequency of extra canals is higher with short blunt roots. Four canals occur in as high as 60% of cases. In most cases the extra canal has a common apex with the original mesiobuccal canal, but a separate foramen has been observed in 12.5% of cases (Fig. 5-2).

96   PRACTICAL ENDODONTICS

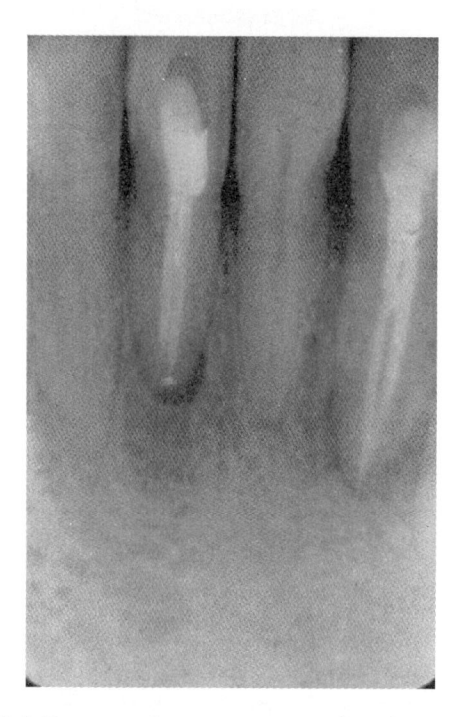

Figure 5-1 Extra canals are more prevalent in mandibular incisors. Note the mandibular central incisor with two separate canals and two openings and the mandibular lateral incisor with two canals converging into a common foramen.

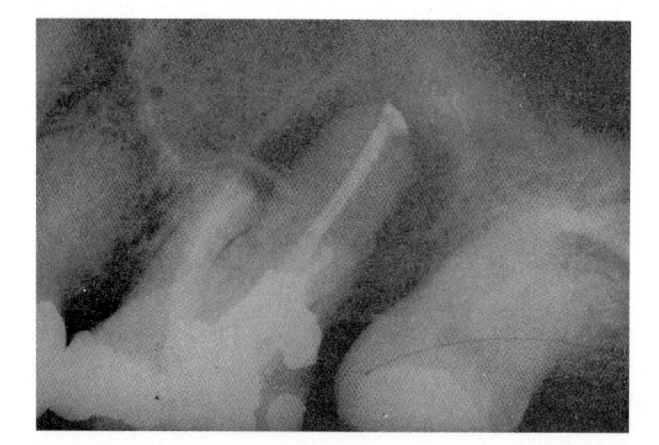

Figure 5-2 Extra canals are often found in maxillary molars. It is the mesial-buccal root that most frequently demonstrates this, as seen in this film.

The Tooth With the Most Developmental Anomalies is the Maxillary Lateral Incisor

1. Dens invaginatus (dens in dente) (Fig. 5-3)
2. Extra root or canal (Fig. 5-4 and 5-5)
3. Enamel defect above cinculum (Fig. 5-6)
4. Palatal groove (Fig. 5-7)

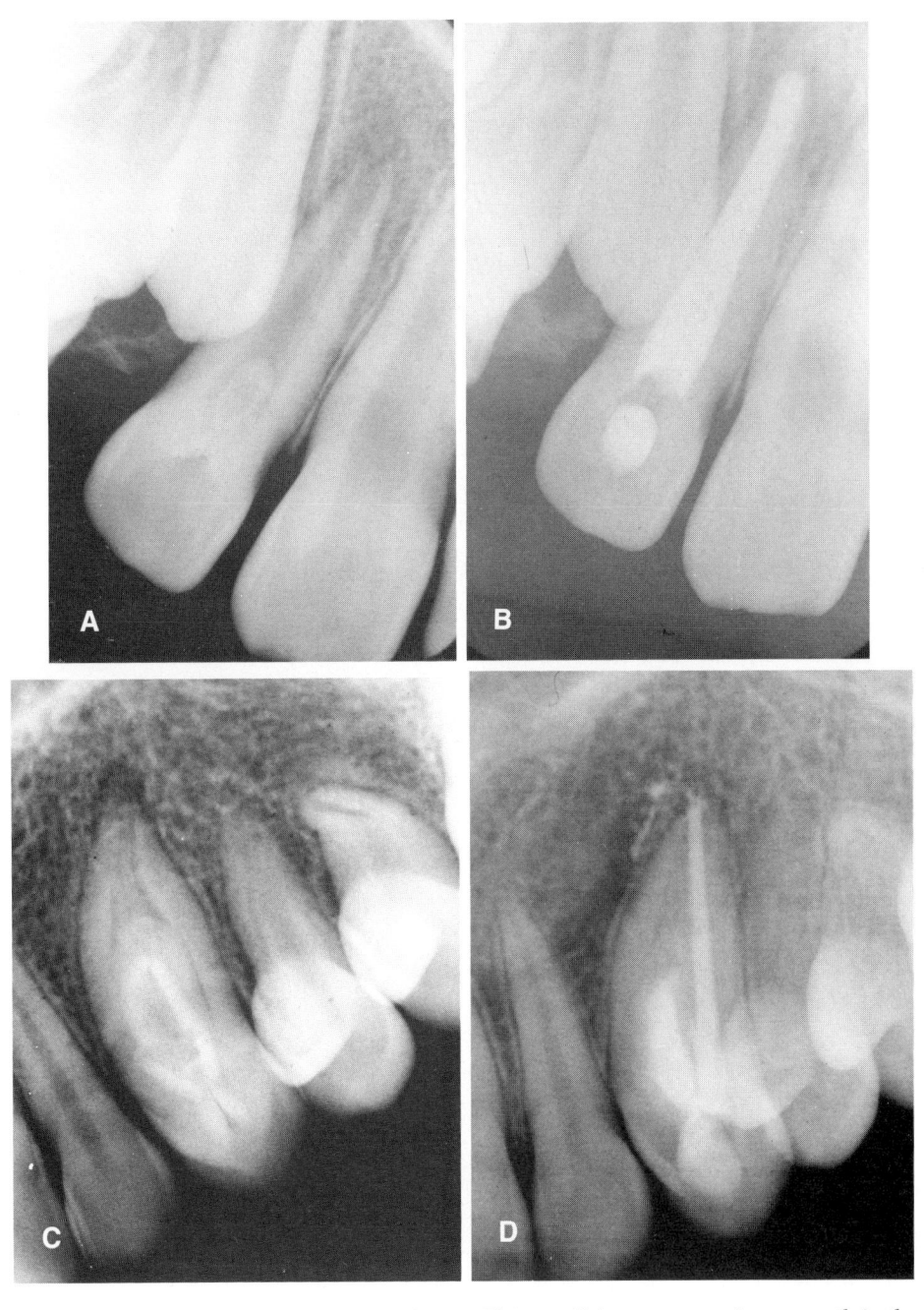

Figure 5-3 Dens Invaginatus (dens in dente). This condition can occur in any tooth in the mouth, but it appears more frequently in the permanent maxillary lateral incisor. **A,** Example of a dens in dente in which pulpal degeneration occurred before complete root formation. **B,** Apexification procedure was performed before complete obturation with gutta percha. **C,** Demonstrates the different variations of dens in dente illustrating anatomy. **D,** Treatment consideration.

98 PRACTICAL ENDODONTICS

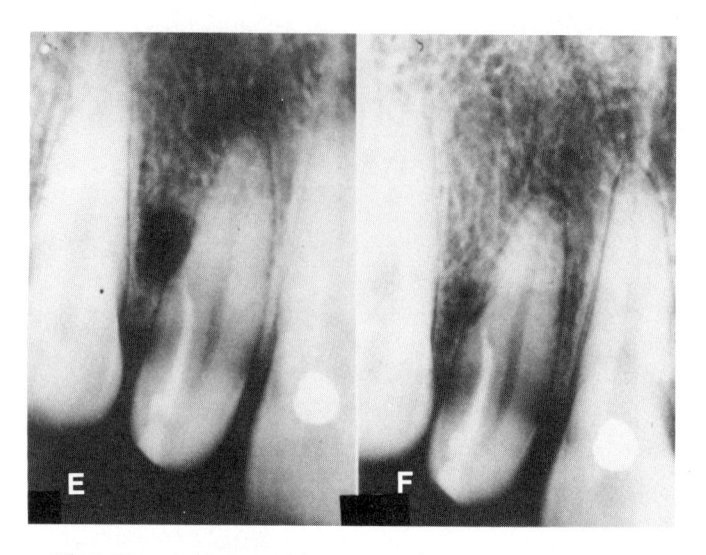

Figure 5-3, *cont'd* **E,** Dens in dente with two canals each having its own pulp chamber. The small side canal on distal was the only canal needing treatment. **F,** Six-month recall showing some resolution of radiolucency.

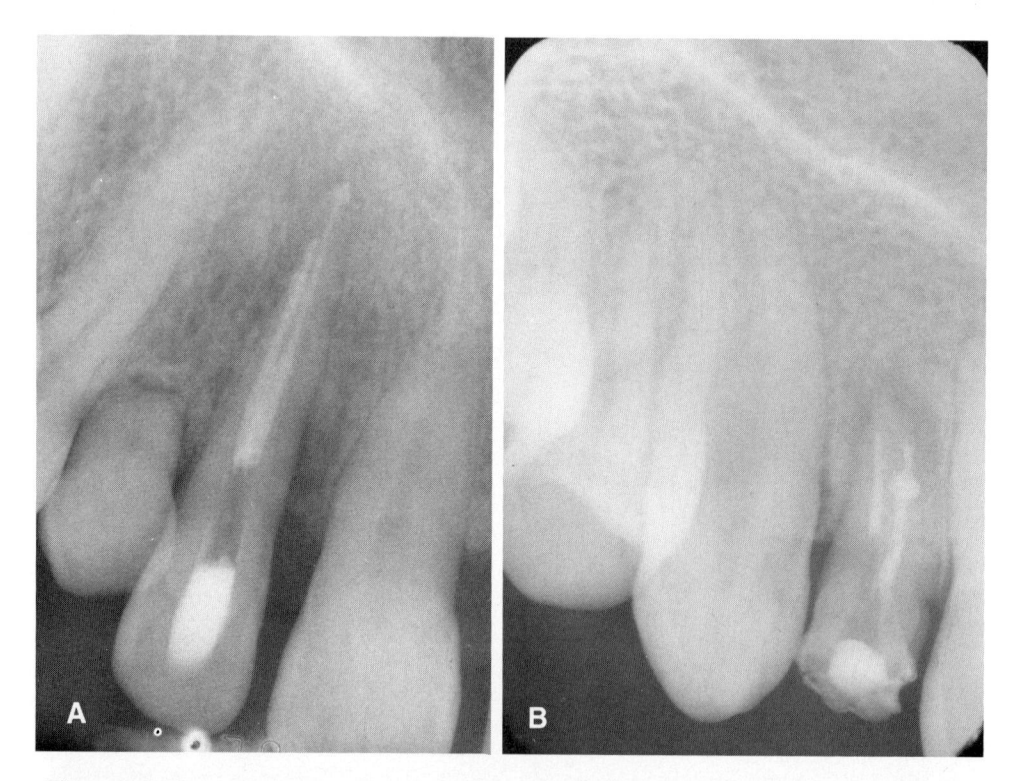

Figure 5-4 Extra canal in maxillary lateral incisor. **A,** Two canals with common apex. **B,** Two canals with two separate apical foramens.

Chapter 5 ♦ Anatomical Variations 99

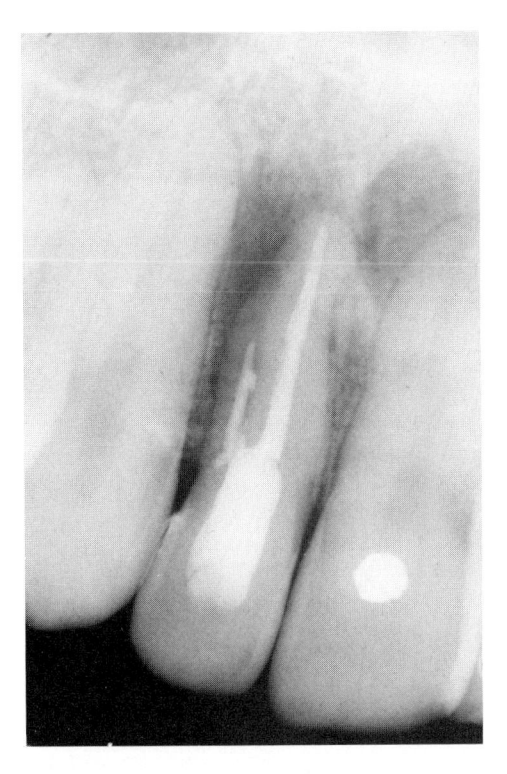

Figure 5-5 Extra root in maxillary lateral incisor.

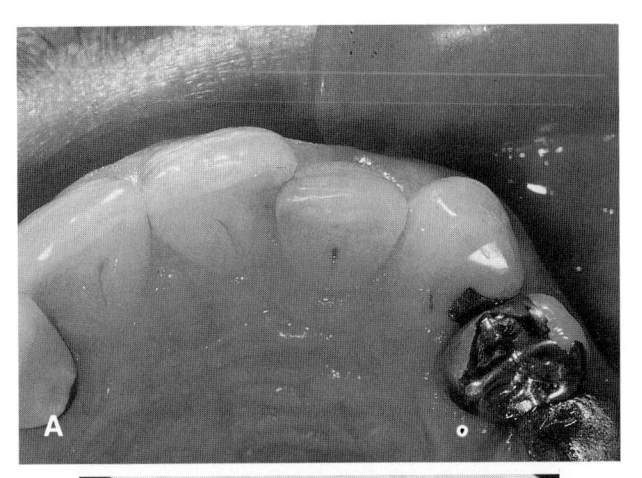

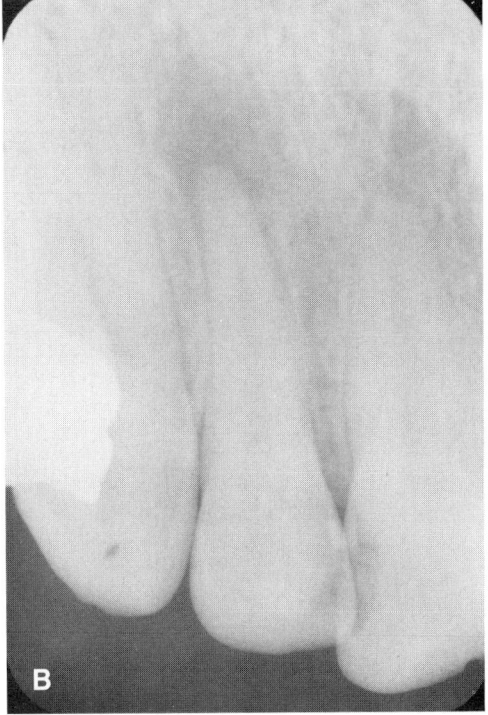

Figure 5-6 Enamel defect above cingulum. **A,** Pit above cingulum extending into pulp. **B,** Radiograph of same tooth showing periapical rarefaction.

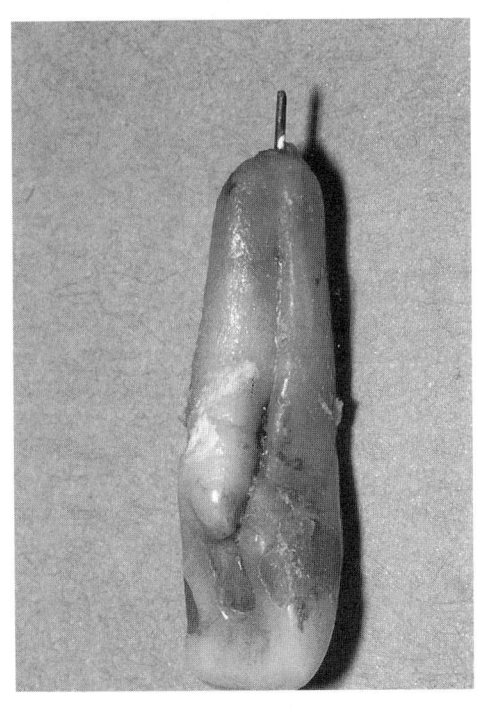

Figure 5-7 Palatal groove defect. This groove can extend as far down the root surface as to the apex. This case demonstrates a misdiagnosis. Root canal therapy had been initiated, although this tooth had been periodontally involved with probably a vital pulp.

TABLE 5-1 ♦ *Classification of invaginated teeth and treatment suggestions.*

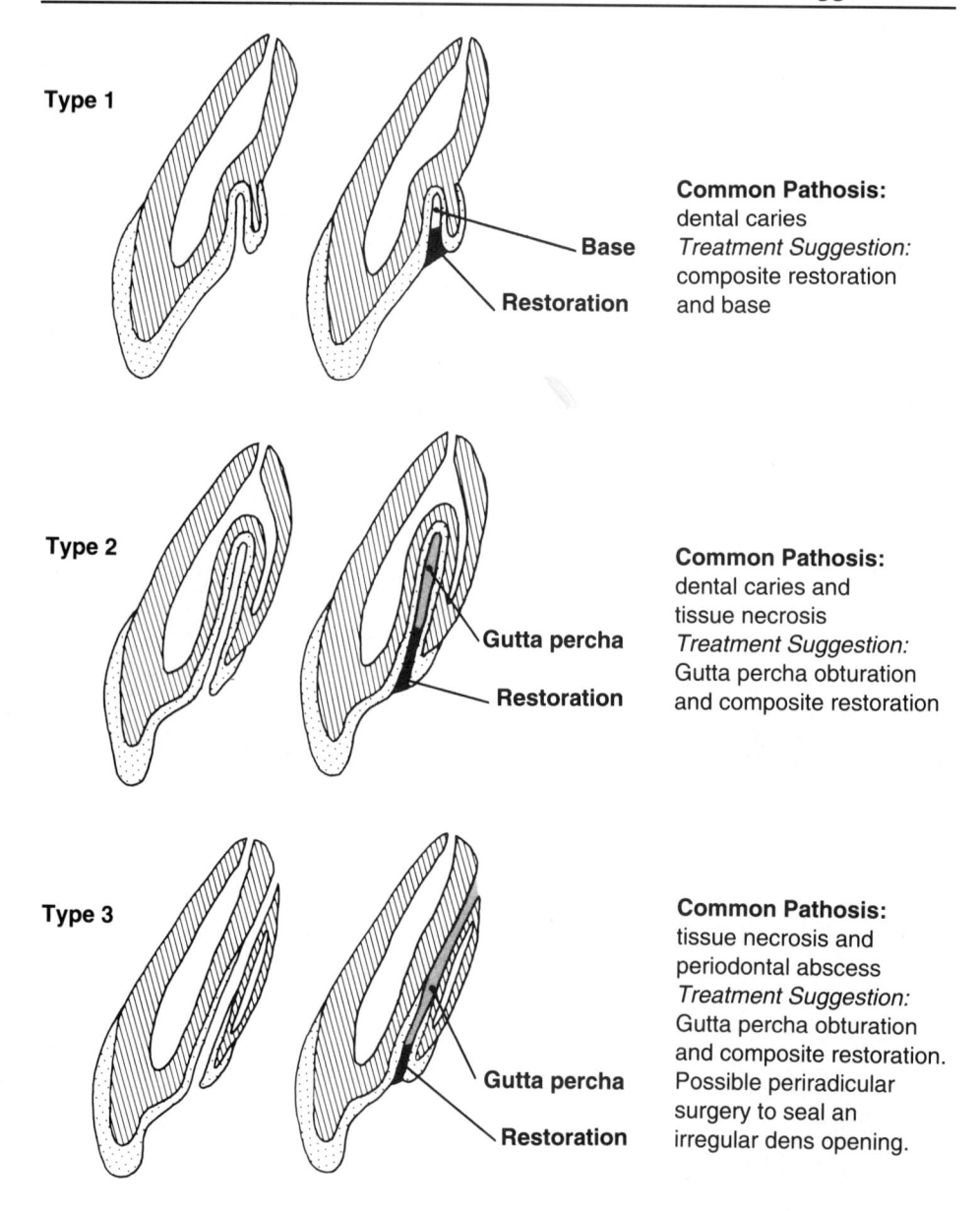

Type 1

- Base
- Restoration

Common Pathosis: dental caries
Treatment Suggestion: composite restoration and base

Type 2

- Gutta percha
- Restoration

Common Pathosis: dental caries and tissue necrosis
Treatment Suggestion: Gutta percha obturation and composite restoration

Type 3

- Gutta percha
- Restoration

Common Pathosis: tissue necrosis and periodontal abscess
Treatment Suggestion: Gutta percha obturation and composite restoration. Possible periradicular surgery to seal an irregular dens opening.

CLUES IN LOCATING EXTRA ROOT CANALS
Radiograph
1. Short crown-root ratio (Fig. 5-8)
2. Sharp change in radiographic density of root canal space (Fig. 5-9)
3. Unclear outline or unusual contour of any root (Fig. 5-10)
4. Dark shadow running nearly parallel to a file in a root canal space (Fig. 5-11)

Clinical
1. Prominent cingulum (Fig. 5-12, *A*)
2. Prominent lingual cusp (Fig. 5-12, *B*)
3. Prominent buccal cusp and wide mesiodistally (Fig. 5-12, *C*)
4. Prominent buccal cusp and wide buccolingual on the mesial side (Fig. 5-12, *D*)
5. Smaller than usual canal (Fig. 5-12, *E*)

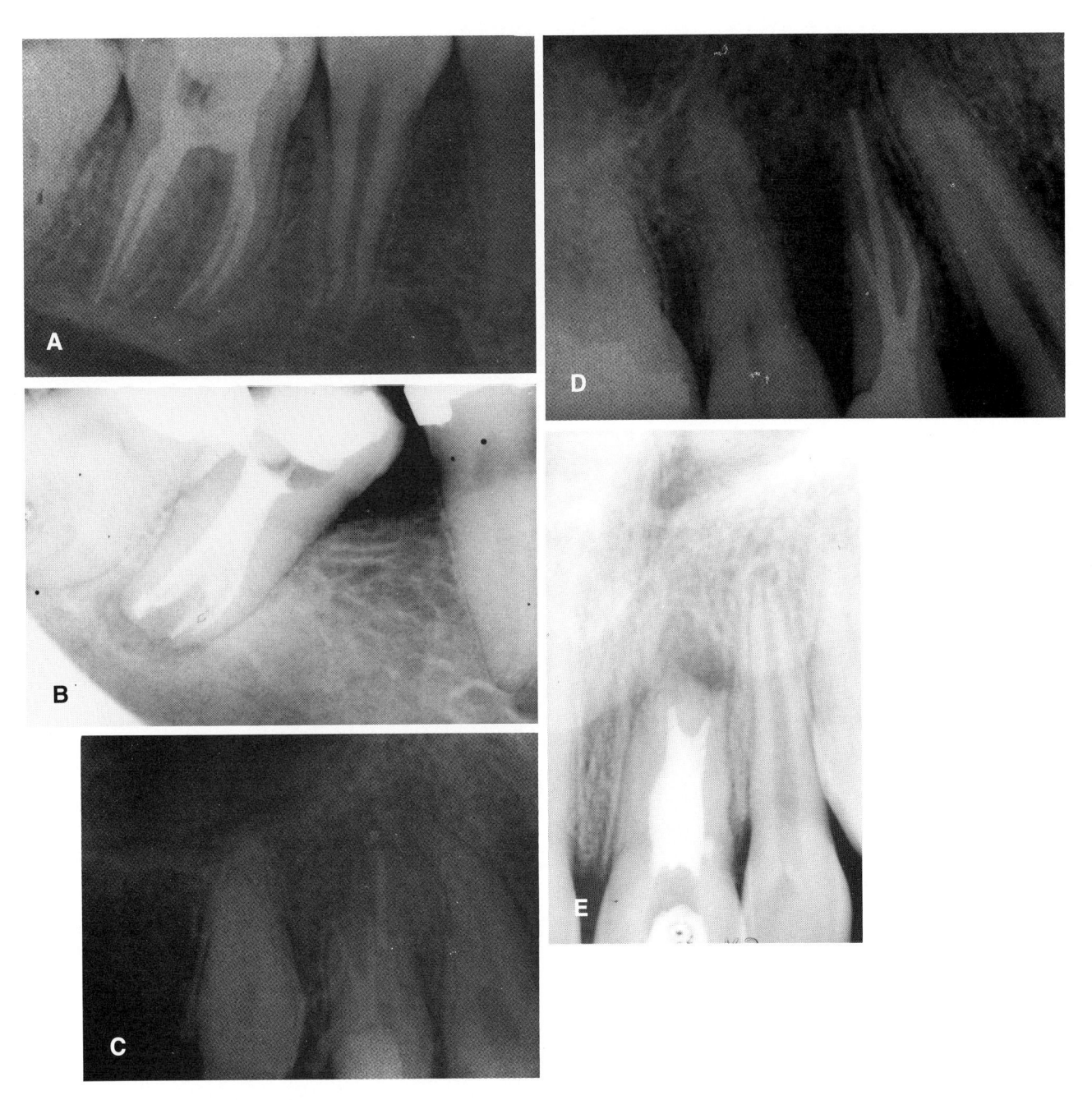

Figure 5-8 Extra canals are more prevalent in short bulky roots, in which there is a short crown-root ratio as seen in **A** and **B,** mandibular molars, **C** and **D,** maxillary premolars, and E, Maxillary central incisor.

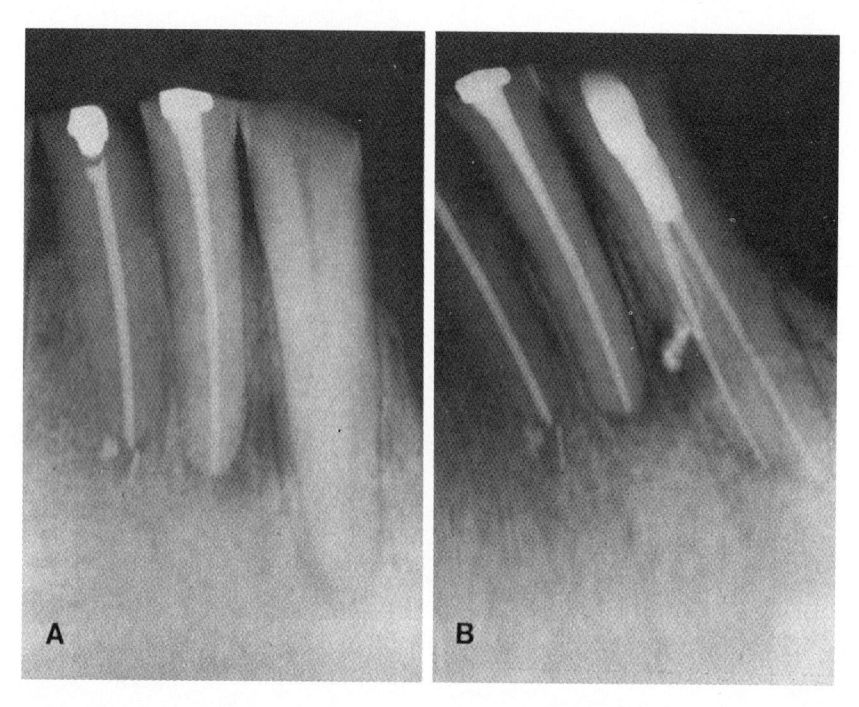

Figure 5-9 Search for a sharp change in the radiographic density of the root canal space as seen in **A**. **B**, Obturation of two main canals and that of a small lateral secondary canal leading to the lateral lesion of the cuspid.

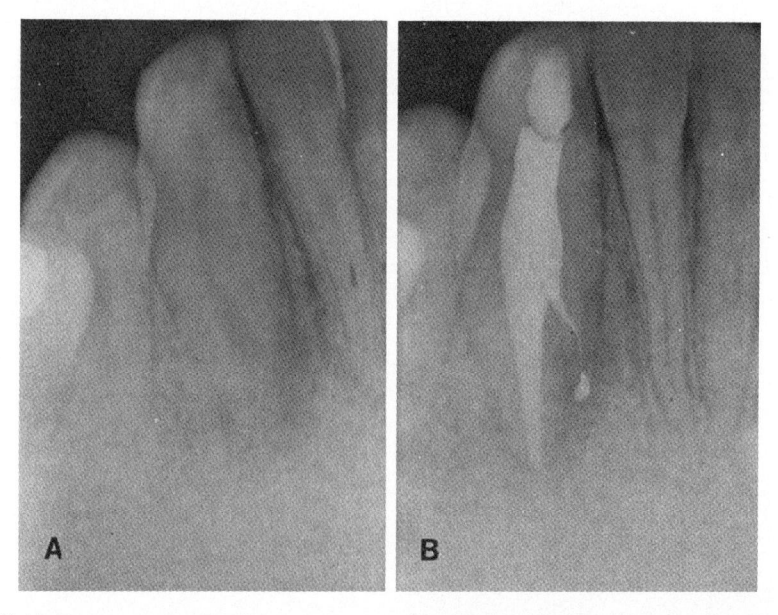

Figure 5-10 Extra canals may be found where unusual contours of a root may exist. **A**, Preoperative and **B**, postoperative films of a mandibular cuspid. Note the unusual configuration of the root at the level of the middle and apical thirds of the root in *A* and the small secondary canal that has been cleansed and obturated in *B*.

Chapter 5 ♦ Anatomical Variations 103

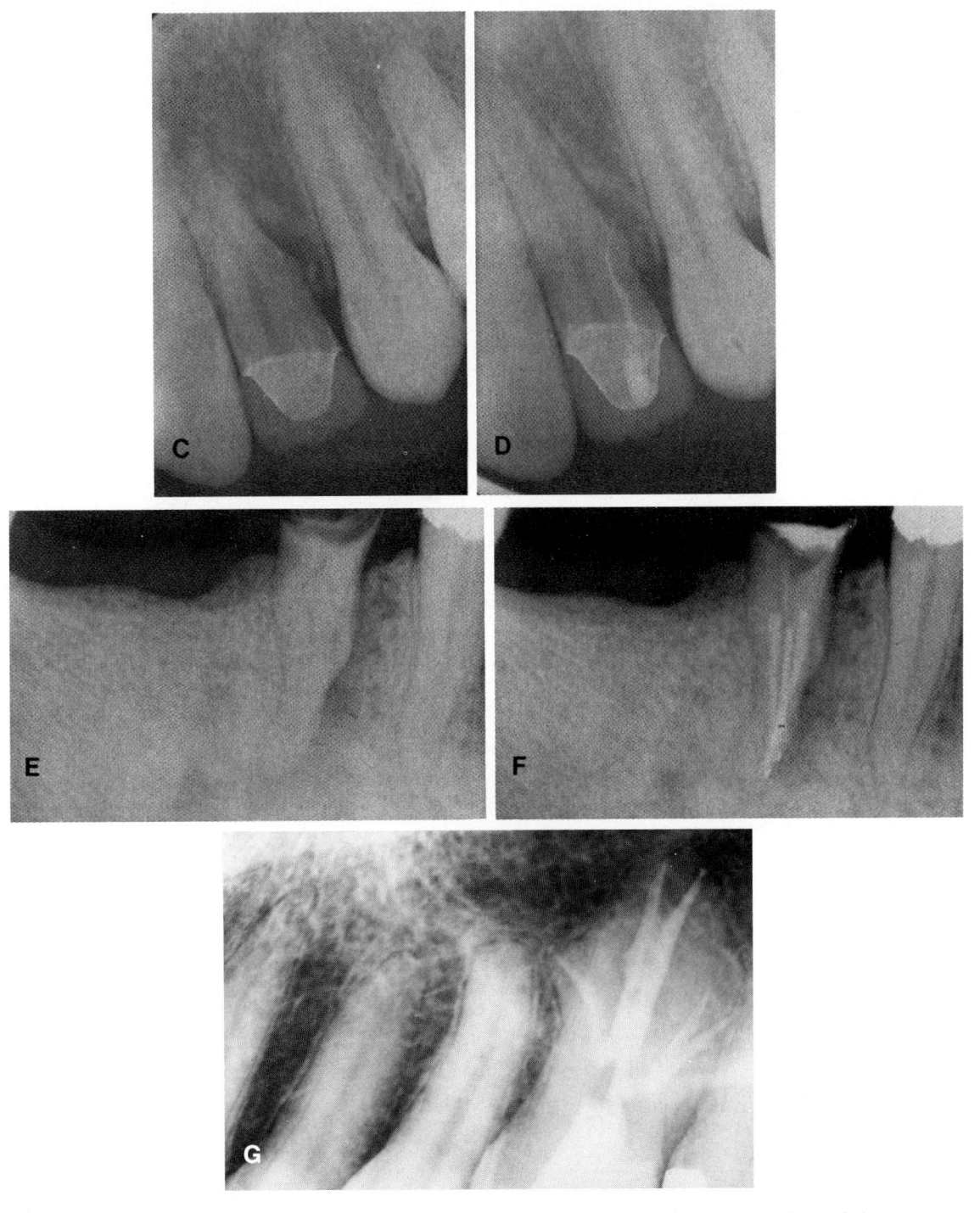

Figure 5-10, *cont'd* **C,** Film showing the unusual contour on the distal surface of the maxillary lateral in an area of a lesion. **D,** Obturation of a small irregular secondary canal directed to that configuration and lesion. **E,** Preoperative and **F,** postoperative films showing extra canals in a tooth that shows an irregular configuration to its shape and surface. **G,** Maxillary first molar with one mesial-buccal canal, two palatal canals, and two distal canals.

104   PRACTICAL ENDODONTICS

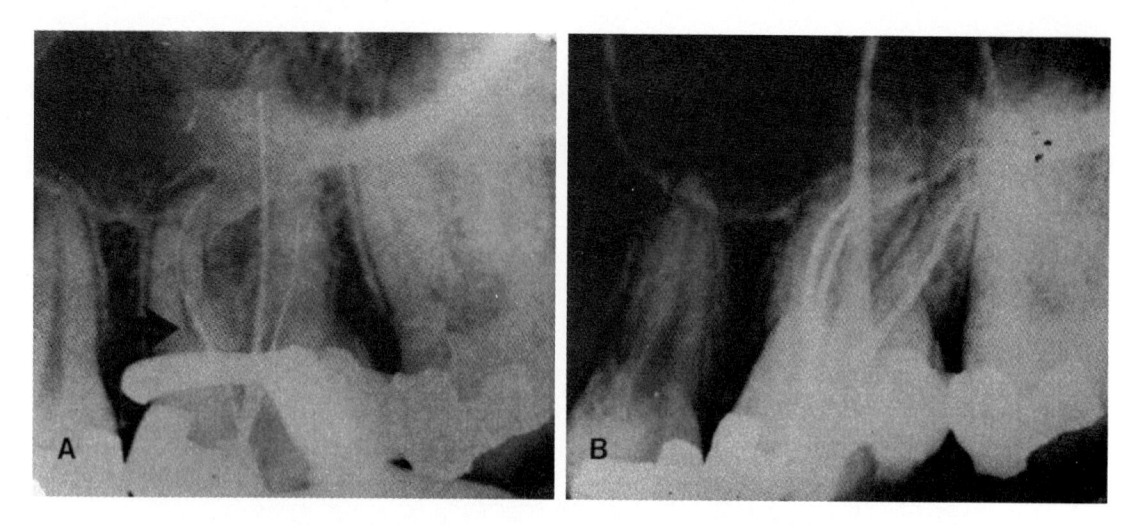

Figure 5-11 **A,** Film showing files in canals establishing working distance. Note dark shadow running nearly parallel to the file in the mesial-buccal root canal space (*arrow*). **B,** Completed therapy film showing the two mesial-buccal canals obturated.

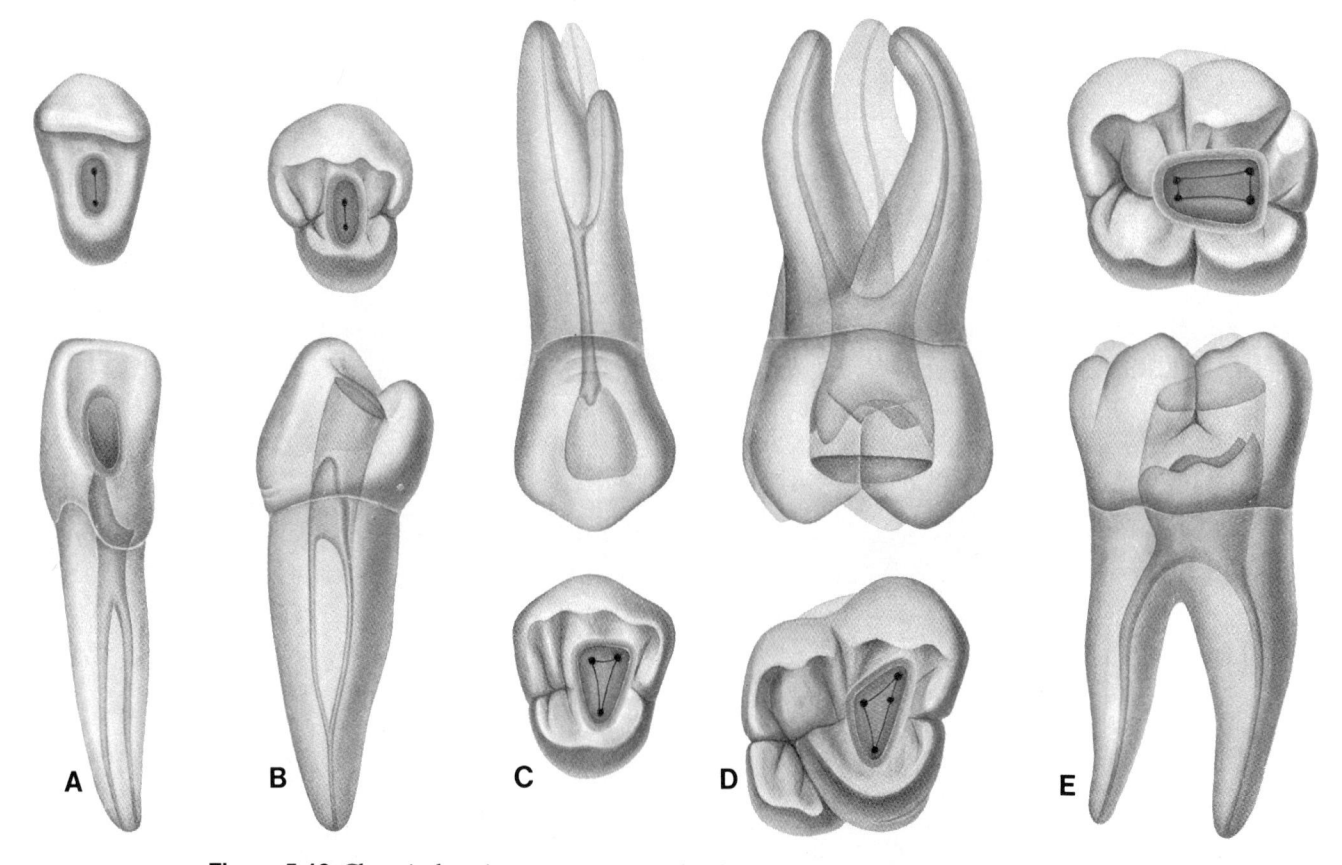

Figure 5-12 Clues in locating extra root canals. Extra canals and extra roots are usually located in the labiolingual plane. **A,** Prominent cingulum of a mandibular incisor; an extra canal may be found lingually. **B,** Prominent lingual cusp of a mandibular bicuspid; extra canal may be found lingually. **C,** Prominent buccal cusp and wide crown mesial-distally; a mesial-buccal canal or root may be found in the maxillary first premolar. **D,** Prominent buccal cusp and wide crown buccal-lingually on the mesial half in the maxillary molar; a second mesial-buccal canal may frequently be found. **E,** Where unusually small canals are seen, an extra canal may be found, as in the distal root of a mandibular molar.

6

Routine Endodontic Therapy

This chapter will deal with the preparation and obturation of the root canal system. All steps must be followed to make the entire canal system receptive to the filling substance. If these steps are followed, the obturation technique can be performed easily.

X-RAY TECHNIQUE

Much information can be gained from a clear, undistorted preoperative radiograph. The size and location of the pulp chamber, the overall length of the tooth,

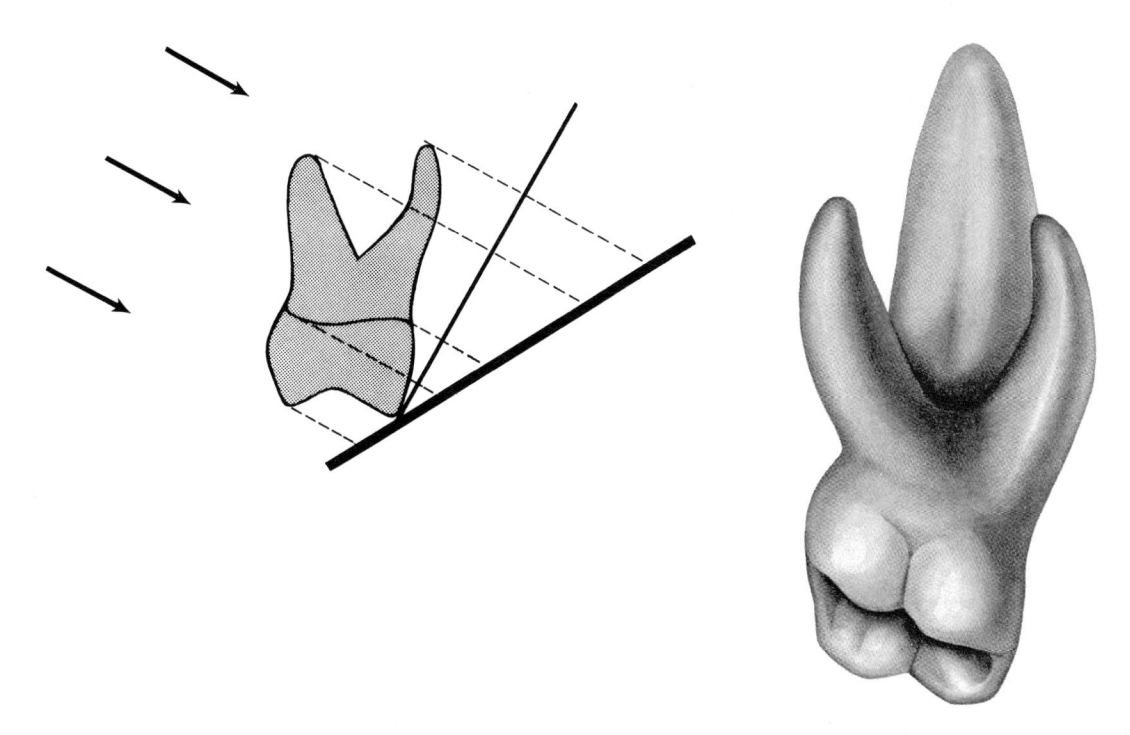

Figure 6-1 Comparison of periapical radiograhic techniques. Bisecting angle technique. The x-ray beam is directed perpendicular to an imaginary plane that bisects the angle formed by the recording plane of the x-ray film and the long axis of the tooth.

105

106 PRACTICAL ENDODONTICS

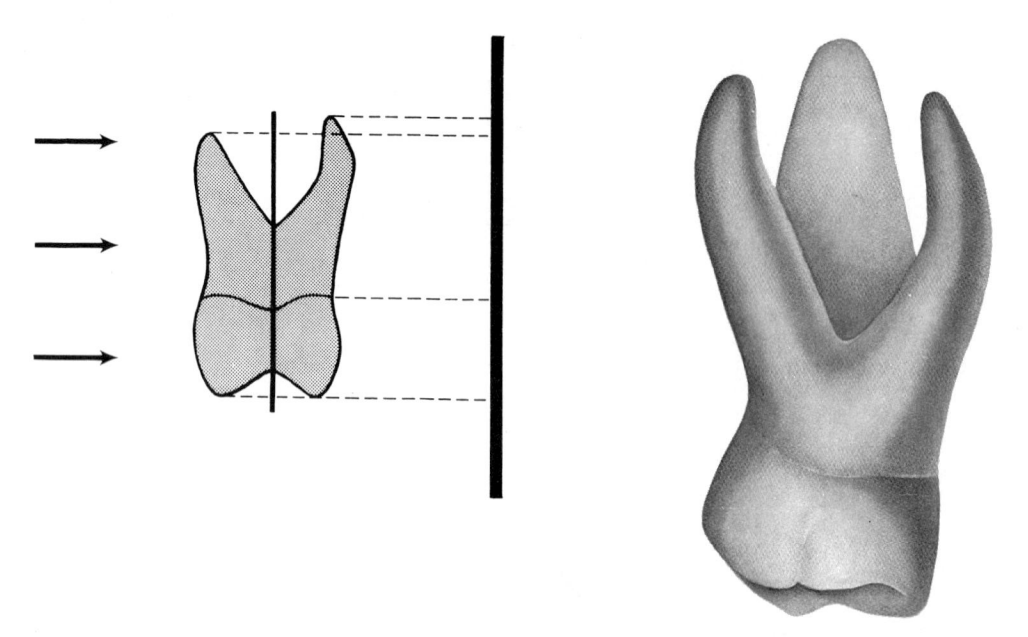

Figure 6-2 Paralleling technique. The x-ray beam is directed perpendicular to the recording plane of the film, which has been positioned parallel to the long axis of the tooth. Notice that there is less distortion than in the bisecting angle technique.

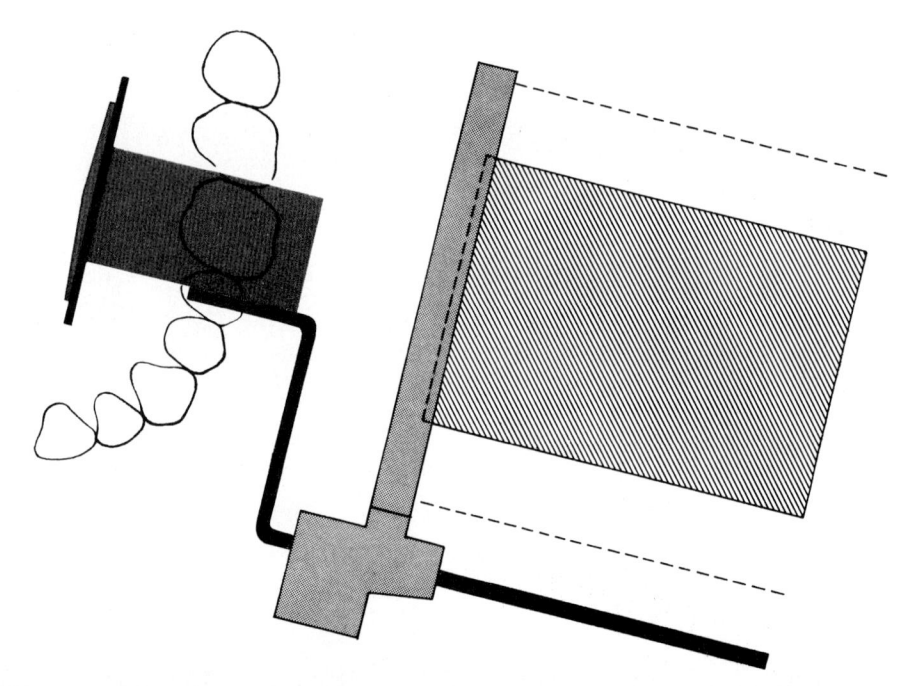

Figure 6-3 XCP film holder. This is an important aid in obtaining radiographs with minimal distortion. It allows the film to be positioned perpendicular to the occlusal surfaces of the teeth and aids in positioning the x-ray cone.

and the anatomy and patency of the root canal system can be visualized.

Purpose: To produce an accurate radiograph so the succeeding films will have the same degree of accuracy for comparison.

Technique: A radiograph is taken with a film in the XCP holder and the patient biting on the XCP block. The long cone is lined up parallel with the XCP mount (Fig. 6-3).

PRETREATMENT

Purpose: To facilitate rubber dam application, to prevent leakage during treatment, and to prevent fracturing of the tooth before final restoration.

Technique: All decay and/or weak restorations are removed, and tooth surfaces are restored. If tooth cannot be restored with an amalgam, composite, or temporary filling, then a copper or stainless steel band or a crown form must be used. The rule is when the crown lacks three or more surfaces of natural tooth structure it must be protected from fracture with a band or crown (Fig. 6-4).

The steps in the preparation of a band or crown form are as follows (Fig. 6-5):
1. Remove all the decay and undermined enamel.
2. Remove the interproximal contacts.
3. If crown form is to be used, reduce the occlusal surface.

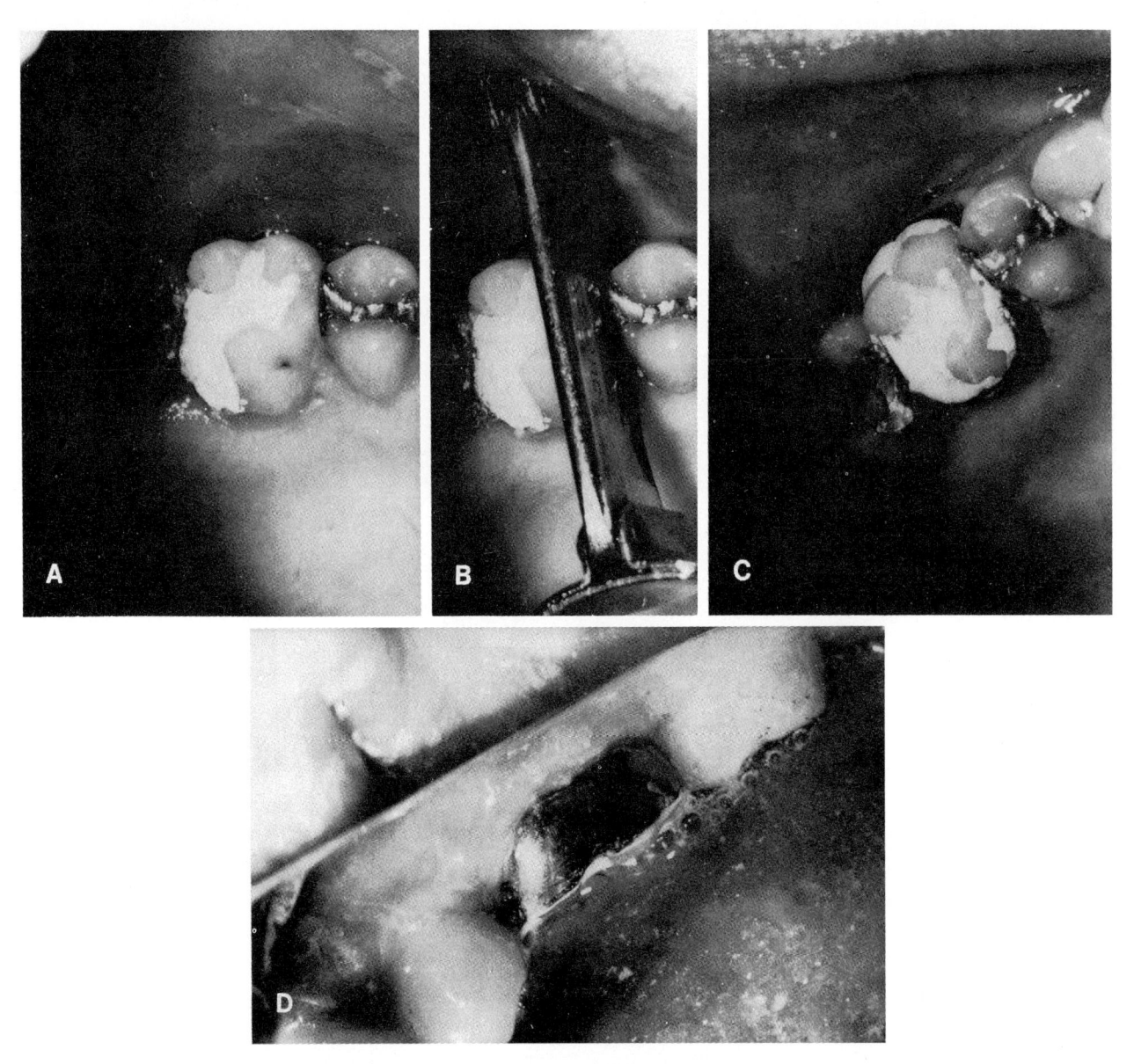

Figure 6-4 **A,** A broken-down molar in which all decay was removed and a temporary restoration placed. **B,** Mizzy hand separator is used to remove the interproximal contacts. **C,** A stainless steel band is cemented in place. An occlusal view. **D,** A buccal view.

108   PRACTICAL ENDODONTICS

4. Typical access opening is made through the preparation.
5. Fill most of the pulp chamber with cotton pellets.
6. Contour and fit a band or crown form.
7. Fill the band or crown form with cement and seal it on the tooth.
8. Place rubber dam and prepare a typical access opening into the crown form or into the cement if a band was used.
9. Remove the cotton pellets from the pulp chamber. The tooth is now ready for endodontic therapy to be performed.

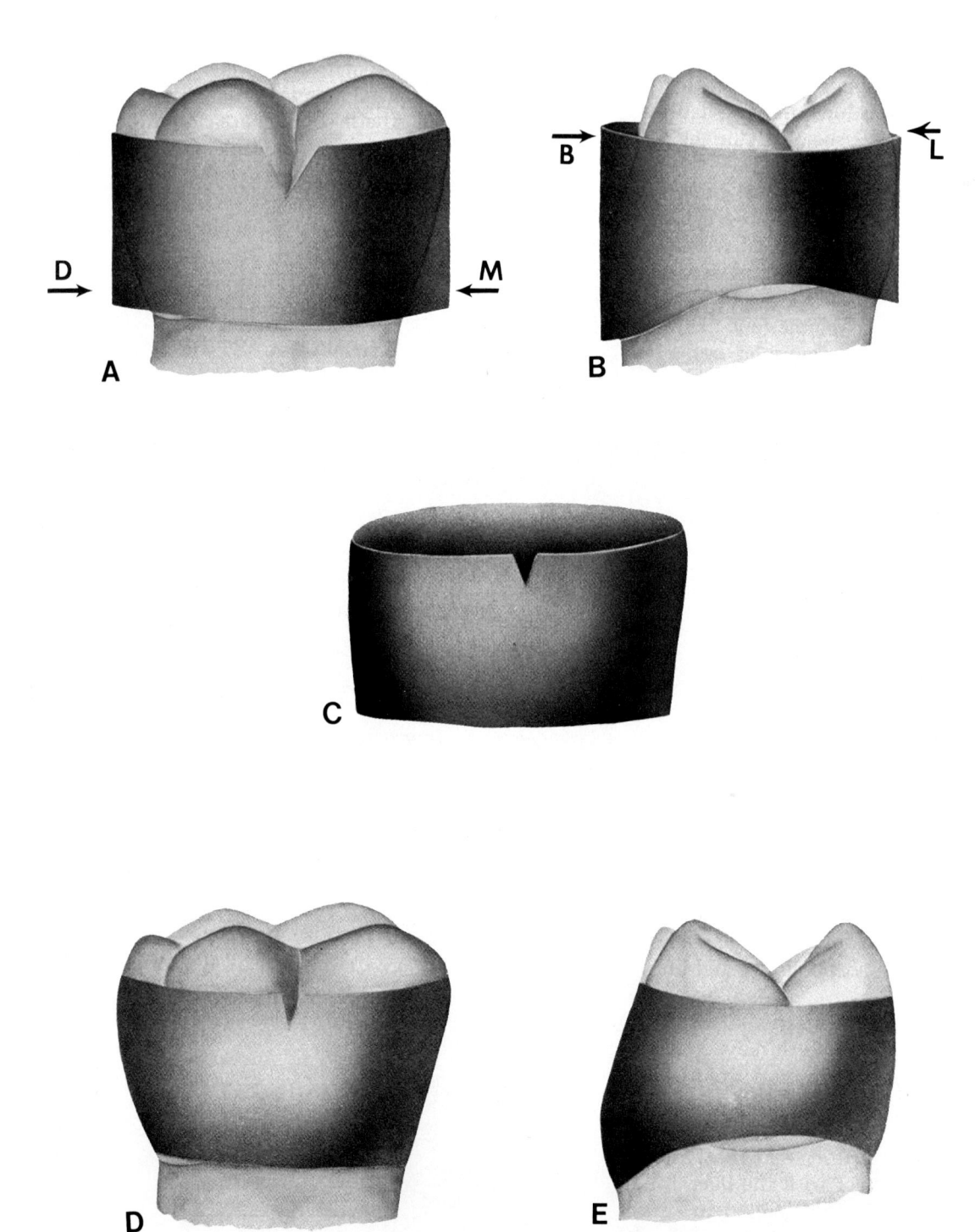

Figure 6-5 The fitting and contouring of a band. **A** and **B,** Stretch, fit, and contour. **C,** Fitted and crimped band. **D** and **E,** Band cemented in place.

ANESTHESIA

Maxilla

Routine Injection: Supraperiosteal Injection—Anesthetic solution is deposited into the tissue overlying the periosteum of the involved tooth (Fig. 6-6, *A*).

Supplementary Injections: Subperiosteal Infiltration—After superficial anesthesia is obtained with the supraperiosteal infiltration, without removing the needle from the tissue, it is retracted slightly and repositioned beneath the periosteum. Using controlled pressure, a small volume (0.5 ml) of anesthetic solution is deposited under the periosteum against the cortical plate of bone. Very little discomfort is experienced during or after injection.

Palatal Infiltration—For posterior teeth only. A few drops of solution (0.25 ml) are injected into the palatal mucosa halfway between the midline of the palate and the gingival margin of the involved tooth (Fig. 6-6, *B*).

Intraseptal Infiltration—An intraosseous injection. Puncture is made through anesthetized gingival papilla. Needle penetrates the thin cortical plate of bone beneath and enters the cancellous bone of the inter-

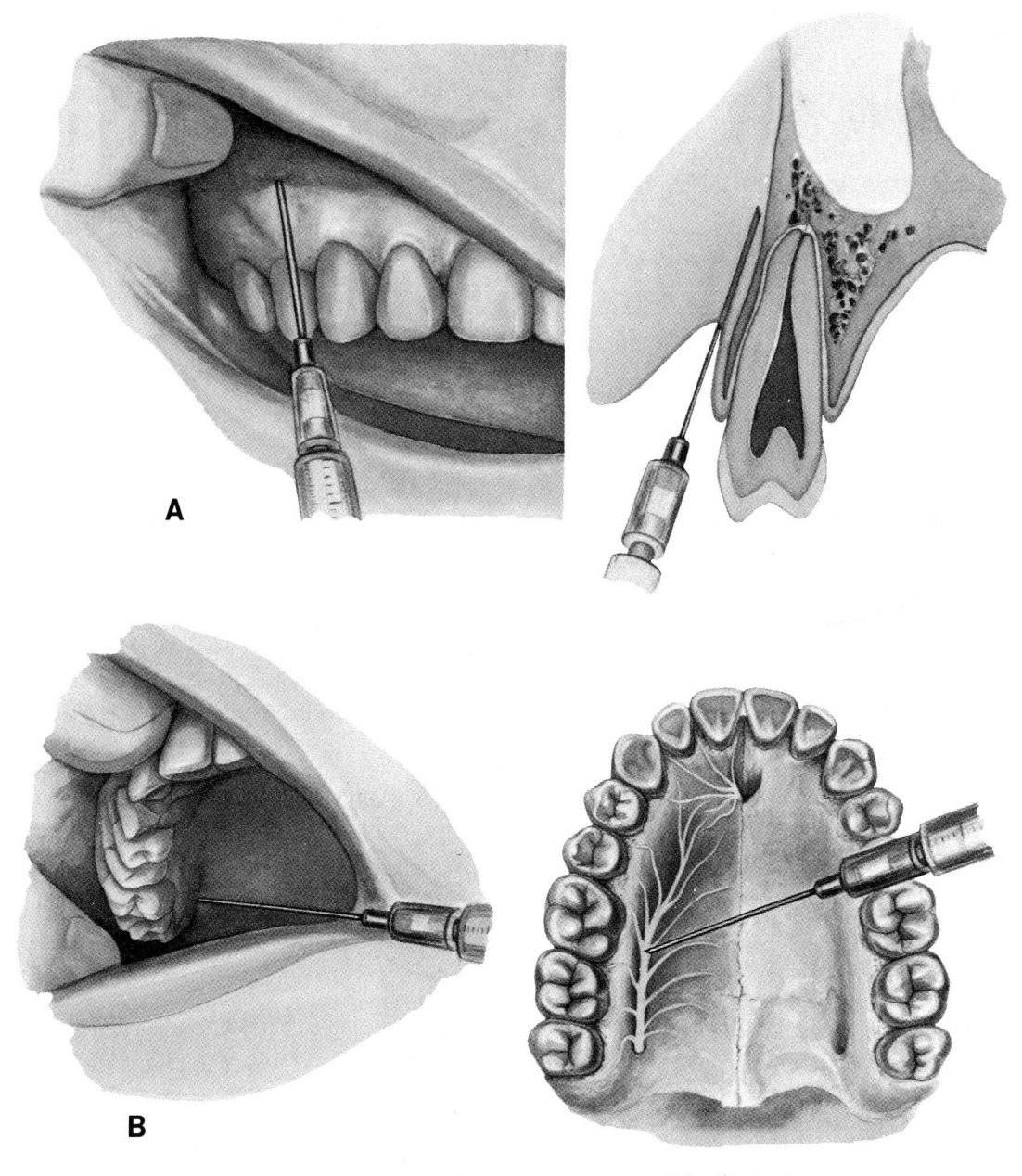

Figure 6-6 Maxillary injections. **A,** Infiltration injection. **B,** Palatal injection.

Table 6-1 ♦ Routine Injections Followed by Supplementary Injections for Profound Pulpal Anesthesia

	Routine Injections	Supplementary Injections
Maxilla		
Incisors and cuspids	Supraperiosteal (infiltration)	Subperiosteal then intraseptal (mesial and distal)
Premolars	Supraperiosteal and palatal (infiltration)	Subperiosteal then intraseptal (mesial and distal)
Molars	Supraperiosteal and palatal (infiltration)	Subperiosteal then intraseptal (mesial and distal)
Mandible		
Incisors and cuspids	Inferior alveolar (mandibular block)	Subperiosteal then intraseptal (mesial and distal)
Premolars and molars	Inferior alveolar (mandibular block) long buccal and mental	Lingual then intraseptal (mesial and distal)
"Injection of Last Resort"	Direct pulpal	In any tooth, when discomfort is evident as pulp is exposed, follow use of injections listed above.

dental septum, where a few drops of anesthetic solution are deposited. Heavy, controlled pressure is required. A short, firm needle is used. Injections are made into the mesial and distal bone septum. Blanching of the surrounding tissue is evidence of intraosseous penetration.

Mandible

Routine Injection: Inferior Alveolar (Mandibular) Block—Supplementary injections are not administered until signs of mandibular anesthesia have become evident, i.e., numbness and tingling at corner of mouth, etc (Fig. 6-7, *A*).

Supplementary Injections: Subperiosteal Infiltration—For anterior teeth only. A small volume (0.5 ml) of anesthetic solution is deposited beneath the periosteum against the cortical plate of bone.

Lingual Infiltration—For posterior teeth only. This injection, together with the buccal infiltration injection described below, is used to anesthetize anastomosing fibers from the cervical plexus. The needle penetrates the thin tissue on the lingual side of the mandible, halfway between the floor of the mouth and the gingival margin of the involved tooth. A few drops of anesthetic solution are carefully deposited beneath this delicate tissue (Fig. 6-7, *C*). (Injection into the *floor of the mouth* is contraindicated.)

Buccal Infiltration—A few drops of solution are injected into the mucobuccal fold, adjacent to the involved tooth.

Intraseptal Infiltration—This is a most important injection in the mandible, as in the maxilla (see above) (Fig. 6-7, *E*).

"Injection of Last Resort"

Direct Pulpal Injection—Used if sensation still exists at time of pulp exposure (explain problem to patient). Tooth is isolated, and any debris in area of exposure is removed. Needle tip penetrates the pulp tissue at the exposure site. A small volume (½ ml) of solution is injected into the pulp chamber quickly, with force. Momentary sensation. May be repeated as deeper pulp tissue is exposed (Fig. 6-7, *F*).

Chapter 6 ♦ Routine Endodontic Therapy 111

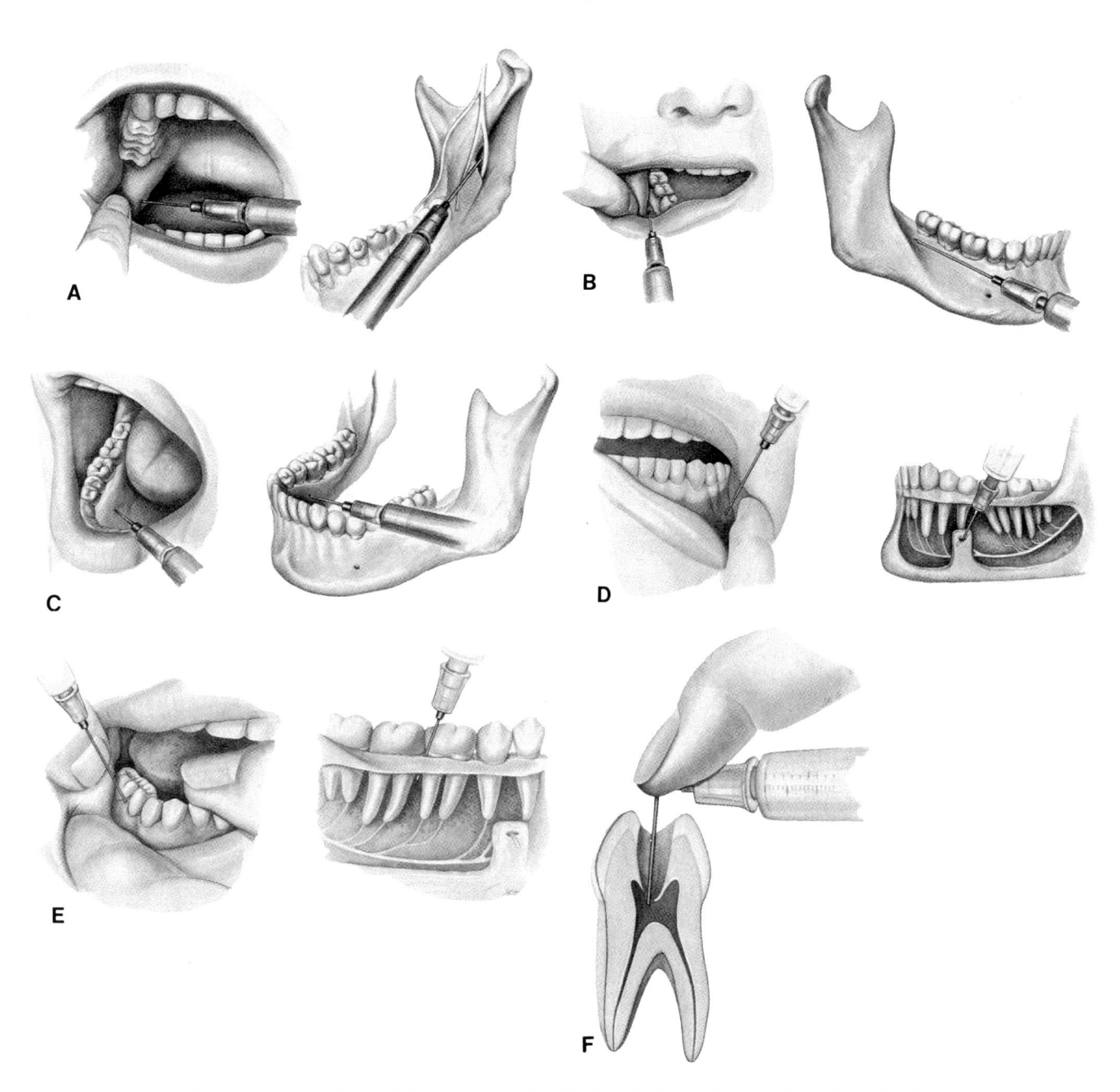

Figure 6-7 Mandibular injections. **A,** Mandibular block injection. **B,** Long buccal injection. **C,** Lingual injection. **D,** Mental injection. **E,** Intraseptal injection. **F,** Intrapulpal injection.

RUBBER DAM

Purpose: It prevents leakage and bacterial contamination and prevents the aspiration of instruments and materials. Facilities working in the canal by restricting tongue movements.

Technique: Place the dam on a winged clamp outside the mouth first and then seat the clamp and dam over the tooth as a unit. After placement, the dam is slipped over the wings of the clamp. The Visiframe can then be used to support the dam.

All the recommended clamps are "winged," allowing clamp placement while attached to the rubber dam. Single tooth isolation is all that is required.

Table 6-2 ♦ *Four Basic Clamps*

Clamp	Used for
Ivory No. 9 (Fig. 6-8)	Upper central Upper cuspid
S.S. White No. 211 (Fig. 6-9)	Lower anteriors Upper lateral
Ivory No. 2 (Fig. 6-10)	Bicuspids
Ivory No. 5 (Fig. 6-11)	Molars

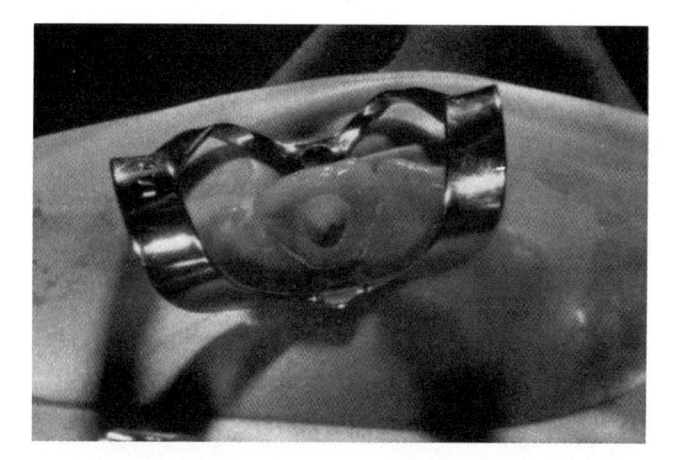

Figure 6-8 Ivory No. 9 clamp around maxillary central incisor. Notice access opening.

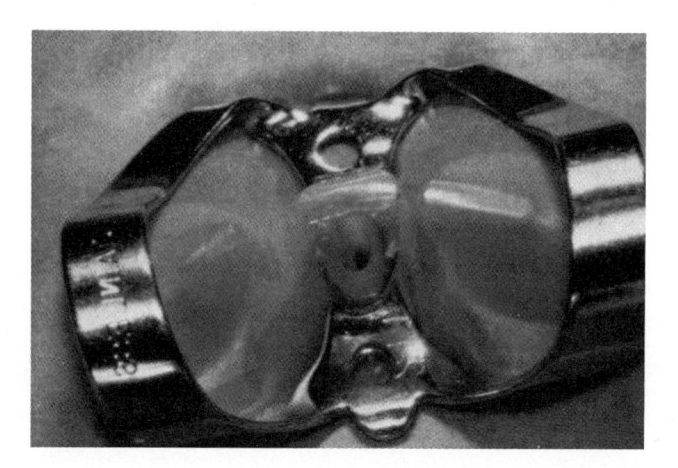

Figure 6-9 S.S. White No. 211 clamp around mandibular central incisor. Notice access opening.

Chapter 6 ♦ Routine Endodontic Therapy   113

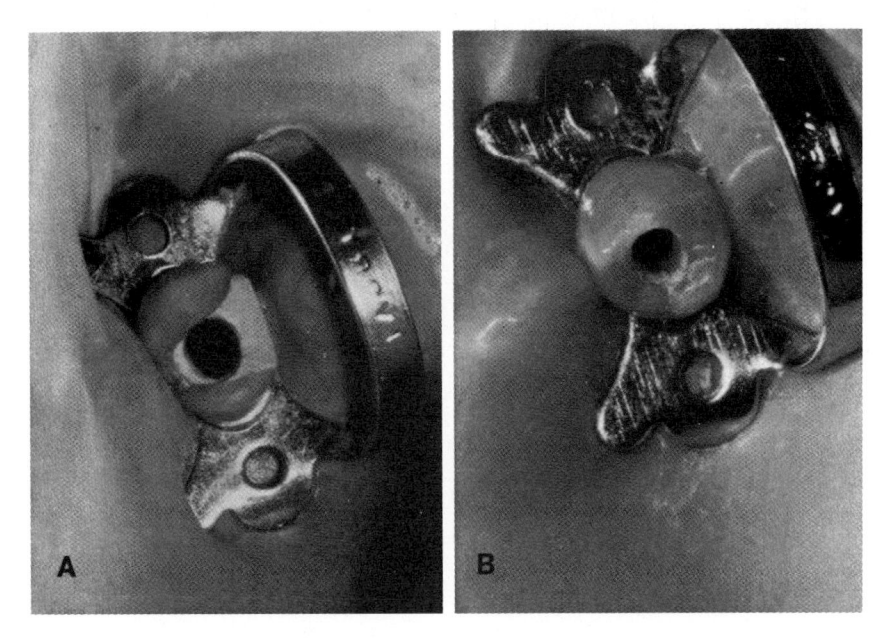

Figure 6-10 Ivory No. 2 clamp around bicuspid. **A,** Maxillary bicuspid. **B,** Mandibular bicuspid. Notice access opening.

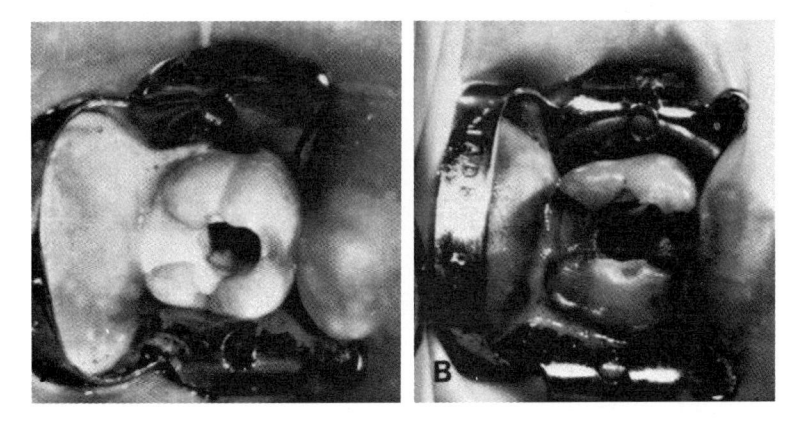

Figure 6-11 Ivory No. 5 clamp around molar. **A,** Mandibular molar. **B,** Maxillary molar. Notice access opening.

ACCESS OPENING

Purpose: Create a straight line pathway from the occlusal surface to the apical foramen with no interfering tooth structure between these two points.

Technique: Access preparation is started by a *penetration* with a high-speed No. 2 or No. 4 round bur. Refinement of the opening and complete removal of the pulp chamber roof is completed using the No. 4, No. 6, or No. 8 long shank, slow-speed, round bur. *Funnelling* of the opening is done with the bur moving outward from the pulp chamber, peeling away the dentinal and enamel triangles (Fig. 6-14). When tooth is out of alignment, access opening should be done before placing the rubber dam.

Four Principles of Correct Cavity Design (Fig. 6-13)

1. *Direct Line Access:* The access cavity must be designed so that instruments may be placed directly into the apical portion of the root canal without being deflected by coronal tissue.
2. *Removal of Debris:* The entire roof of the pulp chamber must be removed by cutting away all the overhanging dentin.
3. *Temporary Seal:* The walls of the access cavity must be flared to provide positive seat for the temporary dressing. If the cavity walls are made parallel or undercut, the temporary seal may become dislodged toward the pulp chamber, so breaking the seal and allowing contamination.
4. *Weakening of the Crown:* The size of the access cavity must not be made so large that the remaining crown of the tooth is unnecessarily weakened. The outline of the cavity is dictated by the shape of the pulp chamber and the direction of the root canals.

Orientation for Access

1. Initial entry should always be directed toward the area of greatest bulk or toward the larger canal.
2. In case of malpositioned teeth, access should be started without the use of a rubber dam until the chamber is located to maximize orientation.
3. Look for bony eminences indicating root position.
4. Study the long axes of adjacent crowns.
5. The outline form of the access opening conforms to the external outline of the crown.

Aids in Locating Canals

1. To locate canals that may not be obvious, look carefully at the floor of the pulp chamber. Dark lines may be seen that course between canal orifices on the pulpal floor. Once any canal is located, the remaining two canals can usually be approached by following these dark lines as they radiate from the located orifice. The presence of these dark lines may be obscured by amalgam staining, secondary and/or reparative dentin on the pulpal floor, caries, or various types of restorations.
2. Another aid in locating obscured canal orifices is to place a drop of iodine on the floor of the pulp chamber. Wait a few minutes and remove the excess iodine by flushing with alcohol. The organic material in the canal orifices will stain darker than the surrounding tooth structure.
3. Use of fiber optic on buccal or lingual surface, either directly or indirectly.

Text continued on p. 130.

Chapter 6 ♦ Routine Endodontic Therapy 115

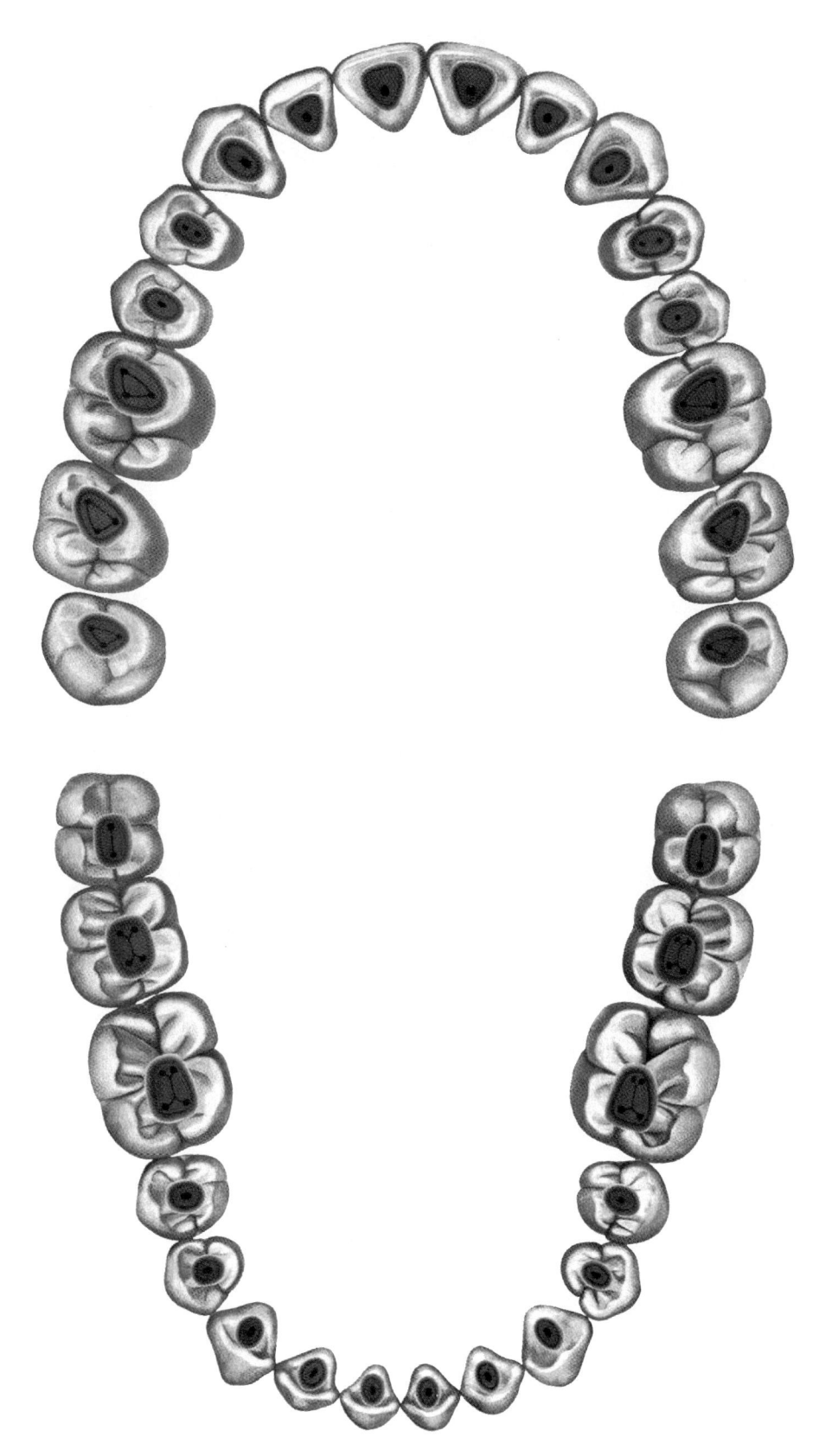

Figure 6-12 Access openings; maxillary and mandibular arch. The pulp chamber anatomy dictates the shape of the access opening.

PREACCESS DISTANCES

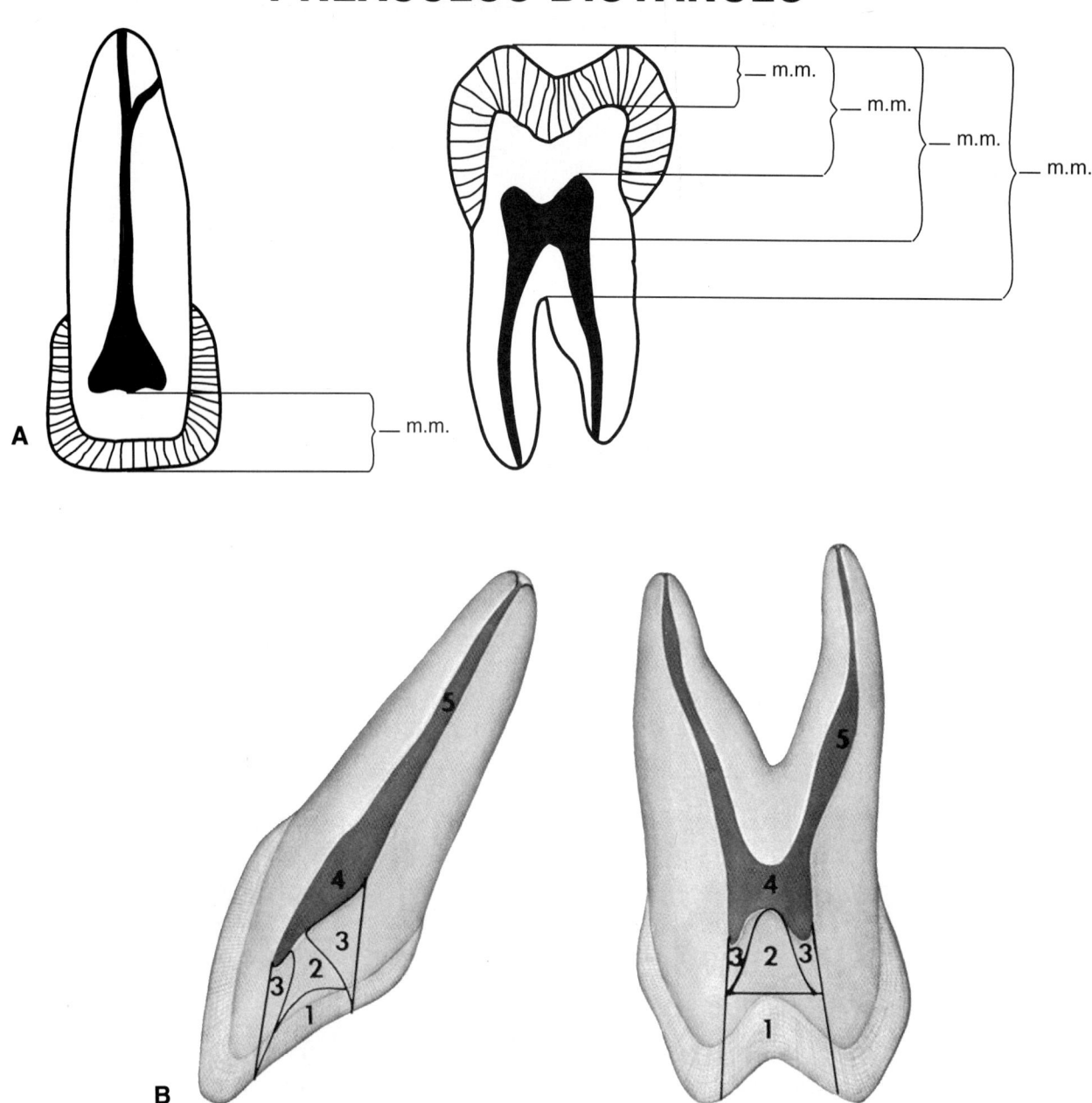

Figure 6-13 A, Pre-access distance. **B,** Basic steps in access openings. **Step 1: Outline form through enamel.** The outline form should be completed through the enamel into the dentin, similar to a class I cavity preparation. All caries, weak restorations, and weak tooth structure should be removed. The initial opening is accomplished using a No. 2 or No. 4 round, high-speed bur. **Step 2: Location and exposure of the pulp chamber.** The refinement of the preparation in the dentin is accomplished using the No. 4, 6, or 8 long-shank, round bur revolving at slow speed. The pulp chamber is being searched for, keeping the floor of the preparation concave. The actual pulp exposure is demonstrated using the endodontic explorer. **Step 3: Refinement of opening and complete removal of pulp chamber roof.** Refinement of the opening and complete removal of the pulp chamber roof is completed using the No. 4, 6, or 8 long-shank, slow-speed, round bur. All cutting is done with the bur moving out from the pulp chamber. **Step 4: Removal of pulp chamber contents.** Removal of the contents of the pulp chamber is completed using the No. 4, 6, or 8 long-shank, slow-speed, round bur, and/or an excavator. Actually a complete pulpotomy is being done before entering the root canal; however, in multirooted teeth, one should not revolve the round burs on the floor of the pulp chamber. **Step 5: Location of the root canal.** Location of the root canal orifice is demonstrated with the aid of the endodontic explorer. (From Serene TP: *Principles of pre-clinical endodontics*, Dubuque, Iowa, 1974, Kendall/Hunt.)

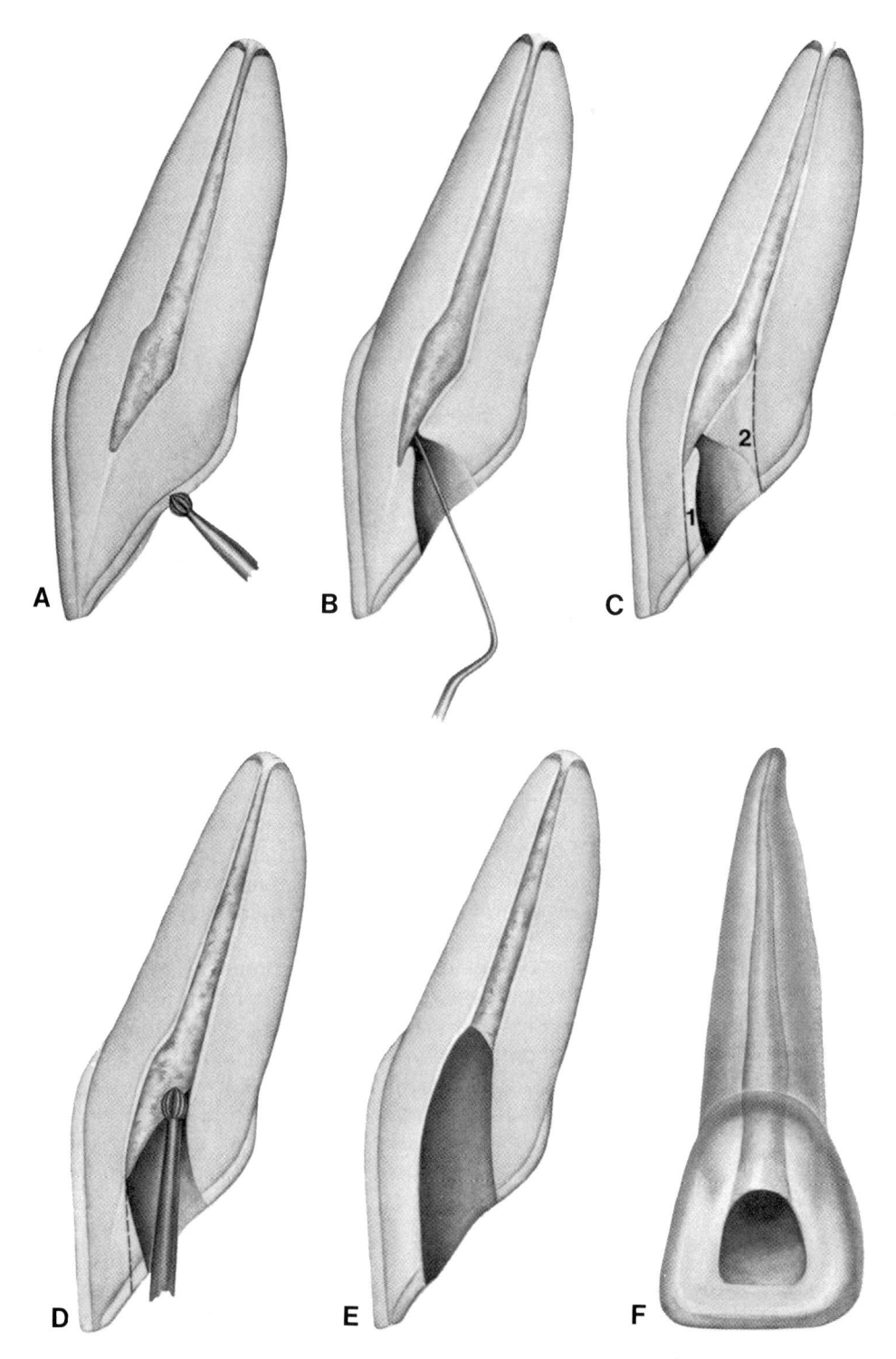

Figure 6-14 Access opening of maxillary anterior teeth. **A,** Initial opening is accomplished using a No. 2 or No. 4 round, high-speed bur. The bur is positioned at approximate right angles to the lingual surface just incisal to the cingulum. **B,** Demonstration of penetration into the pulp chamber with an explorer. **C,** Outline of funnelling that needs to be done. **D,** Removing triangles 1 and 2 by moving the bur outward from the pulp chamber. A No. 4, No. 6, or No. 8 long-shank, slow-speed, round bur is used. The bur is directed parallel to the long axis of the tooth. **E,** Access opening complete. Interproximal view. **F,** Lingual view. Notice the triangular funnel-shaped coronal preparation. Also note the beveled extension toward incisal and apical on occlusal opening.

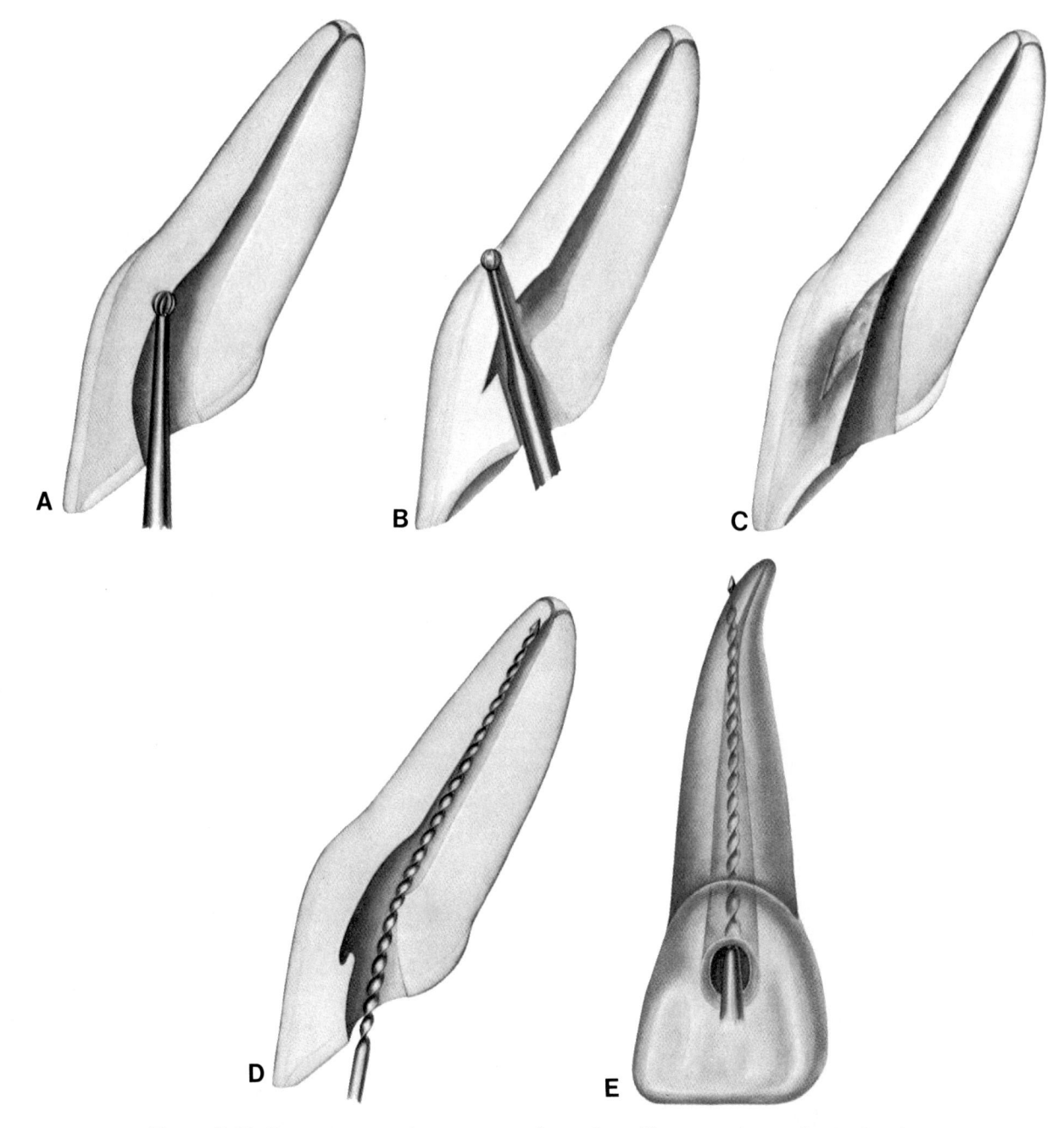

Figure 6-15 Common errors in access openings of maxillary anterior teeth. **A,** *Gouging.* **B,** *Perforation of crown. A* and *B* are caused by not directing the bur parallel to the long axis of the tooth after initial penetration. **C,** *Discoloration.* **D,** *Ledge with inadequate cleansing and shaping of canal.* **E,** *Perforation of root. C, D,* and *E* are caused by failure to remove triangles 1 and 2 (funnelling of access opening).

Chapter 6 ♦ Routine Endodontic Therapy 119

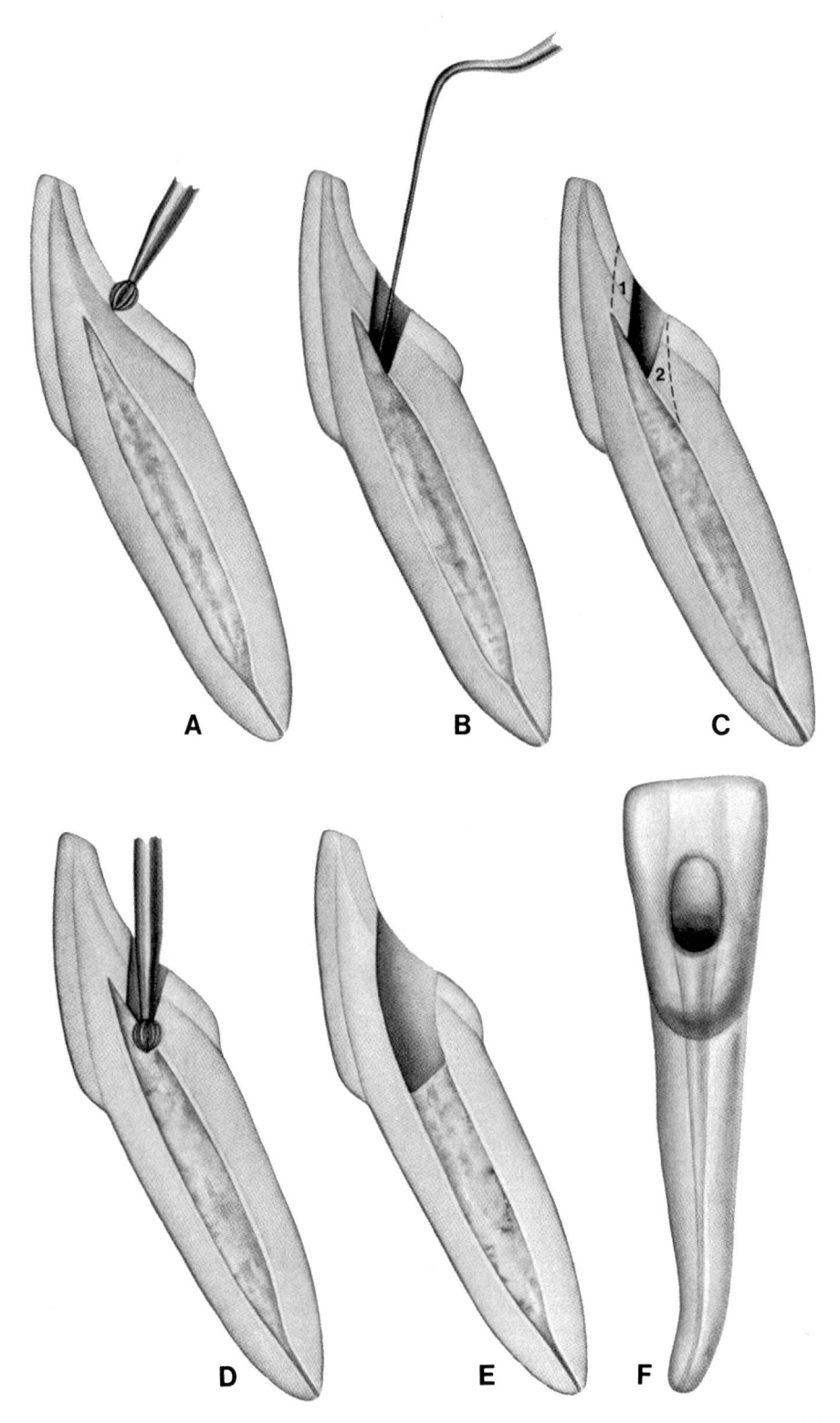

Figure 6-16 Access opening of mandibular anterior teeth. **A,** A No. 2 or No. 4 round bur at high speed is positioned just incisal to the cingulum. The bur is directed approximately at right angles to the lingual surface. **B,** After penetration into the pulp chamber, the opening is confirmed with an endodontic explorer. **C,** Outline form of funnelling that needs to be done. **D,** Removing triangles 1 and 2 by moving the bur outward from the pulp chamber. A No. 4 long-shank, slow-speed, round bur is used. The bur is directed parallel to the long axis of the tooth. **E,** Access opening completed. Interproximal view. **F,** Lingual view.

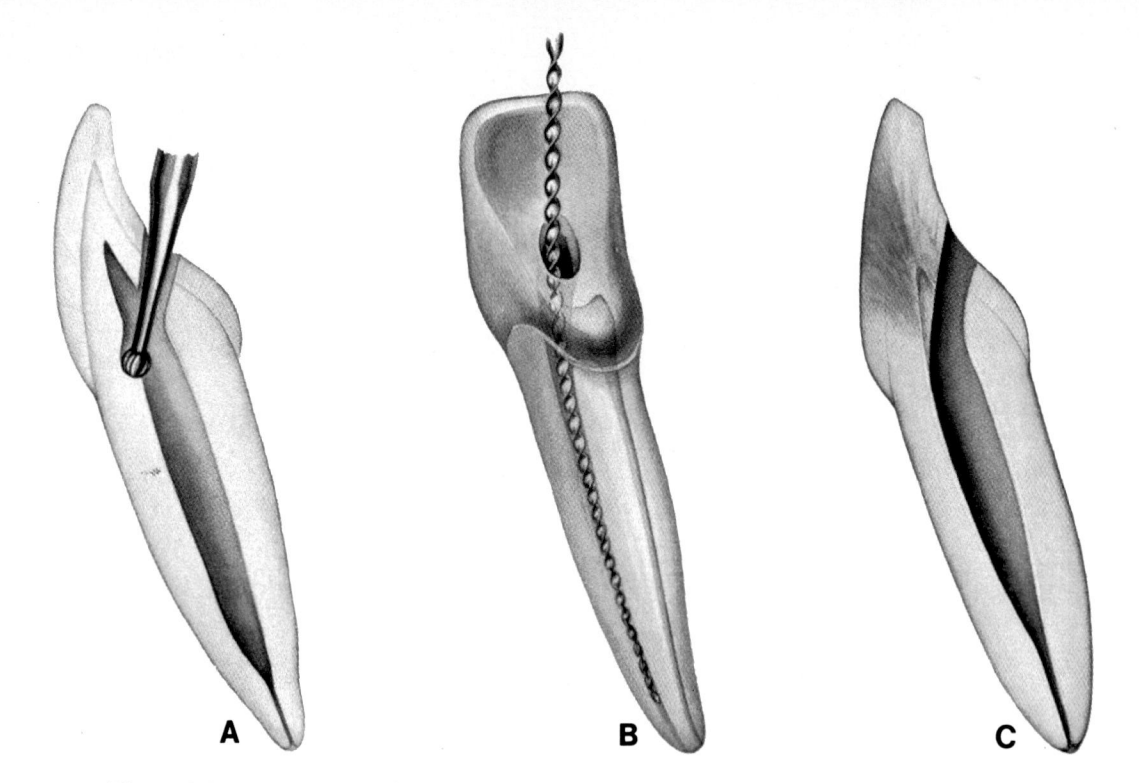

Figure 6-17 Common errors in access openings of mandibular anterior teeth. **A**, *Gouging*-caused by not directing the bur parallel to the long axis of the tooth after initial penetration. **B**, *Missing lingual canal.* **C**, *Discoloration.* B and C are caused by failure to remove triangles 1 and 2 (funnelling of access openings).

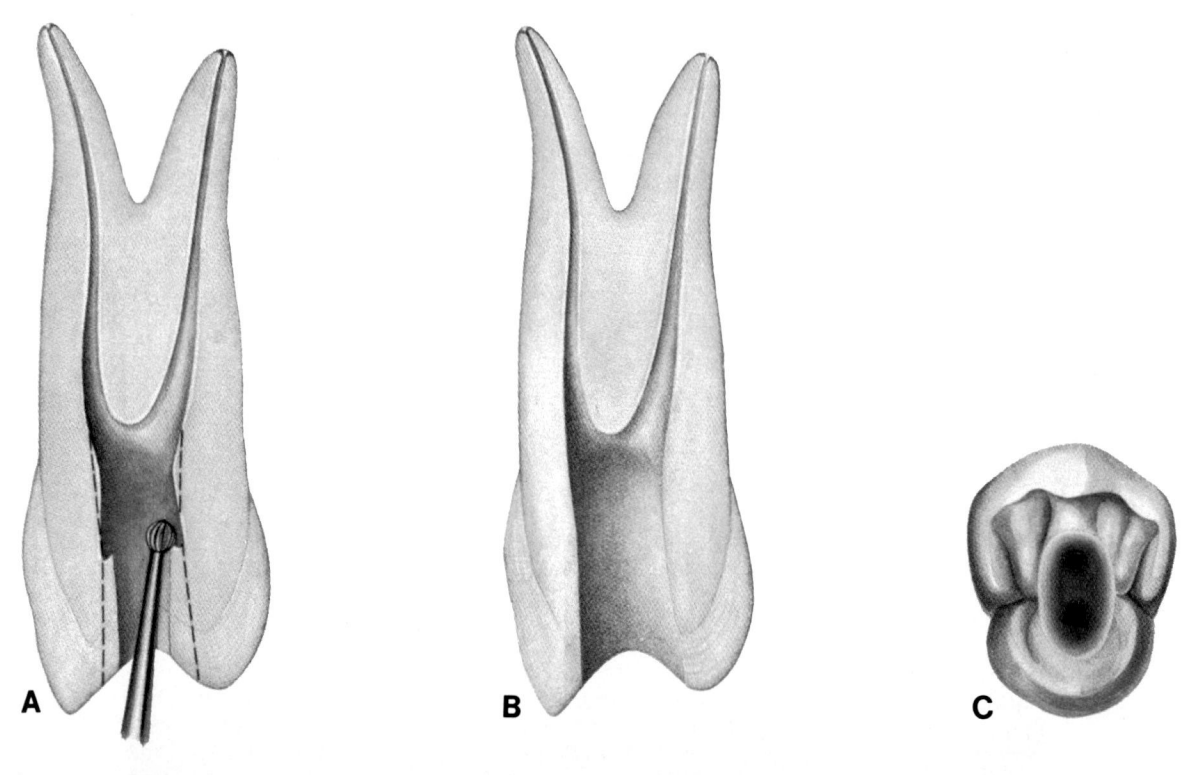

Figure 6-18 Access opening of maxillary bicuspids. Initial penetration is made with a No. 4 high-speed, round bur in the middle of the central groove. The bur is directed at right angles to the occlusal surface of the crown. **A**, Funnelling is done with a No. 4 long-shank, low-speed, round bur. The roof of the pulp chamber is removed by moving the bur in an outward stroking motion. **B**, Access opening complete. Interproximal view. **C**, Occlusal view.

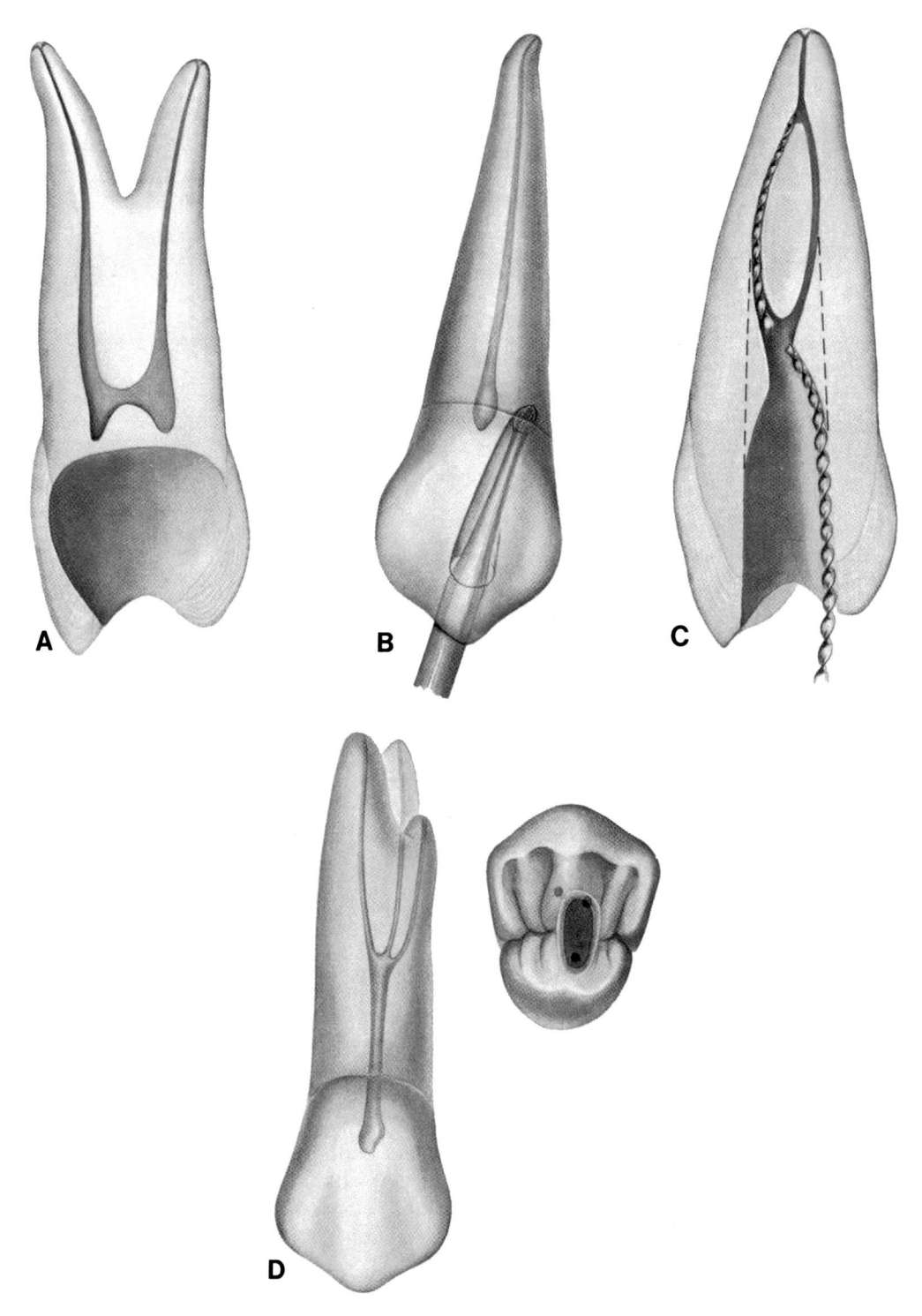

Figure 6-19 Common errors in access openings of maxillary bicuspids. **A,** *Gouging.* **B,** *Perforation.* A and B are caused by not directing the bur parallel to the long axis of the tooth. **C,** *Broken instrument*-caused by failure to remove the dentinal triangles before placing instruments in the canals. **D,** *Missing extra canal*-caused by failure to funnel access opening and not following the outline of the pulp chamber.

122 PRACTICAL ENDODONTICS

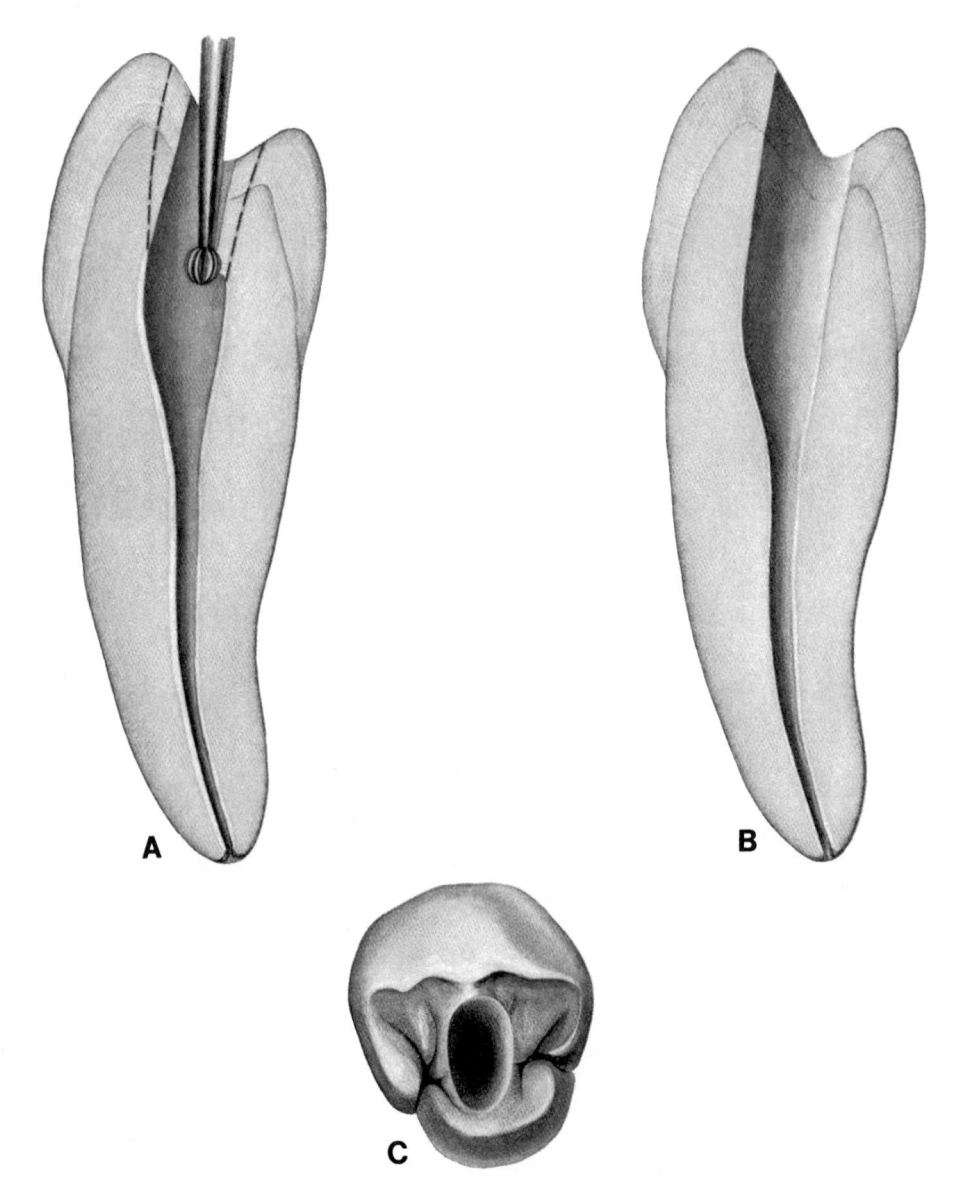

Figure 6-20 Access opening of mandibular bicuspids. Initial penetration is made with a No. 4 high-speed, round bur in the central groove slightly toward the buccal cusp. The bur is directed at right angles to the occlusal surface of the crown. **A,** Funnelling with a No. 4 long-shank, slow-speed, round bur. The roof of the pulp chamber is removed by moving the bur in an outward stroking motion. **B,** Access opening complete. Interproximal view. **C,** Occlusal view.

Chapter 6 ♦ Routine Endodontic Therapy   123

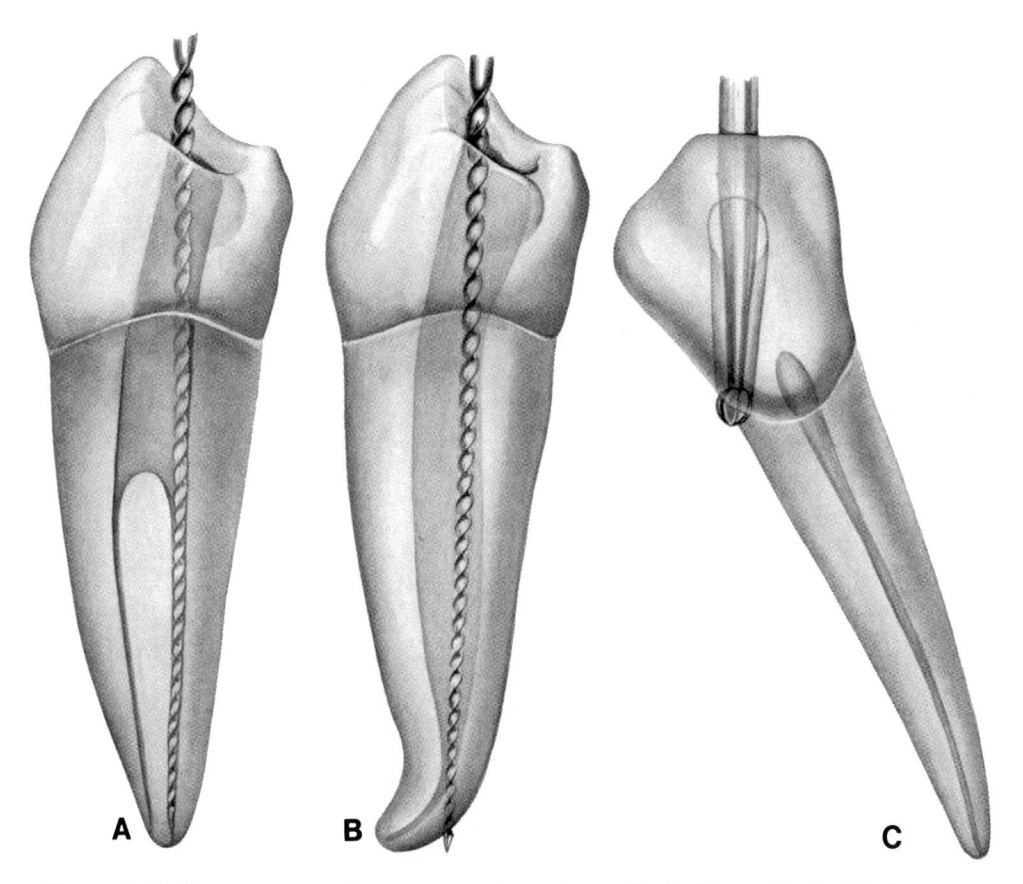

Figure 6-21 Common errors in access openings of mandibular bicuspids. **A,** *Missing extra canal.* **B,** *Perforation of root.* A and B are caused by inadequate funnelling of access opening. **C,** *Perforation of crown-*caused by not directing the bur parallel to the long axis of the tooth.

124 PRACTICAL ENDODONTICS

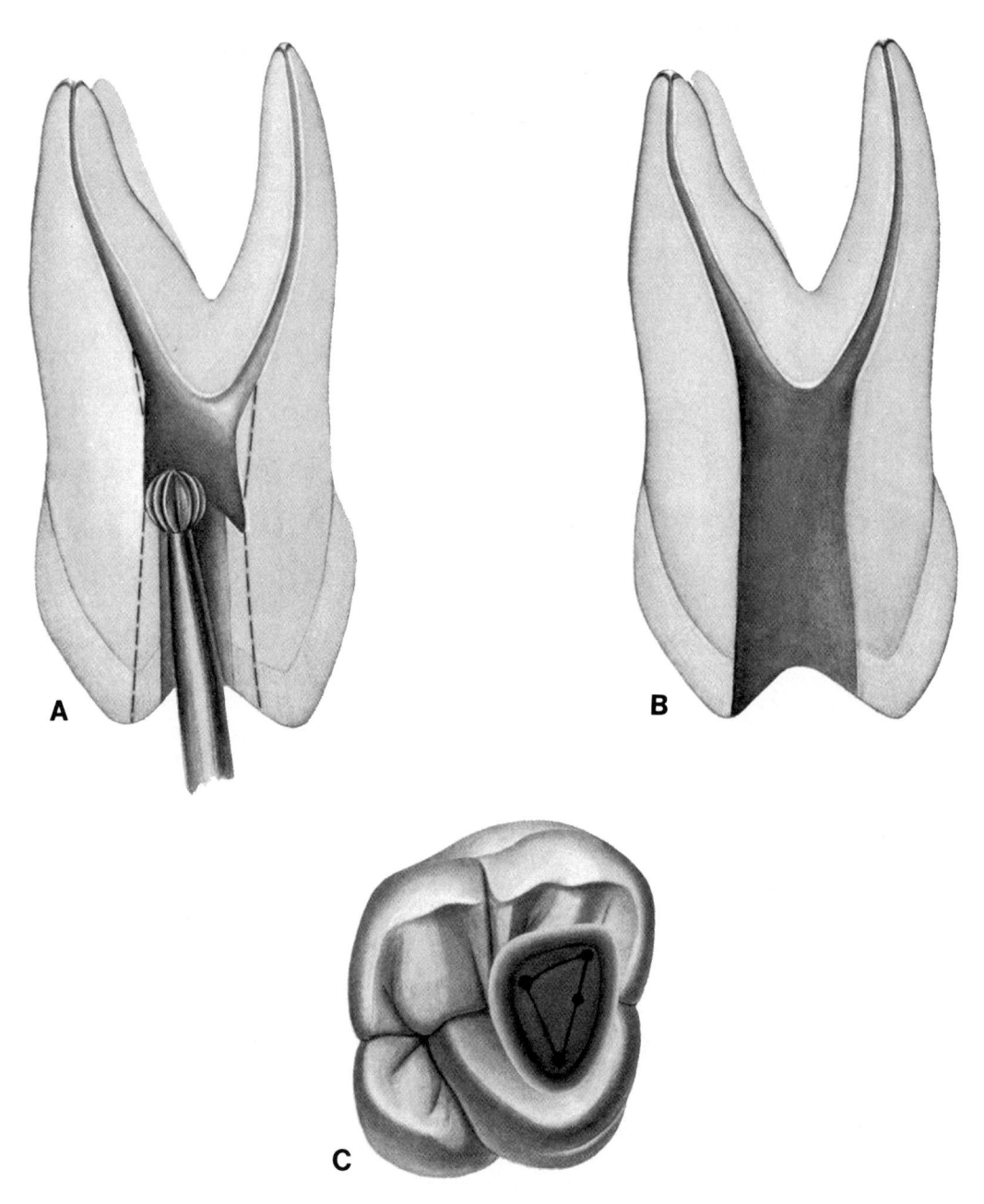

Figure 6-22 Access opening of maxillary molars. Initial penetration is done with a No. 4 or No. 6 high-speed, round bur in the central fossa. The bur is directed at right angles to the occlusal surface of the crown. When penetrating the roof of the chamber, the bur is directed to the palatal canal. **A,** Funnelling with a No. 6 long-shank, slow-speed, round bur. The roof of the pulp chamber is removed by moving the bur in an outward stroking motion. **B,** Access opening complete. Interproximal view. **C,** Occlusal view. Notice that the access opening is entirely within the mesial half of the tooth and forms a triangle. The base of the triangle is toward the buccal and the apex is to the lingual, with a canal orifice positioned at each angle of the triangle.

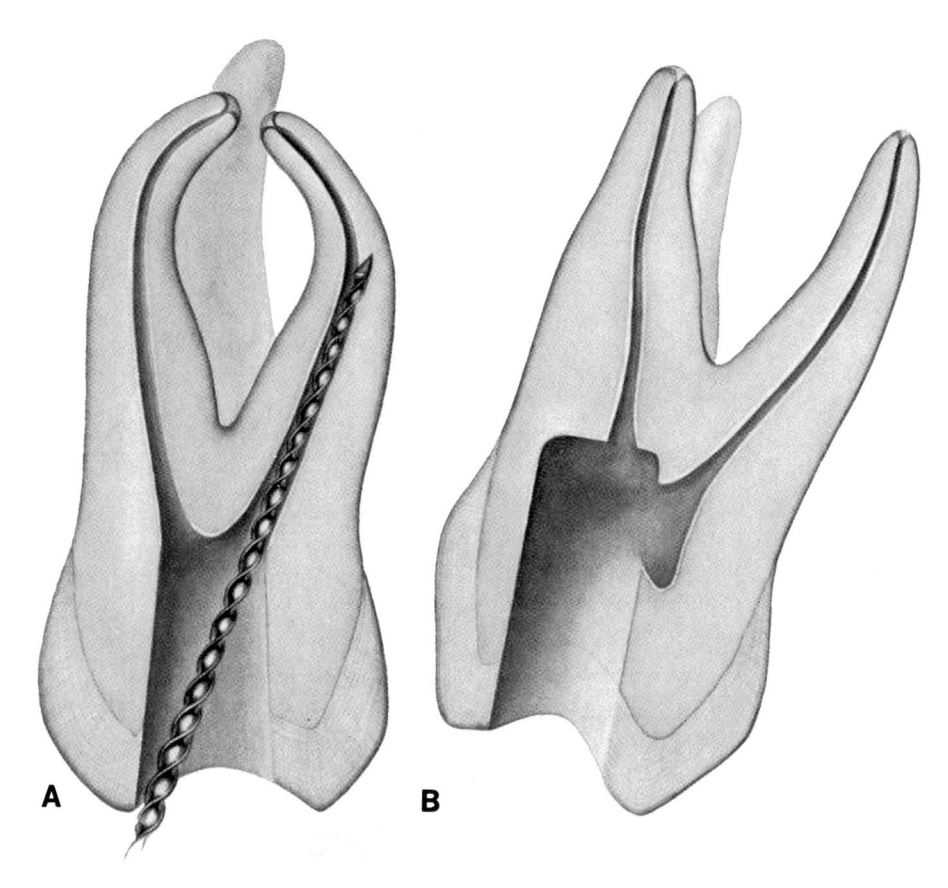

Figure 6-23 Common errors in access openings of maxillary molars. **A,** Ledging-caused by failure to remove dentinal triangle. Another cause is using a large straight instrument in a curved canal. **B,** Gouging. Failure to direct the bur parallel with the long axis of the tooth upon penetration.

126 PRACTICAL ENDODONTICS

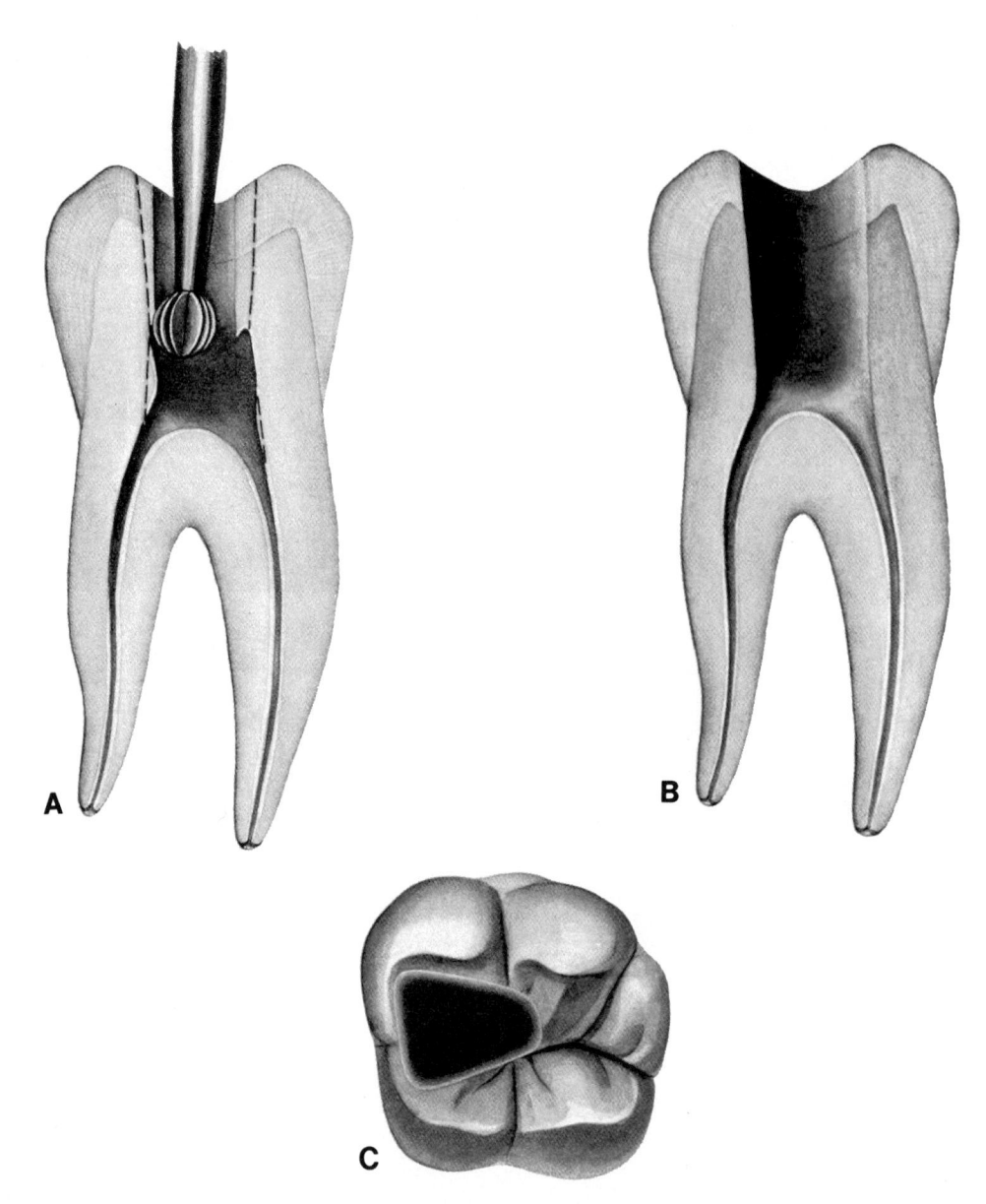

Figure 6-24 Access opening of mandibular molars. Penetration is done with a No. 4 or No. 6 high-speed, round bur in the central fossa. The bur is directed at right angles to the occlusal surface of the crown. When penetrating the roof of the chamber, the bur is directed to the distal canal. **A,** Funnelling with a No. 6 long-shank, slow-speed, round bur. The roof of the pulp chamber is removed by moving the bur in an outward stroking motion. **B,** Access opening complete. Interproximal view. **C,** Occlusal view. Notice that the access opening is entirely within the mesial two-thirds portion of the crown. Buccolingually, it is slightly buccal in relation to the occlusal table.

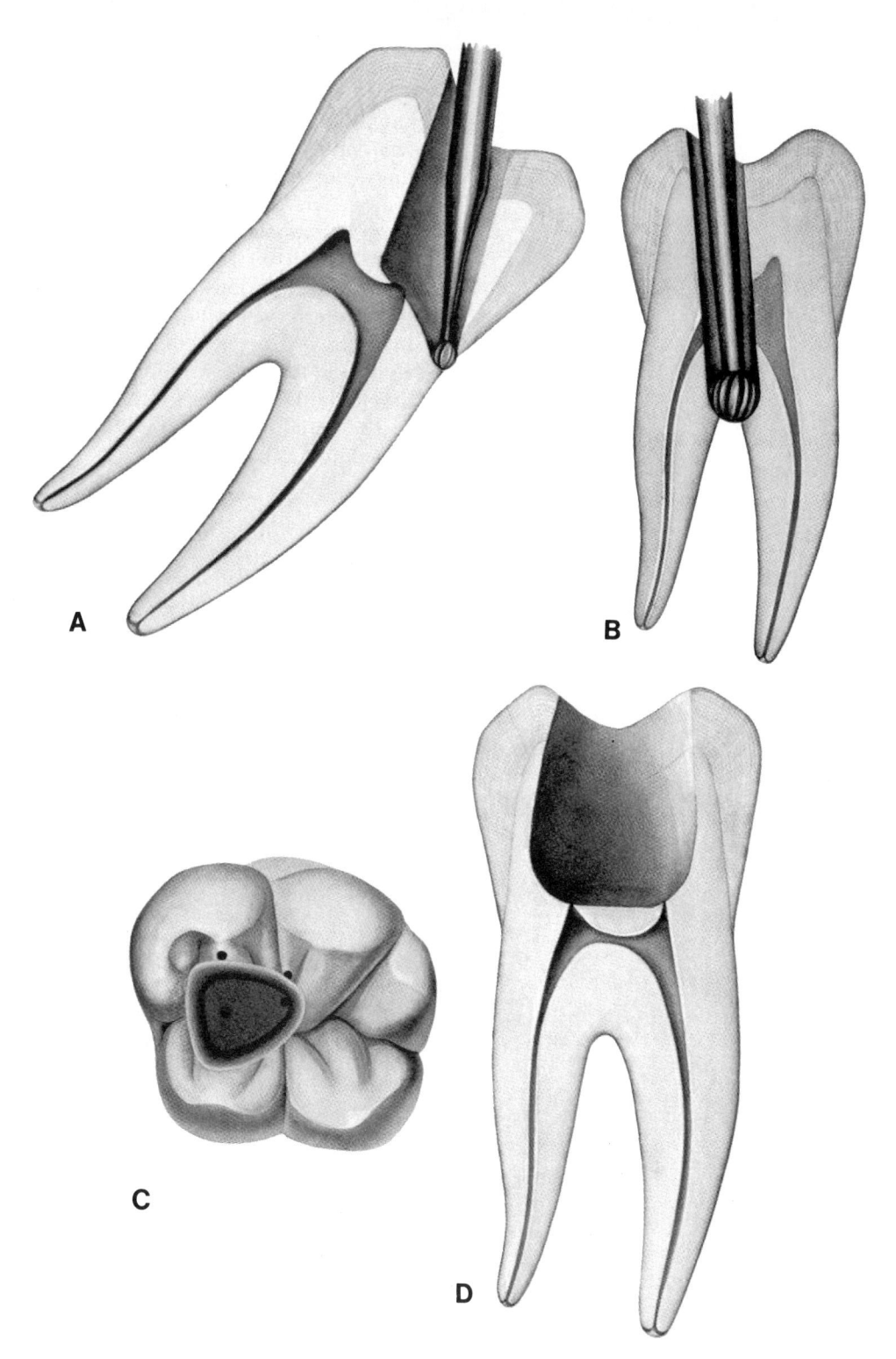

Figure 6-25 Common errors in access openings of mandibular molars. **A,** *Perforation of crown*-caused by failure to direct the bur parallel with the long axis of the tooth. **B,** *Perforation in furcation*-caused by using a long-shank bur at high speed and not realizing the depth of the pulp chamber. The depth of most pulp chambers is approximately 6 mm. **C,** *Faulty cavity preparation*-caused by not following the proper anatomy of the occlusal table. The mesial buccal orifice is present beneath the mesial buccal cusp. The fourth canal is usually located buccally to the distal canal and under the distal buccal cusp tip. **D,** *Gouging and leaving roof of pulp chamber*-caused by not directing bur at right angles to the occlusal table and not penetrating completely. If the opening appears shallow with openings to the canal separated by light-colored dentin, one should suspect that the opening is incomplete. The floor of the pulp chamber in a multirooted tooth is somewhat darker and may have grooves connecting the canal orifices.

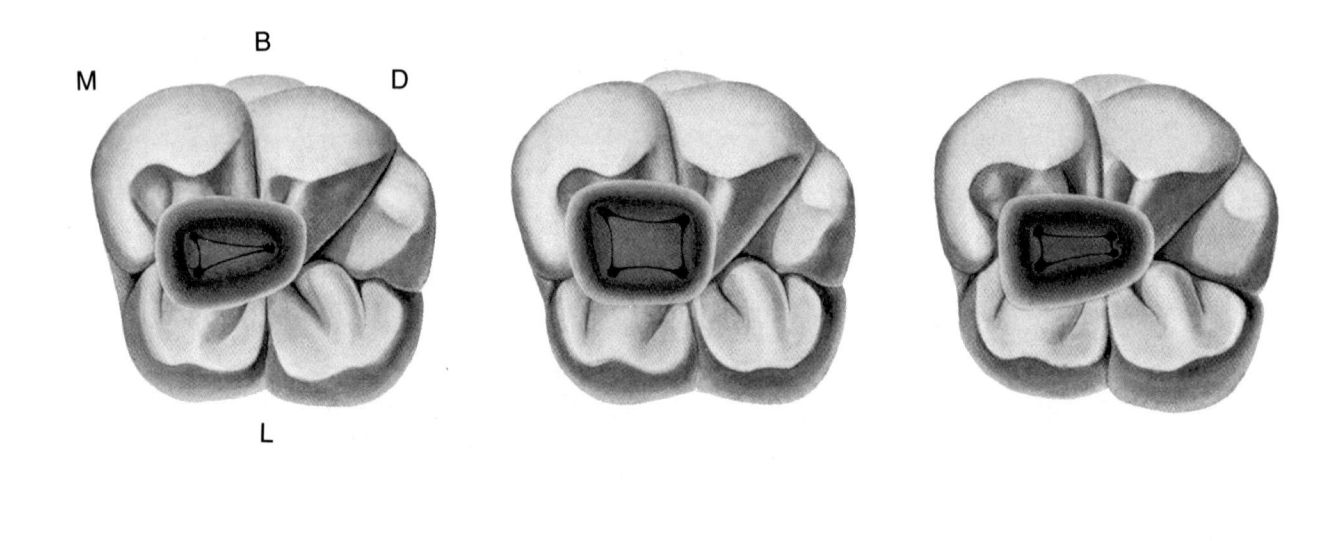

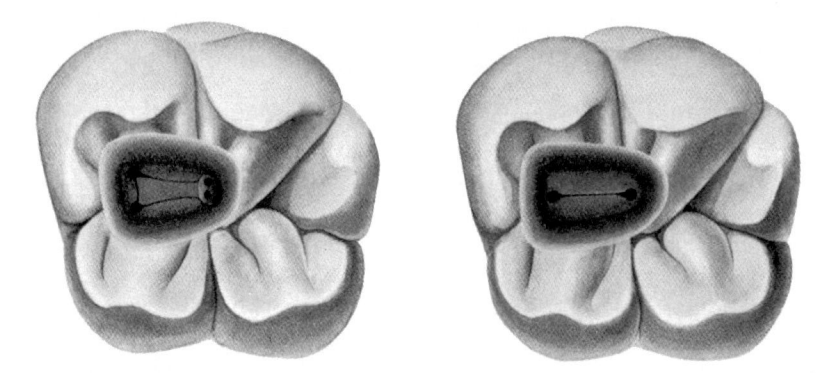

Figure 6-26 Variation of orifices in mandibular molars.

Chapter 6 ♦ Routine Endodontic Therapy   129

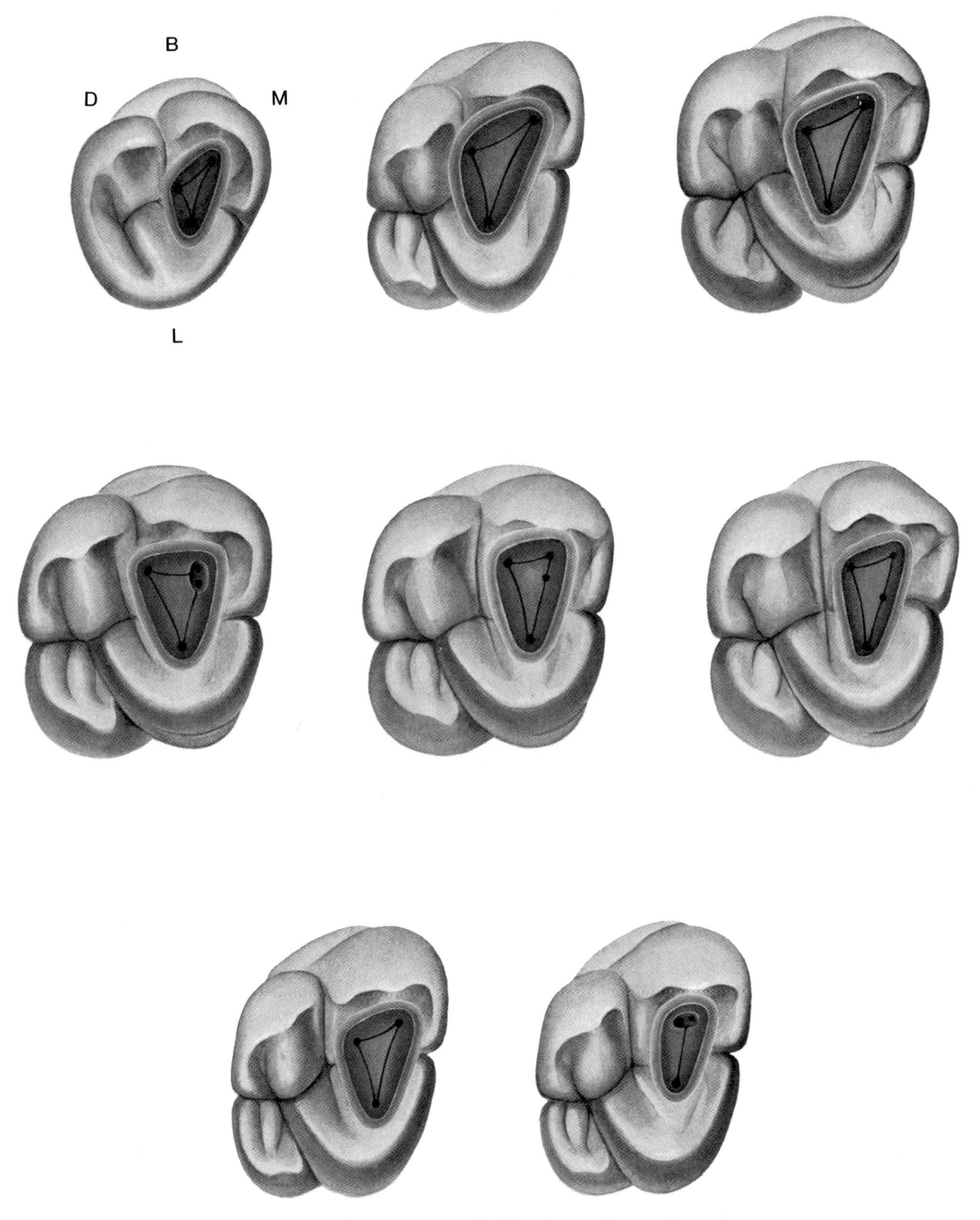

Figure 6-27 Variation of orifices in maxillary molars.

LENGTH DETERMINATION

The tooth length is the distance from the incisal or cusp tip to the apex. The working length is the distance from the incisal or cusp tip to the apical foramen. The difference between the anatomical tooth length and the working length is usually 0.5 mm. The difference between the tooth length and the working length radiographically is 1 mm. Use buccal cusp as a guide on posterior teeth and the incisal edge on anterior teeth.

Apex locators can be a useful aid for tooth length determination. At the present time, the electrical apex locator is a good aid when used with radiographs. Radiography, however, is necessary to visualize the curvature and anatomical complexities within the root.

Purpose: To determine the working length of the canal so that upon cleansing and shaping the canal all instruments will be confined to the canal.

Technique: The working length is established by measuring with a millimeter ruler the preoperative radiograph. A No. 10 file is inserted this distance, and then a No. 15 file is inserted the same length. A confirming radiograph is then taken (Figs. 6-28 and 6-30).

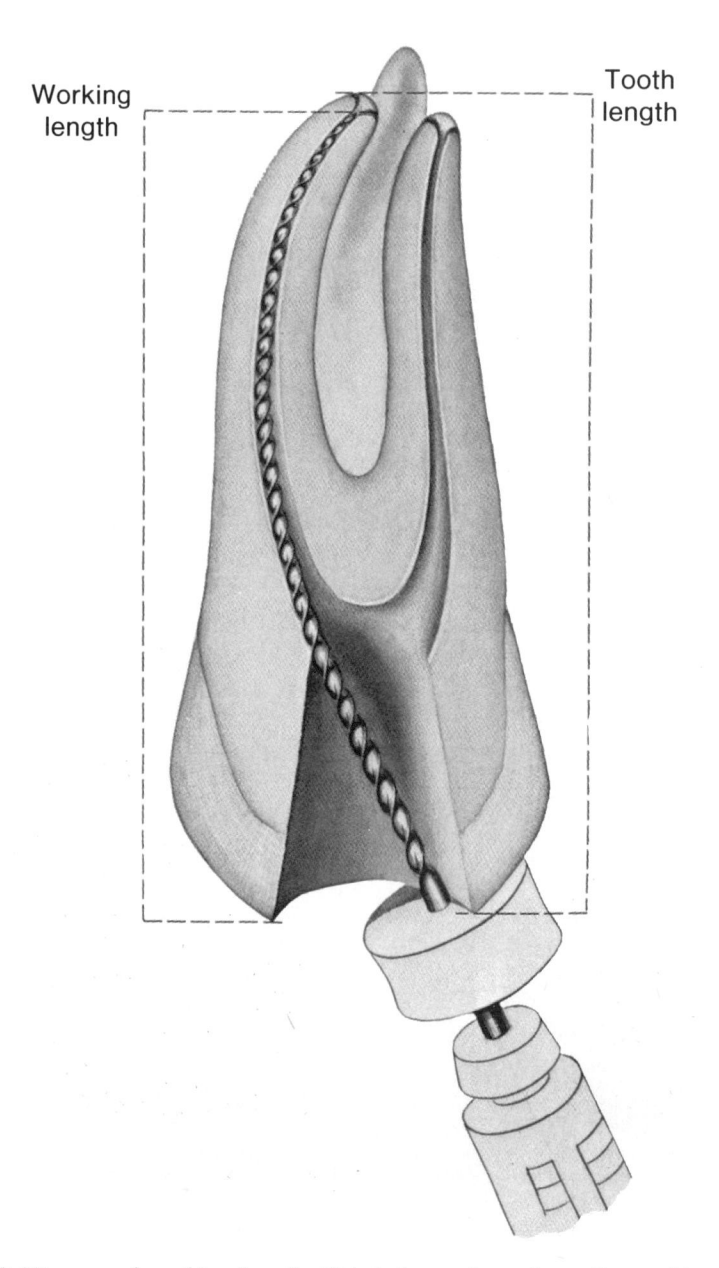

Figure 6-28 Diagram of working length. This is 1 mm from the radiographic apex.

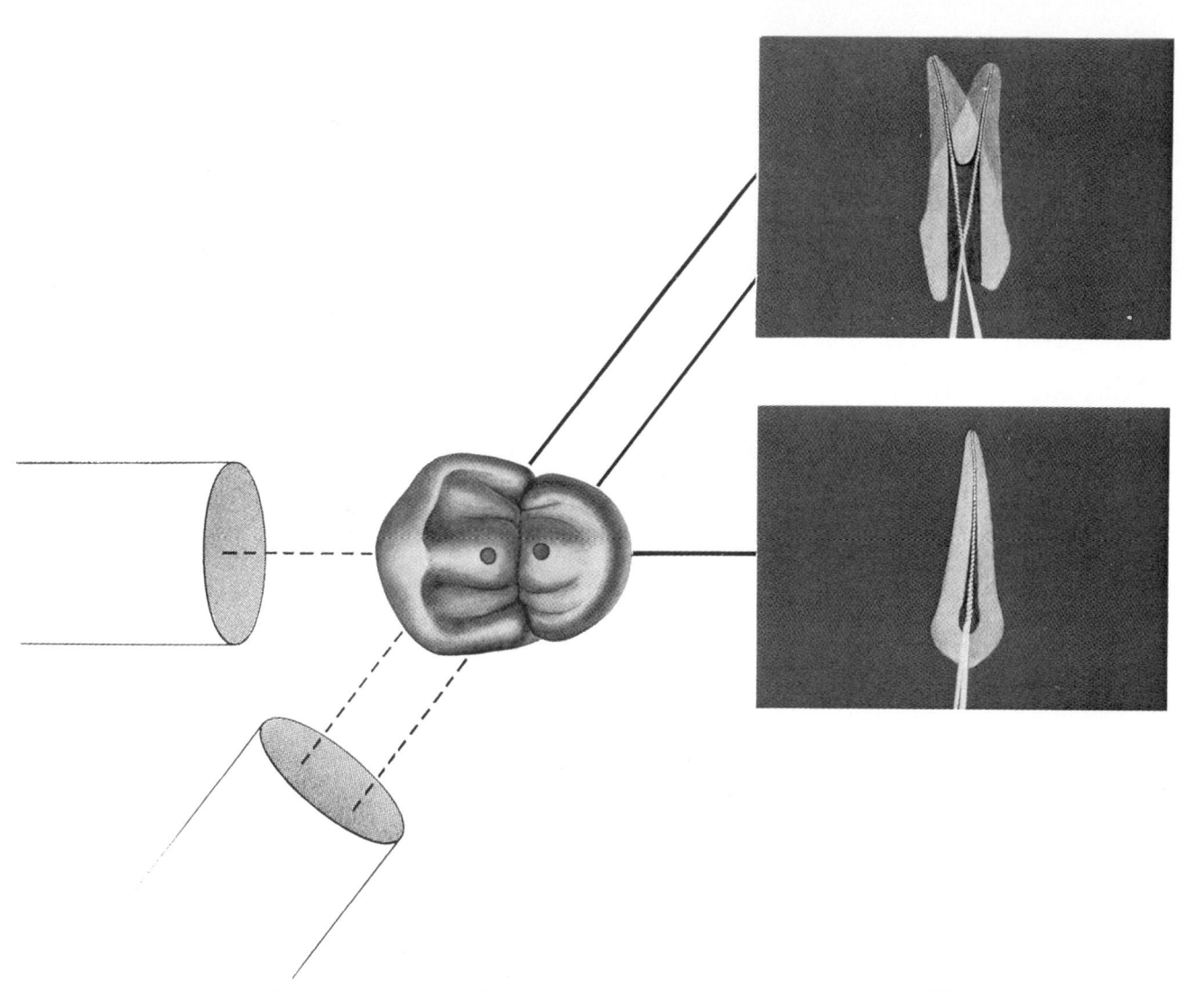

Figure 6-29 *Buccal object rule:* When multicanals are present it often becomes difficult to distinguish the canals on the radiograph. When the x-ray tube is moved to give an angled exposure, the root separates on the film. When the x-ray tube is pointing toward the distal, the canal farther from the film moves in the direction that is directed. Thus, the buccal canal appears distal to the palatal canal.

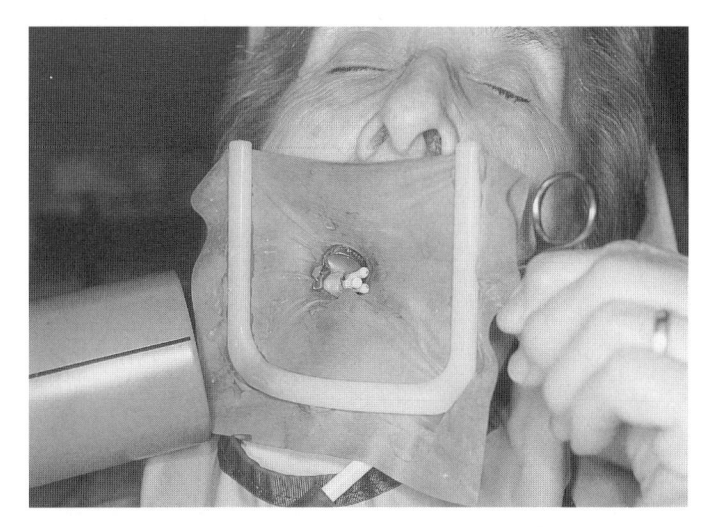

Figure 6-30 Picture of radiograph to be taken of instruments within canals.

132 PRACTICAL ENDODONTICS

PRINCIPLES OF ROOT CANAL PREPARATION (Fig. 6-31)

I. Convenience Form

The convenience form is a straight-line access from the incisal or occlusal surface to the apex. The objective is to prevent overmanipulation or elipticizing of the apical area.

II. Resistance Form

The objective of the resistance form is to preserve the integrity of the natural apical constriction. This helps to prevent overextension of the filling material following condensation.

III. Retention Form

The objective of the retention form is to provide about 2 mm of near parallel walls at the apical end of the root canal preparation to provide tugback or retention of the trial or master cone. The root canal must be tapered from the apical collar to the access cavity to ensure that the retention comes from the apical end.

IV. Extension

The working length of the tooth is usually 1 mm short of the radiographic apex unless it can be demonstrated otherwise. Proper extension of the preparation facilitates complete debridement of the root canals and must be reconfirmed with radiographs. Because all canals are curved to some degree and are straightened proportionately during instrumentation, all canals have the potential of getting shorter as they are filed.

V. Toilet of Cavity

Irrigation and lubrication with sodium hypochlorite solution should be performed before, during, and after the use of each file. The toilet of the cavity is complete when all internal surfaces of the root canal have been completely cleansed and the walls of the canal preparation are smoothed.

RULES FOR CLEANSING AND SHAPING

1. Do not cleanse and shape the root canal until the exact working length has been established.

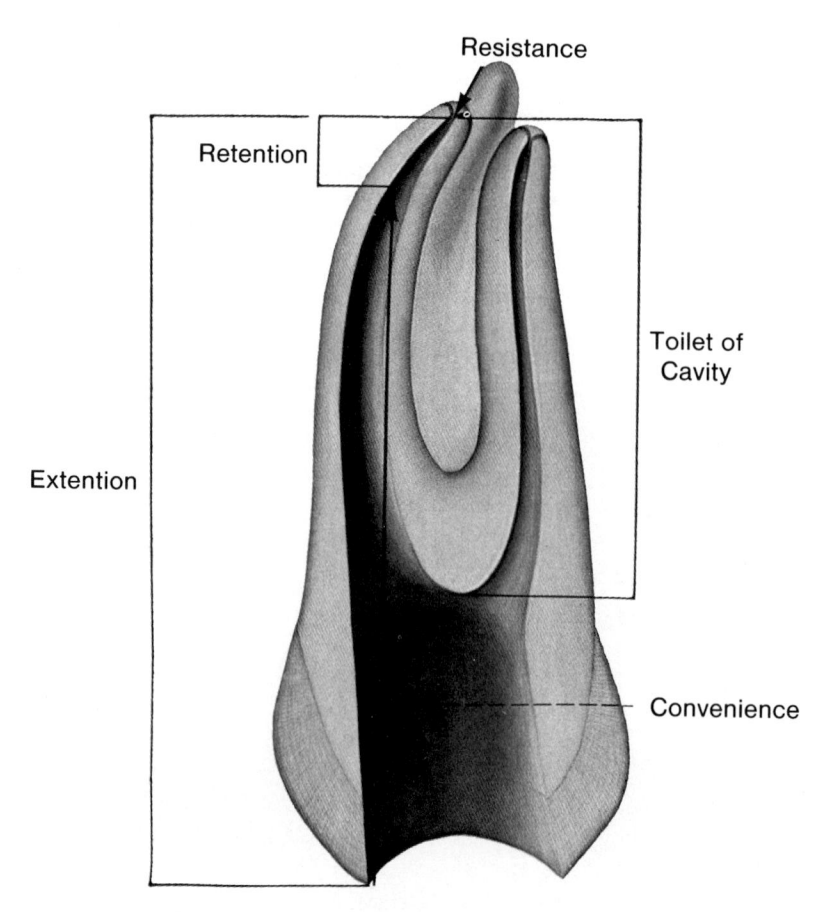

Figure 6-31 Final shaping of root canal preparation. (From Serene TP: *Principles of preclinical endodontics,* Dubuque, Iowa, 1974, Kendall/Hunt.)

2. Place a bend on each instrument before inserting into the root canal.
3. Irrigate before and after the use of each instrument.
4. Instruments should be used in sequence while advancing to a larger diameter.
5. Instruments should be cleaned before reentering the canal.
6. Never force an instrument if it binds.
7. Maintain a patent apical constriction by following each file size, always returning to the original working length with the No. 15 file or the file that first meets resistance.
8. Examine each instrument before placing it into the canal.

CLEANSING AND SHAPING

Purpose: The purpose of the cleansing and shaping procedure is to prepare the canal with a smooth, continuously tapering, funnel-shaped preparation for a three-dimensional filling. This phase of the technique is the key to success in endodontic therapy.

Technique: Root canal debridement is performed in three steps (Fig. 6-32):
1. Initial preparation and establishment of patency in the apical third
2. Preparation of the body of the canal
3. Final shaping of the canal

After the proper access opening and the working length measurement have been established, the cleansing and shaping of the canal can be initiated.

Technique:
1. Gross pulpal tissue should first be removed with a barbed broach. The barbed broach should only be used in the larger canals such as maxillary anterior teeth and in the palatal and distal canals of molars.
2. All files and reamers should be prepared with rubber stops to confine instruments within the root canal. Set stops on instruments to the recorded length. Place a small bend at the apical half of the instrument before inserting into canal.
3. Flood the chamber with a 2.5% solution of sodium hypochlorite. This is performed before, during, and after the use of each file. A 3% solution of hydrogen peroxide is alternated with the sodium hypochlorite. RC Prep can be used in place of the hydrogen peroxide in the narrow canals to aid in the cleansing and lubricating of the canal.
4. Serial filing is now started. This is a procedure of returning to the original working length of the tooth with the No. 15 file or the file that first meets resistance. This must be done continuously throughout the process of serial filing to maintain a patent canal and a smooth transition from one instrument to the next.

The first file used should just barely engage the canal walls when it is carried to the working length. The apex of the canal is filed with the size that first meets resistance and then shaped usually at least two or three sizes larger. The No. 10 or No. 15 file is usually used to initiate the apical preparation. Then the No. 20 and No. 25 file sizes are used in sequence, placing each one to the working length and withdrawing with a pull stroke. The apical preparation should be prepared to at least size No. 25 file in small canals, and larger in anterior teeth, distal canals of mandibular molars, and palatal canals of maxillary molars. The preparation of the body of the canal is performed with reamers or files. The larger instruments are kept away from the apical preparation, but after each larger size instrument the No. 15 file is used to renegotiate the working length. The final shaping of the canal is completed when the canal is shaped to a gradual taper, widest at the occlusal, and the canals have been sufficiently cleansed.

5. After the canal has been cleansed and shaped, irrigate again with sodium hypochlorite and dry the canal with sterile absorbent points.

INTRACANAL MEDICATION

Purpose: Medications are used as an adjunct to meticulous cleansing and shaping of the root canal system. Their sole purpose is to maintain asepsis within the canal between treatments.

Technique: A pellet of cotton is moistened with the medicament, dried in a 2 × 2 gauze sponge, and placed in the chamber. A dry cotton pellet is placed over this, and a temporary filling is sealed into place (Fig. 6-33). When calcium hydroxide is used, it is injected into the pulp chamber and carried into the canal with an absorbent point measured to the canal length (Fig. 6-34).

Any antimicrobial agent that is noninjurious to the patient can be used to maintain asepsis in a properly cleaned canal. The most widely used agents are eugenol, Cresatin, camphorated parachlorophenol, and calcium hydroxide.

Appointments should be no less than 2 days and no more than 2 weeks apart. This time interval permits periapical inflammation to subside, yet is not so long that antibacterial agents will be diluted to ineffectiveness or cavity-sealing agents will begin to leak.

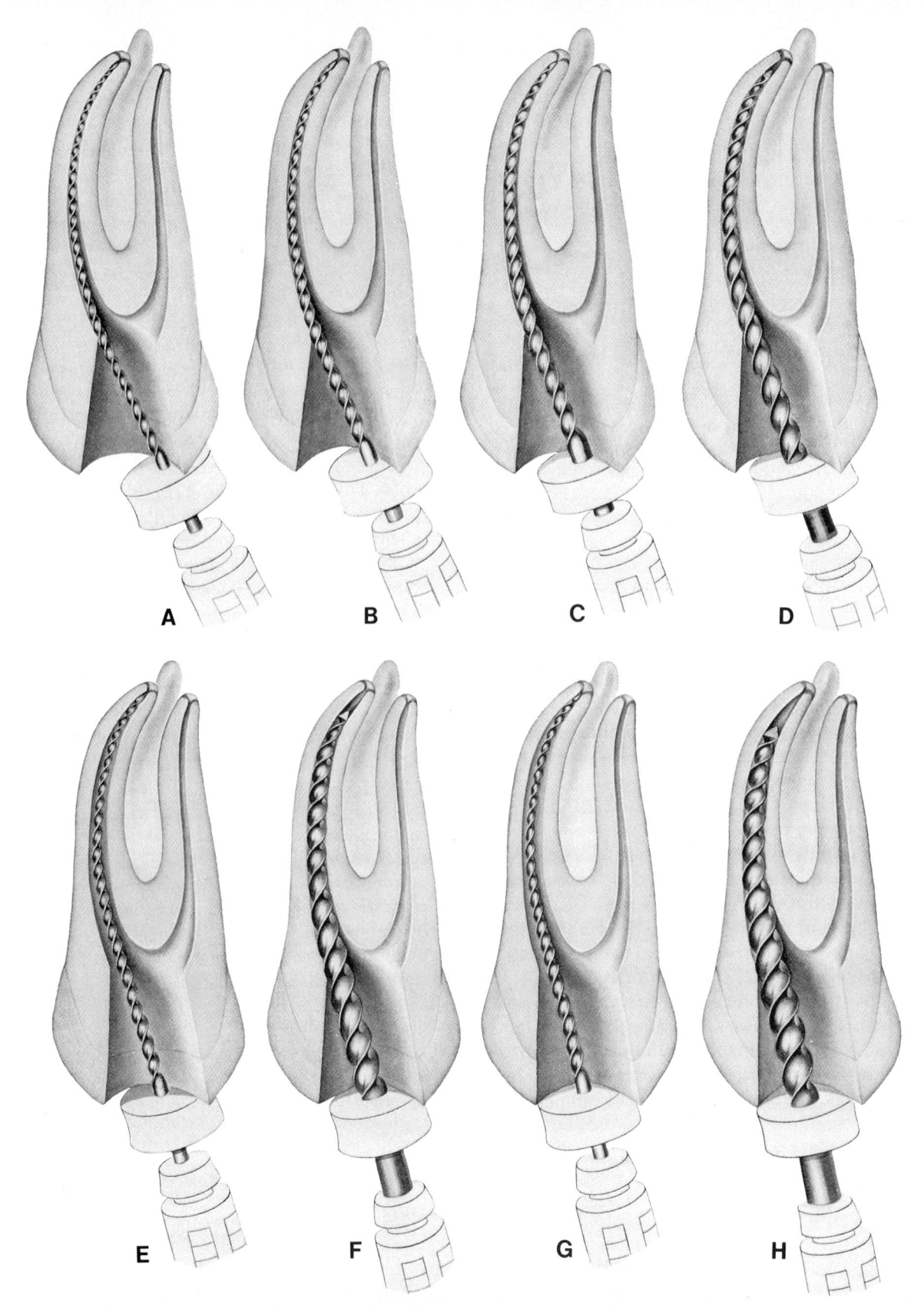

Figure 6-32 Cleaning and shaping the root canal. **A,** No. 15 file to the established working length. **B,** No. 20 file to the established working length. **C,** No. 25 file to established working length. *A, B,* and *C* demonstrate the apical preparation. A small Gates Glidden drill is now used in the coronal third of the canal to widen the orifice and allow free movement of instruments to the apex. **D,** No. 30 file to 1 mm from working length. **E,** No. 15 file to recapitulate. **F,** No. 35 file to 2 mm from working length. **G,** No. 15 file to recapitulate. **H,** No. 40 file to 3 mm from working length.

Continued.

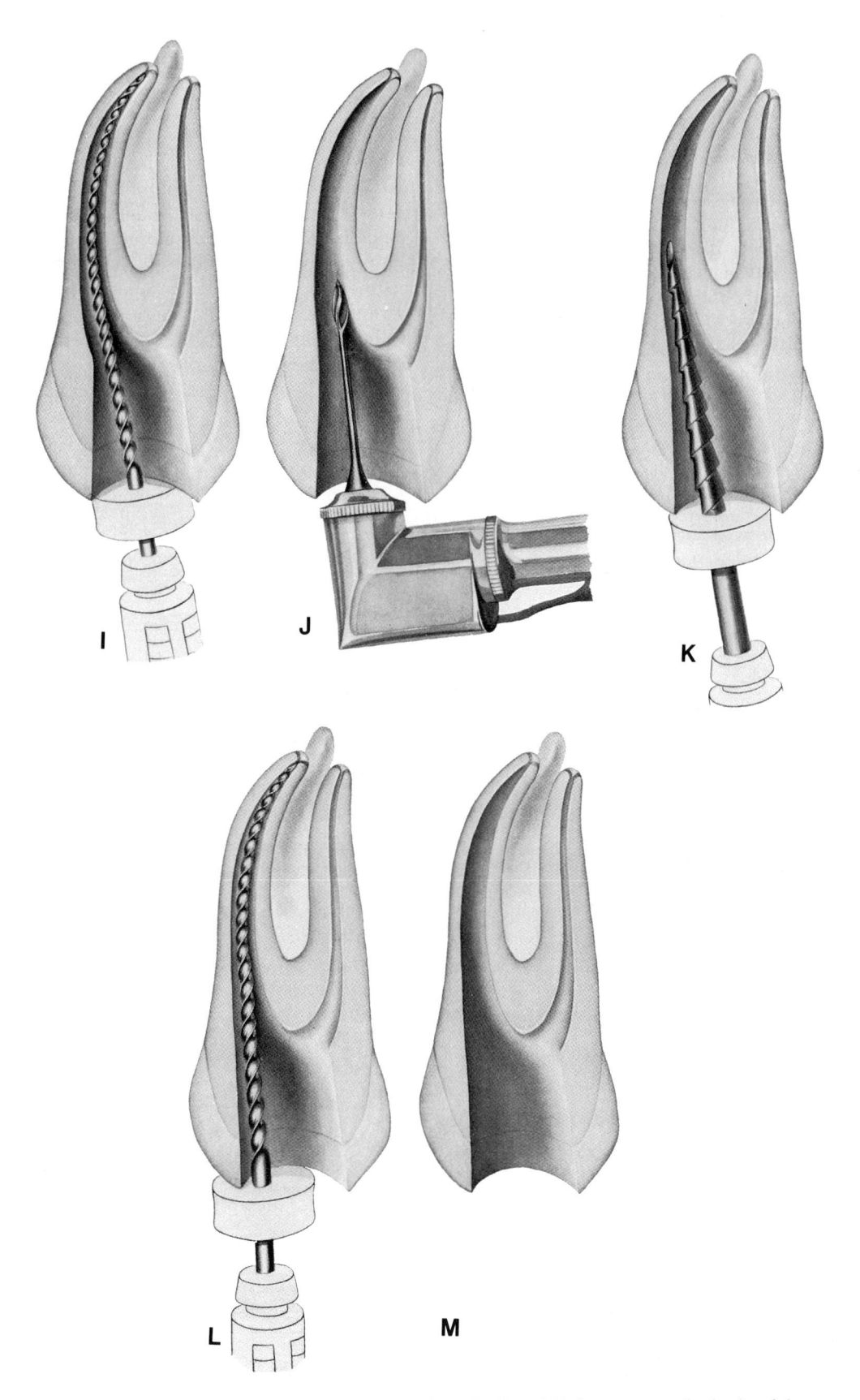

Figure 6-32, *cont'd.* **I,** No. 15 file to recapitulate. *D, F,* and *H* demonstrate the body of the preparation. **J,** A larger size Gates Glidden drill can now be used here in the middle and occlusal third of the canal to increase the body of the preparation. **K,** No. 45 Hedstrom file to remove the rest of the dentinal triangle and smooth the walls of the preparation. **L,** No. 25 file in place to reconfirm the length of the tooth. Notice that the instrument length is now shorter than in **A,** and the instrument is straighter, since the dentinal triangle has been removed. **M,** Final shaping of canal.

136 PRACTICAL ENDODONTICS

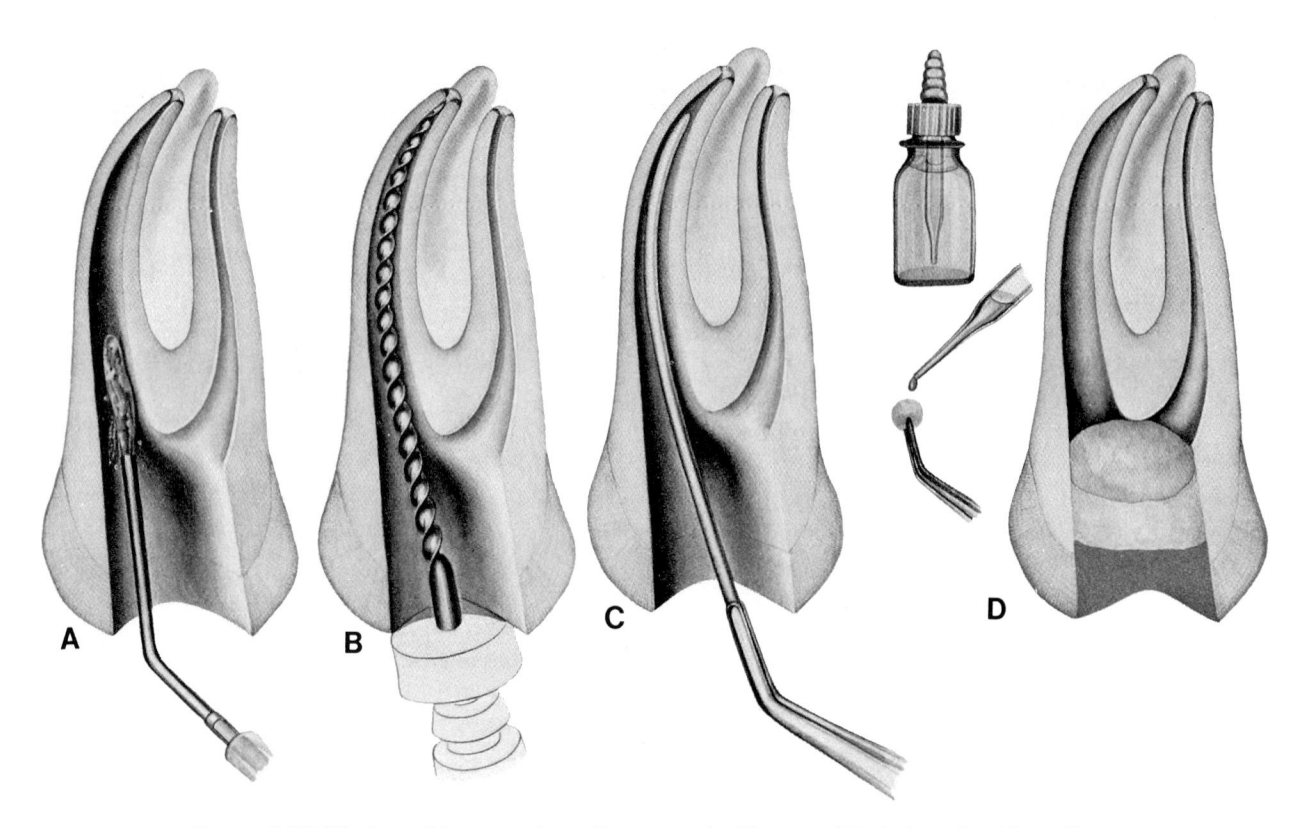

Figure 6-33 Placing of intracanal medicament. **A,** The canal is irrigated with sodium hypochlorite. **B,** The last instrument to apex is placed in canal. **C,** A paper point is used to dry the canal. **D,** A medicament on a cotton pellet is placed in the chamber, a dry cotton pellet is placed on top, and cavit is used to seal the access opening.

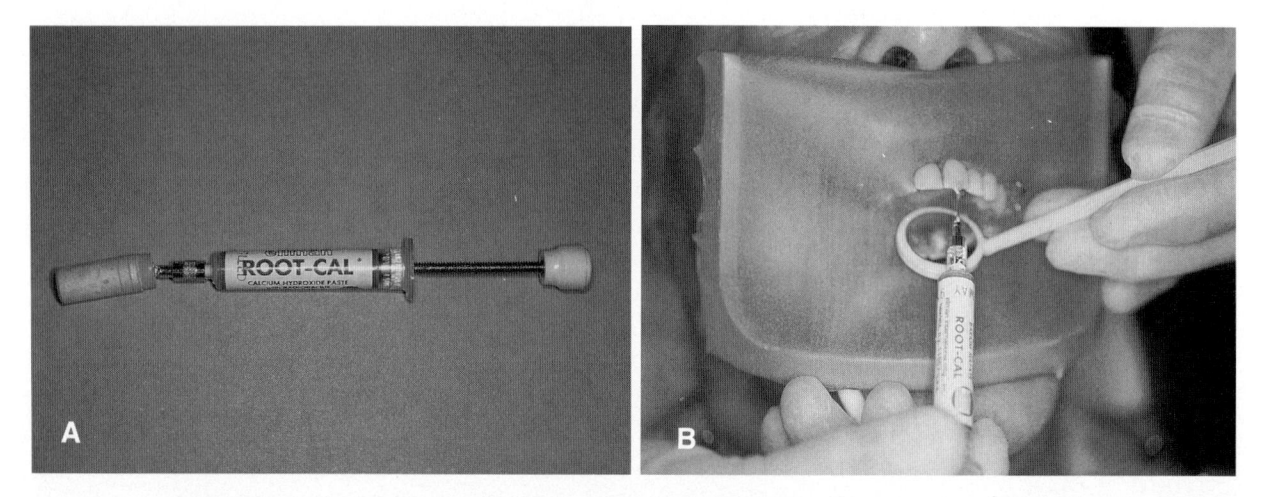

Figure 6-34 Calcium hydroxide as intracanal medicament. **A,** Calcium hydroxide in syringe. **B,** Placement of calcium hydroxide in canal.

OBTURATION

Purpose: To eliminate all of the space in the root canal system so that leakage will be prevented.

Technique: Condensation of gutta percha is achieved to establish a three-dimensional filling (Figs. 6-35 and 6-36).

The following criteria must be met before the canal is ready to be obturated: (a) The tooth should be comfortable. (b) There is no or little exudate in the canal. (c) If a fistula was present, it should be healing. (d) Smooth tapered preparation.

1. Remove the temporary seal.
2. Irrigate with sodium hypochlorite and reinstrument canal with the last size instrument that went to working length of the tooth. Make certain there are no pulpal remnants or necrotic debris remaining.
3. Irrigate and dry the canal completely with sterile absorbent points.
4. Select a standardized gutta percha point that matches the last size instrument taken 1 mm from the radiographic apex. The point should fit tight in apical portion of canal, binding at the apex.
5. Remove the master gutta percha point from the canal with cotton pliers and recheck the length of the point with the original measurement.
6. Take a radiograph. (a) If point fits more than 1 mm short of radiographic apex, choose a gutta percha point one size smaller. (b) If point fits loosely, remove it and cut off 1 mm, and reinsert the point. Continue this procedure until it binds at apical portion of canal and tugback is felt.
7. Mix root canal sealer to a thick creamy consistency on a freshly sterilized slab with sterile spatula. Pick up a small amount of sealer with a No. 15 file and coat the surface of the root canal with a counterclockwise rotary motion.
8. Coat apical half of gutta percha point with sealer and carry the point gently and smoothly to desired position in the tooth, obtaining a snug fit.
9. Dip the No. 15 finger plugger into a dappen dish filled with chloroform and then insert it along the side of the gutta percha point and, with an apical motion, condense the point against the walls of the canal, making room for an additional point.
10. Take a radiograph. (a) If the point fits accurately in the apical portion, the canal may be further sealed with additional gutta percha points. (b) If the gutta percha point is beyond the apex, remove it. Reshape the canal, this time creating a proper apical constriction.
11. Additional gutta percha points are condensed into the canal by first creating space with the finger spreaders. Beginning with No. 15, then No. 20, and if possible No. 25.

    If a No. 25 finger spreader was last used, place a No. 25 gutta percha point in the space it created. If a No. 15 or a No. 20 was last used, then place an X-fine gutta percha point into the space, first cutting the tip of the point so it most accurately resembles the space created by the last finger spreader.

    This process of condensing accessory gutta percha points is continued until the entire canal is packed tightly and no additional gutta percha points can be added.
12. Heat the heat carrier red hot and remove the excess gutta percha in the pulp chamber to a level of 1 mm below the gingival line.
13. Condense the gutta percha apically with pluggers, making sure that when the plugger selected is placed in the canal it does not touch the dentinal wall but is totally within gutta percha.
14. Remove all traces of gutta percha and root canal sealer from the pulp chamber by wiping the chamber with chloroform.
15. Place a cotton pellet in the pulp chamber and cavit as a temporary filling until the final restoration can be done.

138 PRACTICAL ENDODONTICS

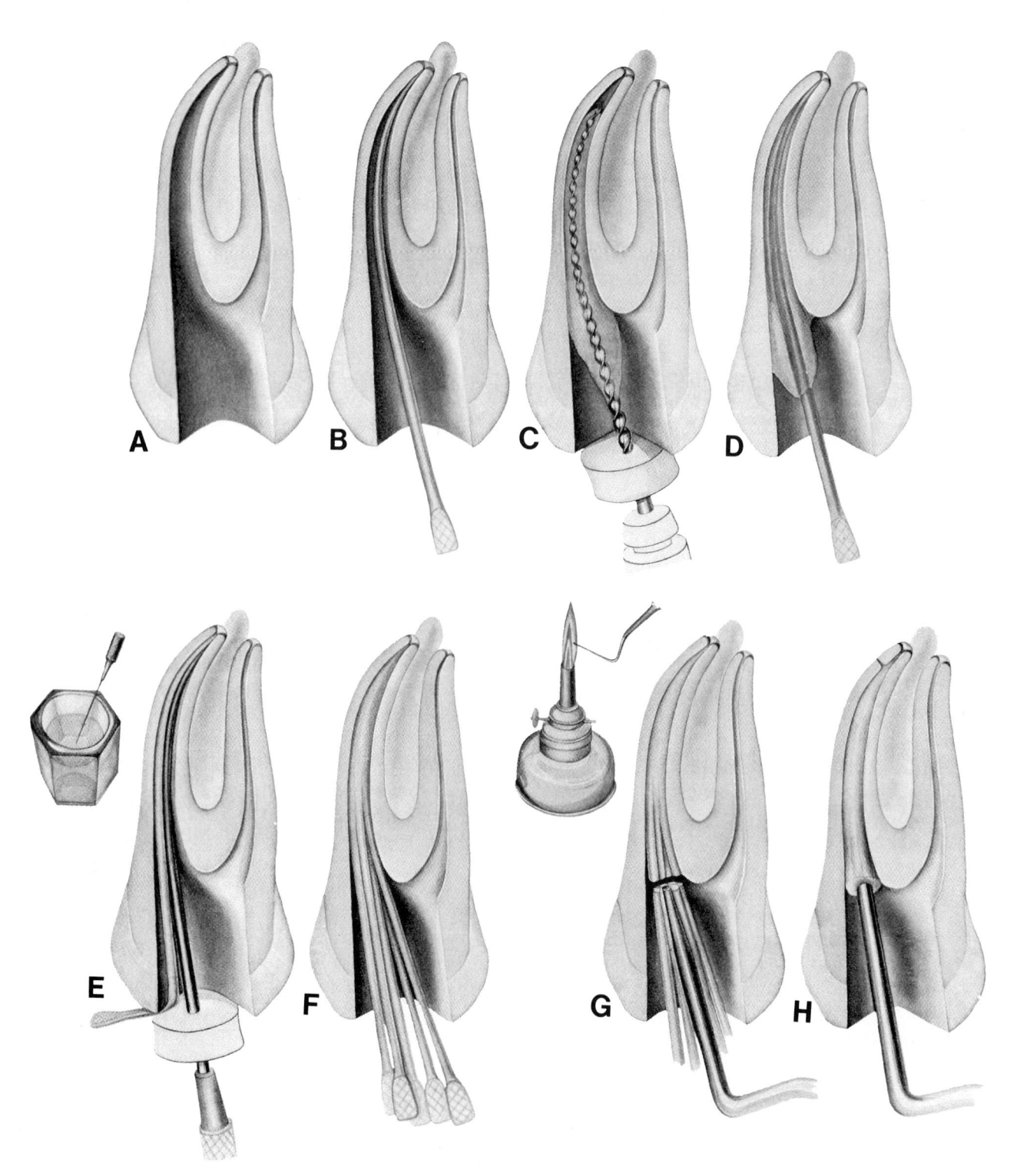

Figure 6-35 Obturation using a modified lateral condensation technique. **A,** Final shaping of canal. **B,** Fitting primary gutta percha cone one millimeter from radiographic apex. **C,** Placing root canal cement in canal with a No. 15 file. **D,** Primary gutta percha cone cemented in place. **E,** Placing a finger spreader in chloroform and then in the canal to make room for auxiliary gutta percha points. **F,** Canal packed with auxilliary gutta percha points until no more cones can be placed. When the spreader cannot be inserted more than 4 mm beyond the orifice of the canal, a sufficient number of auxiliary cones have been added. **G,** Hot instrument used to remove excess gutta percha below cervical line. **H,** Cold plugger used to pack gutta percha apically. *Note:* The Analytic Technology Touch 'n Heat instrument can be substituted for the heat carrier.

Chapter 6 ♦ Routine Endodontic Therapy 139

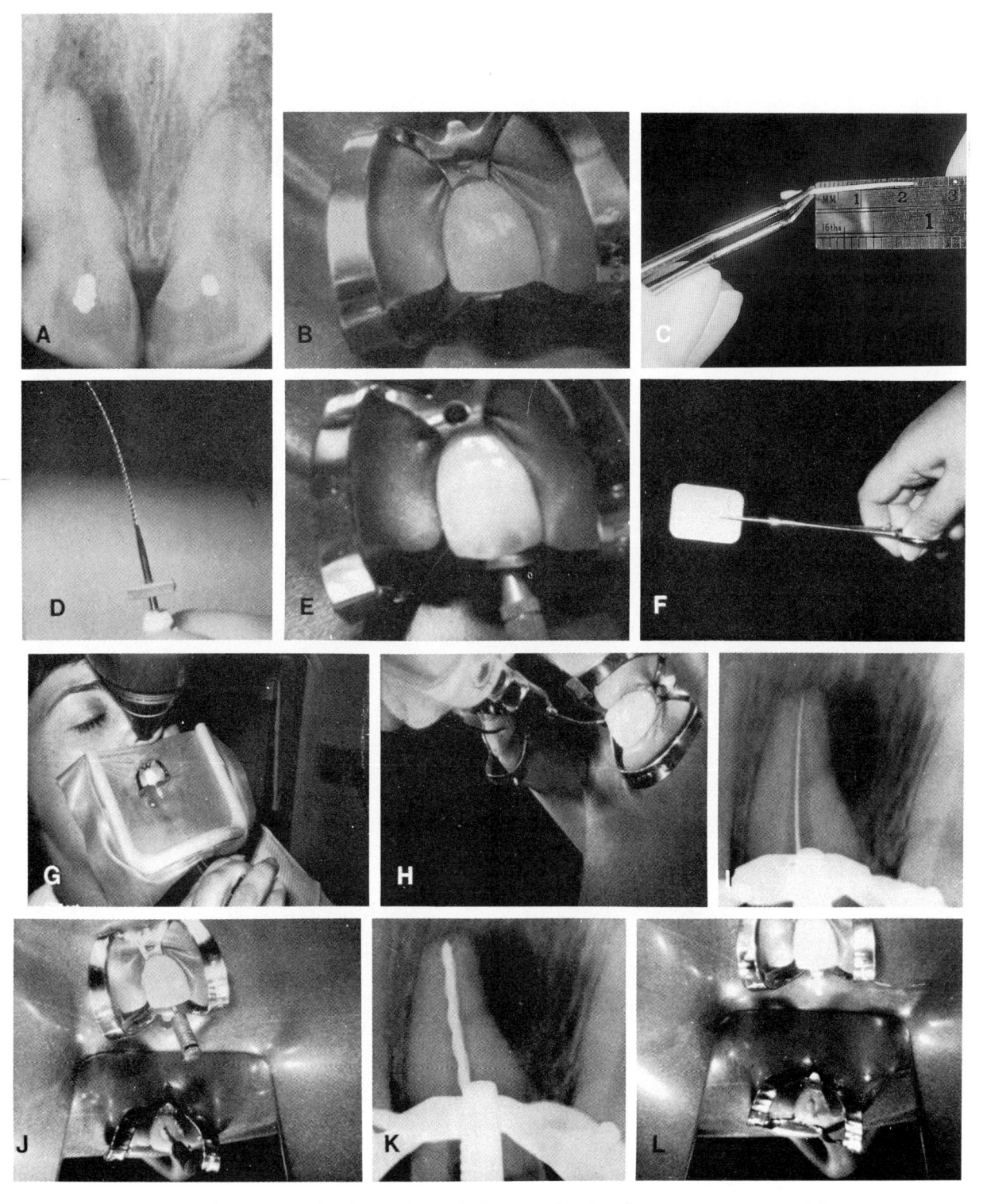

Figure 6-36. A series of radiographs and photographs that demonstrate root canal therapy from the start of the procedure to completion. **A,** Preoperative radiograph showing area of radiolucency on lateral aspect of central. **B,** Rubber dam and No. 9 Ivory clamp in place. **C,** Placing of rubber stopper on file at tentative measurement. **D,** Precurving file. **E,** File placed in canal. **F,** Film attached to hemostat. **G,** Radiograph taken of instrument in canal. Patient holds the hemostat with the film attached, and the x-ray cone is positioned over the tooth. **H,** Canal is flooded with sodium hypochlorite. **I,** Radiograph of instrument in place. **J,** Canal being cleansed and shaped. **K,** Radiograph of last instrument taken to apex. **L,** Paper point used to dry the canal.

Continued.

140 PRACTICAL ENDODONTICS

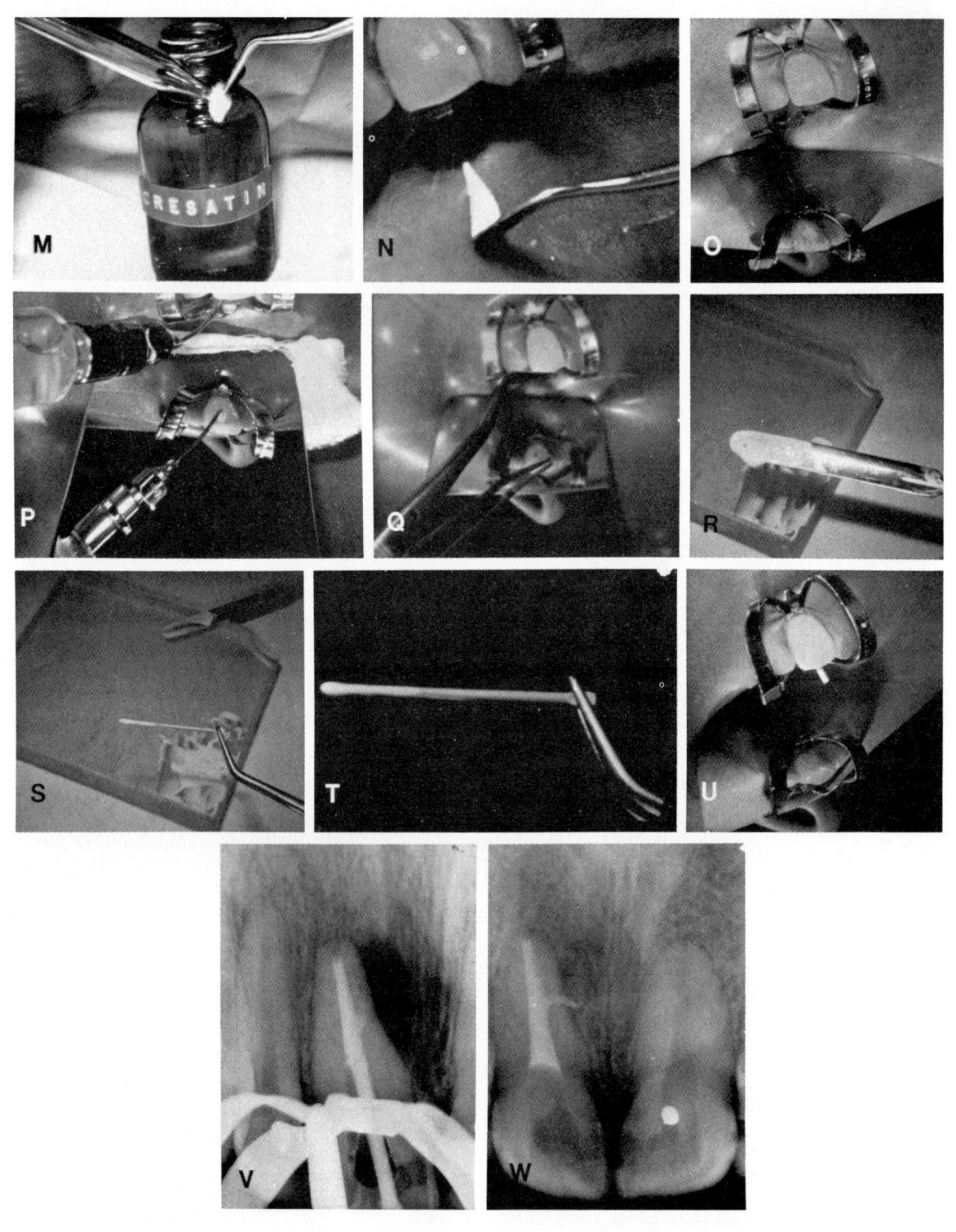

Figure 6-36, *cont'd* **M,** A drop of Cresatin placed on a cotton pellet. The cotton pellet is then dried in a 2 × 2 gauze sponge. **N,** Cavit placed as temporary seal. **O,** Access opening sealed with cavit. **P,** Canal being irrigated with sodium hypochlorite after cavit and cotton removed. **Q,** Paper point used to dry the canal. **R,** Root canal cement mixed on glass slab. **S,** Cement placed on primary gutta percha cone. **T,** Gutta percha cone with cement. **U,** Primary gutta percha cone cemented in place. **V,** Radiograph of gutta percha cone cemented. Lateral condensation is now started. **W,** Six-month postoperative radiograph demonstrating healing. (Courtesy of Dr. Gerald Sacks.)

7

Low Temperature Thermoplasticized Gutta Percha (Ultrafil)

Although gutta percha has been used in dentistry for some 150 years, it is only recently that gutta percha has been able to be thermoplasticized at a low temperature (70° C) and injected into the root canal. This chapter will be devoted to the use of thermoplasticized gutta percha "Ultrafil" for filling root canals. The injected gutta percha gives a dense homogeneous fill with consistency and has sealing properties similar to lateral condensation. The evolution of the Ultrafil System produced a number of viscosities of gutta percha that gives the operator an added degree of versatility and a number of techniques for filling routine root canal teeth with open apices, apexification, apexogenesis, sharp curves, lateral canals, large canals, internal resorption, or unusually C-shaped canals, perforations, separated instruments (see Fig. 11-8, *E* and *F*), ledged, irregular and calcified canals, and retrograde fillings.

The last part of this chapter will be devoted to the coreless Trifecta technique, which uses the high viscosity, Successfil gutta percha combined with Ultrafil.

ADVANTAGES OF ULTRAFIL THERMOPLASTICIZED GUTTA PERCHA

1. Flow properties (thermoplastic)
2. Varied viscosities
3. Fast
4. Can be molded (moldable)
5. Can be compacted
6. Can be laterally condensed
7. Requires minimal pressure during condensation
8. Uniform and dense
9. Increased patient comfort
10. Disposable cannules
11. Versatile
12. Easy backfill method
13. Adheres to dentin walls
14. Flows into lateral and accessory canals

The Ultrafil System consists of a heater, Ultrafil syringe, and disposable cannules of gutta percha with a 22-gauge needle attached (Fig. 7-1).

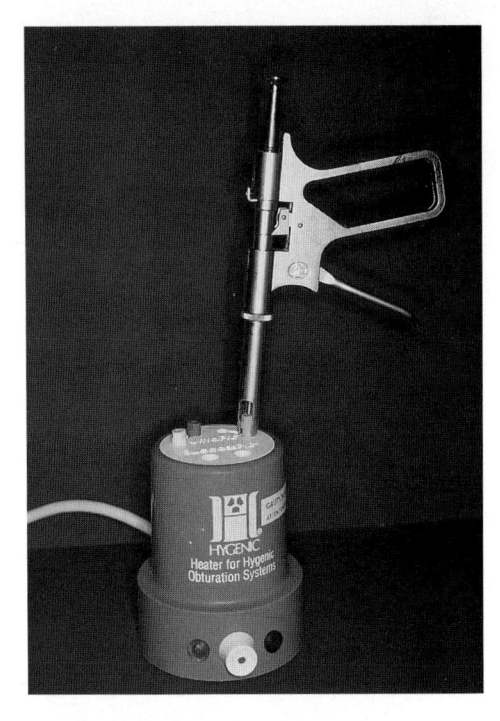

Figure 7-1 Ultrafil System with heater, syringe, and cannules.

142 PRACTICAL ENDODONTICS

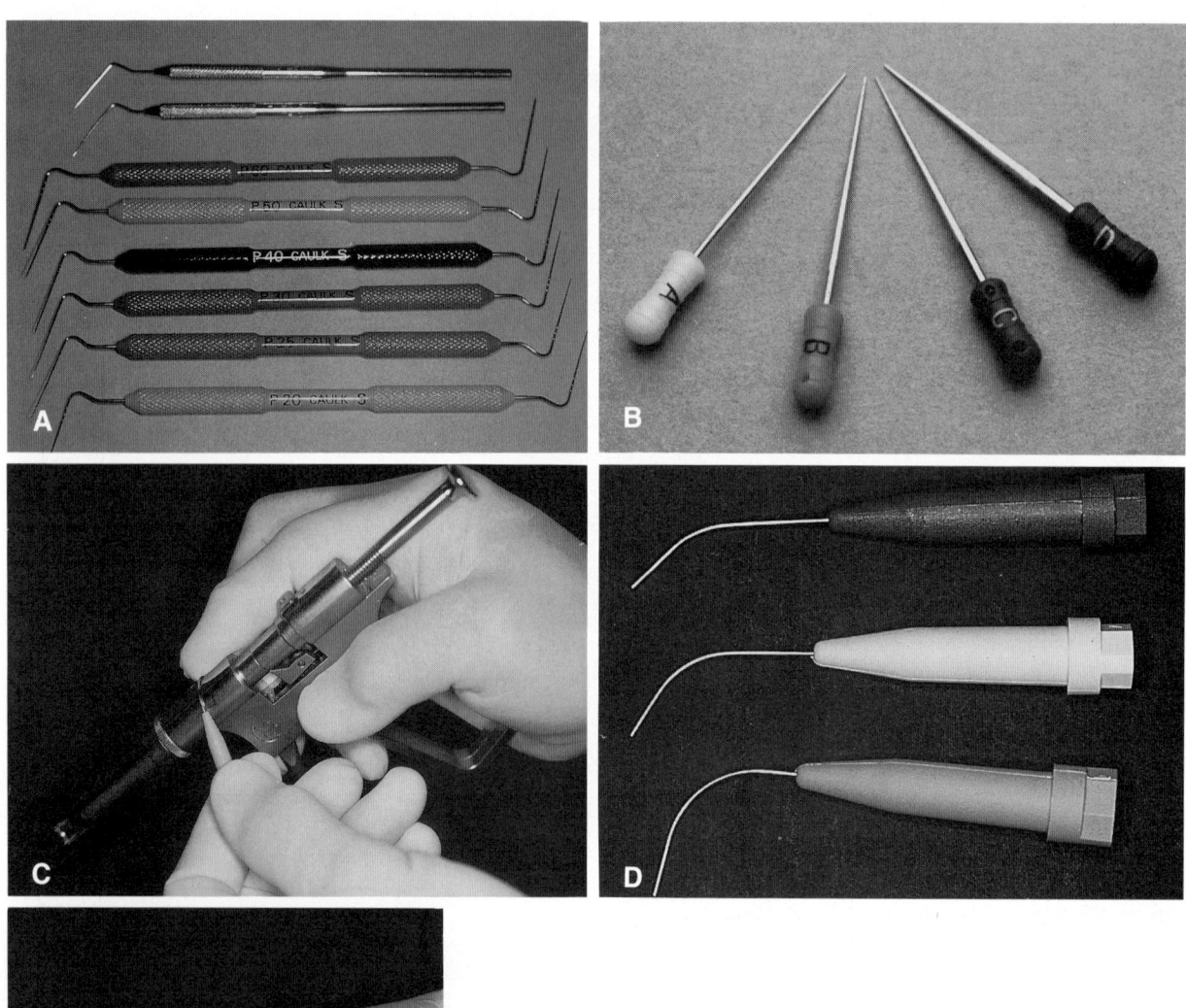

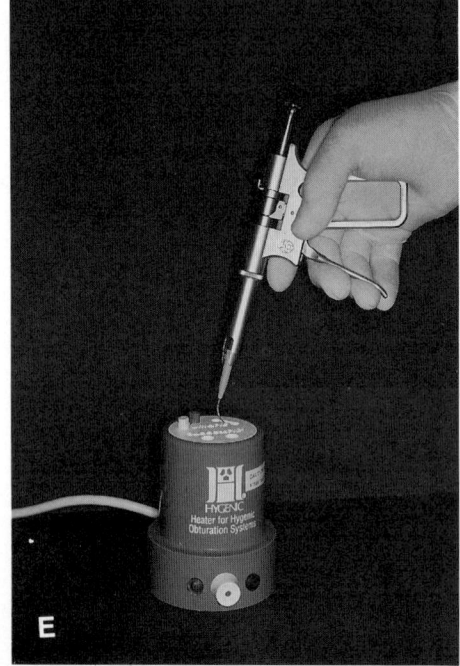

Figure 7-2 **A** and **B**, Examples of spreaders and pluggers that can be used. **A**, M - Plugger/ Spreader 20-60 (Caulk - Dentsply); D11 and D11T spreaders (Premier). **B**, Finger pluggers (Caulk - Dentsply). **C**, Needle is placed over the barrel of the syringe and curved to desired angle. **D**, Several needles curved at different angles. **E**, Cannules are placed in slotted holes in heater to receive curved needle.

ADJUNCT HAND INSTRUMENT ARMAMENTARIUM (Fig. 7-2, *A* and *B*)

1. Spreaders
2. Pluggers
3. Finger pluggers

CANNULES

The cannules are prefilled with gutta percha and a 22-gauge needle is attached. Each cannule contains enough gutta percha to fill at least one molar. To facilitate injection in posterior and some anterior teeth the needles of the cannule are precurved before placing them in the heater. Place the cannule needle over the midbarrel of the syringe and bend the needle to the barrel shape (Fig. 7-2, *C* and *D*). The cannule is placed in the preset heater at 90° C for 15 minutes (Fig. 7-2, *E*). The heater is prepared with a slot to receive the curved needle. There is approximately 1 minute working time with the gutta percha after it is removed from the heater and placed in the injection syringe. During this time the temperature will drop to around 70° C and will be ready for injection.

TYPES OF GUTTA PERCHA

There are three types of injectable gutta percha identified by their colored cannules.
1. Regular set - White cannule (setting time 30 minutes)
2. Firm set - Blue cannule (setting time 4 minutes)
3. Endoset - Green cannule (setting time 2 minutes) (Fig. 7-3)

The Regular Set and Firm Set have the same high flow properties but different setting times. The Firm Set is much faster setting, approximately 4 minutes. This quality makes it more readily condensable with pluggers. The Endoset with the highest viscosity has much less flow, sets in 2 minutes, and is readily compacted. It is used primarily when compaction is desired.

THERMOPLASTICIZED INJECTING TECHNIQUES

1. Injection of entire canal
2. Master cone and injection
3. Injections and vertical condensation (compaction)
4. Injection and lateral condensation
5. Trifecta and Successfil technique
6. Retrograde surgery

CANAL PREPARATION

After the working length is established, the canal is prepared in the routine manner by stepping back the file in 1-mm increments to approximately 1 to 2 sizes higher than the first instrument that binds at the dentocemental junction (Fig. 7-4). This procedure is called *telescoping, funneling,* and/or *incremental filling.* The integrity of the foramen is maintained to act as a natural barrier to prevent extrusion of the filling material. To test for an apical stop, place a No. 15 file to

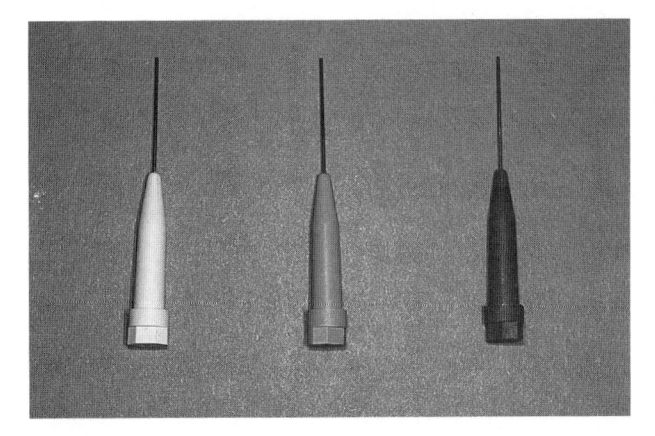

Figure 7-3 Regular set (*left*), Firm set (*middle*) and Endoset (*right*) with 22-gauge needle attached.

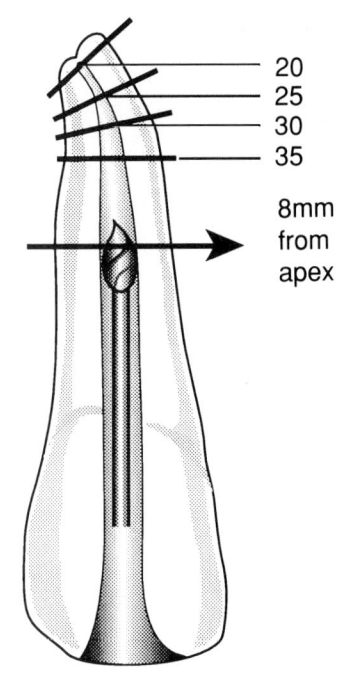

Figure 7-4 The gingival third is prepared to a No. 2 Gates Glidden drill approximately 8 to 10 mm from the working length. The apical third is prepared by backstepping in 1-mm increments beginning with the first instrument that binds at the foramen.

144 PRACTICAL ENDODONTICS

the working length. If the file passes through the foramen a stop is not present.

The body consists of the gingival and middle third. It is prepared with No. 1 and No. 2 Gates Glidden drills to approximately 6 to 8 mm from the working length to receive the Ultrafil needle (22 gauge), which is approximately the size of a No. 70 file or No. 2 Gates Glidden drill (Fig. 7-4).

When the foramen is incomplete or iatrogenically opened in excess, an apical barrier is necessary to contain the gutta percha in the canal. Dentin chips can be backfiled to form a stop, dry calcium hydroxide can be carried to the foramen to act as a barrier, or a gutta percha master cone can be used as the apical plug (Fig. 7-5, *A*).

TECHNIQUE FOR ULTRAFIL INJECTION OF THE ENTIRE CANAL WITH REGULAR SET OR FIRM SET

The low viscosity allows the Regular set and Firm set gutta percha to be used for injection of the entire canal when an apical stop is present, and to flow into lateral and accessory canals, narrow and curved canals, around separated instruments, and internal resorption.

Syringe Preparation

- The cannule is taken from the heater and placed in the injection syringe.
- A slight amount of gutta percha is extruded to determine the flow (Fig. 7-5, *B*).
- The cannule is replaced in the heater for several seconds (Fig. 7-6).

Technique For Injection Of The Entire Canal

1. Coat the canal wall with sealer using a No. 25 reamer or lentulo (Fig. 7-7, *C*).
2. Insert the needle into the canal at least 8 to 10 mm from the working length. May vary 7 mm or more (Fig. 7-7, *D*).
3. Inject the gutta percha by squeezing the trigger with light continuous pressure.
4. Release the trigger to re-engage plunger.

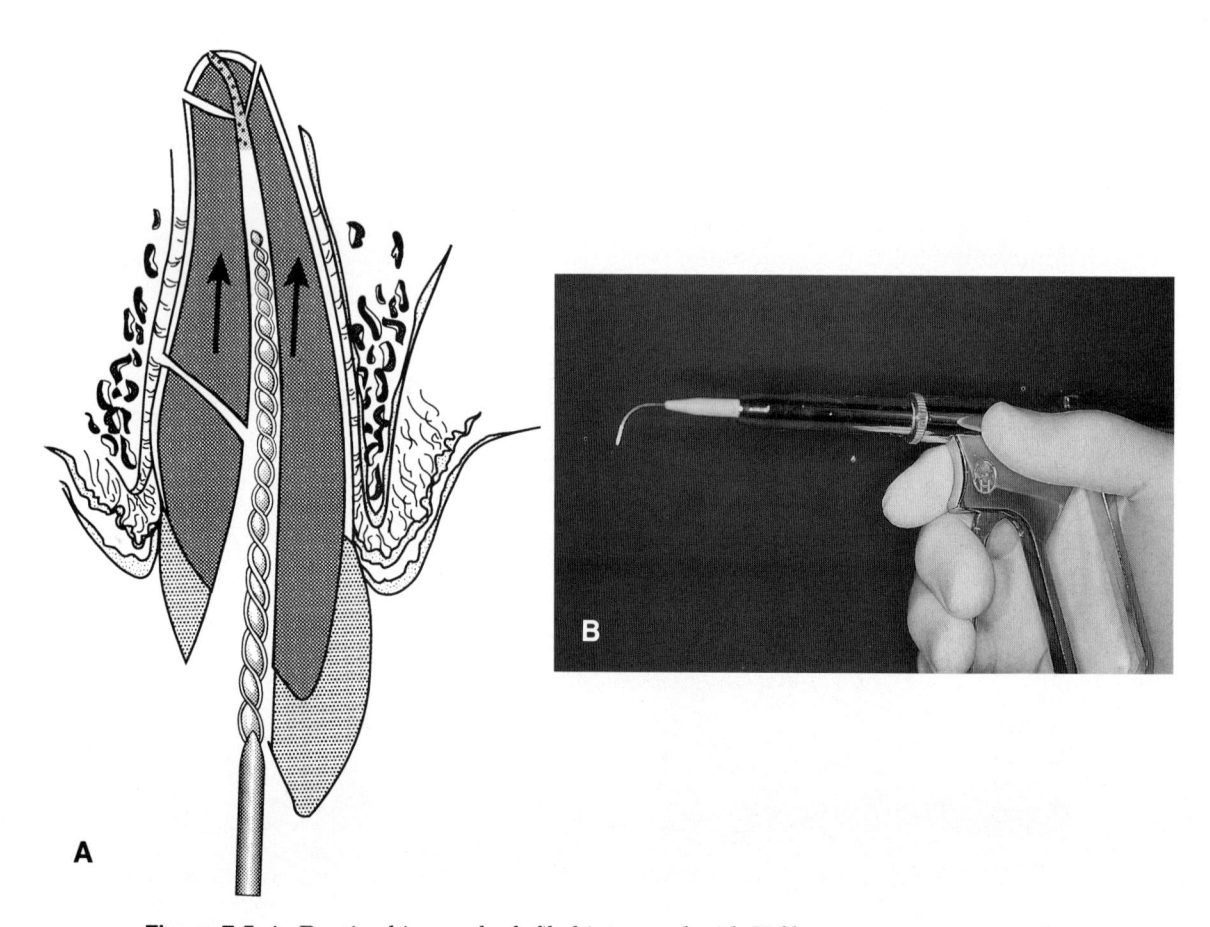

Figure 7-5 A, Dentin chips are back filed into canal with K-file or a master cone can be used. **B,** A slight amount of gutta percha is extruded to determine flow before injection.

5. Squeeze the trigger again and continue as above in no. 3 and no. 4. You will feel the needle being "pushed" out of the canal.
6. Allow the needle to be pushed out of the canal by the backflow (Fig. 7-7, *E*). Continue to inject as necessary until the gutta percha is in the chamber. It usually takes two or three squeezes of the trigger. Remove excess gutta percha from the pulp chamber with a spoon excavator and a cotton pellet moistened with alcohol. The gingival third is condensed with a large plugger (Fig. 7-7, *F*).
7. For multi-rooted teeth, repeat the procedure for each canal. It may be necessary to replace the cannule into a heater for a few seconds with the syringe attached to reheat the gutta percha. A radiograph is taken to determine adequate flow and the possible presence of voids. If necessary the gutta percha is condensed with a D11T spreader dipped in sealer. The D11 spreader is then used to make room for the insertion of the needle (1 or 2 mm) and the canal reinjected.

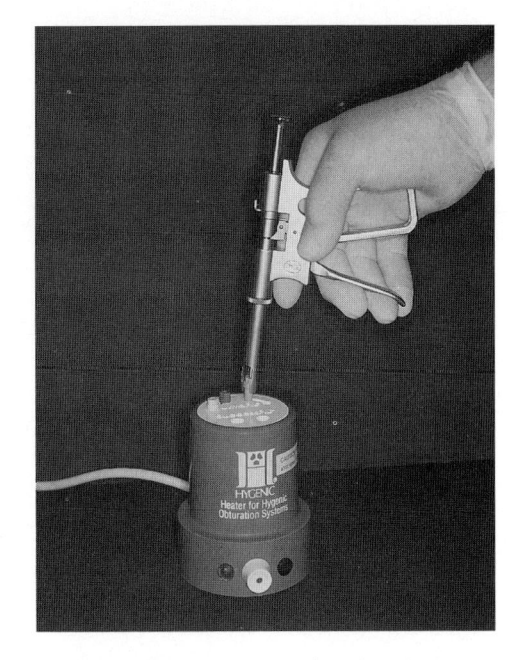

Figure 7-6 Syringe replaced in heater.

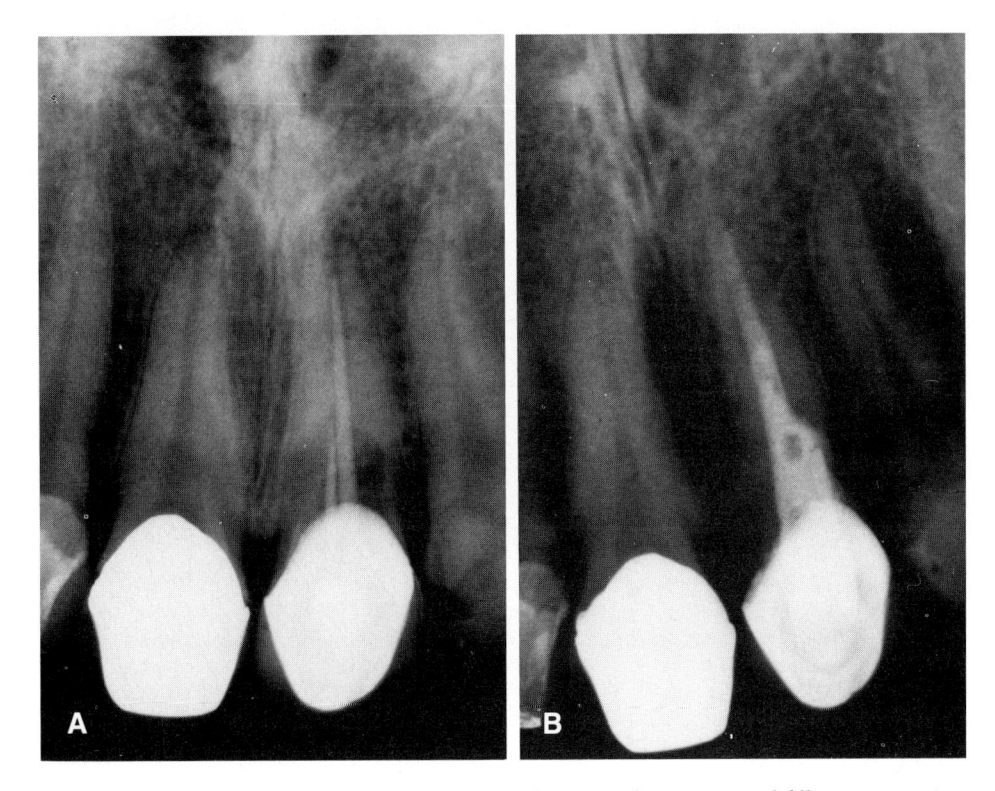

Figure 7-7 A, A radiograph of tooth No. 8 with incomplete root canal filling, resorption in the gingival third and no apparent apical stop. **B,** The gutta percha filling was removed and with large pluggers a dry mix of calcium hydroxide and water was sealed in the canal for 1½ years to aid in obtaining an apical stop and to control the resorption.

Continued.

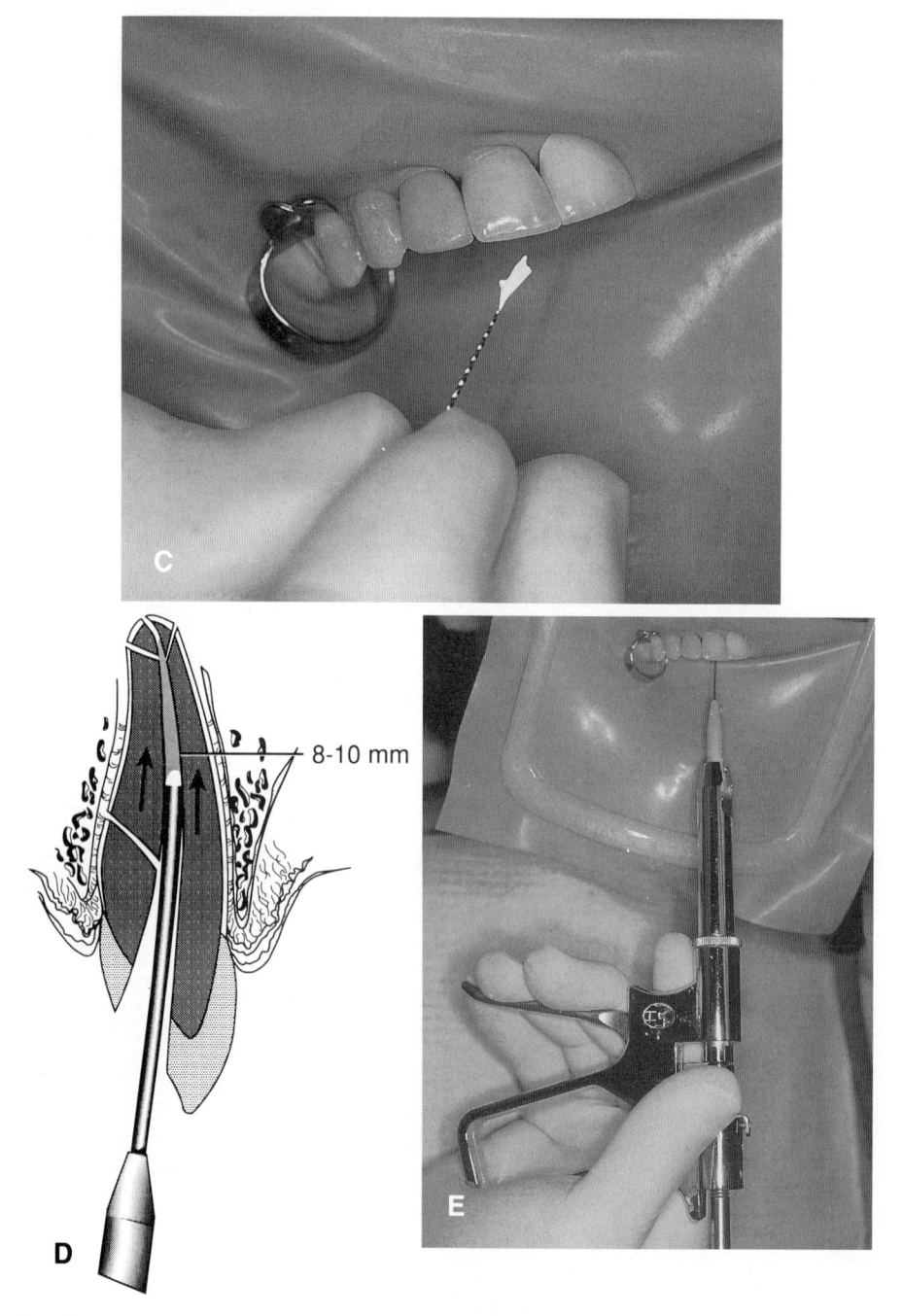

Figure 7-7, *cont'd* **C,** The calcium hydroxide was removed and sealer was carried into the canal with a No. 25 reamer. **D,** The injection needle was placed in the canal approximately 10 mm from the working length and injected with Firm set Ultrafil. **E,** Needle is pushed out of canal by the gutta percha and canal being filled.

Continued.

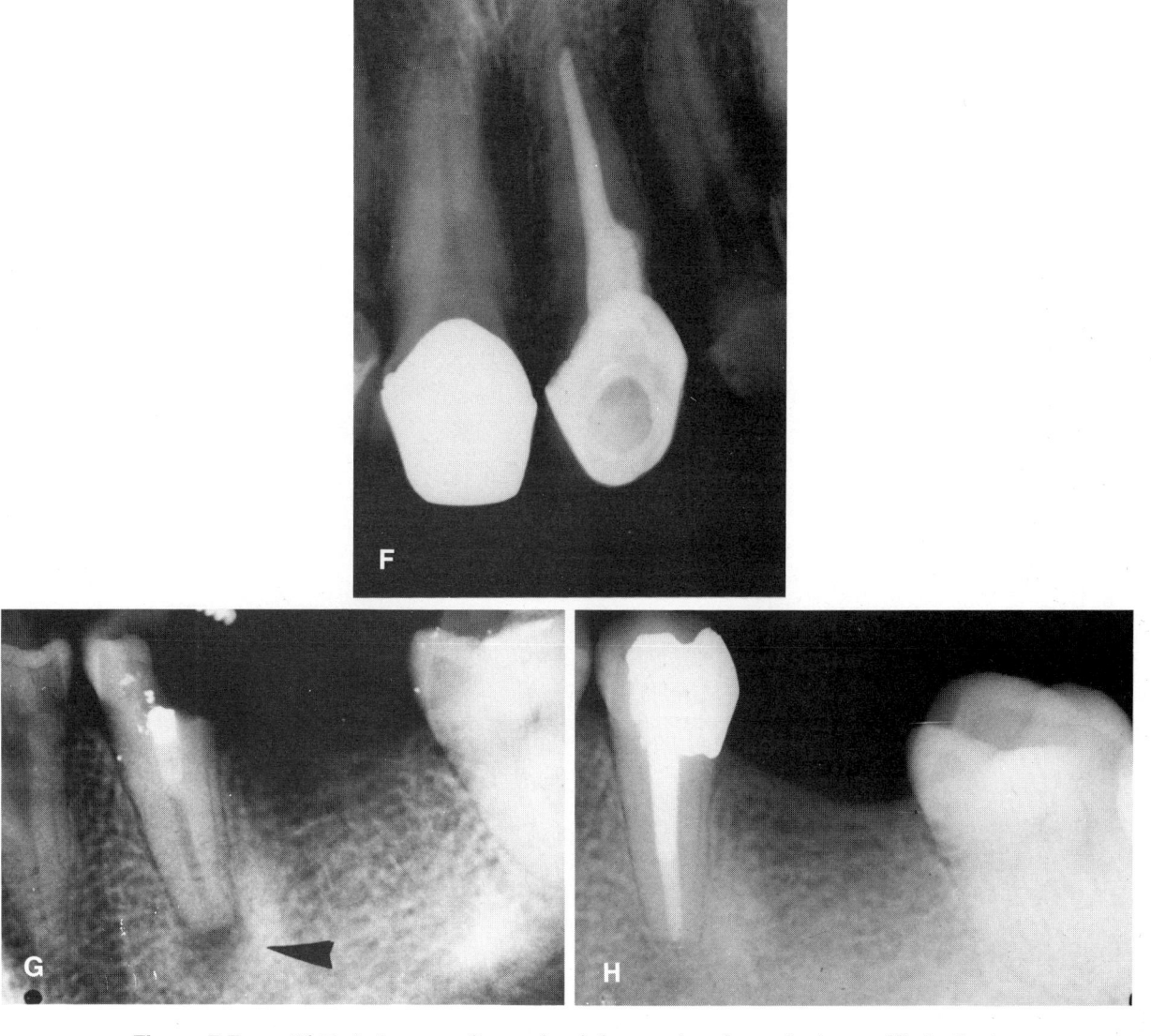

Figure 7-7, *cont'd* **F,** A 5-year radiograph of the canal and resorbed area filled. **G,** A mandibular bicuspid with an apical periodontitis. **H,** A 1-year postoperative showing repair, following injection with sealer and Regular set Ultrafil. (Courtesy of Dr. Elie Maalouf, University of St. Joseph, Beyrouth, Liban.)

INJECTION AND MASTER CONE: REGULAR SET AND FIRM SET

This technique can be used in any case at the discretion of the operator or when an apical barrier is not present and the foramen is compromised by over instrumenting the canal. The master cone acts as a barrier. Either the Regular set (white) or the Firm set (blue) can be used. They both have the same flow properties.

1. Fit a master cone into the canal with tugback in the apical third (Fig. 7-8, *A* and *B*).
2. Place a small amount of sealer in the canal with a No. 25 reamer or lentulo (Fig. 7-8, *C*).
3. Reinsert the master cone gently but firmly into the canal and laterally condense the master cone with a D11T spreader (dipped in sealer) (Fig. 7-8, *D*) followed by the D11 (Fig. 7-8, *E*). The wider diameter of the D11 allows room for insertion of the needle (Fig. 7-8, *F*).
4. Insert the needle into the space made by the D11 spreader about 1- to 3-mm into the canal (Fig. 7-8, *E* and *F*).
5. Inject until the gutta percha begins to flow out of the canal and pushes the needle out. One half to one squeeze is usually sufficient (Fig. 7-8, *G*). In teeth with multiple canals the needle should be removed as soon as the injected gutta percha is visible so as not to have excess gutta percha block the other canals. Excess gutta percha can be removed with a spoon excavator or double-ended explorer.

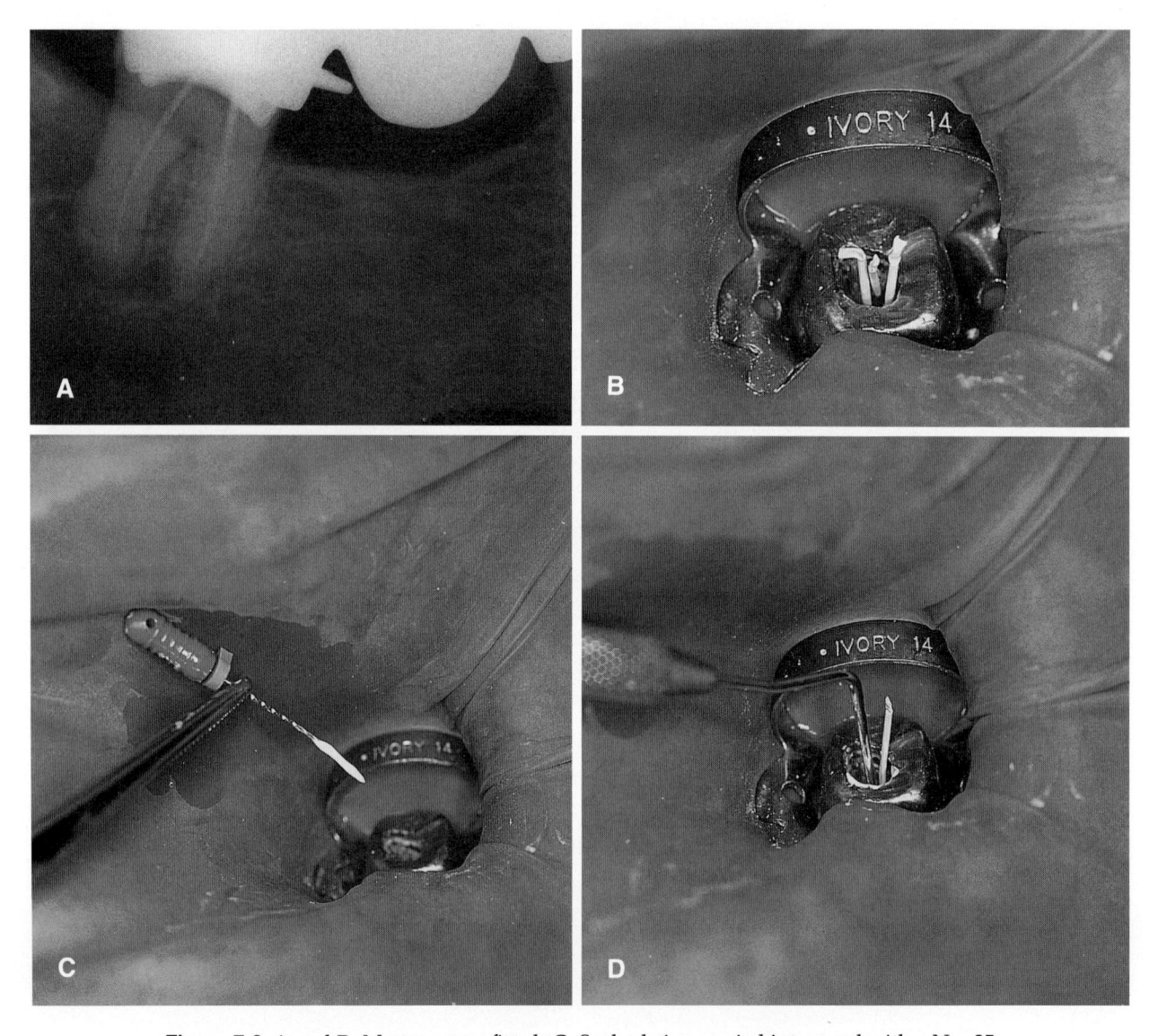

Figure 7-8 *A* and *B*, Master cones fitted. *C*, Sealer being carried into canal with a No. 25 reamer. *D*, Master cone is condensed laterally with a D11T spreader.

Continued.

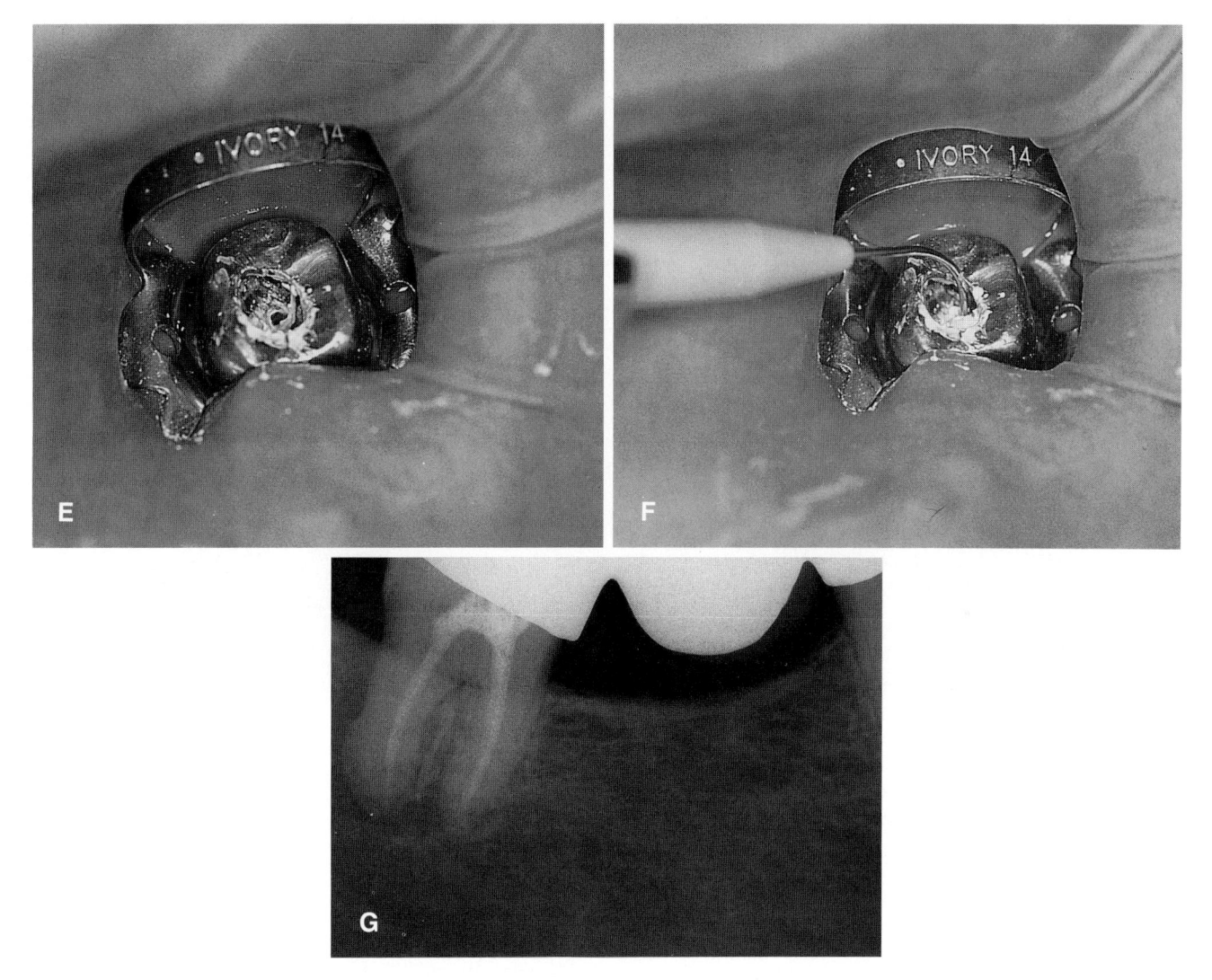

Chapter 7 ♦ Low Temperature Thermoplasticized Gutta Percha (Ultrafil) 149

Figure 7-8, *cont'd* **E,** Opening made by lateral condensation with D11 spreader. **F,** The canal is injected with Firm set gutta percha until the backflow is visible. **G,** The completed filling.

INJECTION AND VERTICAL COMPACTION: ENDOSET

This technique is selected at the discretion of the operator when an apical stop is present, in teeth with internal resorption, and in teeth with large canals and apexification.

1. Pre-fit gutta percha pluggers to approximately 2 to 3 mm from the apical foramen (Fig. 7-9).
2. Place sealer in the canal with a No. 25 reamer (Fig. 7-8, C).
3. Insert needle into the canal several millimeters and inject Endoset (approximately one squeeze) of the gutta percha (Fig. 7-10).
4. Using the prefitted plugger, compact the gutta percha vertically to the working length (Fig. 7-11, A and B).
5. Take radiograph to determine if foramen is sealed (Fig. 7-11, C and D).
6. Backfill and compact as needed to fill the entire canal (Fig. 7-12).

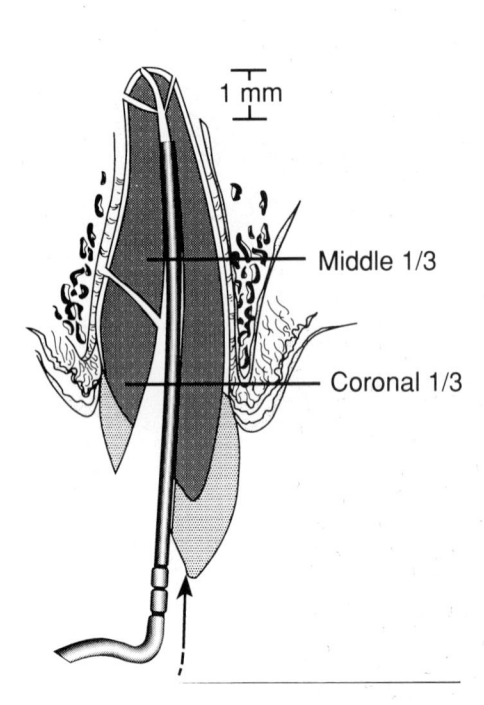

Figure 7-9 Pre-fit plugger.

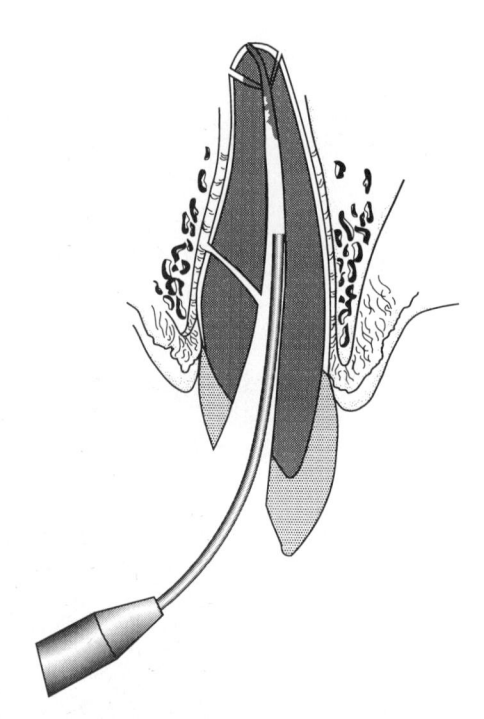

Figure 7-10 Needle is inserted into canal and several millimeters (1 to 1½ squeezes) of Endoset gutta percha are injected.

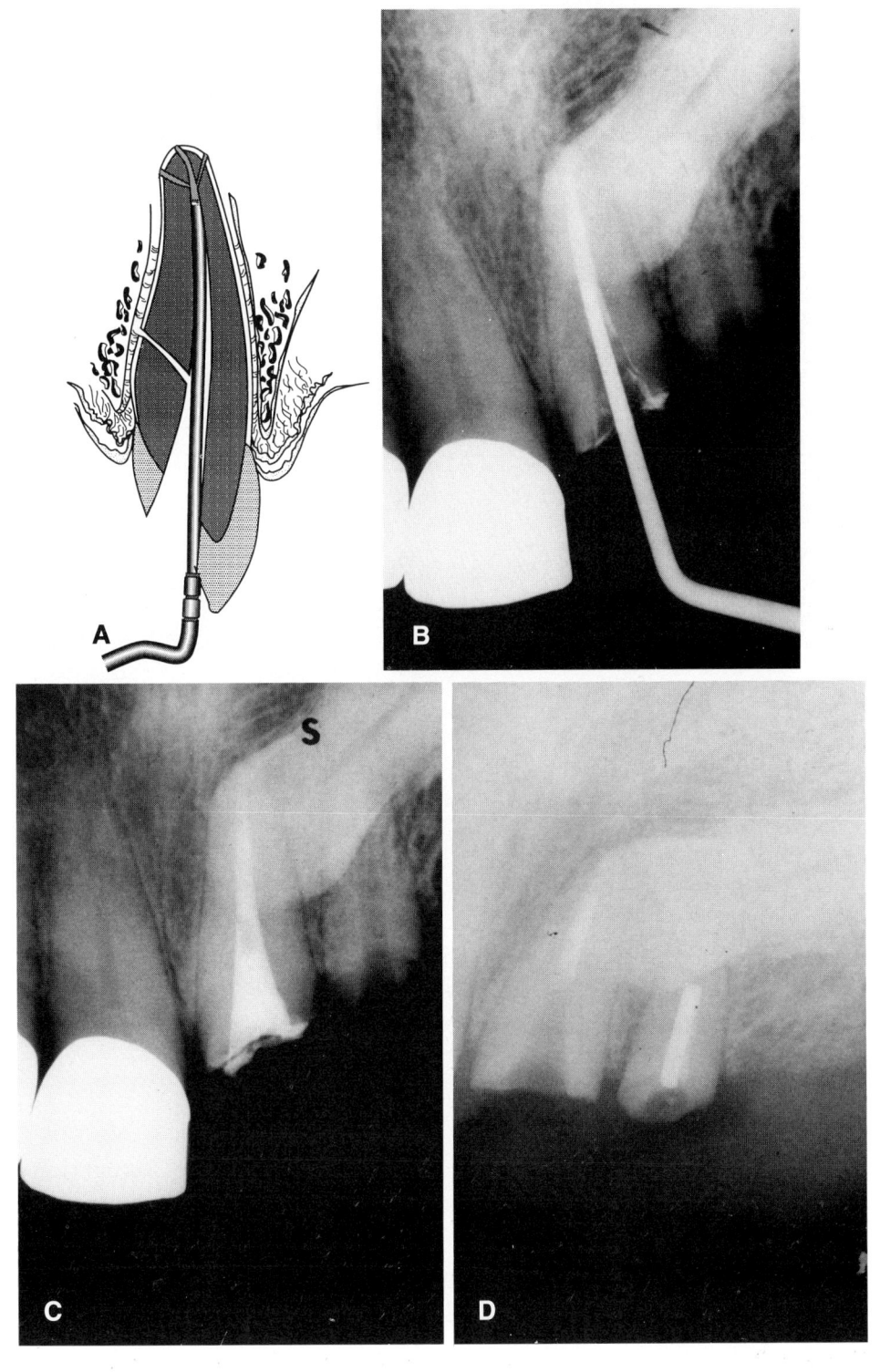

Chapter 7 ♦ Low Temperature Thermoplasticized Gutta Percha (Ultrafil)   151

Figure 7-11 **A** and **B**, A No. 60 prefitted plugger is used to vertically compact the gutta percha. About 1½ squeezes high viscosity fast setting Endoset was injected into the apical third. **C**, The canal with sealer(s) was reinjected with one squeeze and compacted. **D**, The canal was prepared for a post.

152 PRACTICAL ENDODONTICS

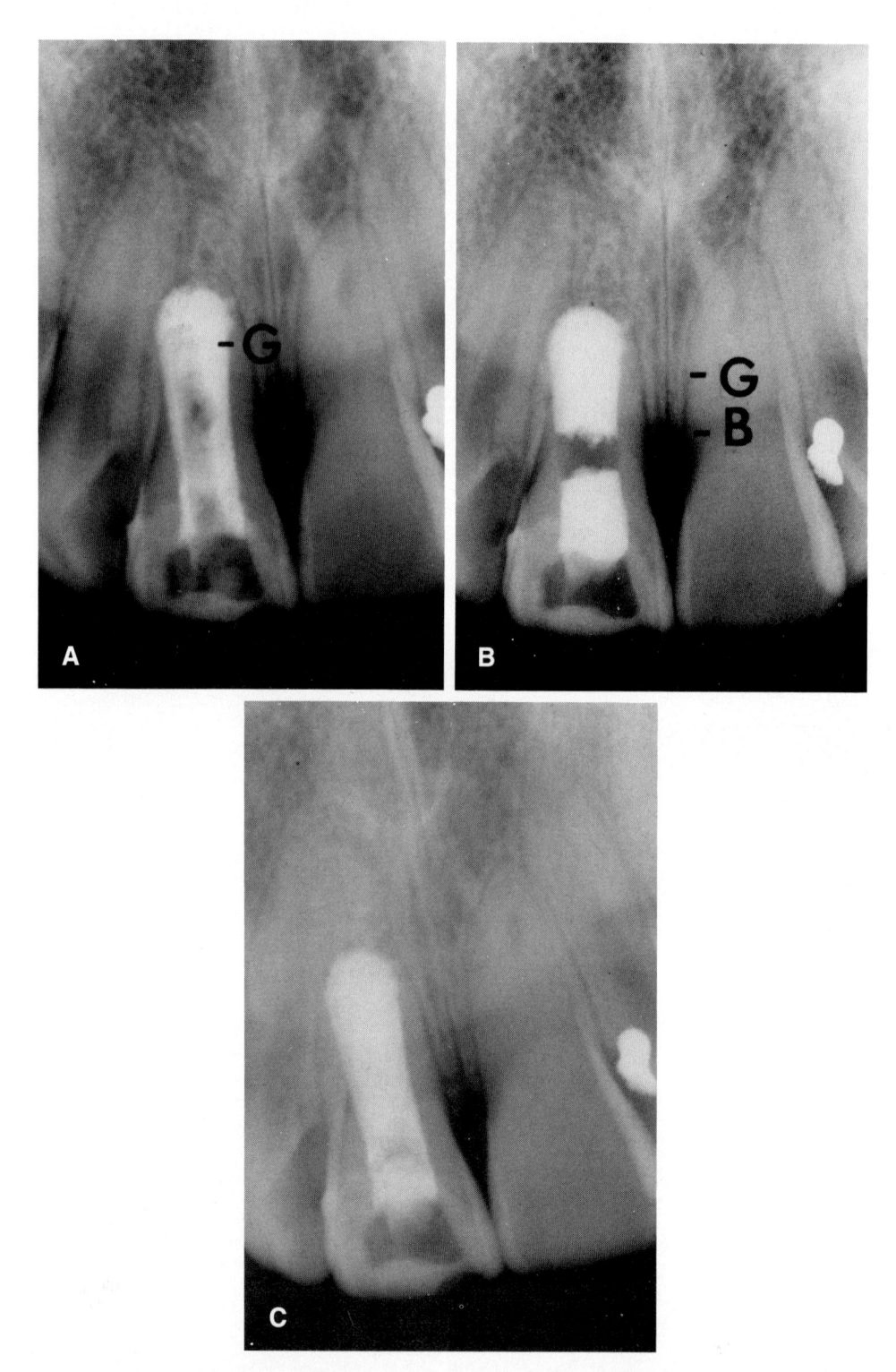

Figure 7-12 A, Endoset gutta percha (green cannule) was injected into the apical third of tooth No. 9 that had undergone apexification. The needle was inserted 3 to 4 mm from the apex. The gutta percha was vertically compacted with a prefit plugger. **B,** The middle of the canal was injected with the Firm set (blue cannule) and compacted apically. **C,** The gingival portion of the canal was injected with Firm Set and compacted.

INJECTION AND LATERAL CONDENSATION: FIRM SET OR REGULAR SET

This technique is also selected at the discretion of the operator when an apical stop is present and it allows the operator to laterally condense the gutta percha.
1. Place small amount of sealer in canal (Fig. 7-8, C).
2. The needle is placed 8 to 10 mm from the working length. Inject Firm set or Regular set into the entire canal (see Fig. 7-7, D).
3. Tooth No. 13 is filled with Firm set Ultrafil (Fig. 7-13, A).
4. A D11T spreader dipped in sealer is used to condense (Fig. 7-13, B).
5. The canal is laterally condensed and reinjected (Fig. 7-13, C).
6. Six months recall shows radiolucent area decreasing (Fig. 7-13, D).

TRIFECTA TECHNIQUE: SUCCESSFIL, FIRM SET, AND ENDOSET

The Trifecta technique utilizes two viscosities of gutta percha Ultrafil and Successfil. Successfil gutta percha is provided in a l-cc syringe and is carried into the canal on a K-file. Its very high viscosity (minimal flow) make it possible to place the Successfil gutta percha precisely to the working length. The combination of the two types of gutta percha provide flow with apical control. The foramen and several millimeters of the canal are filled with the high viscosity Successfil gutta percha and the remaining portions of the canal are filled with a lower viscosity injectable gutta percha Regular set or Firm set.

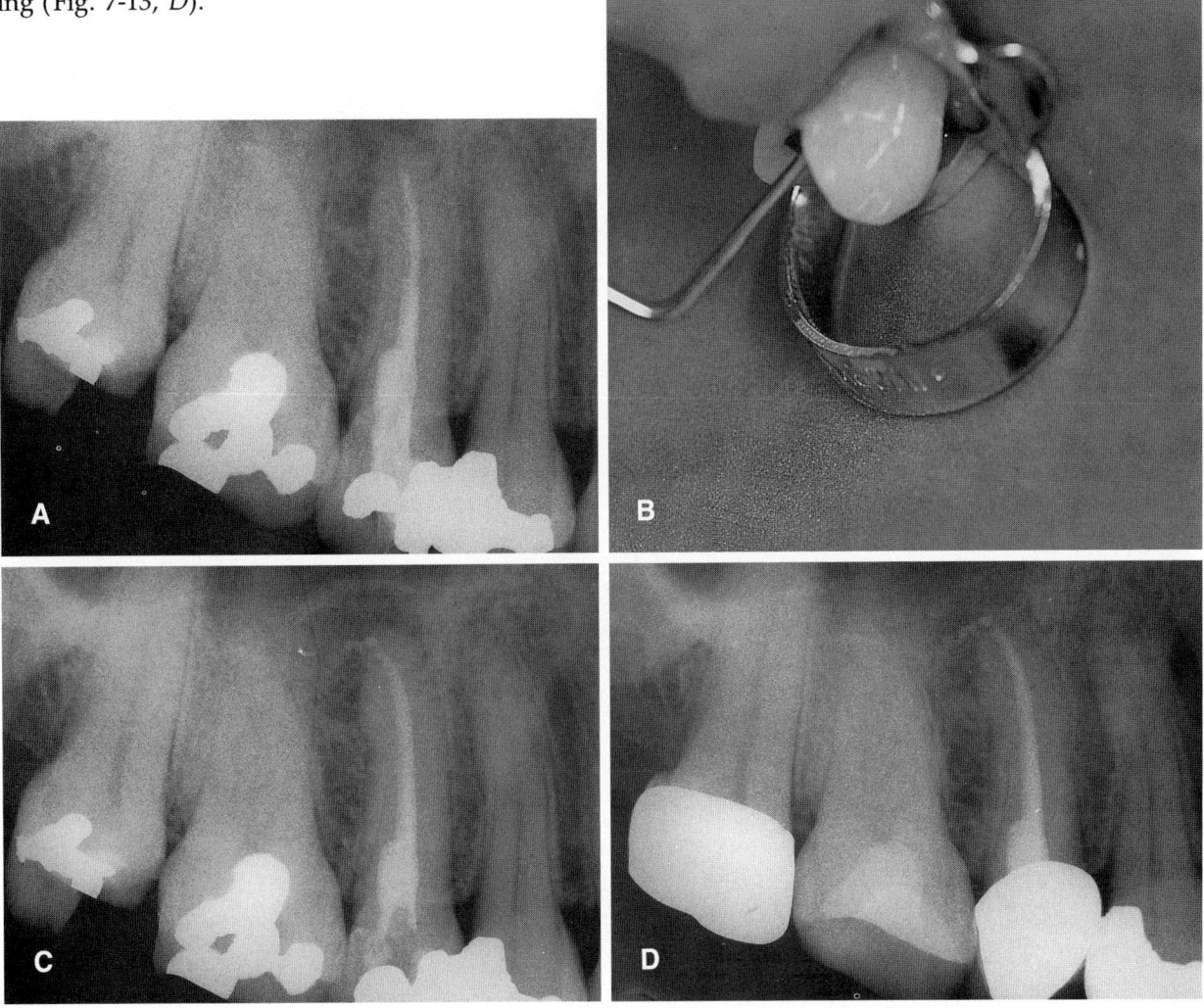

Figure 7-13 The injection needle was placed into canal and injected with Firm set Ultrafil (see Fig. 7-7, D). **A,** Tooth No. 13 is filled with Firm set Ultrafil. **B,** A D11T spreader is used to condense laterally and vertically. **C,** Canal laterally condensed and reinjected. Note the apical movement of the filling. **D,** Six months postoperative showing radiolucent area decreasing.

Armamentarium (Fig. 7-14)

- Successfil gutta percha syringe (1 cc)
- Successfil heater
- Set of K-files No. 15 to No. 40

Technique

This technique can be used at the discretion of the operator.

1. The canal is prepared in the usual manner.
2. Prefit hand or finger plugger in the apical third 1 mm short of working length, one in the middle third, and one in the coronal third (Fig. 7-15).
3. Select a K-file one size smaller than the last file used in the canal and set a stop at the working length (Fig. 7-16, A and B).
4. Place small amount of sealer in canal (Fig. 7-17).
5. Insert the file 2 to 3 mm into the syringe and inject coating 2 to 3 mm of the tip (Fig. 7-18).
6. Without twisting, insert the instrument to the working length. Immediately twist counterclockwise and remove the file, leaving the gutta percha at the apex (Fig. 7-19).
7. Condense using the prefit hand or finger plugger in the apical ⅓ (Fig. 7-20).
8. Inject Ultrafil Regular set or Firm set into the canal until filled (Fig. 7-21).
9. If compaction is desired use Endoset and condense with plugger prefit to middle third of the canal and recondense as needed (Figs. 7-22 and 7-23).

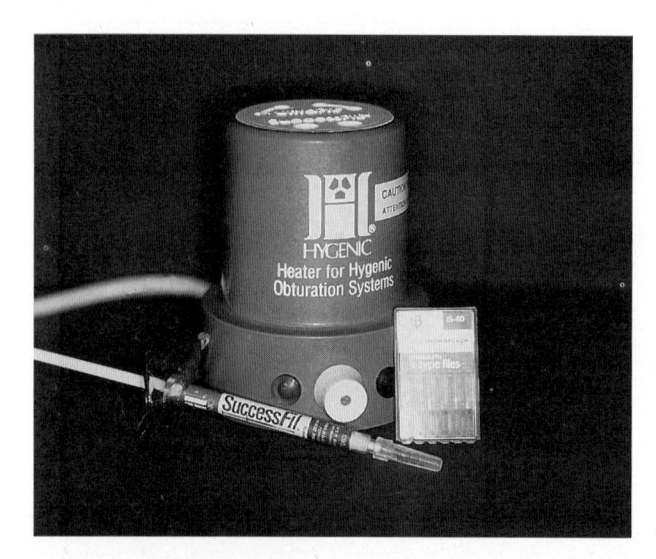

Figure 7-14 Armamentarium for Trifecta technique: syringe, heater, and K-files.

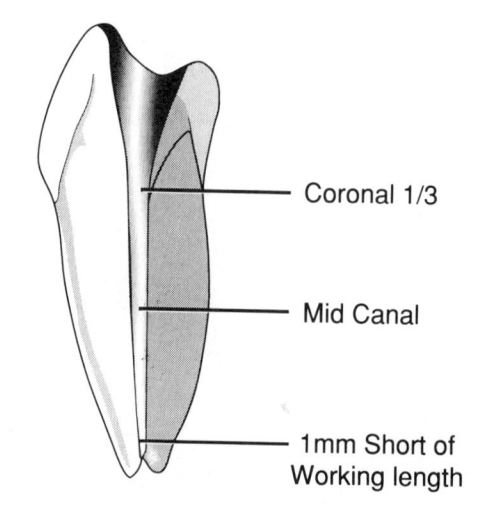

Figure 7-15 Pluggers are prefit for apical, middle, and gingival third.

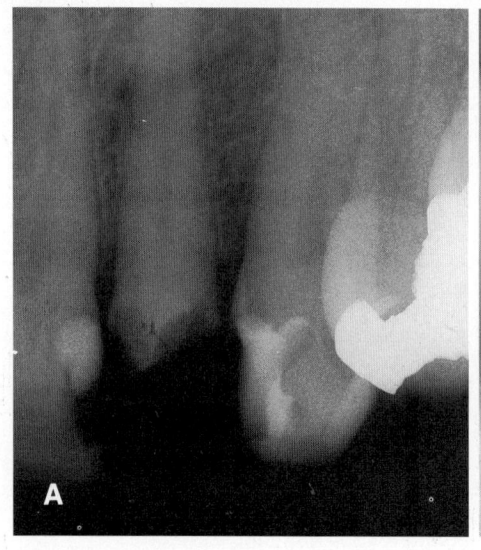

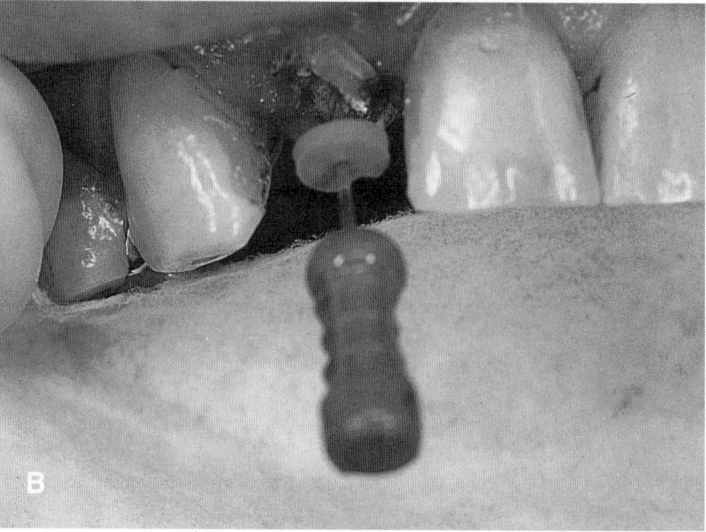

Figure 7-16 **A,** Radiograph of tooth No. 7 with fractured crown with narrow apex. **B,** A K-file 1 size smaller than the last file used in the canal.

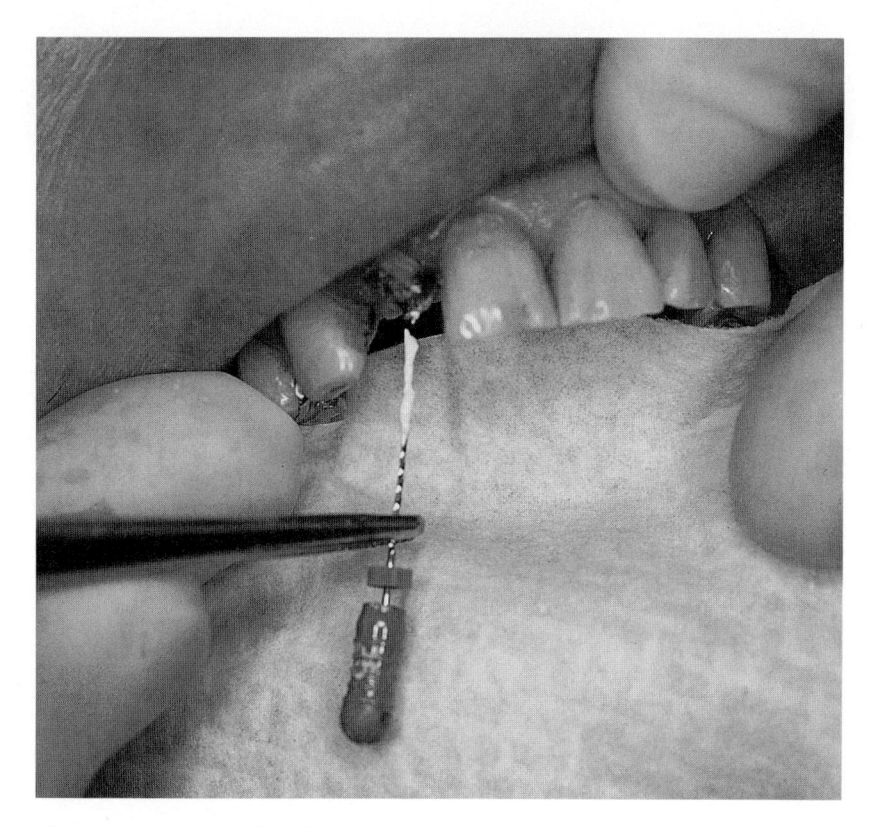

Chapter 7 ♦ Low Temperature Thermoplasticized Gutta Percha (Ultrafil) 155

Figure 7-17 Sealer placed in canal with reamer.

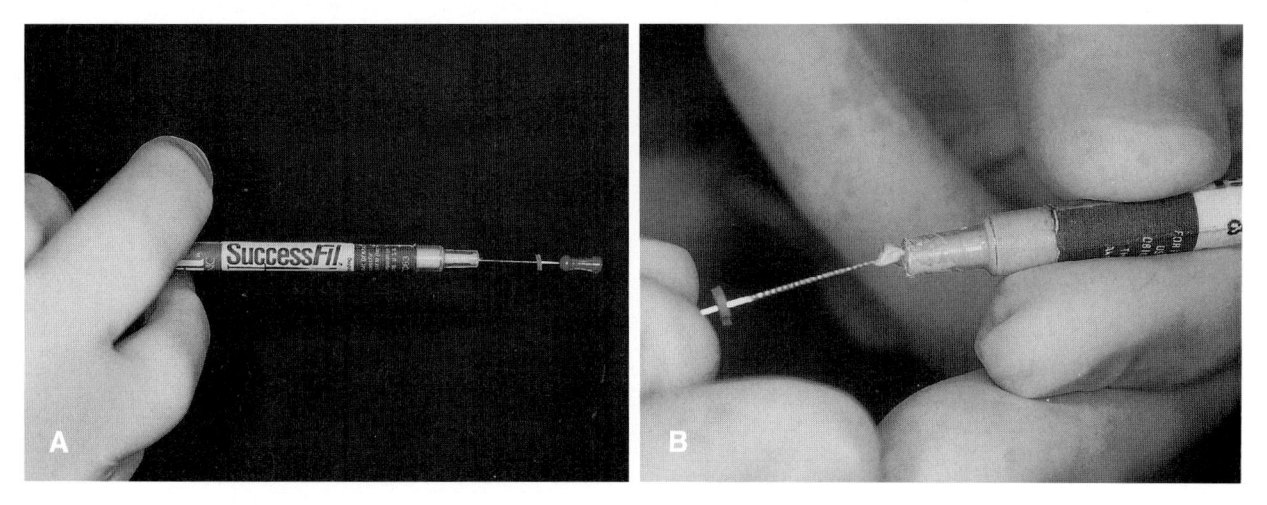

Figure 7-18 A, K-file placed in heated syringe 2 to 3 mm. **B,** K-file is injected with 2 to 3 mm of gutta percha.

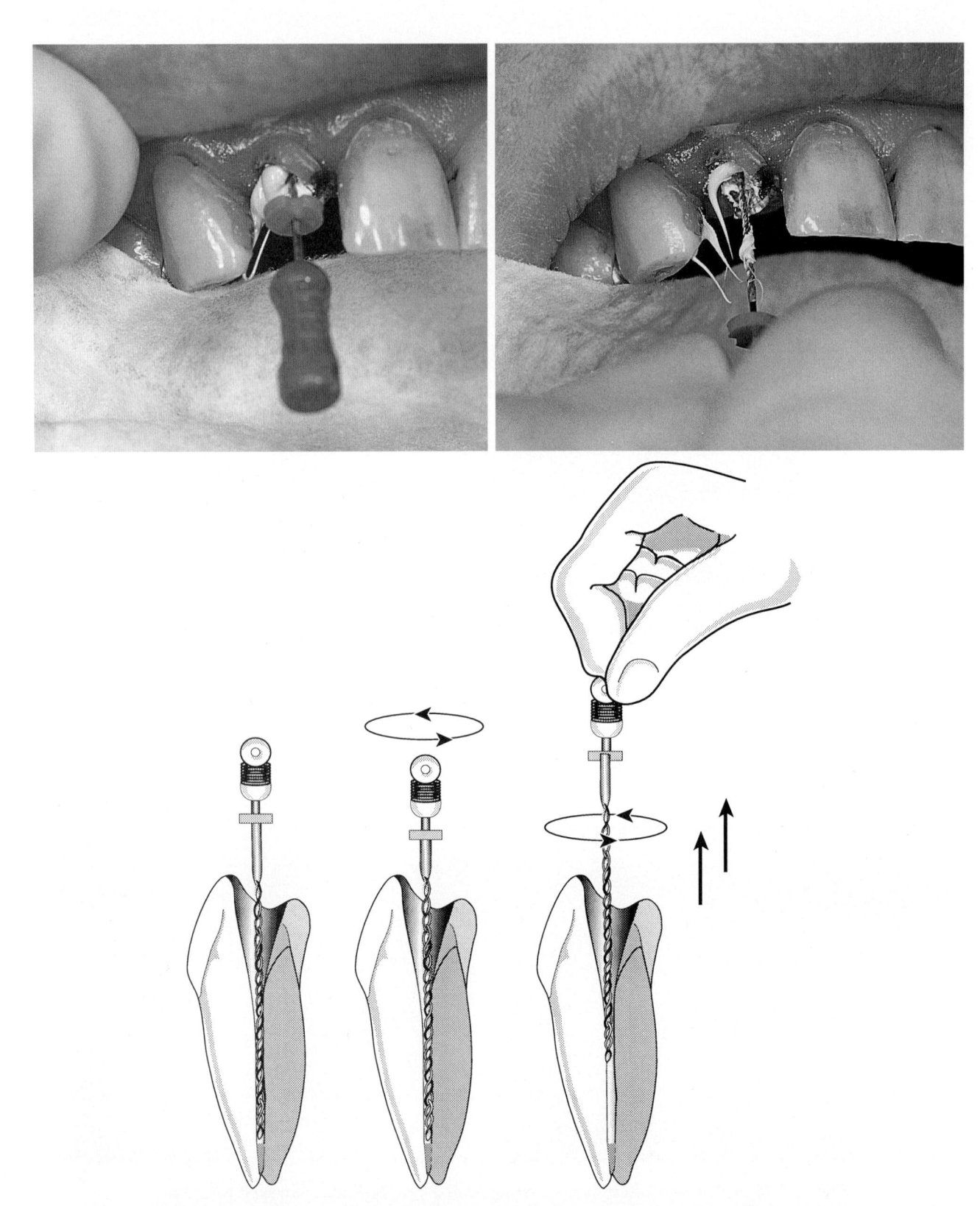

Figure 7-19 Without twisting, immediately insert instrument with the gutta percha–coated tip into the canal to the working length. Immediately twist instrument counterclockwise, leaving gutta percha in the apex.

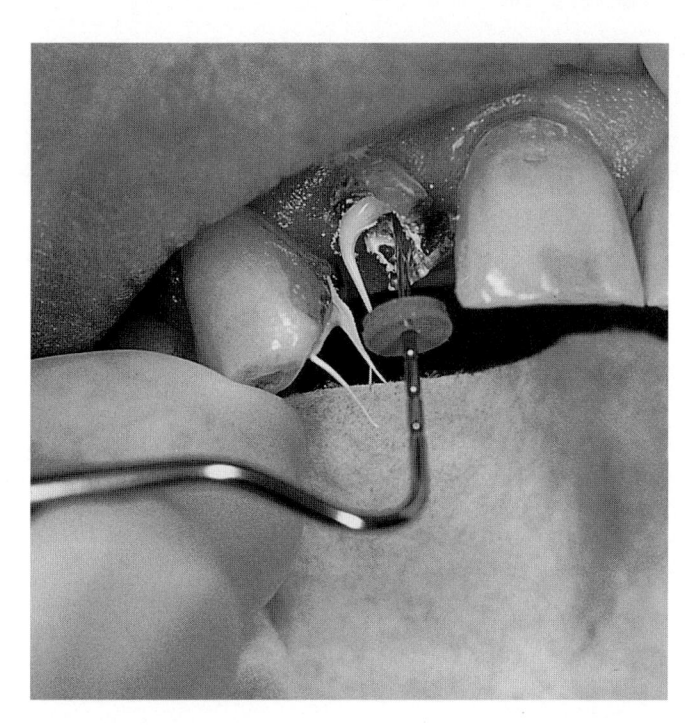

Figure 7-20 Gutta percha condensed with prefit plugger in apical third. The gutta percha is condensed with short up and down strokes.

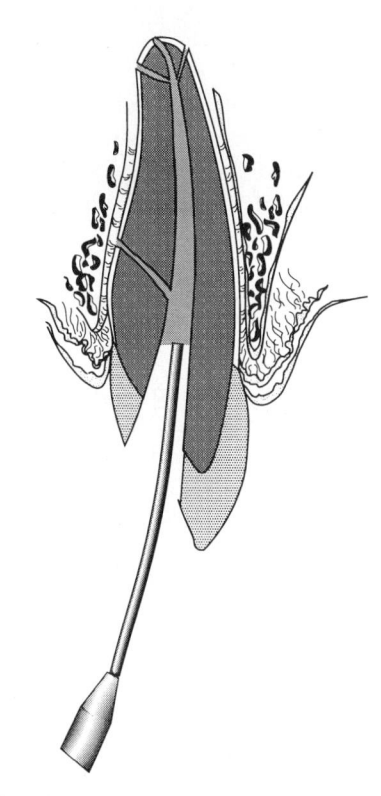

Figure 7-21 Regular set or Firm set is injected into canal.

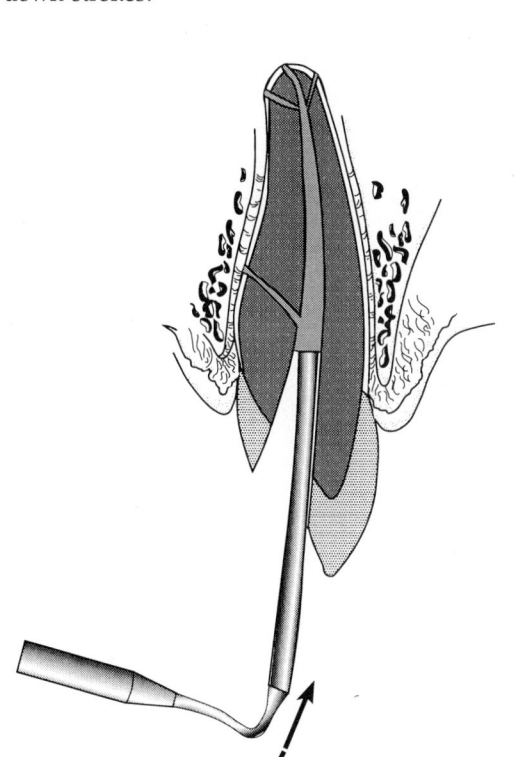

Figure 7-22 The gutta percha is condensed in the middle third and gingival third with the prefit pluggers.

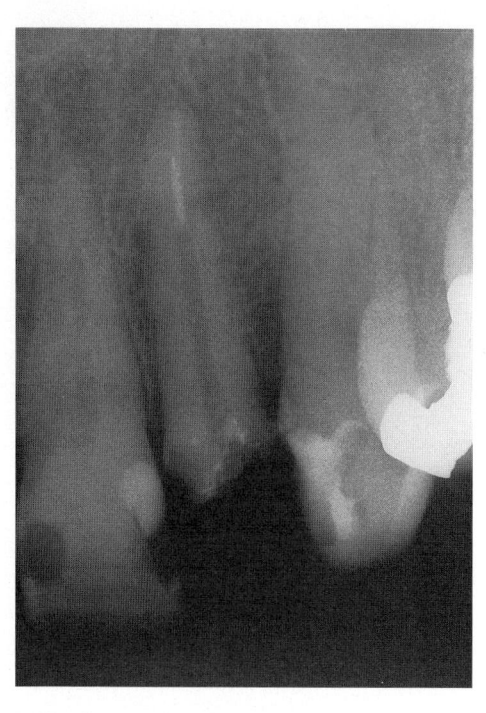

Figure 7-23 The canal was prepared for a post.

RETROGRADE FILLINGS WITH FIRM SET AND ENDOSET

The Firm set and Endoset gutta percha have relatively fast setting times that have proven to be well-suited for retrograde restorations (Fig. 7-24). The technique is outlined in Chapter 12, Surgical Endodontics (see Fig. 12-16).

Factors That Enhance The Flow Of Gutta Percha

- *Heat:* The optimum flow temperature is 70° C and is determined by a preset, thermostatically controlled heater at 90° C and allows for heat loss immediately before injection.
- *Viscosity:* As gutta percha is heated the viscosity is decreased and the flow is increased.
- *Canal diameter:* The canal should be enlarged to receive a 22-gauge needle in the gingival third. The smaller the canal, the greater the apical flow.

Factors that Affect the Flow Adversely

- *Air entrapment:* A tight-fitting needle may cause air entrapment and short fillings.
- *Oversize canals:* May cause backward flow of gutta percha around needle and cause filling to be short.
- *Debris:* May cause deflection and early backflow, causing short fillings and voids.
- *Moisture:* Cools the gutta percha and restricts flow.
- *Heat loss:* The canals should be injected within 60 to 70 seconds after removal of cannula from heater.

Factors that Control Flow

- *Apical constriction:* The narrowness of the apical foramen restricts the flow.
- *Amount* of gutta percha injected.
- *Depth* of needle insertion.
- *Apical barrier:* Should the foramen be compromised or overinstrumented, an apical stop can be made with dentin filings, calcium hydroxide, a master cone, or Successfil.

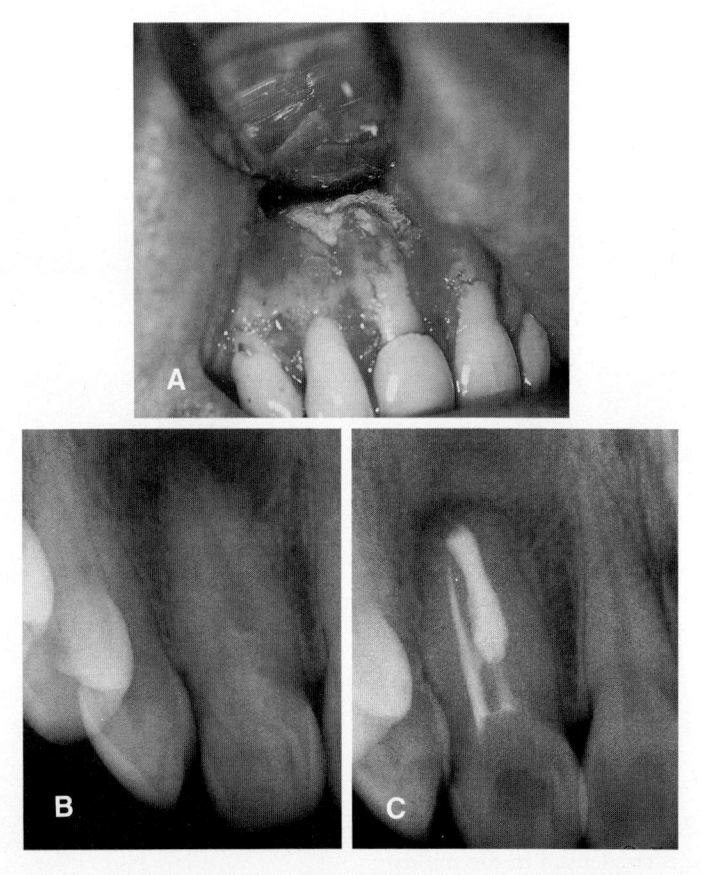

Figure 7-24 **A,** A retrograde Endoset Ultrafil gutta percha filling. Note lack of excess filling material. **B,** A maxillary lateral incisor with an apical periodontitis and dens in dente. **C,** Following surgery the large main canal is filled with Endoset. The secondary distal canal is filled with Firm set. The narrow central canal is filled with Regular set.

8

Comparison of Other Filling Techniques

The primary goal in root canal therapy is the cleansing and shaping of the root canal system. Once this has been accomplished, it makes little difference which technique is used in the obturation of the root canal. This chapter will deal with alternative methods of filling canals. Each one of these techniques can be used routinely. Cases will be presented, however, to show the advantages of the specific technique used in the given situation.

VERTICAL CONDENSATION WITH WARM GUTTA PERCHA (Fig. 8-1)

The warm gutta percha technique is useful in (Fig. 8-3):
1. Filling auxiliary canals
2. Filling internal resorption

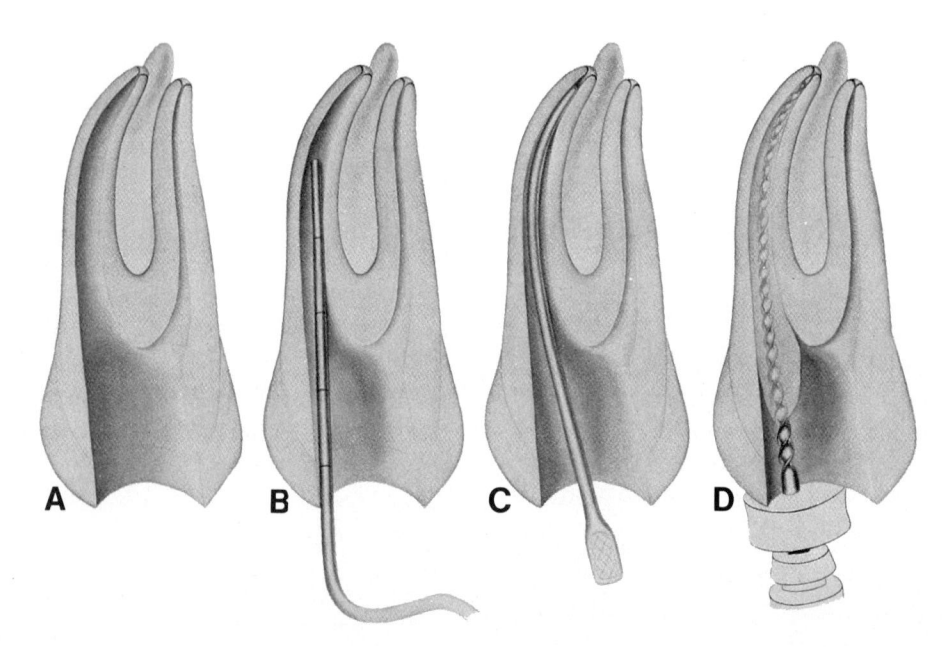

Figure 8-1 Warm gutta percha technique. **A,** Root canal cleansed and shaped. **B,** Fitting of plugger in apical third. Plugger must fit loosely and not touch any part of the dentinal wall. All pluggers being used in the apical, middle, and coronal third of the canal must be selected ahead of time to make sure they fit loosely. **C,** Fitting of gutta percha cone. The gutta percha cone is fitted until it binds 2 mm at radiographic apex and tugback is felt. **D,** Root canal cement is placed in the canal with a No. 15 file. The walls of the canal are coated with cement. **E,** The fitted gutta percha cone is cemented in place. **F,** A heat carrier heated red hot is used to remove excess gutta percha down to orifice of the canal. **G,** While the gutta percha is still warm, a cold plugger is used to condense the gutta percha vertically. The plugger used was selected before the gutta percha was fitted and was determined to fit loosely at the coronal third of the canal. The plugger must be in the gutta percha at all times and not touch the walls of the canal. **H,** A heat carrier heated red hot is stabbed into the gutta percha and quickly removed. **I,** A cold plugger that was fitted in the middle third of the canal is used to condense the gutta percha vertically. **J,** A heat carrier is again heated red hot, stabbed into the remaining gutta percha, and quickly removed. **K,** A cold plugger that was fitted in the apical third of the canal is used to condense the gutta percha vertically. **L,** Approximately 5 mm of gutta percha should remain after condensation. The rest of the canal is filled to the desired height with segments of gutta percha. A heat carrier is heated red hot, and a segment of gutta percha is attached to the heat carrier and placed into the canal and twisted off the carrier. **M,** A cold plugger fitted in the apical third is used to condense the gutta percha vertically. This procedure is repeated until the total canal is filled to 1 mm below the orifice or, if post space is desired, left to the desired length.

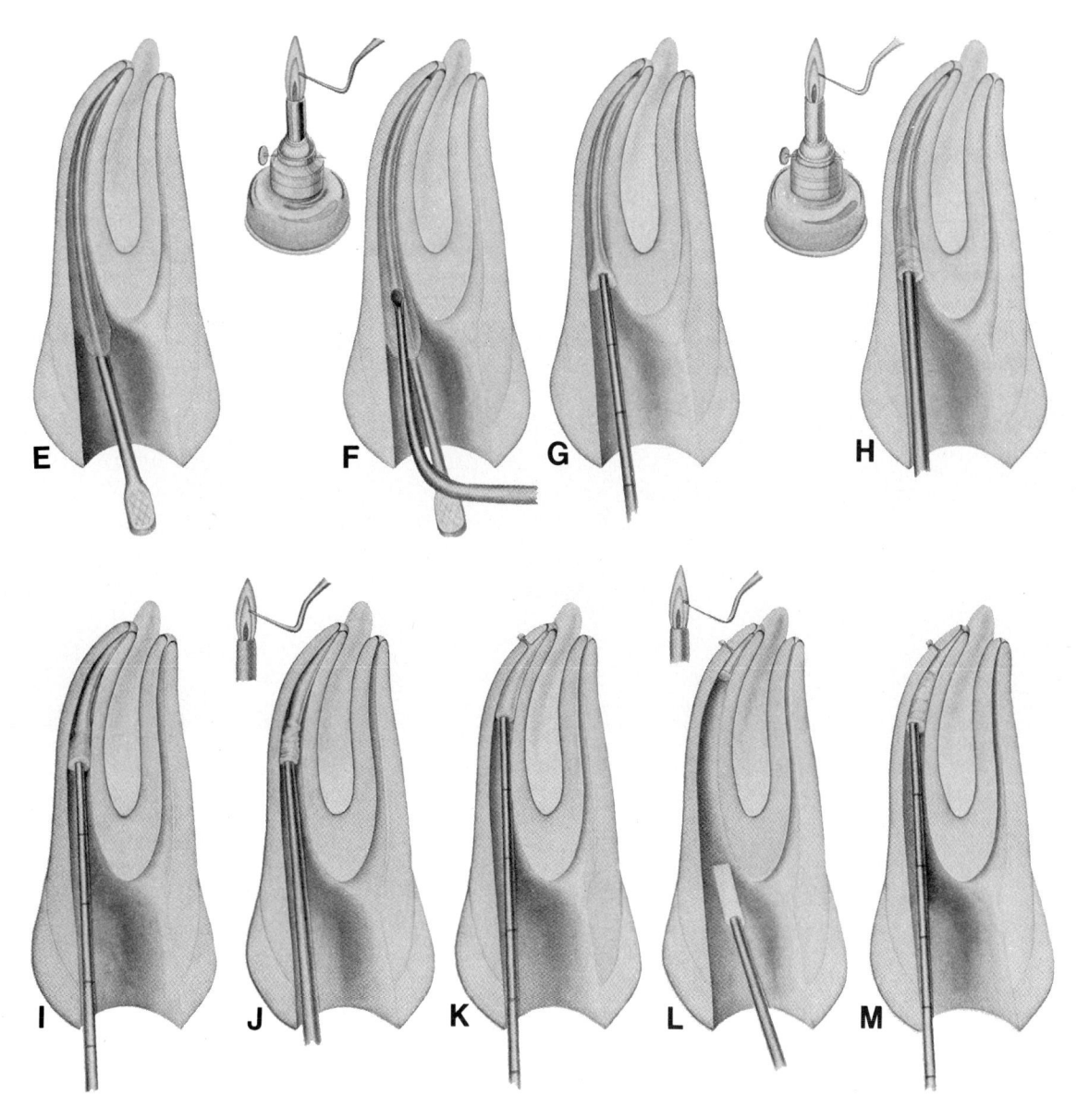

Chapter 8 ♦ Comparison of Other Filling Techniques   161

Figure 8-1, *cont'd* For complete legend, see opposite page.

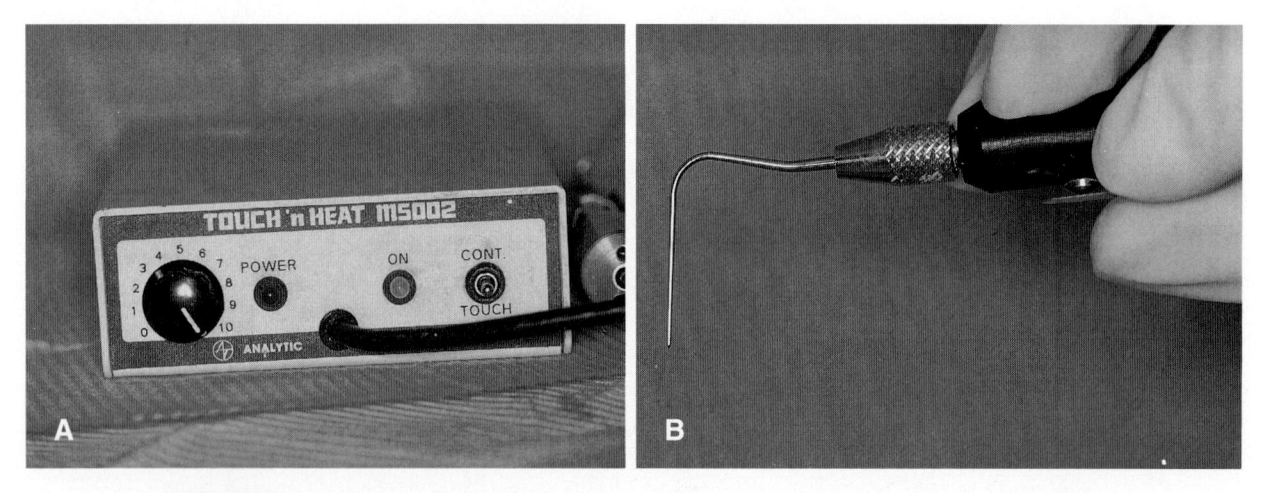

Figure 8-2 Touch 'n Heat instrument (Analytic Technology) can be substituted for the flame and heat carrier instrument. **A,** Touch 'n Heat device. **B,** Heat tip carrier. (Analytic Technology Corp., Redmond, WA.)

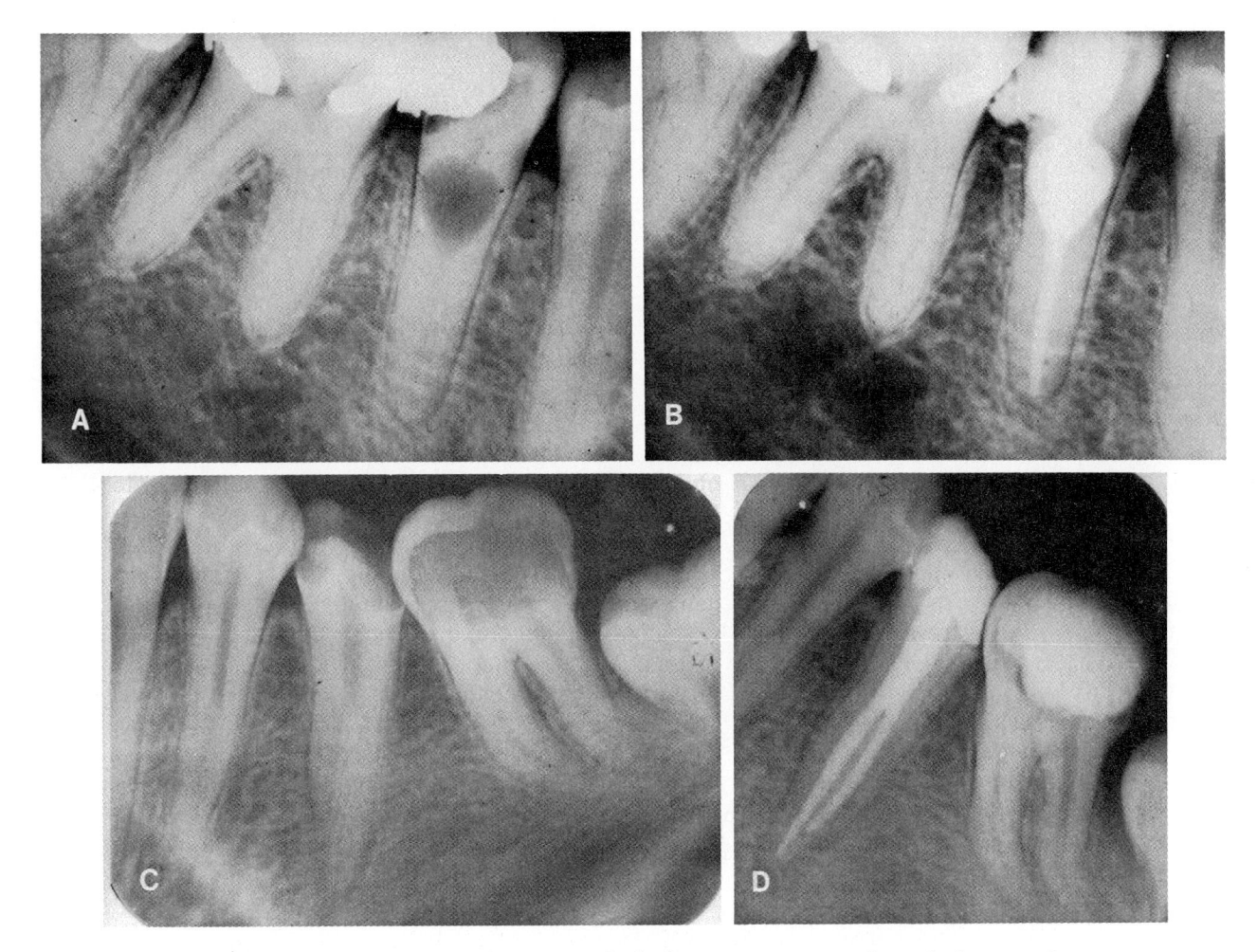

Figure 8-3 Two examples of cases in which the warm gutta percha technique can be extremely useful. **A,** Internal resorption in coronal third of canal. **B,** Root canal filled with the warm gutta percha technique. **C,** A bifurcated root canal in the middle third of the root. **D,** Root canal filled with the warm gutta percha technique.

VERTICAL CONDENSATION WITH CHLOROPERCHA (Figs. 8-4 and 8-6)

The chloropercha technique is useful in the following (Figs. 8-5 and 8-7):
1. Filling auxiliary canals
2. Unusual canal curvatures
3. Anatomical anomalies
4. Bypassing a ledged canal
5. Bypassing a broken instrument

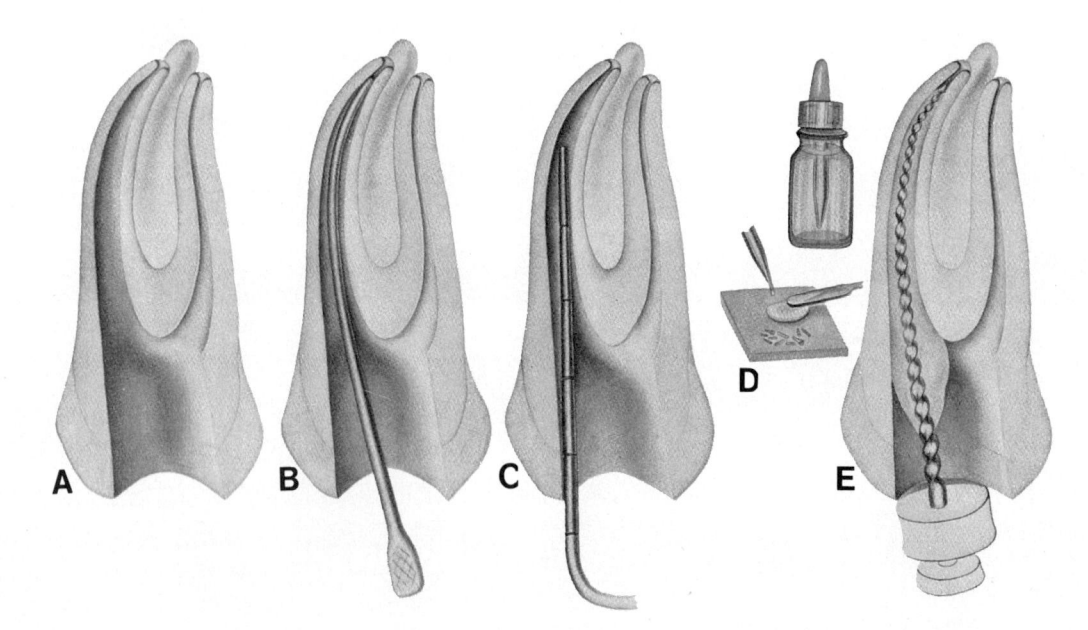

Figure 8-4 Vertical condensation with chloropercha. **A**, Root canal cleansed and shaped. **B**, Fitting of gutta percha cone 2 mm from radiographic apex and feeling tugback. **C**, Fitting of plugger in apical third. Plugger must fit loosely and not touch any part of the dentinal wall. All pluggers being used in the apical, middle, and coronal third of the canal must be selected ahead of time to make sure they fit properly. **D**, Chloroform and segments of gutta percha are mixed together to a creamy consistency. **E**, The chloropercha cement is placed in the canal by using a No. 15 file. **F**, A heat carrier is heated red hot, and a segment of gutta percha is attached to the heat carrier. **G**, The gutta percha segment is carried into the canal and twisted off. **H**, A cold plugger that was prefitted in the apical third of the canal is used to condense the gutta percha vertically. **I**, The heat carrier is again heated red hot, and another segment of gutta percha is attached to the heat carrier. **J**, The gutta percha segment is carried into the canal and twisted off. **K**, A cold plugger that was prefitted in the middle third of the canal is used to condense the gutta percha vertically to the last segment of gutta percha. **L**, The heat carrier is heated red hot, and another segment of gutta percha is attached to the heat carrier. **M**, The gutta percha segment is carried into the canal and twisted off. **N**, A cold plugger that was prefitted in the coronal third of the canal is used to condense the gutta percha vertically to the last segment of gutta percha. This procedure is continued until the whole canal is filled to the desired height.

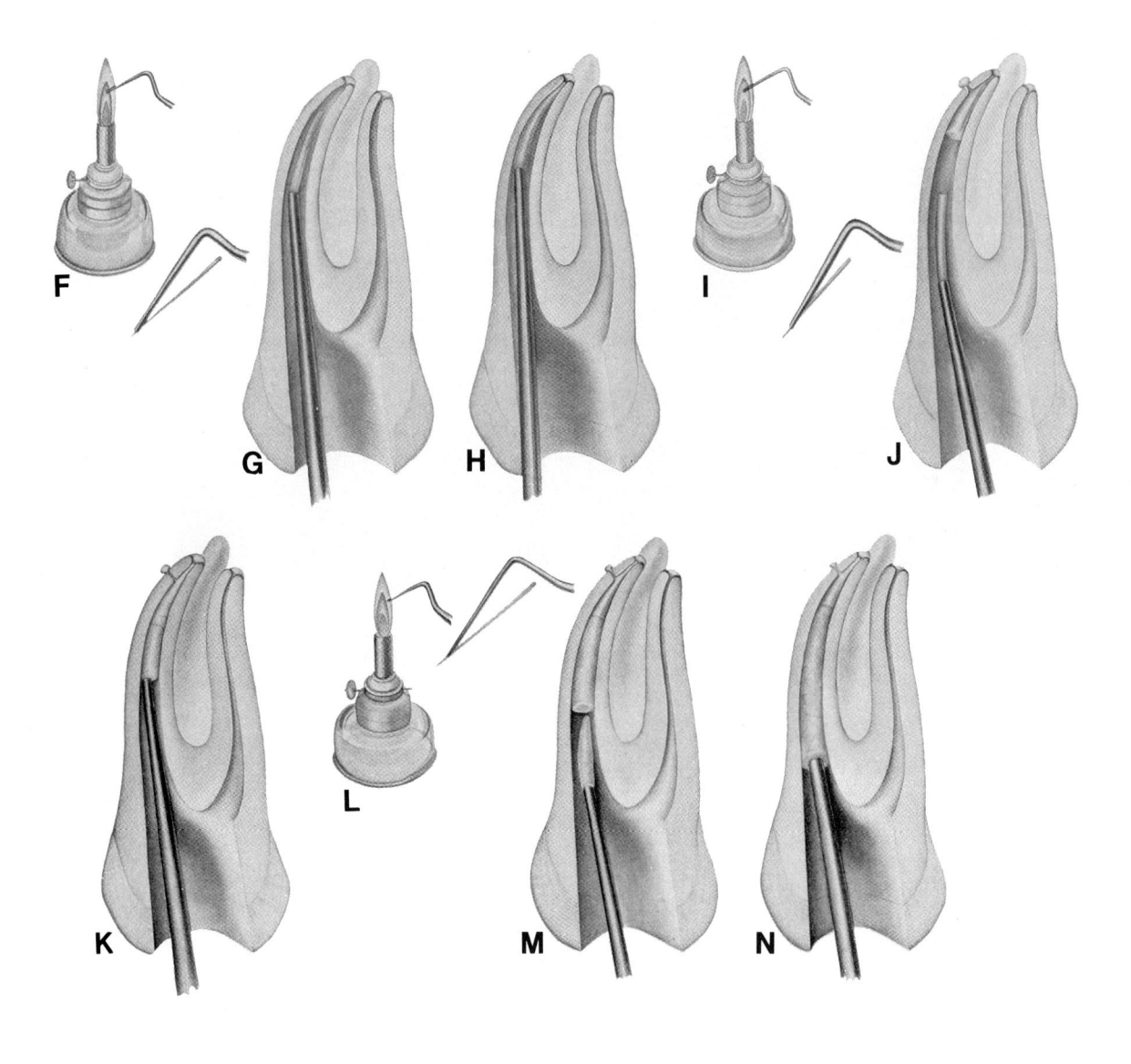

Chapter 8 ♦ Comparison of Other Filling Techniques 165

F

G

H

I

J

K

L

M

N

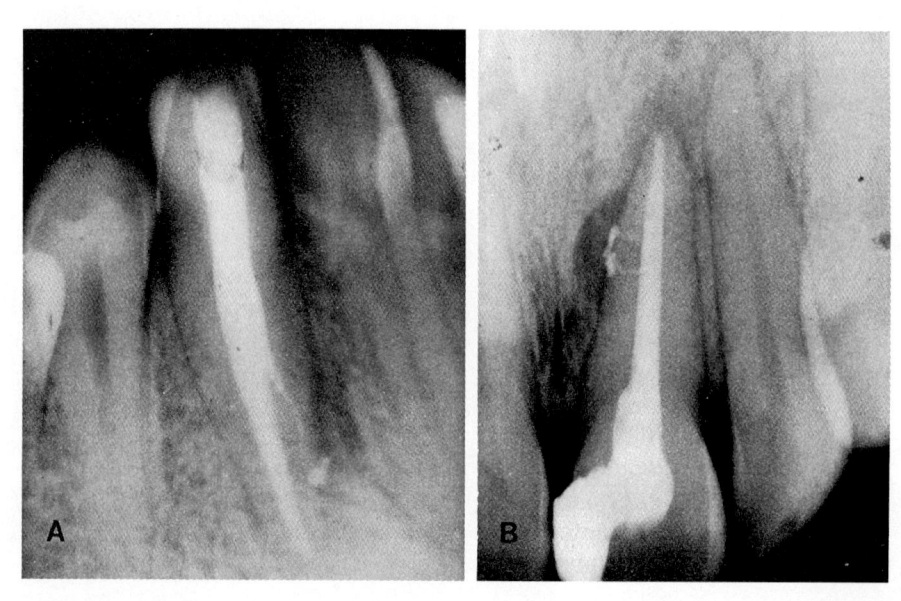

Figure 8-5 Examples of cases in which the chloropercha technique can be extremely useful. **A,** A mandibular cuspid with an accessory canal. **B,** Maxillary central with two accessory canals in the middle third of root. Accessory canals were anticipated because of lateral lesion.

Chapter 8 ♦ Comparison of Other Filling Techniques 167

LATERAL CONDENSATION WITH CHLOROPERCHA

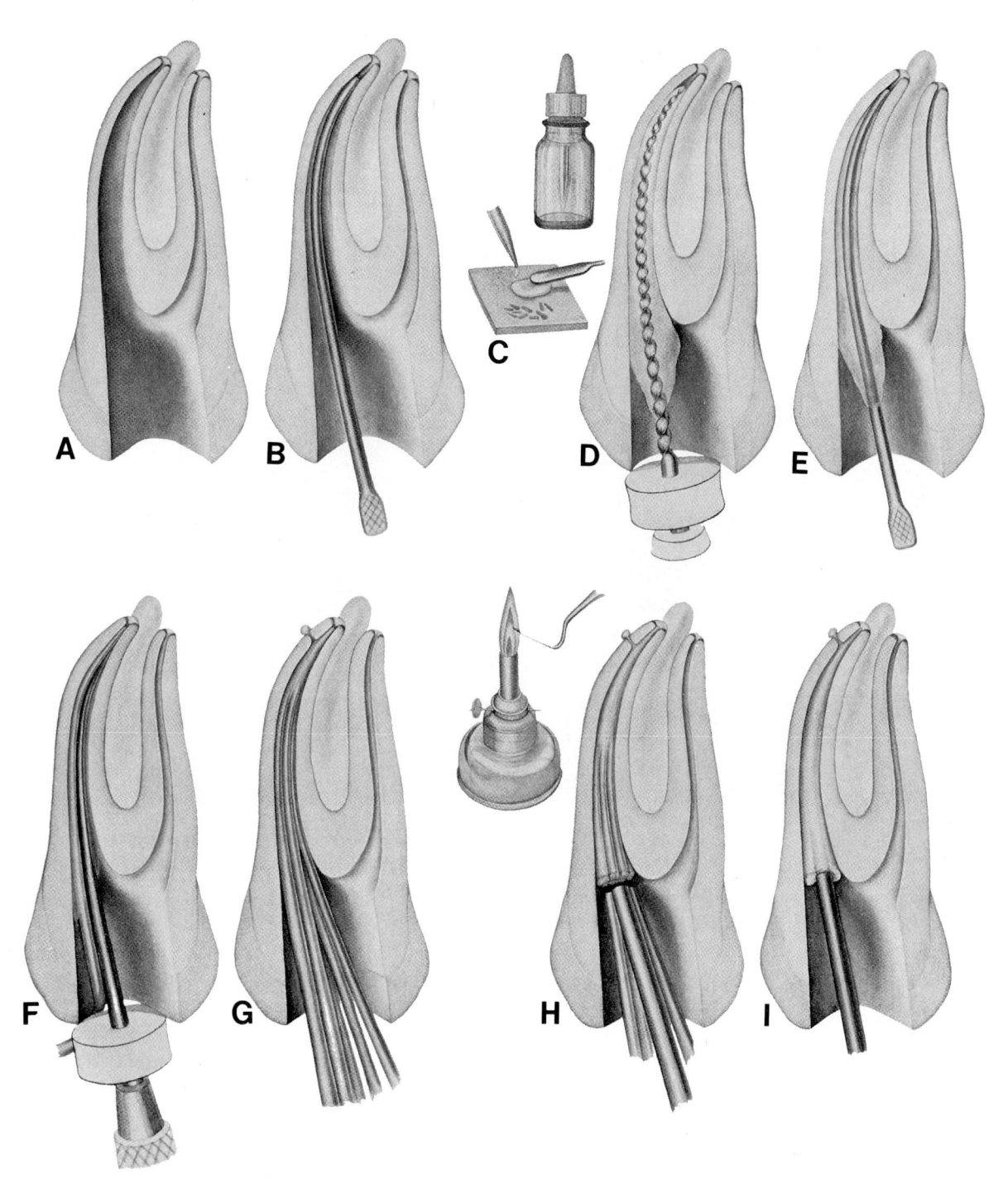

Figure 8-6 Lateral condensation with chloropercha. **A,** Root canal cleansed and shaped. **B,** Fitting of gutta percha cone 2 mm from radiographic apex and tugback felt. **C,** Chloroform and segments of gutta percha are mixed together to a creamy consistency. **D,** The chloropercha cement is placed in the canal by using a No. 15 file. **E,** Fitted gutta percha cone is positioned in place. **F,** A finger spreader is used to condense the gutta percha laterally. **G,** Accessory gutta percha cones are packed into the canal after the finger spreader is used until no more room is left for any more gutta percha cones. **H,** A hot heat carrier is used to remove the excess gutta percha below the level of the orifice. **I,** A cold plugger is used to condense the gutta percha apically.

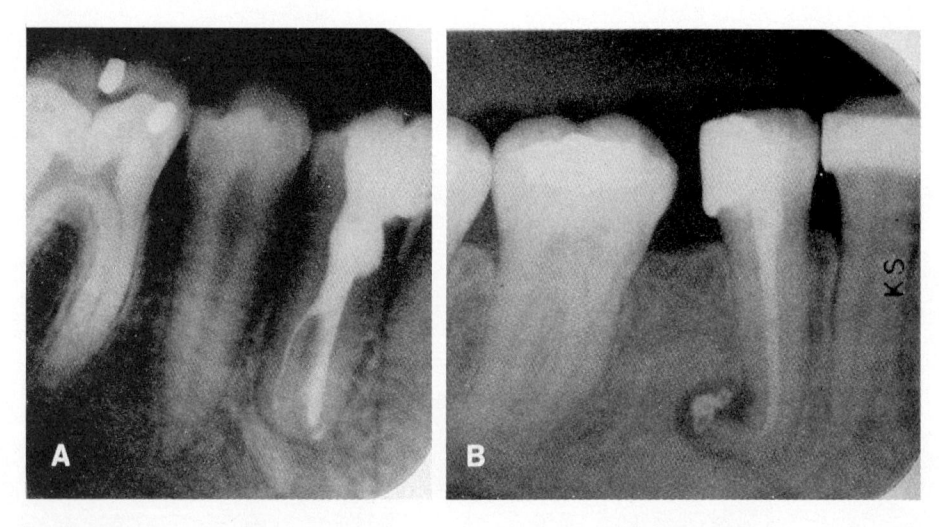

Figure 8-7 Two examples of cases in which the chloropercha technique can be extremely useful. **A,** A mandibular first bicuspid with two canals that bifurcate at the apical third. **B,** A mandibular second bicuspid with a severely curved canal.

CUSTOMIZED GUTTA PERCHA POINT (Fig. 8-8)

The customized cone technique is useful in the following (Fig. 8-9):
1. Large canal
2. Canal with irregularities

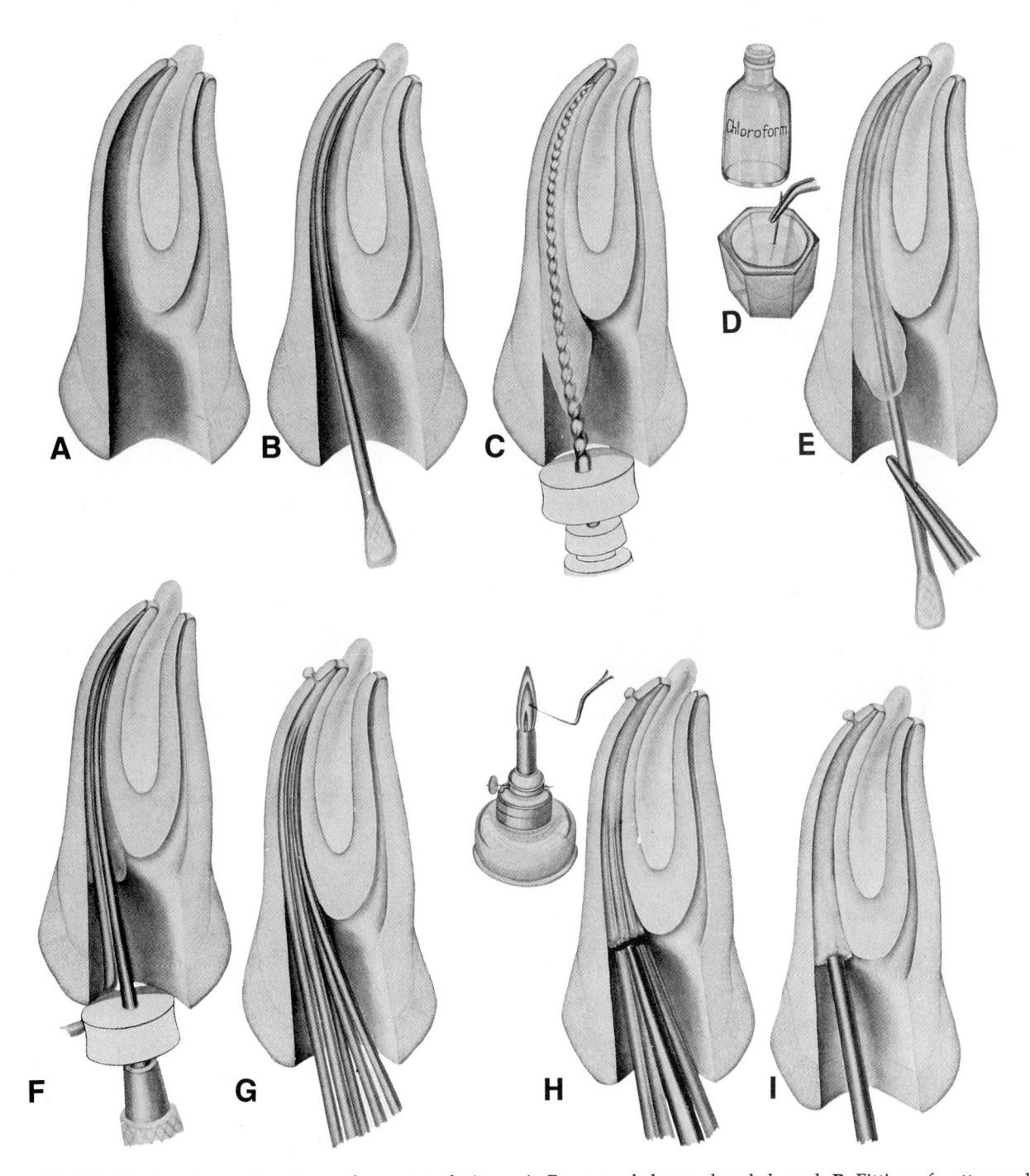

Figure 8-8 Modified customized gutta percha cone technique. **A,** Root canal cleansed and shaped. **B,** Fitting of gutta percha cone 2 mm from radiographic apex, where tugback is felt. **C,** The cement is placed in the canal by using a No. 15 file. **D,** Fitted gutta percha cone is placed in chloroform for 5 seconds. **E,** Softened gutta percha cone is then placed in the canal until it binds. **F,** A finger spreader is used to condense the gutta percha laterally. **G,** Accessory gutta percha cones are packed into canal after finger spreader is used until no more room is left for any more gutta percha cones. **H,** A hot heat carrier is used to remove excess gutta percha below the level of the orifice. **I,** A cold plugger is used to condense the gutta percha apically.

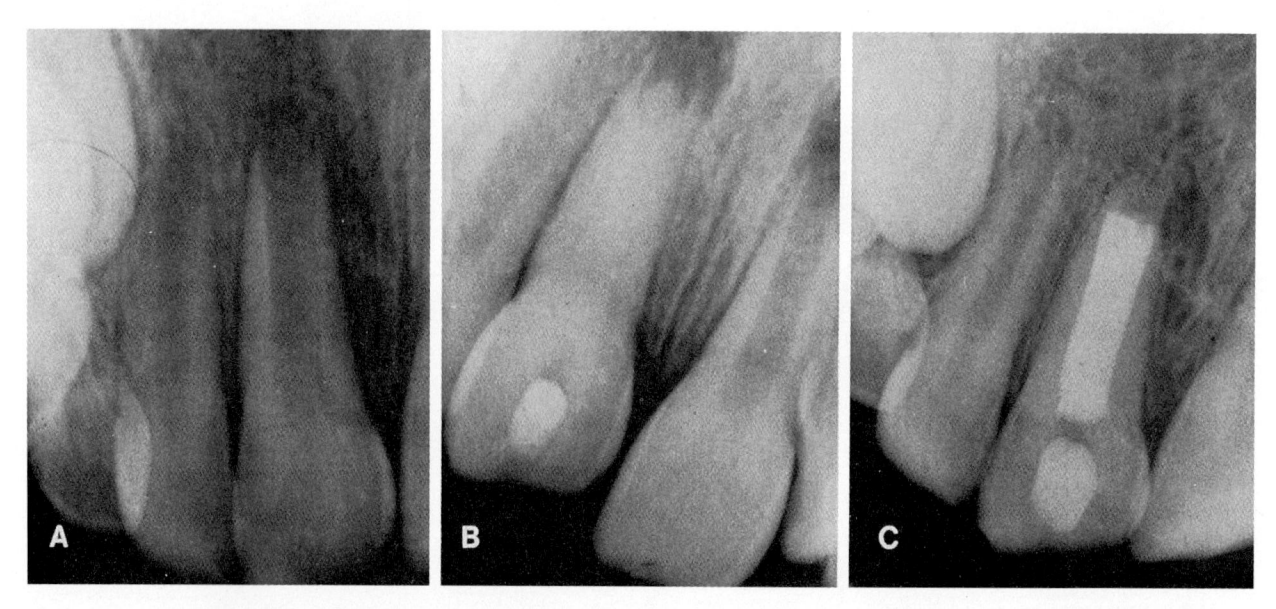

Figure 8-9 Example of a case in which the customized gutta percha cone technique can be extremely useful. **A,** A maxillary central incisor with a wide open apex that never had developed because of devitalization of the pulp. **B,** Apexification procedure using calcium hydroxide in the root canal space. **C,** Filling the root canal after the apex had formed using the customized gutta percha cone technique.

9

Restoration of the Endodontically Treated Tooth

After root canal therapy, the tooth is restored with a build-up to replace the missing tooth structure and a final coronal restoration to surround the root to protect it from fracture while restoring it to near natural function and aesthetics. A full-crowned, posterior endodontically treated tooth is 2 to 3 times stronger than a posterior tooth restored without a crown.

RESTORATIVE COMPONENTS

1. Post/dowel (optional) (Fig. 9-1, *A*)
2. Core (amalgam, glass ionomer, composite resin, gold) (Fig. 9-1, *B*)
3. Core retention (pins, slots, posts, adhesives)
4. Crown (provides the coping or ferrule effect) (Fig. 9-1, *C*)

POSTS

The main function of posts is retention and support of the core. They also minimally reinforce existing tooth structure and distribute occlusal forces along the root. Prefabricated posts are becoming the most popular posts used today. They have improved strength and greater retention when used with the newer adhesives, are easy to place, have less chance of root fracture, lessen the amount of tooth structure lost (thus providing increased ferrule), have better core framework for increased core retention, allow for immediate crown preparation, and have ease of temporization.

POST SIZE

Use the smallest diameter post possible. The post should only minimally alter the final shape of the root canal (Fig. 9-2). This increases tooth strength and reduces the chance of root fracture and post perforation. Wider posts do not improve retention or tooth strength. Once the gutta percha is removed with heat, make post space with a Peeso drill one size larger than the largest Peeso that fit passively in the canal. This Peeso is usually the same number size as the last size Gates Glidden bur used in the canal. Suggested post sizes are:

Peeso	Diameter	Teeth
2	0.9 mm	Mandibular incisors
3	1.1 mm	Premolar (with 2 canals)
		All molar canals
4	1.3 mm	Maxillary lateral incisor
		Premolars (with only one canal)
5	1.5 mm	Maxillary central incisor/cuspids

POST SELECTION GUIDELINES

1. Posts should be long enough to reach half the root length in bone.
2. Posts should be small sizes that minimally alter the final root canal diameter.
3. Posts should be made of strong material so the small diameter posts do not bend.

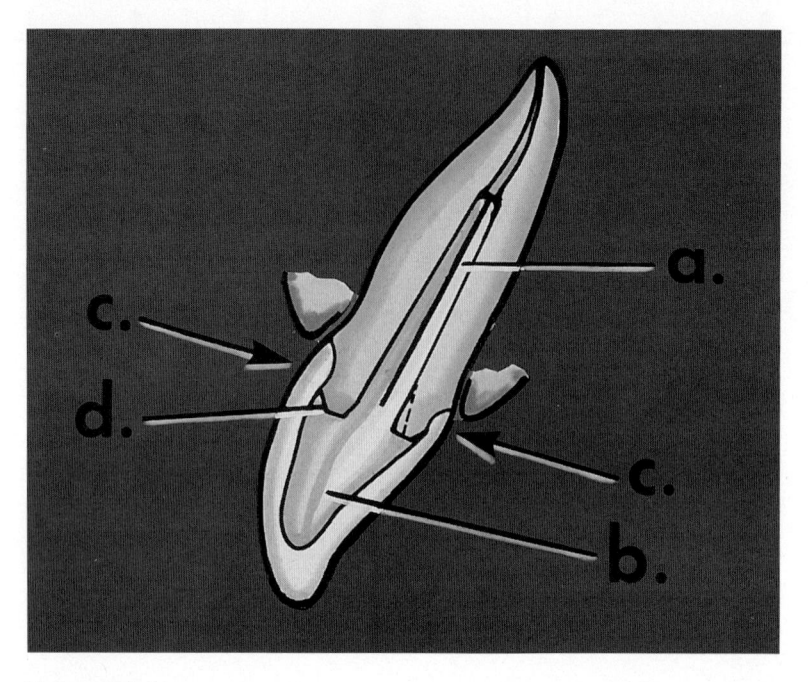

Figure 9-1

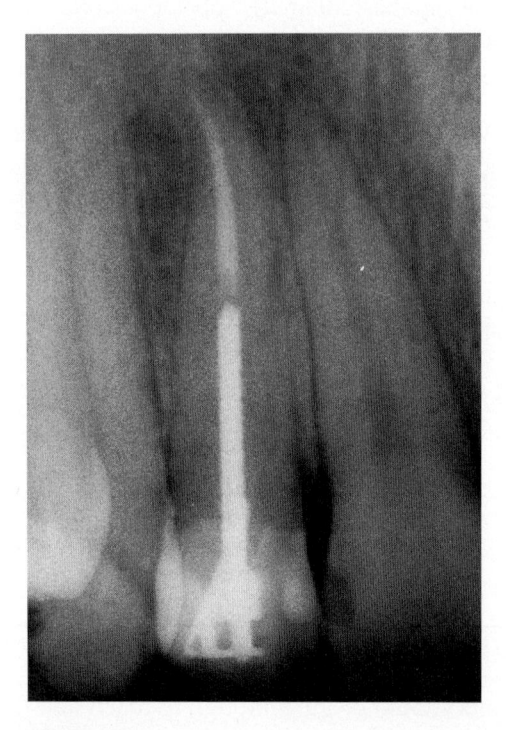

Figure 9-2

4. Posts should be parallel, etched (roughen), and vented.
5. Posts should fit passively.
6. Post sizes should be standardized to fit in corresponding Peeso drill holes.
7. Posts should have a retentive core frame to support and retain the core.

A few of the better post systems on the market today that meet these requirements are the Versadowel (Western Dental Specialty), Ad Post (J Morita), BCH Post (3M), ParaPost (Whaldent), and Beta Post (CTH Inc). Of these systems, the Versadowel system (Western Dental, 800-848-4880) is the only one that is cast and has the most ideal core frame. There are three differnt core frame designs that fit and support the coronal core material and remaining tooth structure of incisors, premolars, and molars. The Versadowel is cast from a stronger stainless steel than other stainless steel posts, which are cut out of a weaker steel blank. Thus smaller sizes can be used, which results in less tooth loss.

The Versadowel comes in four sizes, corresponding to standard Peeso reamer sizes No. 2 to 5. The three different series (Fig. 9-3), from *left* to *right*, the "A" series was designed to fit and support the remaining coronal tooth structure of anterior teeth. Note the framework is thin enough that the metal does not show through. The "U" series is a universal design for placement in posterior teeth. The "M" series is intended for palatal and distal canals in molars. For ease of placement, the Versadowel can be quickly modified to fit within any remaining coronal tooth structure.

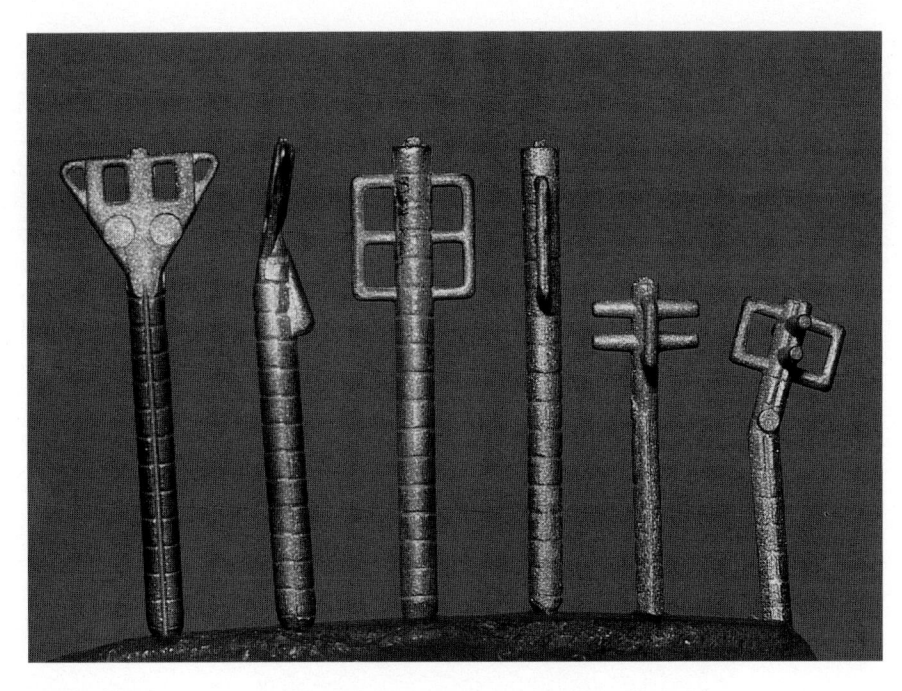

Figure 9-3

TECHNIQUE

Initial Preparation

Remove all carious dentin and unwanted preexisting restorative material to ensure direct line access for the dowel (Fig. 9-4, *A* and *B*). This will include removal of incisal overhangs that sometimes restrict proper placement (Fig. 9-4, *C*).

Gutta Percha Removal and Peeso Selection

Gutta percha can be removed with a hot heat carrier and or a Peeso reamer. The apical seal will not be lost with either technique as long as 5 to 7 mm of gutta percha remains at the apex. Conservation of remaining tooth structure is essential in maintaining the overall strength of the tooth. Canal shape and diameter dictates the size of the Peeso reamer to be used as well as the preparation length. The correct Peeso reamer is selected by comparing sizes over the final radiograph and selecting one that slightly enlarges the canal. If Gates Glidden drills were used to shape the canal, then select a Peeso that is one number size smaller than the last Gates used. For example, a No. 4 Gates Glidden drill is the same size as a No. 3 Peeso reamer. The preselected Peeso reamer is introduced at full speed down the canal through the gutta percha. The dental assistant directs a steady stream of water at the orifice to improve cutting efficiency. Increments of gutta percha are removed from the canal by using the Peeso in an up and down motion while the water clears debris from the flutes (Fig. 9-4, *D*). Rubber stops can be placed on the Peeso for length control, ensuring that the post is at least one half the root length in bone. A lingual antirotational notch can be put in at this time (Fig. 9-4, *E*).

Dowel Selection

Select a dowel that corresponds to the same number Peeso reamer used and place in the canal (Fig. 9-4, *F*). A Boley gauge can be used to measure the excess coronal height and remove it from the apical end of the post (Fig. 9-4, *G*). Modify the dowel length and coronal frame with a wire cutters or high speed bur to customize the dowel to the tooth (Fig. 9-4, *H* and *I*). Place the dowel into the canal (Fig. 9-4, *J* and *K*) and take a radiograph to ensure the dowel fits to the depth of the gutta percha and that the apical portion of the gutta percha was not accidentally removed during Peeso preparation. Remove the dowel with a mosquito hemostat or locking plier and have ready for placement.

Prepare Canal Walls

Prepare the dentin for cementation with glass ionomer cement with a dentin conditioner (polyacrylic acid 10%) by placing it on a cotton-wrapped No. 40 broach (Fig. 9-4, *L*). Resin cements use a different etching agent (read manufacturer's instructions). Scrub the walls for 10 seconds and then have your assistant flush the canal for 30 seconds with the water syringe while you continue to scrub the walls (Fig. 9-

174 PRACTICAL ENDODONTICS

4, *L* and *M*). This will simultaneously wash the polyacrylic acid from the cotton and remove the remaining acid from the canal. Dry the canal with an air syringe and paper points (Fig. 9-4, *N*).

Cement

The choice of cements is up to the practitioner. Zinc phosphate cement has stood the test of time and is still used. Glass ionomer is becoming more popular as a post cementing medium because it is radiopaque, nonstaining, quick set, and relatively strong; it adheres to dentin and the dowel; it is biocompatible; it has low solubility after initial set; and it is used as both a cement and core material. Also glass ionomer cements offer the advantage of fluoride release and has the same expansion/contraction ratio as dentin eliminating the danger of recurrent caries. Once the pulp tissue has been removed, the remaining root is more vulnerable to decay. Resin cements such as Panavia (J Morita) are also becoming popular because they have the highest retention of all the post cements.

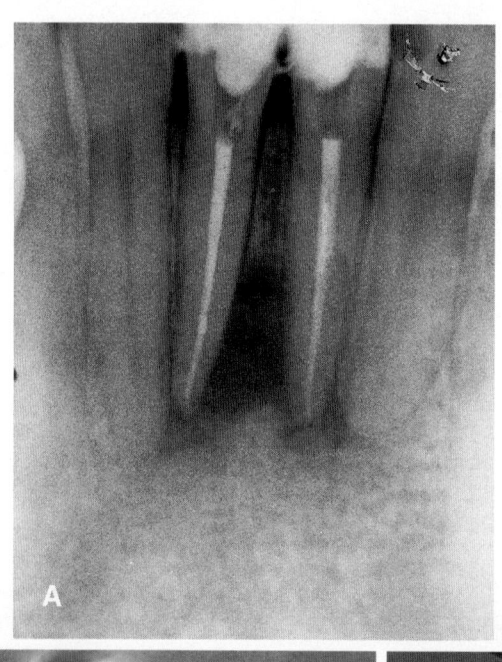

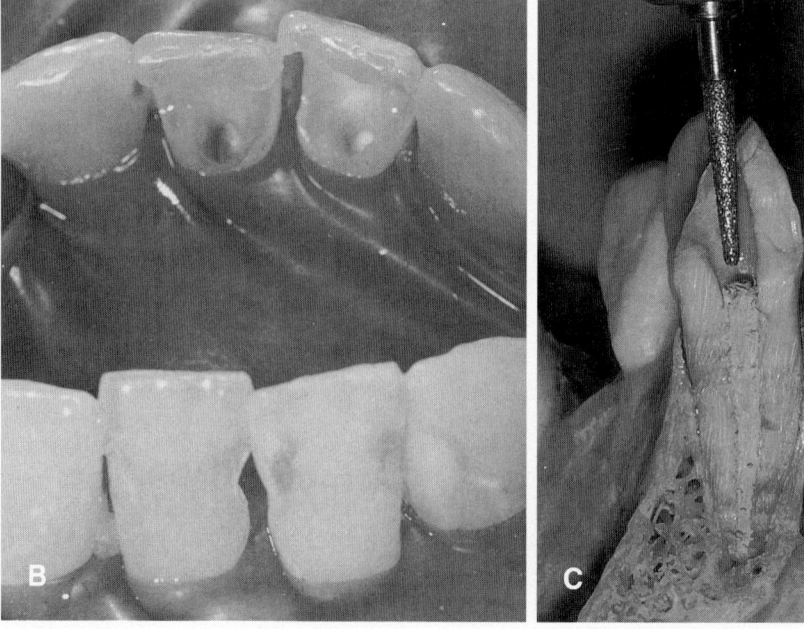

Figure 9-4, A-C

Cement Placement

Mix a reinforced glass ionomer cement such as Chelon Silver (Premier) and place it into a Centrix needle syringe tip, rubber bung placed, and loaded into a Centrix syringe. The tip is placed to the apical portion of the post preparation and injected while moving coronally filling up 80% of the canal (Fig. 9-4, *O* and *P*). Cements can also be placed with a large Lentulo Spiral.

Dowel Placement

Immediately place the dowel into the canal (Fig. 9-4, *Q*). Adjust post to proper position, remove excess cement (Fig. 9-4, *R*), and allow cement to set for 4 to 6 minutes.

Core Selection

Listed below are the strengths and weaknesses of each core material. Generally, composites and gold are used in anterior teeth. When the tooth is an abutment for a long bridge or there is little tooth retention or support, then amalgam or composites are used. Glass ionomer is usually used in a high caries patient, in subgingival defects, or in teeth with good coronal support.

- Cast Gold: High cost; multiple appointments; radiopaque; biocompatible; post/core/crown can be same material; high strength; technique sensitive.
- High Copper Spherical Amalgam: Low cost; fast set; radiopaque; early strength; high plasticity; ease of placement; low marginal seepage; greater chance of electrolytic reaction between post and

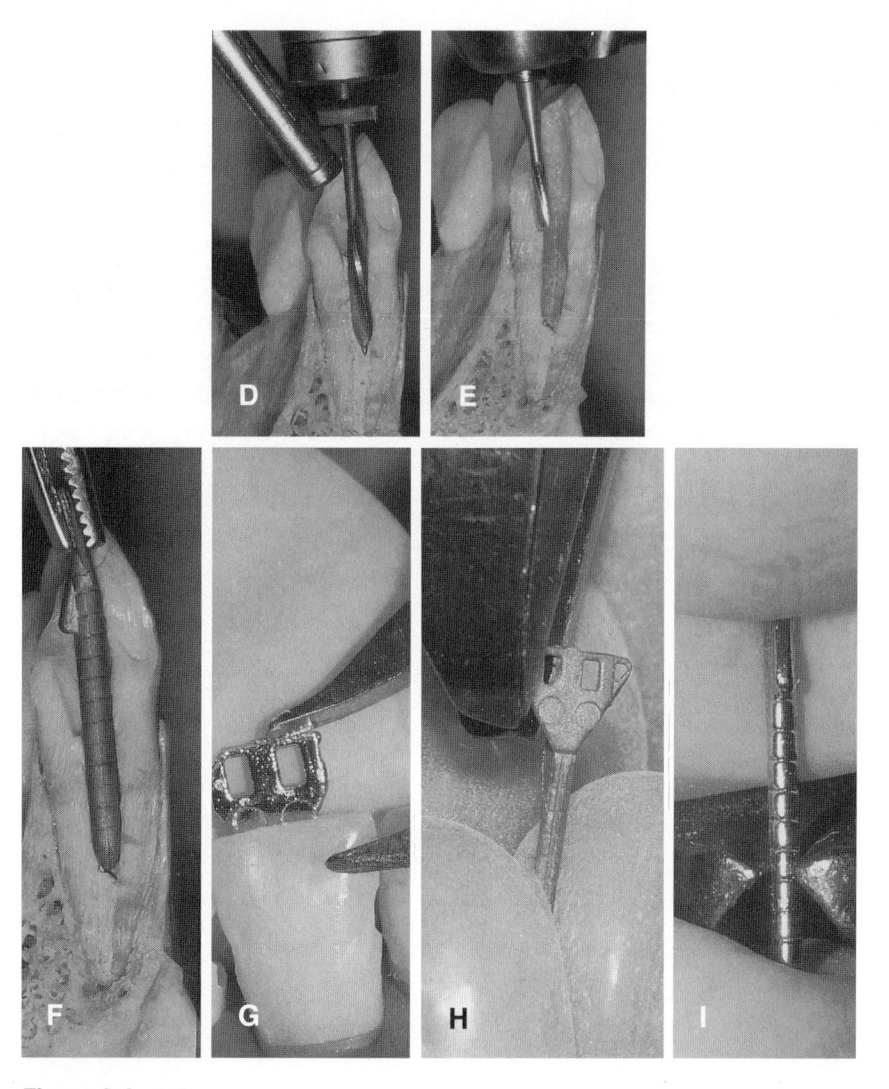

Figure 9-4, D-I

crown. *Suggested products:* Tytin (Kerr) or Valient (Caulk).
- Composite Resins: Fast set; low cost; early strength; easily syringed; high marginal seepage; can be made radiopaque; reduced electrolytic reaction. *Suggested products:* FluoroCore (Caulk) or Core Paste (Denmat). They have high compressive and tensile strength and are both dual curing.
- Reinforced Glass Ionomer: Caries resistant; biocompatible; easily placed and quickly prepared; adheres to cement, post, and dentin; can serve as a restoration for a period of time; strong if supported by remaining tooth structure and dowel frame; some are radiopaque; is initial water sensitive. *Suggested products:* Miricle Mix (GC) or Ketec Silver (Premier).

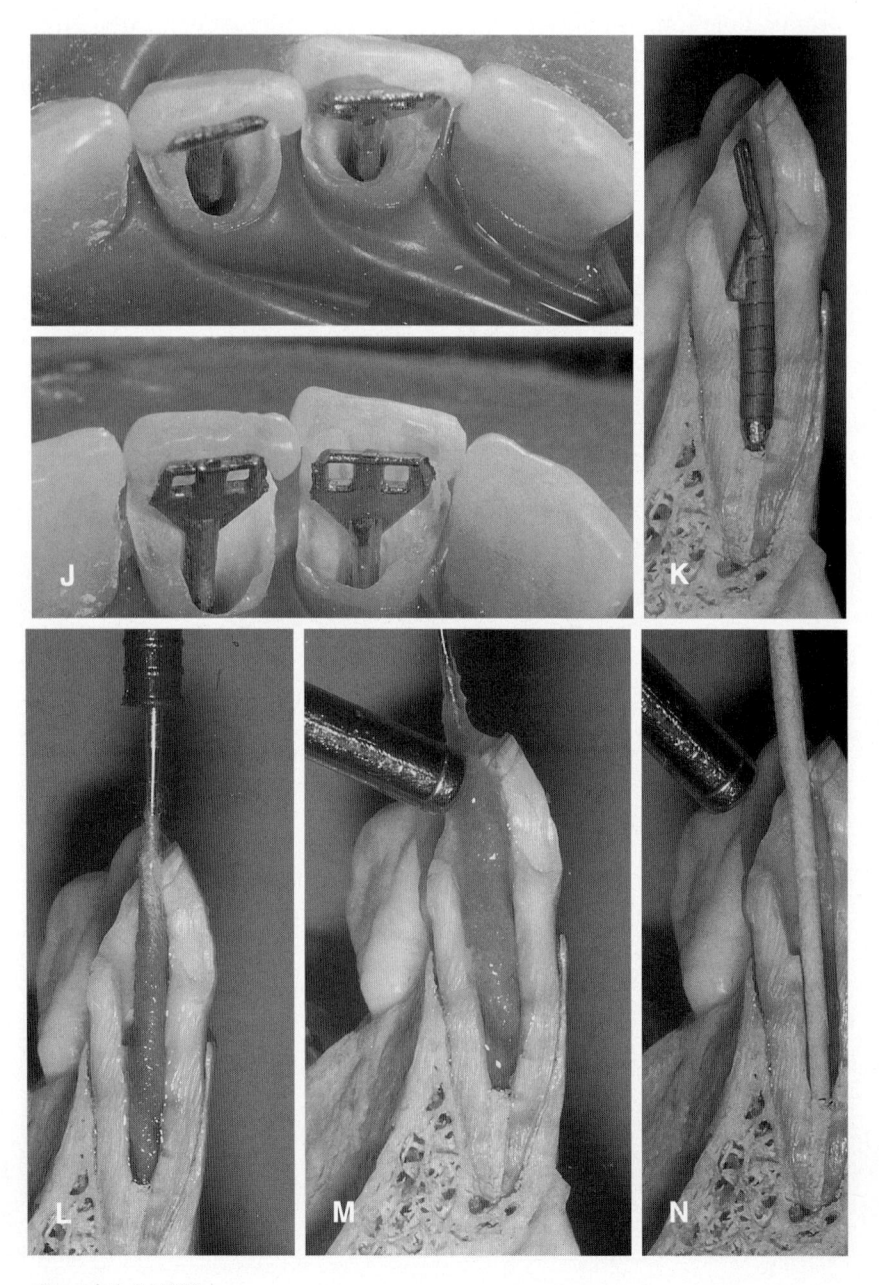

Figure 9-4, J-N

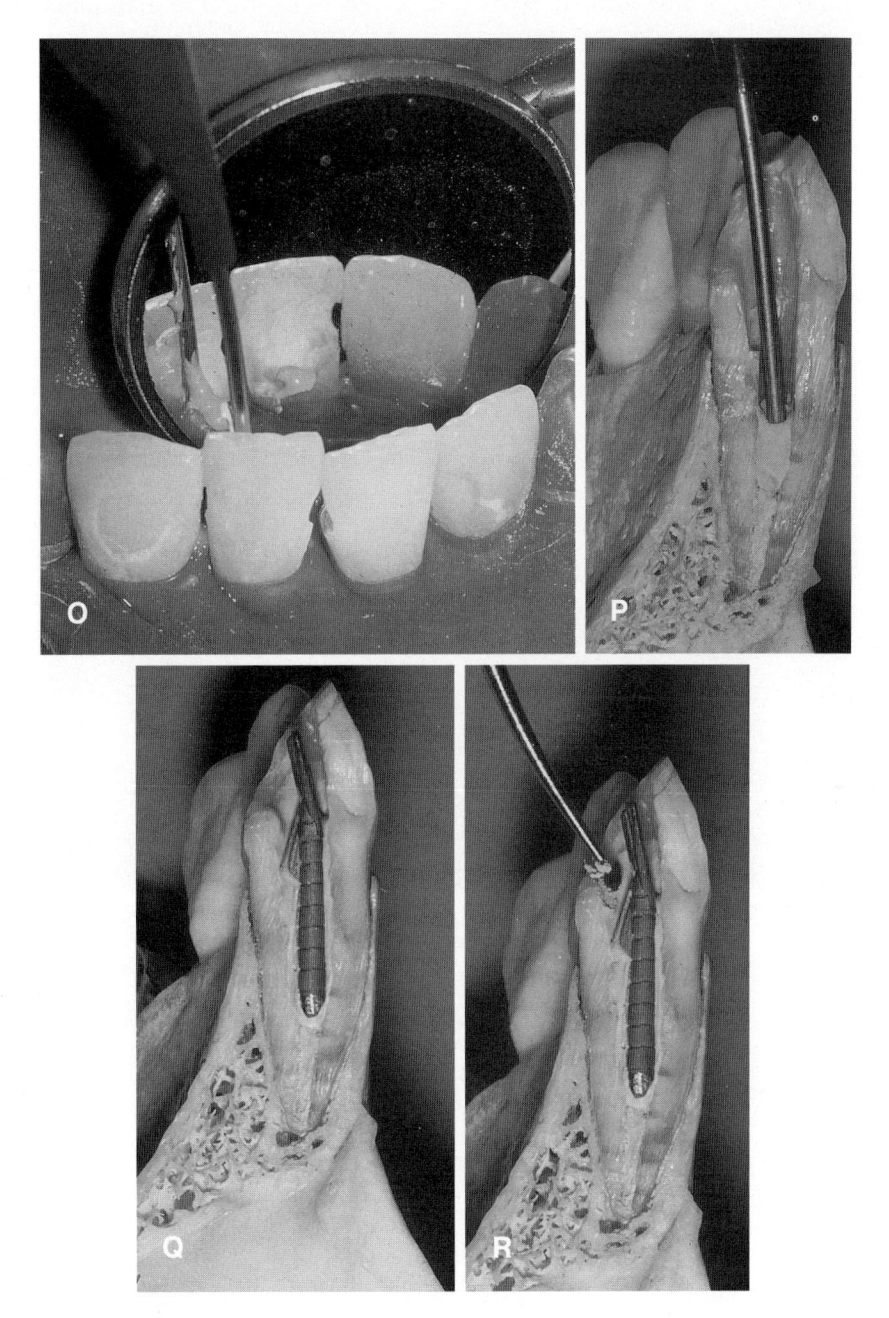

Chapter 9 ♦ Restoration of the Endodontically Treated Tooth 177

Figure 9-4, O-R

PLACEMENT OF THE CORE

If reinforced glass ionomer is to be used for the core, mix another batch of glass ionomer and load it into the shorter plastic Centrix syringe tips and inject around the dowel frame and fill the coronal cavity preparation. Capsulated Ketec Silver can also be used to build up the core. After the glass ionomer core has hardened, the core may be prepared for a crown. In either case plant a light polymerization glaze over the glass ionomer to protect it from fluids for the next 24 hours. When an amalgam or composite core is to be used as a build-up material, the post cement is allowed to set for 4 to 6 minutes. In this case, the lingual was etched (Fig. 9-4, *S* and *T*) and the composite was placed as a final restoration (Fig. 9-4, *U-W*).

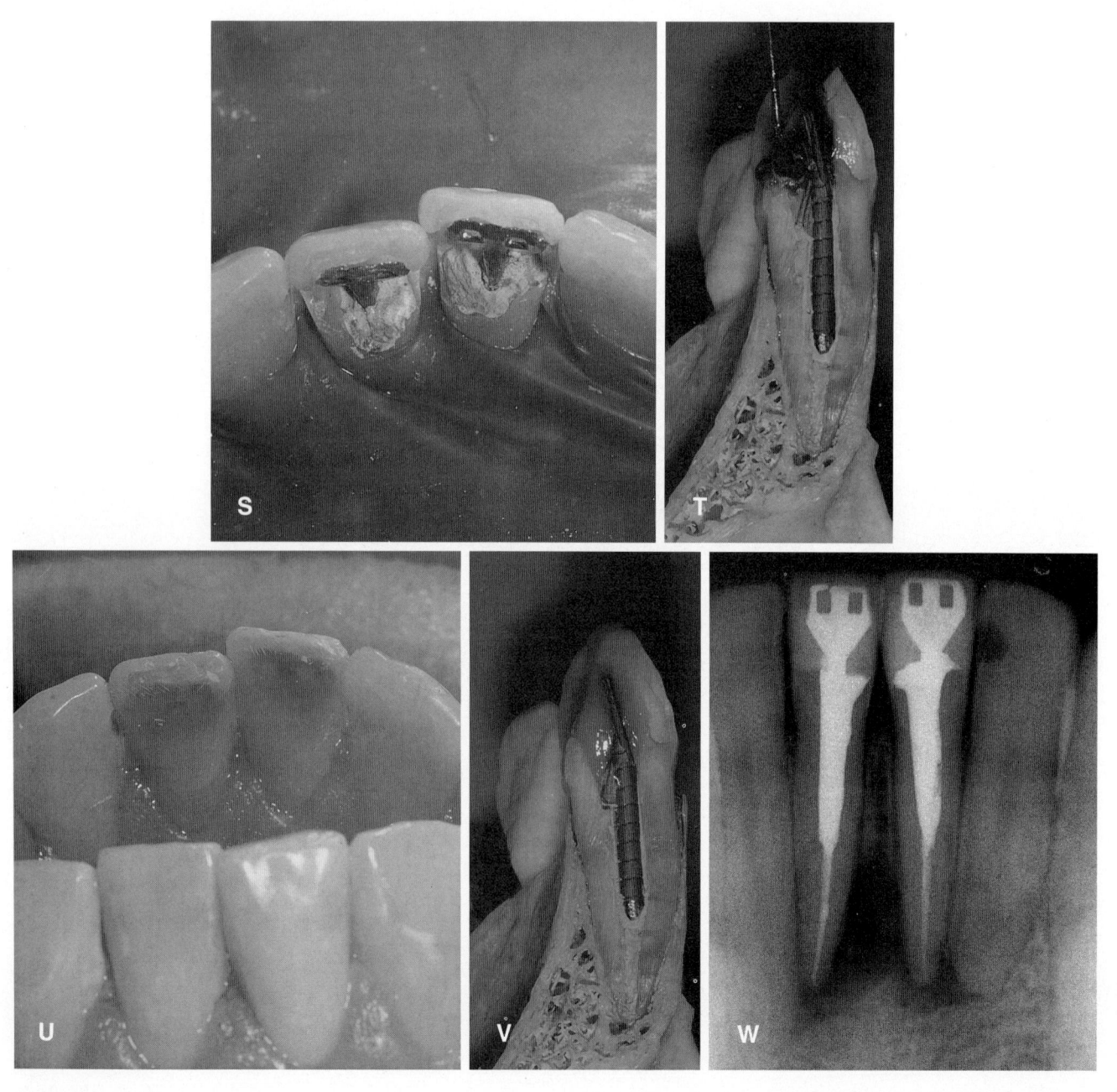

Figure 9-4, S-W

Combination of Materials

There are times when two different core materials are used to build up a tooth (Fig. 9-5). This is particularly true with subgingival fractures or when decay dictates that a glass ionomer is placed subgingivally (Fig. 9-5, *B*) for its anticarious effect and biocompatibility with gingival tissue and a second core material such as composite (Fig. 9-5, *C*) or amalgam is placed supragingivally for its strength and or aesthetics.

When using a posterior Versadowel in a premolar, a glass ionomer is placed followed by the post (Fig. 9-6, *A-C*). Once set, the enamel and dentin are etched and core build-up is placed (Fig. 9-6, *D-G*). Because this case had enough tooth structure, a more aesthetic composite core material was used such as APH (Caulk) or Herculite (Kerr).

To expedite placement of the resin or glass ionomer core, plastic Coreforms (Kerr) can be used. Once hardened, only minor alteration of the preparation will be needed. Also plastic celluloid crown forms can also be used for anterior build-ups and temporary crowns. A temporary post can be made with a paper clip with coronal loop and a bend along the shaft for mechanical retention and placed in the canal. A celluloid crown form filled with a temporary acrylic (Snap or Jet acrylic) and placed over the tooth. It is trimmed and interim cemented to place (Fig. 9-7).

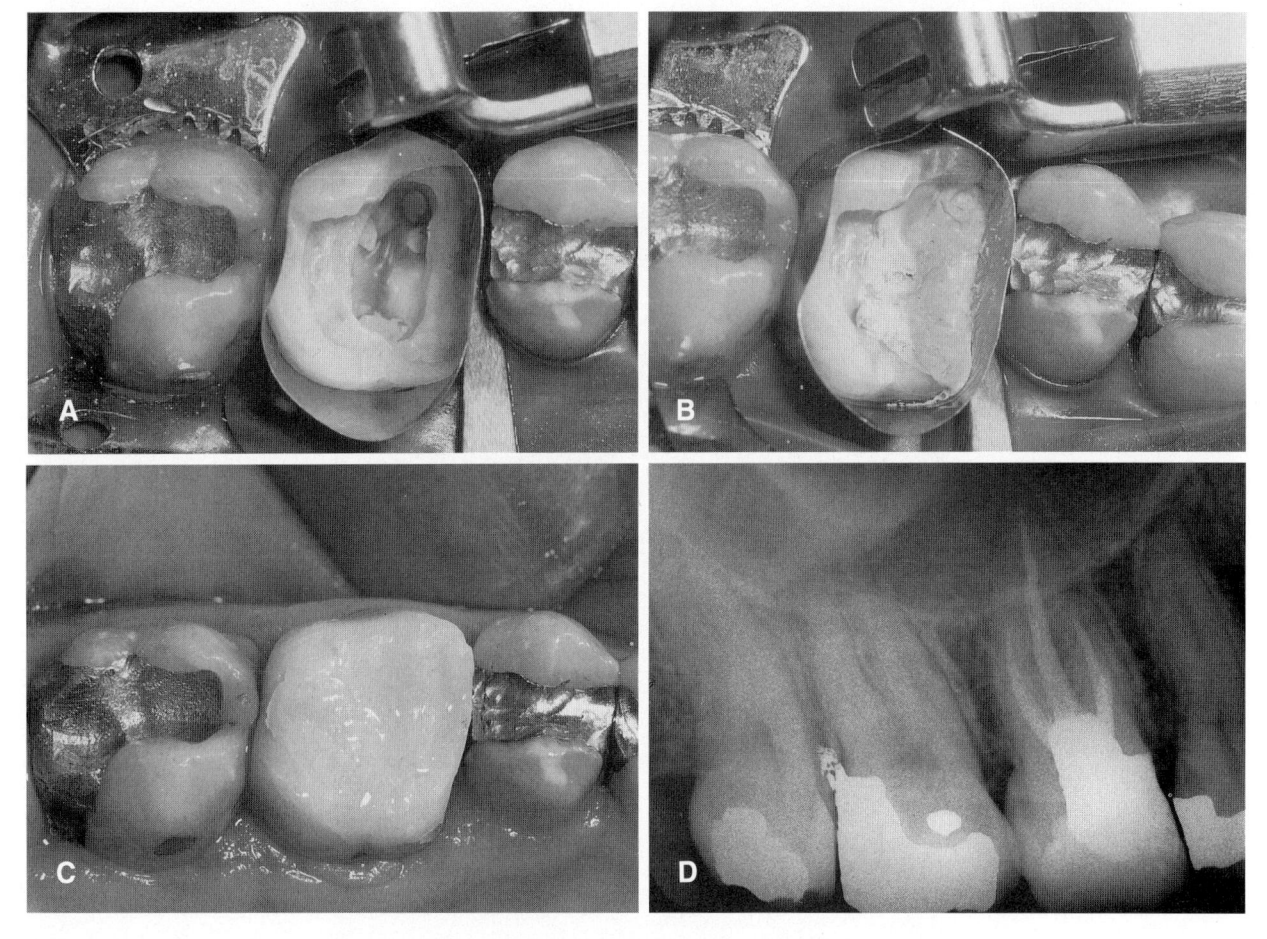

Figure 9-5, A-D

180 PRACTICAL ENDODONTICS

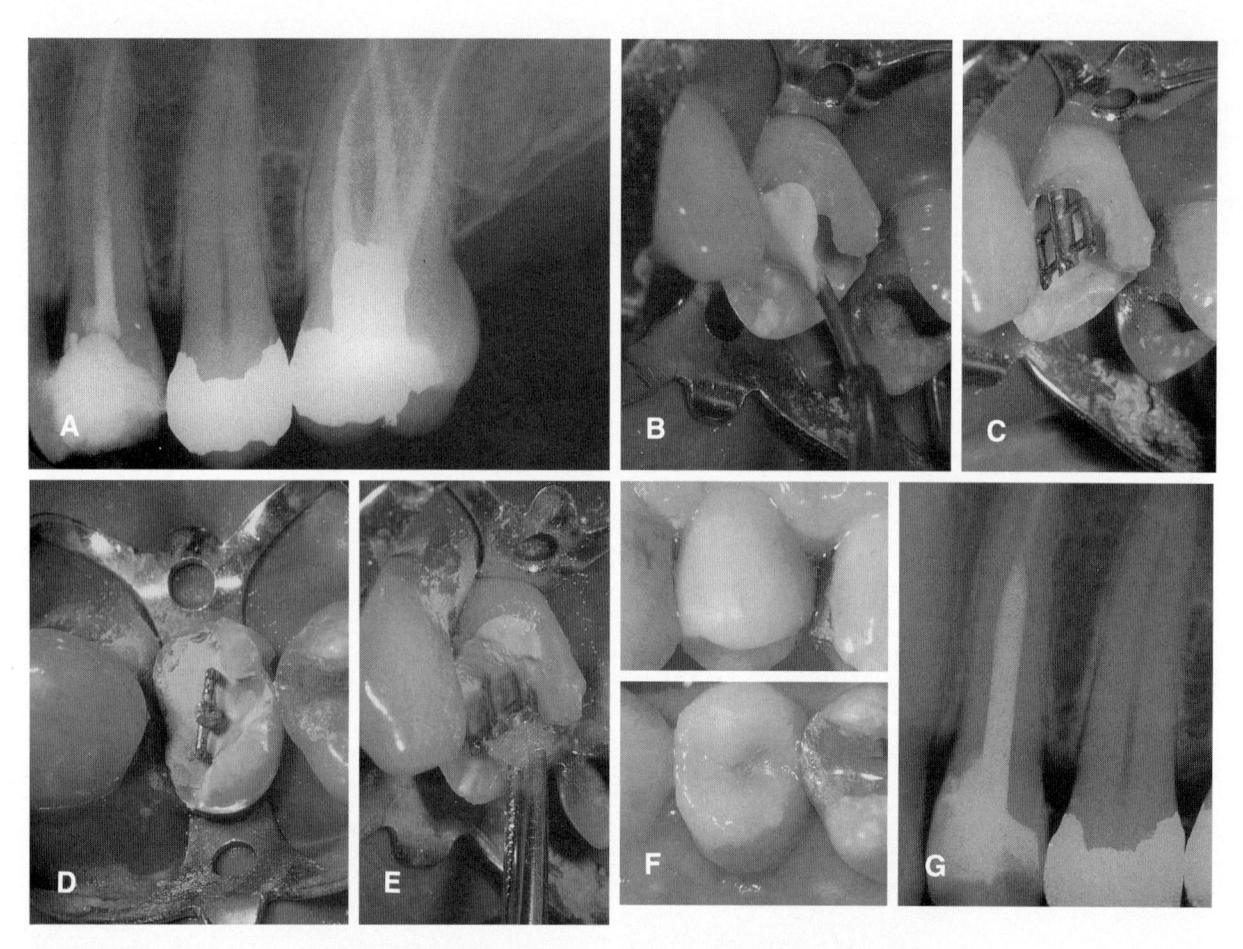

Figure 9-6, A-G

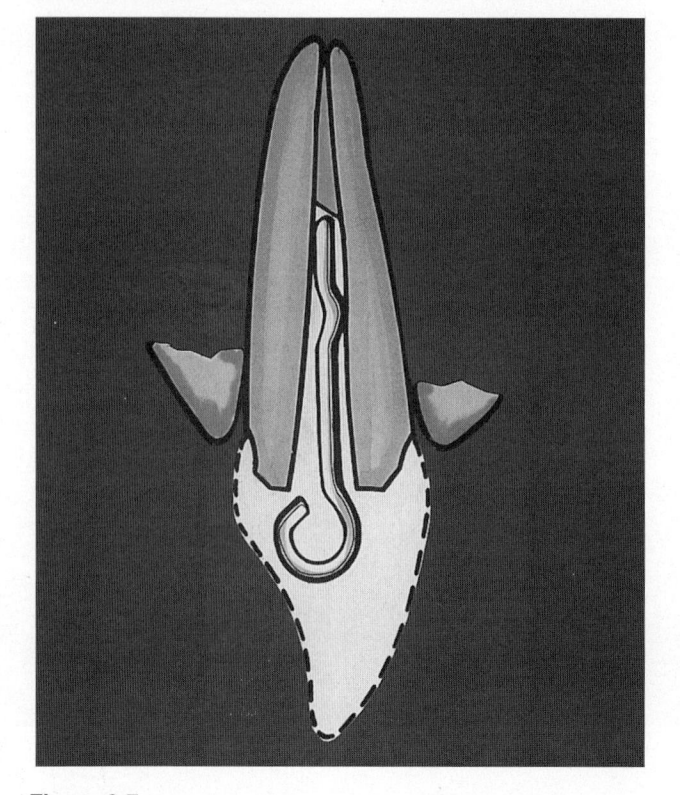

Figure 9-7

ADDITIONAL CORE RETENTION

Pins and slots have been used for many years to help hold the core to the tooth structure. With the advent of stronger dentin adhesive materials such as Allbond II (Bisco), pins are often not needed. The stronger bonding agents allow the use of smaller posts because of increased adhesive strength of the core material to tooth structure, the core shares the lateral and occlusal loads which were before all placed on the posts. These adhesives reduce perculation and increase retention of composite resins. Once etched with phosphoric acid for 20 seconds, rinse with water and dry. Then a bonding agent is placed followed by the core material.

CAST POST AND CORE TECHNIQUE

Fabrication of cast posts is very technique sensitive. When done properly, they are very successful. First remove all interfering coronal tooth structure. Use a Parapost drill to remove the gutta percha from the canal (Fig. 9-8, *A*). If a pin is needed, use the Parapost pin paralleling device (Fig. 9-8, *B*). Fit the Parapost plastic dowel in the canal along with the pin (Fig. 9-8, *C* and *D*) and verify that the Kerr Core Form fit over the post/pin and tooth (Fig. 9-8, *E* and *F*). Using GC Pattern Resin and Duralay resin (Reliance Manufacturing Co.), "salt and pepper" the resin around the plastic dowel (Fig. 9-8, *G* and *I*). Fill the Core Form with Duralay resin and place over the tooth (Fig. 9-8, *J* and *K*). Cut away the plastic shell (Fig. 9-8, *L*) and prepare the tooth and plastic core. Use correct water/powder ratio in your investment so the final cast gold post and core fit passively into the root (Fig. 9-8, *M* and *N*). Remove any temporary cement from the canal (Fig. 9-8, *P*) and irrigate and dry the canal. Smooth down the sprue area and remove any bubbles from the casting (Fig. 9-8, *Q* and *R*). Verify the post passively seats to place (Fig. 9-8, *S* and *T*) and make a light notch on the buccal incisal edge for proper orientation during cementation. Mix the cement (Fig. 9-8, *U*) and place it into the canal with a lentulo or Centrix needle syringe and GENTLY put the post to place. Take a radiograph of the final post/core/crown (Fig. 9-8, *V*).

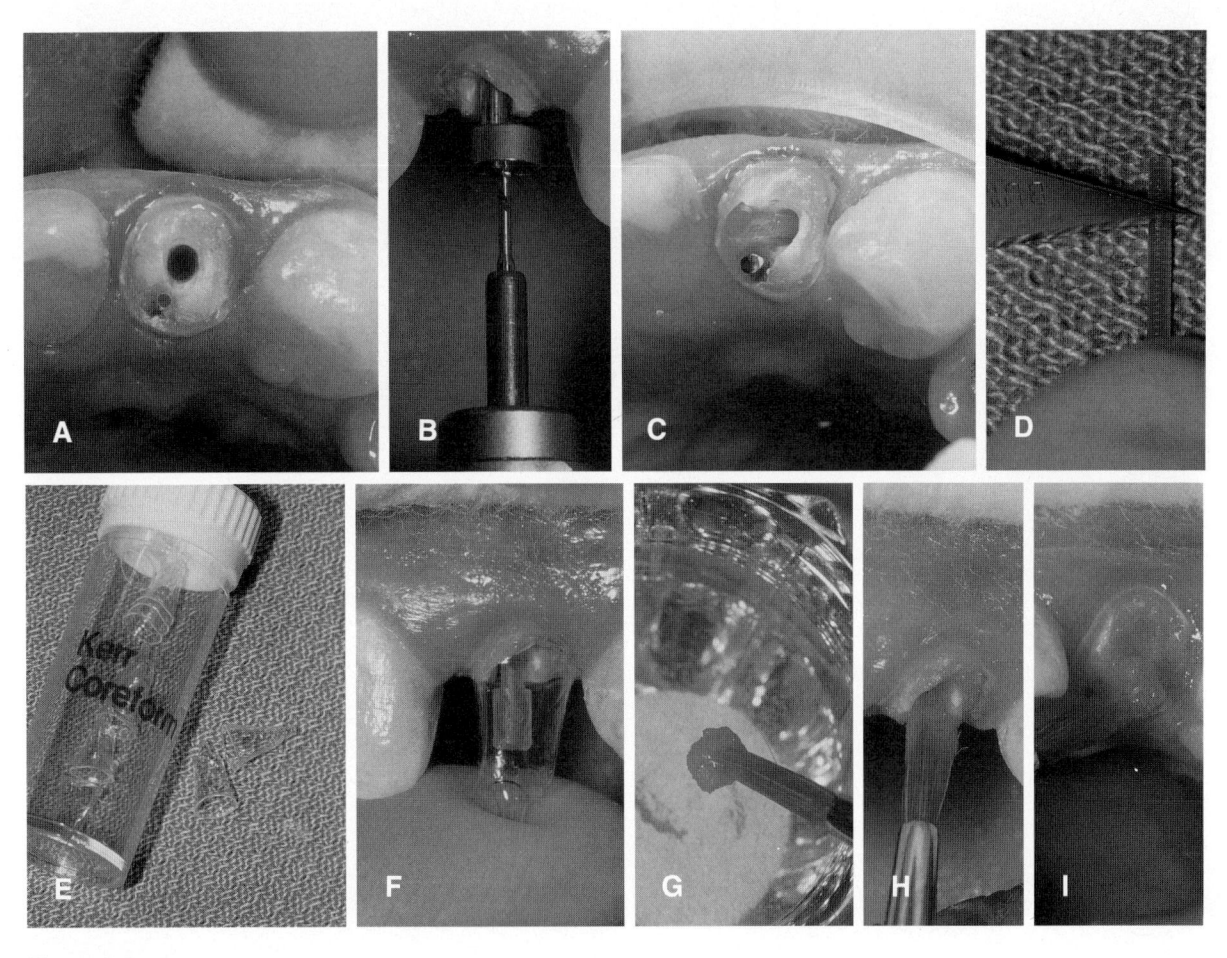

Figure 9-8, A-I

Figure 9-8, J-V

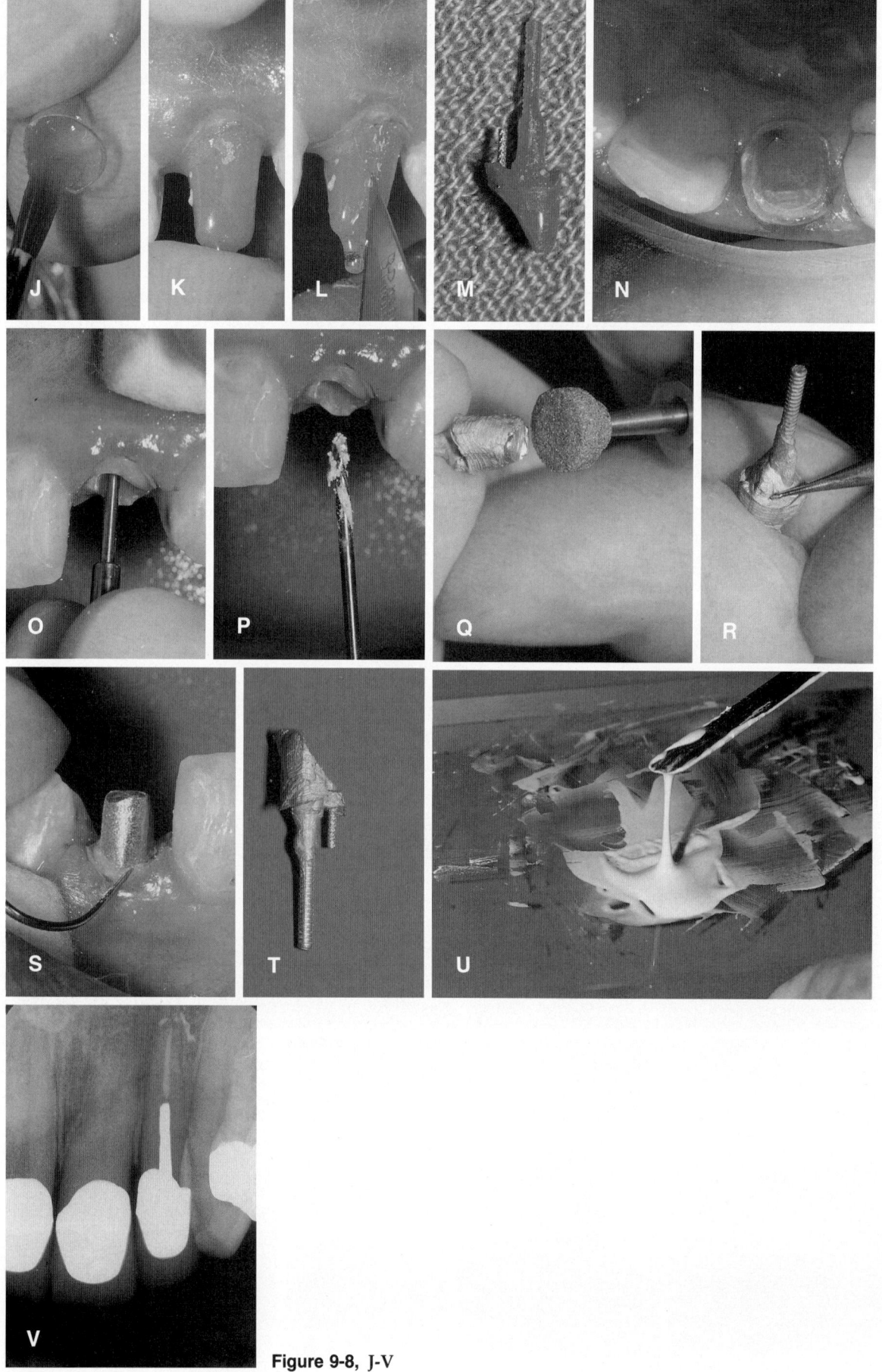

TREATMENT OF THE DEVASTATED TOOTH

Restoring the endodontically treated tooth varies with the situation, but the more we know about the various post and core systems, the more we can be innovative and creative in obtaining the best results in complicated cases. Many times it is difficult to obtain ideal results when treating a compromised tooth. We realize that all core materials leak over time and there is always a possibility of recurrent decay. This may be particularly true when repairing subgingival defects with a core material that is not covered with a gold margin on sound tooth structure. Instead of extracting a tooth, we can make simple repairs and have a tooth that is now caries free and possibly in function for many years; more importantly, we leave long-term options available to the patient.

An example is a mandibular molar with recurrent caries under the old crown down to the gingiva (Fig. 9-9, *A*). In the past, multiple pins and post may have been needed to obtain a secure build-up. Now, after the root canal is done, two small strong Versadowels are cemented in the mesial and distal canals (Fig. 9-9, *B*), dental adhesive placed followed by an amalgam build-up (Fig. 9-9, *C* and *D*). The core is now an interim restoration and will later be prepared as an abutment for a new bridge.

In another case, recurrent caries destroyed the crown of this maxillary premolar (Fig. 9-10, *A* and *B*). Ideally this tooth should be extracted and a new bridge made from molar to the cuspid. Because of financial considerations the patient opted to save the tooth and bridge. All caries were removed and the root canal was completed. The universal Versadowel was cemented in the root with glass ionomer (Chelon Silver) and excess cement was placed subgingivally as part of the core material (Fig. 9-10, *C*). A dentinal adhesive is placed (All Bond II), followed by a composite build-up (Fig. 9-10, *D* and *E*).

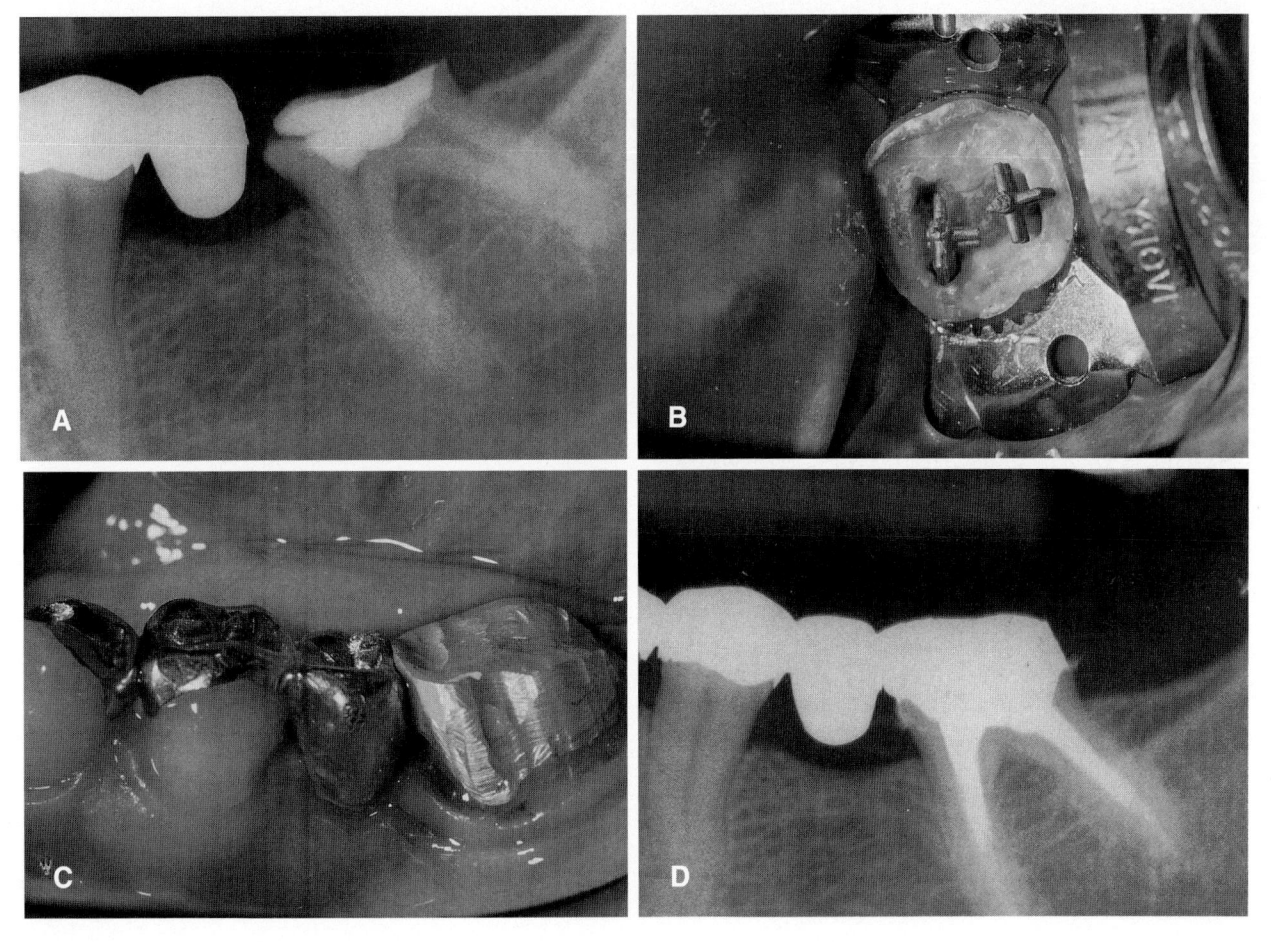

Figure 9-9, A-D

184 PRACTICAL ENDODONTICS

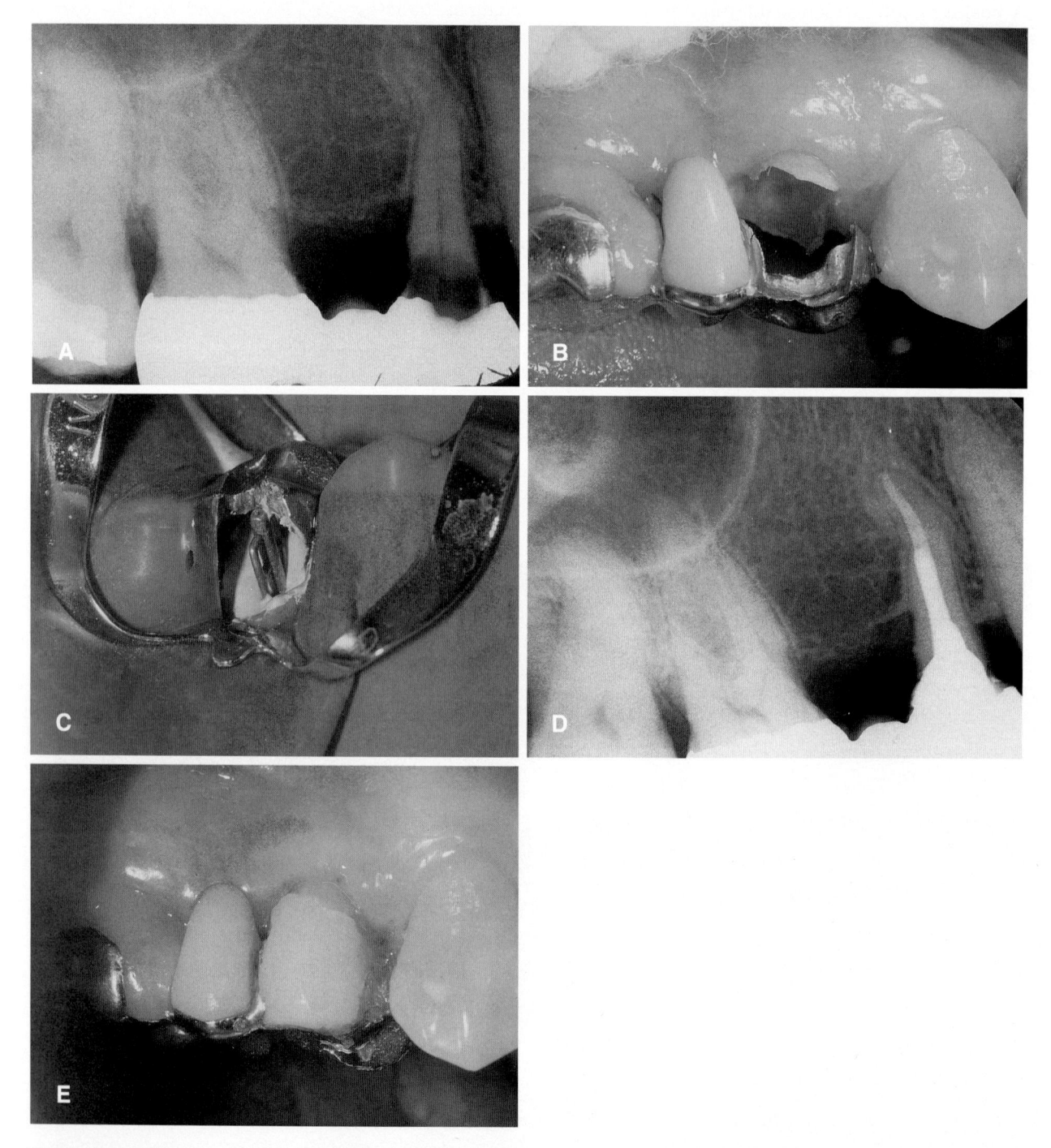

Figure 9-10, A-E

10

Endodontic Complications and Emergencies

This chapter will deal with preventing and treating endodontic emergencies and complications.

POSTOPERATIVE DISCOMFORT

Postoperative discomfort may be caused by the following:
1. Incomplete cleansing and shaping (Fig. 10-1, *A*)
    Prevention: All the principles of cavity preparation (convenience form, resistance form, retention form, extension, and toilet of cavity) must be satisfied before the cleansing and shaping is considered complete.
    Treatment: Refer to Chapter 5 under "Cleansing and Shaping the Root Canal System."
2. Inadequate length control (Fig. 10-1, *B*)
    Prevention: One must have a good preoperative radiograph taken with the long cone technique to measure the tentative working length of the canal. Overinstrumentation into the periodontal ligament can lead to an apical periodontitis. Underinstrumentation, leaving tissue in the canal, could also lead to an apical periodontitis. The working length must be established at 1 mm short of the radiographic apex before any instrumentation of the canal is performed. All instruments entering the canal must have stops at the determined working length. Another radiograph must be taken before the cleansing and shaping is considered complete to reaffirm the working length of the canal.

    Treatment: One must go back and reaffirm the working length. Analgesics and nonsteroidal antiinflammatory drugs may have to be prescribed to relieve any periapical inflamation. If swelling occurs, an antibiotic is indicated.
3. Transportation of the foramina (Fig. 10-1, *C* and *D*)
    Prevention: All instruments entering the canal at the apical ⅓ must be precurved. The apical foramen must not be violated. Large instruments must be kept away from the apex.
    Treatment: Try to renegotiate the main canal starting with a No. 10 file. Prescribe analgesics to relieve any postoperative symptoms.
4. Overmedication (Fig. 10-1, *E*)
    Prevention: Dry the cotton pellet containing the medicament in a 2 × 2 gauze sponge before placing into the pulp chamber. No paper point with the medicament should be left in the canal between appointments.
    Treatment: Remove the cotton pellet containing the medicament and irrigate the canal with sodium hypochlorite. Dry the canal and place a mild medicament, such as eugenol or Cresatin, on a cotton pellet and dry in a 2 × 2 gauze sponge. Place in the pulp chamber with a dry cotton pellet on top and temporary seal. Take tooth slightly out of occlusion.

ENDODONTIC EMERGENCIES

A drug treatment plan must be considered ahead of time when certain symptoms exist. The choice of medication prescribed must be based on the type of symptoms and the degree. The box at right is an example of such a list of drugs that can be used orally during endodontic therapy. Each practitioner must have his or her own list of drugs that work effectively for him or her in a given situation.

Table 10-1 outlines the management of endodontic emergencies.

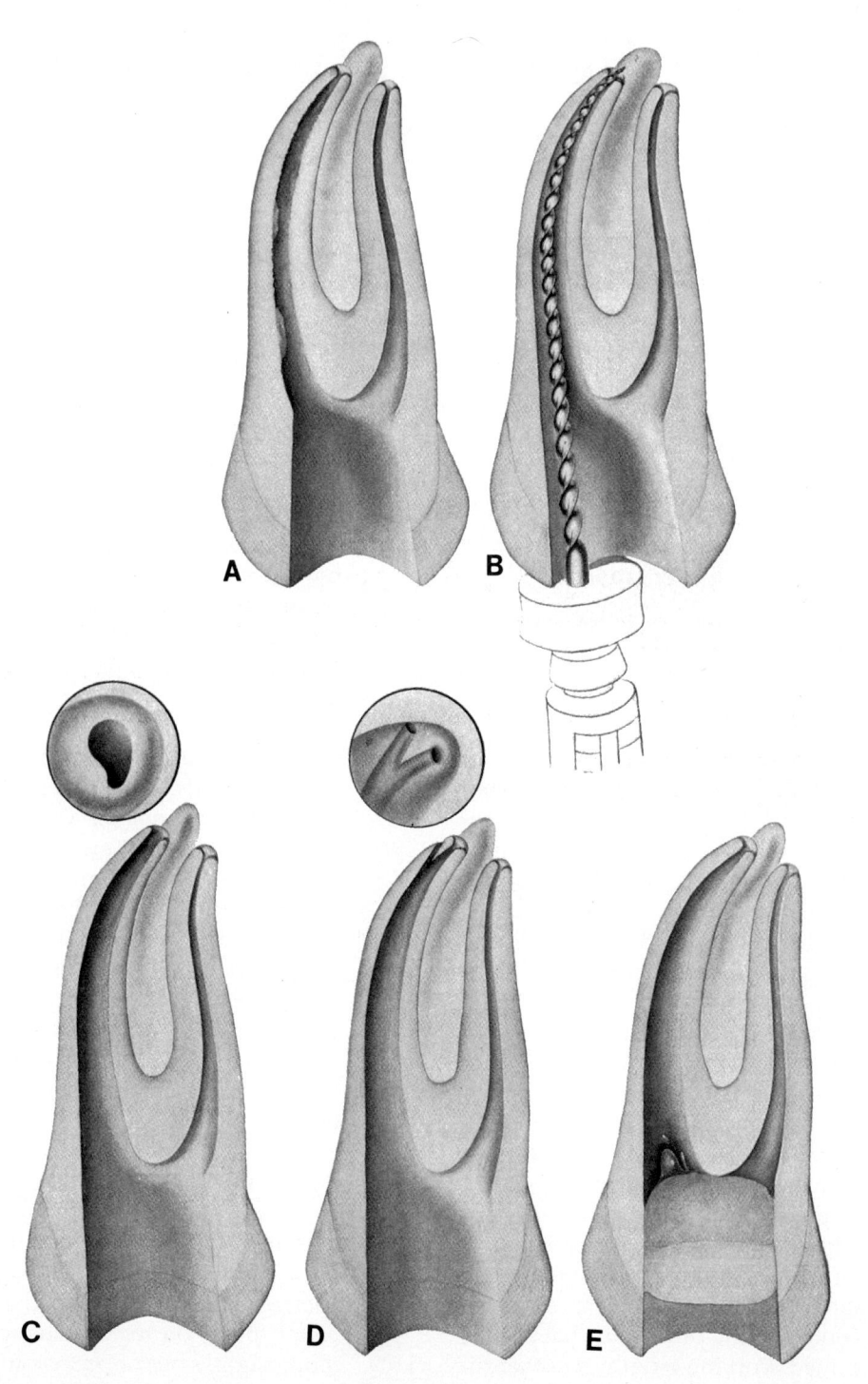

Figure 10-1 Causes of postoperative discomfort. **A,** Incomplete cleansing and shaping of canal. **B,** Inadequate length control. **C,** Transportation of the foramina. **D,** Transformation of the foramina by direct perforation. **E,** Overmedication.

Sample Drug Treatment Plan for Use during Endodontic Therapy

Analgesics

1. Mild Pain
   - A. Aspirin
   - B. Ibuprofen (Motrin)
   - C. Naproxen sodium (Anaprox)

   Allergic to aspirin:
   - D. Tylenol
   - E. Percogesic

2. Moderate Pain
   - A. Fiorinal with codeine No. 3 or No. 4
   - B. Hydrocodone (Vicodin)

   Allergic to aspirin:
   - C. Tylenol with codeine No. 3
   - D. Tylox

   Allergic to codeine:
   - E. Diflunisal (Dolobid 500 mg)

   Allergic to aspirin and codeine:
   - F. Darvocet-N-100

3. Severe Pain
   - A. Oxycodone (Percodan)

   Allergic to aspirin:
   - B. Percocet

Antibiotics

1. Penicillin 500 mg
2. Amoxicillin 500 mg
3. Erythromycin 500 mg
4. Clindamycin (Cleocin 150 mg)
5. Cephalexin (Keflex 500 mg)
6. Metronidozole (Flagyl 500 mg) and Penicillin (500 mg)

Steroids

Three tablets per day for first 2 days and then 2 tablets the 3rd day and 1 tablet the 4th day
1. Decadron 0.75 mg

Table 10-1 ♦ *Management of Endodontic Emergencies*

Symptoms	Recommended Treatment
1. Pulp vital-an intermittent sensitivity to cold (reversible pulpitis)	Remove irritating factor, place calcium hydroxide as base and new restoration. Observe over 6 weeks.
2. Pulp vital-tooth sensitive to cold over a prolonged period of time or sensitive to heat: pain is spontaneous (irreversible pulpitis)	Give profound pulpal anesthesia, emergency pulpotomy, place calcium hydroxide in pulp chamber, and seal access opening.
3. Non-vital pulp with pain and tenderness to percussion with no swelling (acute abscess)	Open canal, irrigate, medicate with calcium hydroxide, and seal access opening.
4. Non-vital pulp with pain and swelling with exudate	Open into canal, irrigate, and place calcium hydroxide after drainage subsides. Place patient on hot saline rinses, antibiotics, and analgesics.
5. Non-vital pulp with pain and swelling with no exudate	Open into canal, irrigate, place calcium hydroxide, and seal access opening. Place patient on antibiotic therapy.
6. Non-vital pulp with fluctuant swelling of soft tissue	Open into canal, irrigate, place calcium hydroxide, and seal access opening. Do incision of fluctuant tissue and place patient on hot saline rinses.
7. Traumatic injuries	
a. Horizontal fractures	Stabilize tooth for 6 to 8 weeks and test for vitality over a 6-month period.
b. Displaced teeth	Bring tooth back into proper occlusion and alignment and stabilize for 6 to 8 weeks. Test for vitality over a 6-month period.
c. Avulsed teeth	Replace tooth into socket as soon as possible, stabilize, and give tetanus and prophylactic antibiotics when indicated. One week after replantation calcium hydroxide is placed in the canal after the canal is cleansed and shaped. The calcium hydroxide is changed when indicated. Patient must be followed over a 6-month period. When no evidence of root resorption is seen, the canal is then obturated with gutta percha.

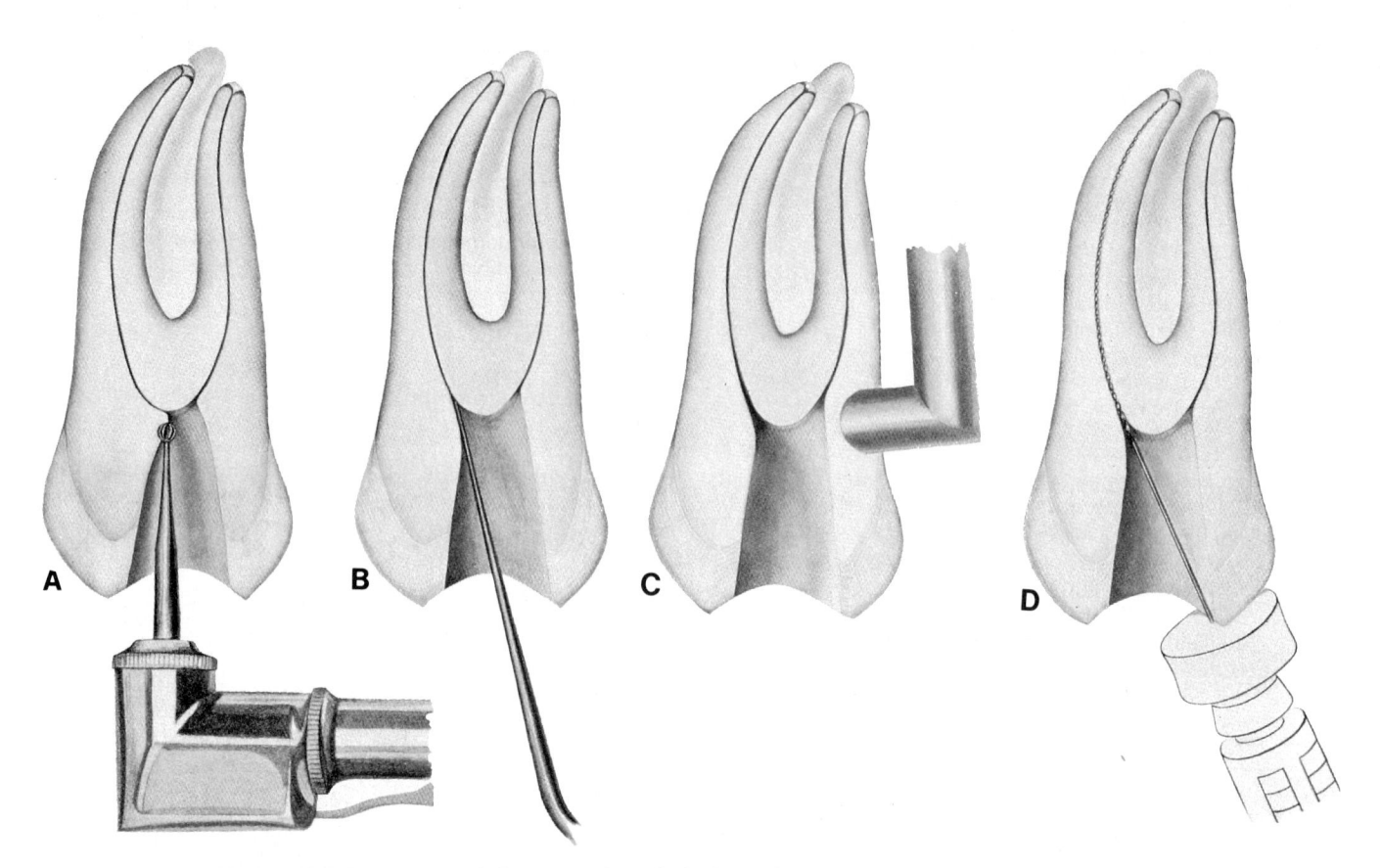

Figure 10-2 Locating and cleansing the calcified canal. **A,** A normal access opening is made through the roof of the pulp chamber. A No. 2 long-shanked, low-speed bur is used to cut downward where the orifice is usually found to the average pulp depth. **B,** Locate the orifice with a DG-16 explorer. This instrument is used as a probe. **C,** A fiber optic light can be used in locating the outline of the pulp floor. The light is usually placed on the lingual surface of the tooth. **D,** Once the orifice is located, a No. 8 or No. 10 file or reamer is used to open the coronal portion of the canal. Sodium hypochlorite and RC Prep are used to soften the dentin and allow the instruments to ease their way into the canal.

ENDODONTIC COMPLICATIONS

1. Calcified canal (see Figs. 10-2 and 10-3)
2. Broken root canal instrument (see Figs. 10-4 and 10-5)
3. Ledge formation (see Figs. 10-6 and 10-7)
4. Perforation (see Figs. 10-8 and 10-9)
5. Ellipticaton (see Fig. 10-10)

Calcified Canal

Although the pulp chamber and the canal calcification may be apparent on the radiograph, in most cases the remnants of the canal still remain. One should always try to negotiate the canal before subjecting the patient to surgery. In many canals, by using a chelating agent (such as RC Prep) and very fine reamers (such as a No. 8 or No. 10) along with a DG-16 explorer, one can open into these canals. Only as a last resort should the patient be subjected to an amalgam retrofilling or an intentional replantation procedure (Fig. 10-2 and 10-3).

Broken Root Canal Instruments

Instrument breakage in endodontics is a problem. Any time such fine delicate instruments as the file, reamer, and broach are used in a curved, narrow, or tortuous canal, one runs the risk of instrument breakage. Dentists who say they have never broken a root canal instrument have not done many root canals. However, just because the instruments do break does not release one from responsibility to the patient. It is up to the dentist to keep this breakage to a minimum by taking certain precautions. The following list of precautions should be observed:

1. Use stainless steel instruments rather than carbon steel. Stainless steel is less likely to break.
2. Instruments should be used in size sequence.
3. Examine each instrument before placing it into the canal. If the flutes are not spaced equally, it is an indication that the instrument has been strained and should be discarded. If the instrument is dull, it will tend to lodge against the dentin and break.

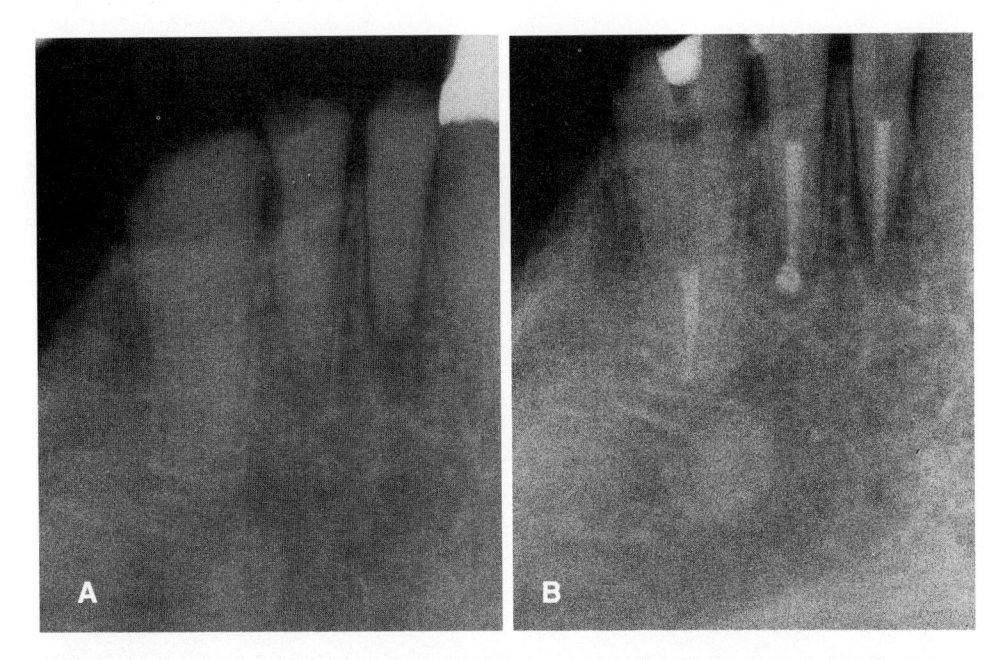

Figure 10-3 Radiographs of calcified canal therapy. **A,** Mandibular anterior teeth appear radiographically without a canal. Although there appears to be no canal on the radiograph on all these teeth, a nonsurgical approach in treating these teeth endodontically should be attempted. **B,** All canals were found and treated.

4. Do not use a fine instrument more than two times.
5. A file should be used in a push-pull motion. The reamer should be used with a ¼ to ½ degree turn. It is the rotation of the instrument in the canal to bite into the dentin that breaks the instrument.
6. An instrument should be cleaned before placing it back into the canal because the debris could retard cutting, and, therefore, predispose the instrument to breakage.
7. An instrument should never be placed into a canal unless the canal is well irrigated. A wet canal will facilitate cutting and thereby prevent breakage.
8. Stops should be placed on all instruments before entering a canal at an exact distance of tooth length.

Periapical surgery or tooth extraction is not always indicated after instrument breakage. If the instrument is fractured and protrudes through the apex, this could cause a periapical inflammation. An amalgam retrofilling is then the treatment of choice after filling the canal with gutta percha to the instrument fragment. If the instrument is fractured within the confines of the canal, then filling the canal with gutta percha down to the instrument fragment is the procedure of choice. Sometimes the chloropercha technique works well here. The softened gutta percha can get around the instrument fragment more easily (Figs. 10-4 and 10-5). The patient should be aware of the broken fragment and the tooth should be kept under observation. The prognosis is not favorable in those cases in which an area of rarefaction is present

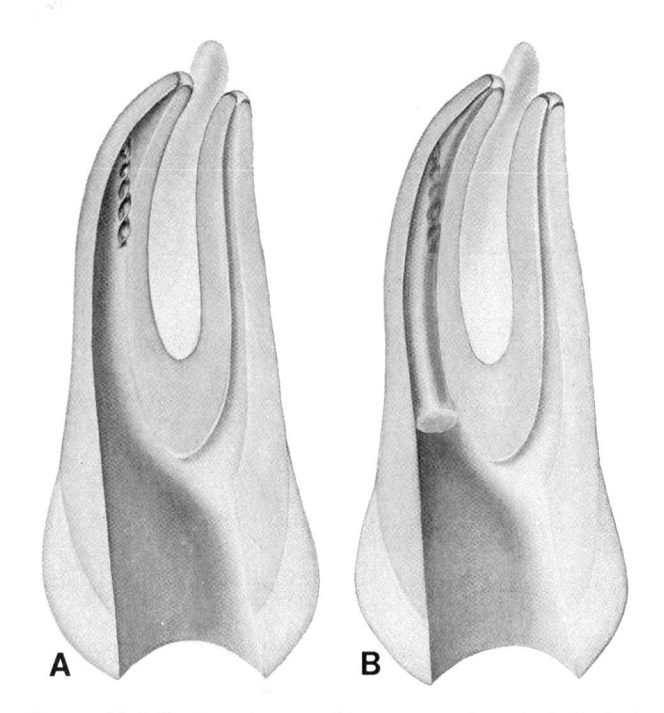

Figure 10-4 Broken root canal instrument in apical third of canal. When instruments break in the root canal, they are often difficult to retrieve. If the instrument cannot be removed, an attempt is then made to bypass the instrument. If this is unsuccessful then the cleansing and shaping of the root canal is continued to the point of the obstruction, as in **A.** The root canal can then be obturated with a chloropercha technique trying to condense gutta percha around and pass the instrument, as in **B.**

190   PRACTICAL ENDODONTICS

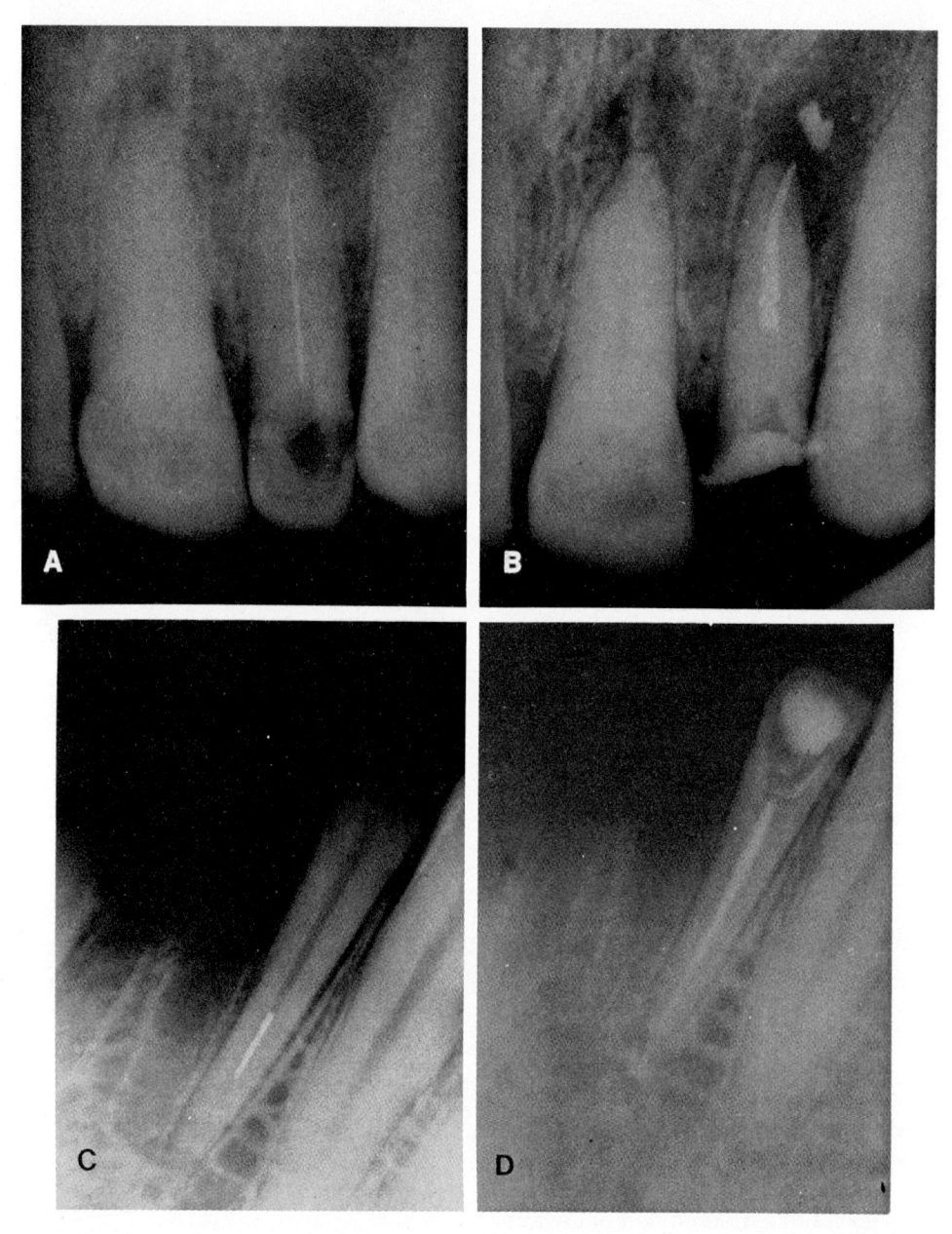

Figure 10-5 Broken root canal instrument. **A,** A broken file in the maxillary lateral incisor. Because the file was close to the pulp chamber, a Stiglitz forcep was used to attach to it and retrieve it from the canal. **B,** The root canal was then cleansed, shaped, and obturated. **C,** When an instrument is broken off in the apical and middle third of the canal, the instrument becomes difficult to remove. In this case, the instrument was bypassed with a No. 10 file. The apical preparation could not be prepared any larger for fear of perforating the root. Gutta percha was then able to be condensed around the instrument and to the apex, as shown in **D**. **E,** Radiograph of radiolucency around the mesial root of a mandibular first molar. **F,** A broken instrument in the mesial-buccal root. An unsuccessful attempt was made to bypass the instrument. The canal was cleansed and shaped to the obstruction, and gutta percha was condensed to this point. **G,** Six-month postoperative radiograph showing healing taken place. **H,** A preoperative radiograph of a maxillary lateral incisor that required root canal therapy. **I,** Upon treating this tooth endodontically, a No. 30 file was broken at the apex, **J,** The instrument was able to be bypassed, and the canal was filled around the obstruction.

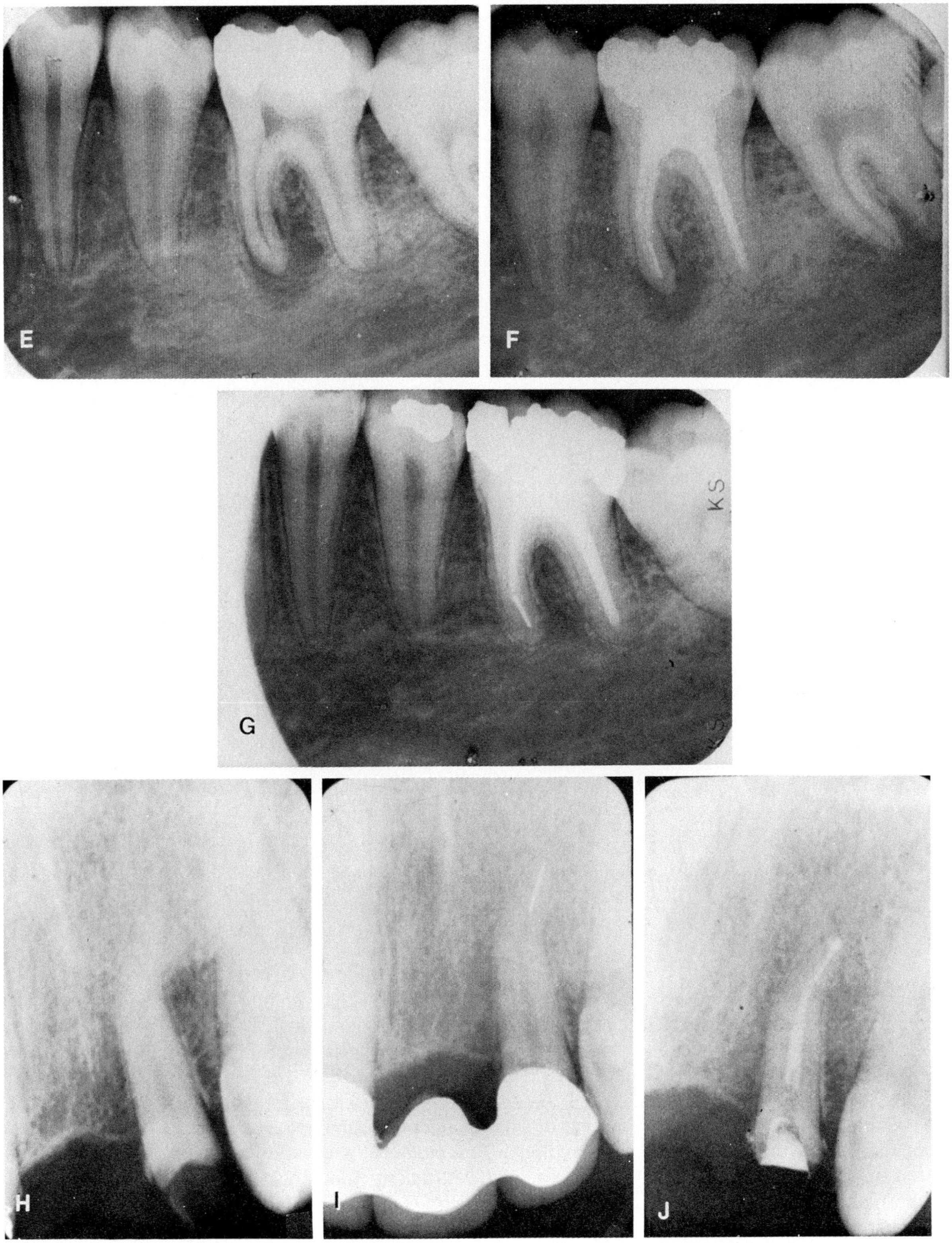
E
F
KS
G
H
I
J

192 PRACTICAL ENDODONTICS

and an instrument is broken in the canal. The prognosis is more favorable if normal bone structure is present before treatment and breakage of the endodontic instrument.

Sometimes access is easier by removing the dentinal triangle, especially around a curve canal. A No. 8 or No. 10 file should be used to try to negotiate past the ledge. A bend is placed on the tip of the instrument, and the file is inserted into the canal. It is placed at the area of obstruction and then rotated and pushed beyond the ledge. The ledge is filed without withdrawing the instrument. It is used as a rasp against the canal wall containing the shelf. When the instrument is no longer cutting, remove it and repeat the same sequence with a No. 15 file, etc. If the No. 10 file stops at the ledge and will not go to the working length, then withdraw the file a few millimeters, rotate it, and then advance the instrument. If the ledge still cannot be bypassed, it may be necessary to file the canal to the ledge and fill to that point. A retrograde filling may be indicated later if healing does not take place.

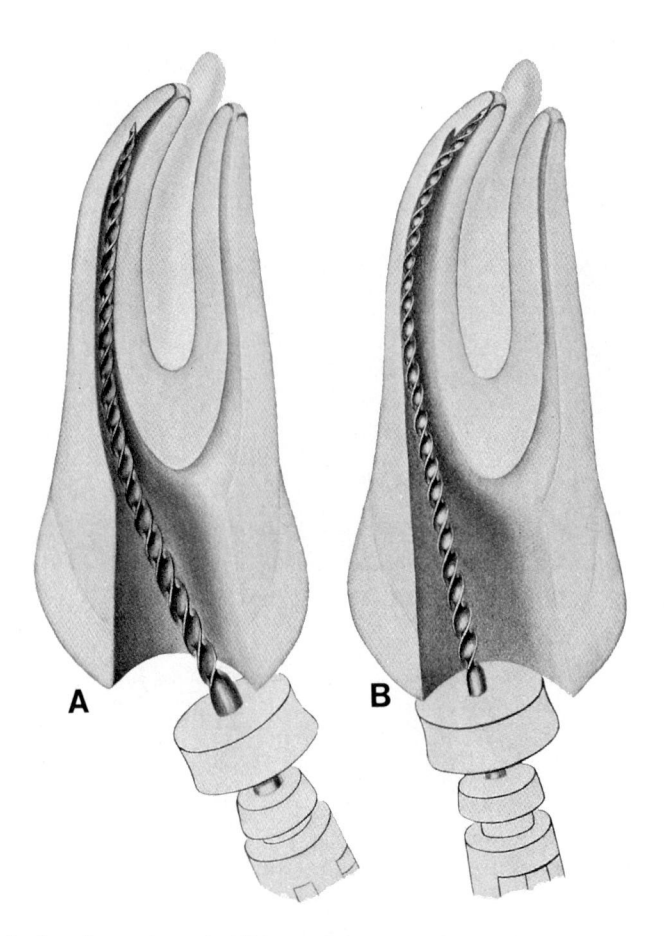

Figure 10-6 Ledge formation. **A,** Using a No. 30 or larger instrument that cannot be precurved can lead to a ledge formation in the apical portion of the canal. Also, if the dentinal triangle is obstructing the orifice, one would be more prone to ledge because the access would not be direct. **B,** When a ledge has been created, the access opening should be reevaluated.

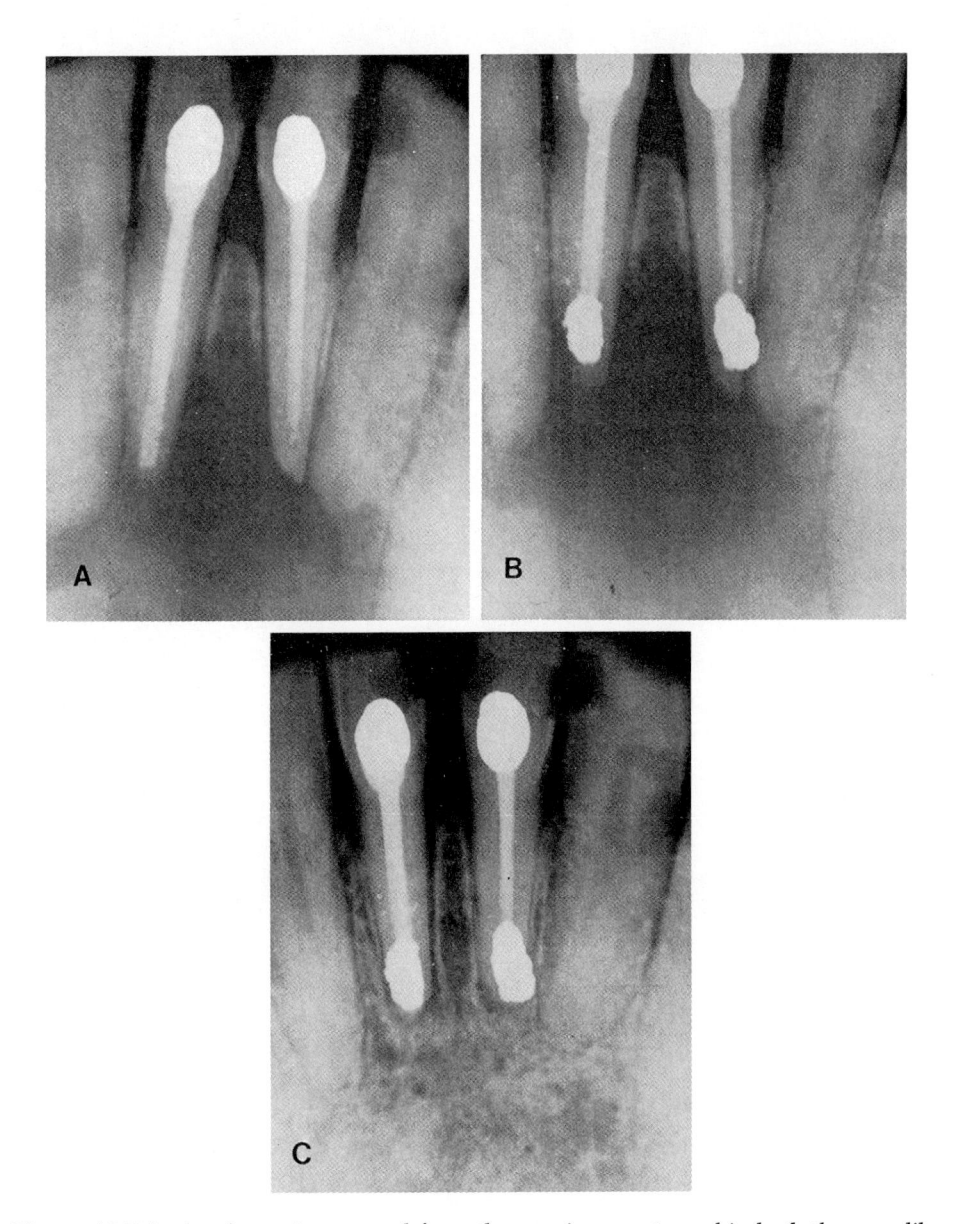

Figure 10-7 Ledge formation created from the previous root canal in both the mandibular central incisors. **A,** Preoperative radiograph of large area of radiolucency around the mandibular central incisors. Retreatment of both of these teeth by a nonsurgical approach was unsuccessful. Two canals were found in both of these teeth with a ledge created in the middle third of the lingual canal. **B,** A retrograde amalgam was placed at the apices of both mandibular central incisors. **C,** Eight-month postoperative radiograph showing complete healing taken place.

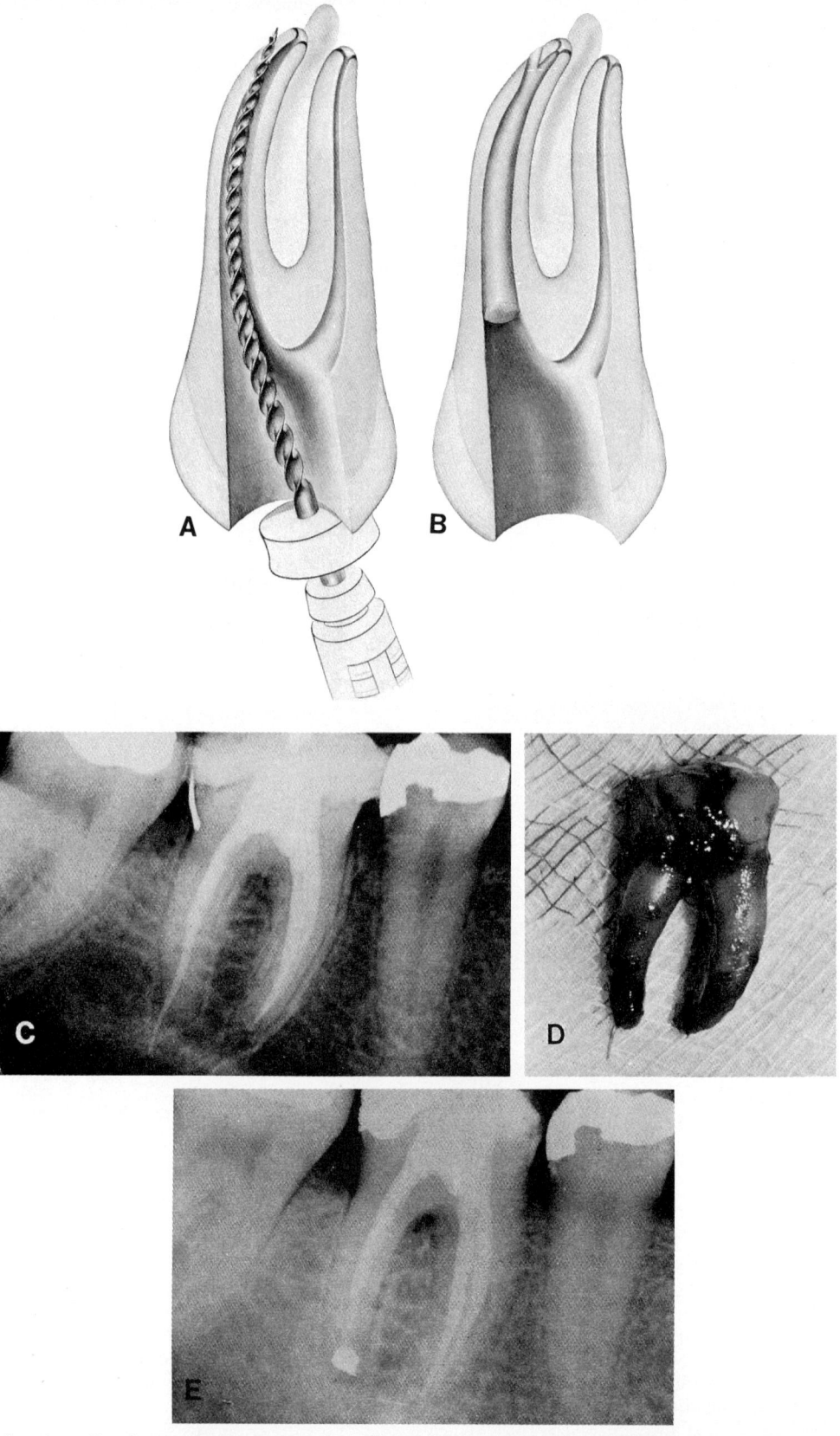

Figure 10-8 Perforation. Careless access preparation and/or using large instruments in the apical area can lead to a perforation. Some signs of a perforation are continual hemorrhage in a canal and constant sensitivity. **A,** Perforation in apical third of canal. **B,** When the original canal can be renegotiated, the main canal can be obturated and the perforation handled like a lateral canal. **C,** When the main canal cannot be negotiated, a surgical procedure must be performed. In this case, a retrograde amalgam would be difficult to perform on the distal root. An intentional replantation procedure was performed. **D,** Photograph showing the tooth extracted and the overextension of gutta percha a few millimeters from the true apical foramen. The excess gutta percha was removed, and the apical foramen was sealed with a zinc-free amalgam. **E,** Radiograph shows the tooth replanted.

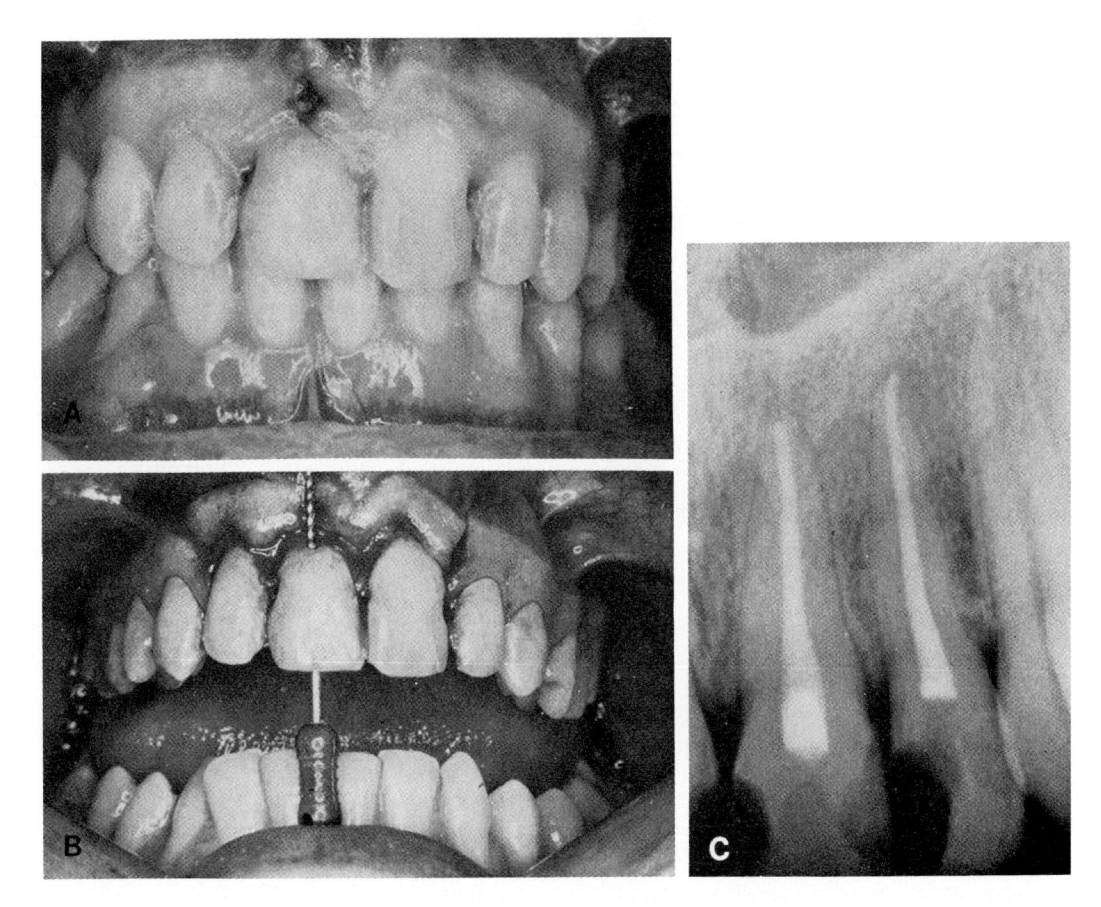

Figure 10-9 Perforation at cervical area of maxillary right central incisor. **A,** An incorrect access opening leading to a perforation of the labial cervical area of the maxillary right central. An area of inflammation can be seen at the attached gingiva above the crown. **B,** Two vertical incisions were made distal to teeth adjacent to the involved tooth. A reamer is placed through the perforation to demonstrate the location of the perforation. **C,** Radiograph demonstrating the sealing off of the perforation with an amalgam and completion of root canal therapy.

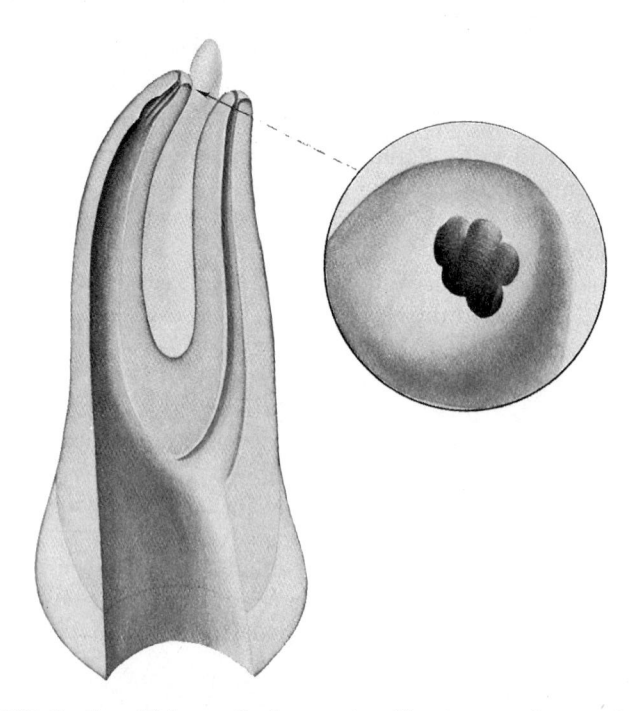

Figure 10-10 Elliptication. This results from using files in a turning motion or filing the lateral walls of the canal with lateral pressure. When large inflexible files are used at the apex, the result sometimes is straightening of the canal. The problem with the ellipticated canal is that the apical foramen has not been debrided and is difficult to fill because the canal has greater diameter than it does a few millimeters more coronally.

POSTOPERATIVE FAILURES

Persistent Periapical Lesion

Recall examination of every endodontically treated tooth should be conducted on a 6-month interval. Only in this way can these cases be reevaluated.

If an area of rarefaction does not heal or show any evidence of some healing by 1 year, then one must evaluate this problem. The vitality of the adjacent teeth should be examined and the tooth should be examined for traumatic occlusion. Retreatment should always be considered in these cases.

If an area is getting smaller but is not completely healed after a 1-year follow-up and if the canal looks well obliterated and the tooth is completely asymptomatic, it is best to leave this case alone. An explanation for the incomplete radiographic healing could be an apical scar, especially if a surgical procedure had been performed. One must always compare the preoperative and postoperative radiographs to evaluate a case effectively.

A persistent radiolucency laterally around the root is sometimes seen. This could be due to a lateral canal. Retreatment in this case should always be considered.

An extra canal should be suspected whenever an apparently well-filled tooth shows a persisting or enlarging periapical radiolucency. Lower anterior teeth, the distal roots of mandibular molars, and the mesiobuccal roots of maxillary molars often have undiscovered extra canals. Retreatment is indicated to search for these extra canals.

Restorative Failure

Crown and/or root fracture is a problem after the tooth has been treated endodontically. To avoid such failures, posterior teeth should be protected with a full crown or an overlay for cusp protection. Anterior teeth with large restorations should be protected with a crown. In certain cases, a dowel and a core should be added for greater support.

11

Nonsurgical Retreatment

A high percentage of success is achieved with the nonsurgical approach for retreatment and is preferable to surgical treatment. Nonsurgical retreatment encompasses the basic approach to endodontics of cleaning, shaping, and three-dimensional obturation (Fig. 11-1).

This chapter outlines techniques for the removal of separated instruments, posts, various root canal fillings (e.g., silver cones, gutta percha, paste fillings and cements) and objects such as broken burs and orifice enlargers. The use of small files (No. 6, 8, 10, or 15), a lubricant RC Prep (urea peroxide), Soluset,

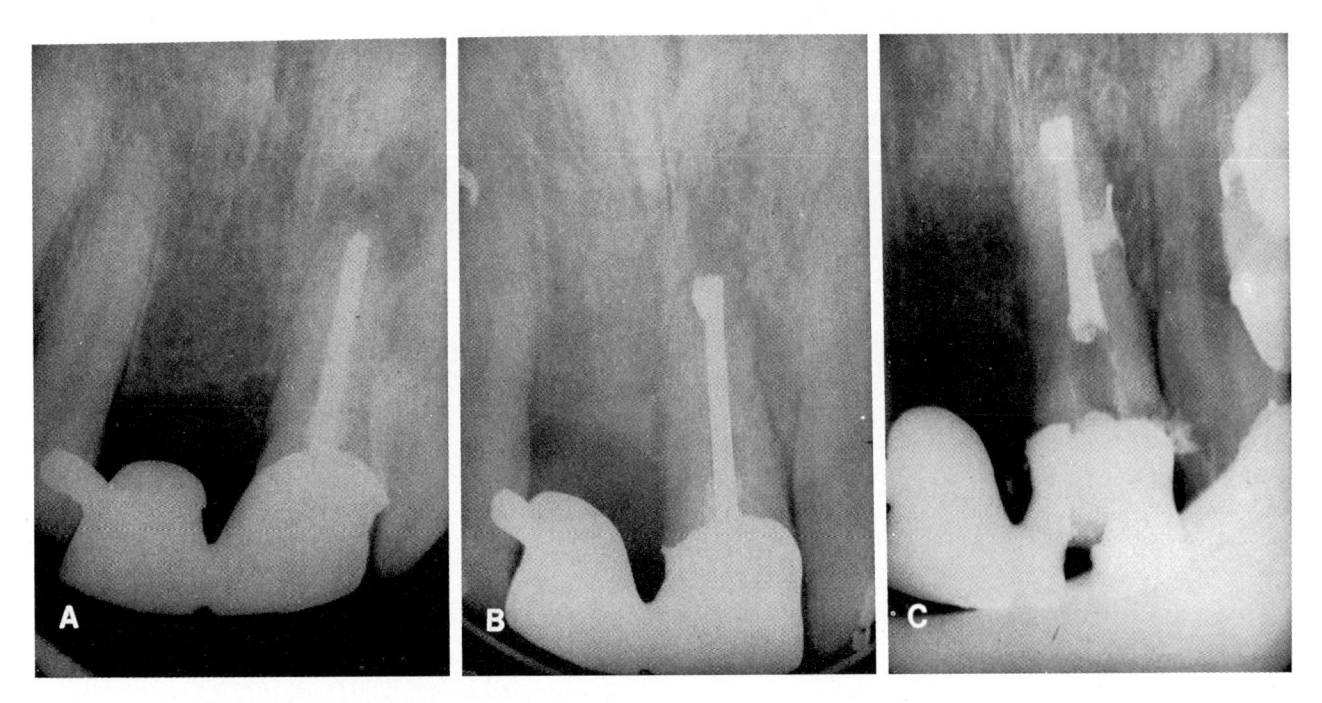

Figure 11-1 Retreatment by a nonsurgical approach is always preferable to surgery. **A**, A radiograph of a maxillary central incisor that had a silver point in the canal. The patient presented with an acute abscess. **B**, An unsuccessful attempt was made to remove the silver point through the crown. A retrograde amalgam procedure was then preformed. This procedure failed and the patient presented 3 months later with a large intraoral swelling above the same tooth. **C**, The bridge was removed and the silver point was then able to be removed. The canal was then cleaned, shaped, and filled by using warm gutta percha technique. Notice the large lateral canal on the distal aspect of the root; a lateral lesion can now be seen.

198 PRACTICAL ENDODONTICS

ultrasound files and scaler, and various silver point retriever pliers are invaluable aids in removing objects from the root canal (Fig. 11-2). The operator must be careful not to remove excessive amount of supporting dentin and tooth structure in an attempt to retrieve the object. If the tooth is rendered nonrestorable the efforts are futile for both the patient and the dentist. The techniques discussed will be those that are considered conservative.

SEPARATED INSTRUMENTS

When an instrument is separated in the canal it should be identified and located with a radiograph. Separated instruments are classified according to their location in the canal (Fig. 11-3):
  a. Protruding in the pulp chamber
  b. Gingival third
  c. Middle third
  d. Apical third
  e. Beyond the apical foramen

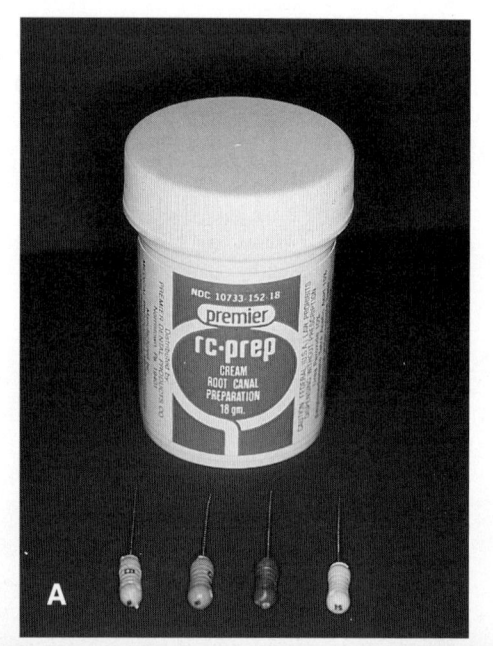

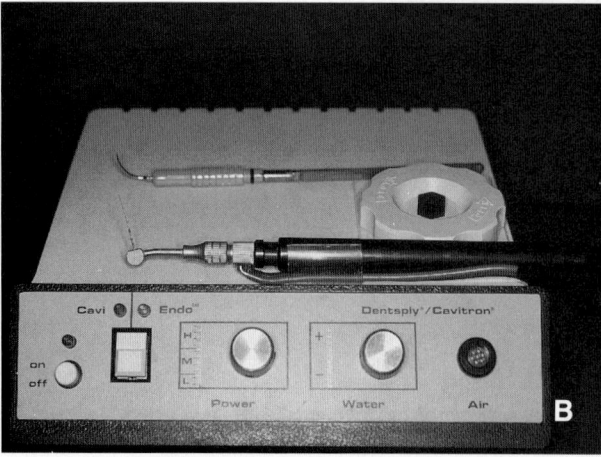

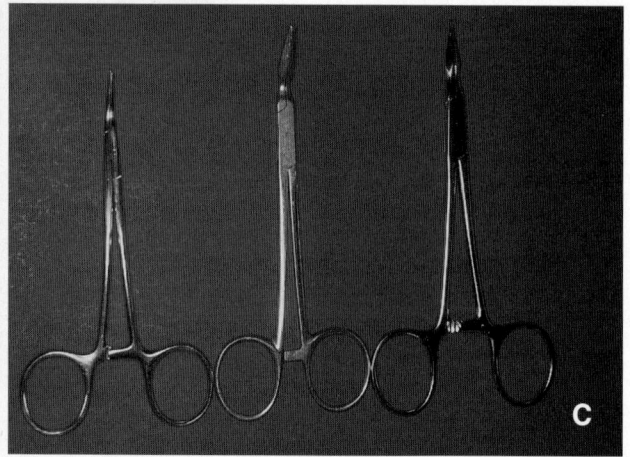

Figure 11-2 **A**, The No. 6, 8, 10, and 15 files with the use of RC Prep as a lubricant to aid in bypassing instruments. **B**, The instruments can be vibrated loose out of the canal with the ultrasound (Caviendo-L.D. Caulk) files and scalers. **C**, Various angled and small beaked silver cone pliers are used to reach into the chamber and canal to retrieve the separated instruments.

Chapter 11 ♦ Nonsurgical Retreatment   199

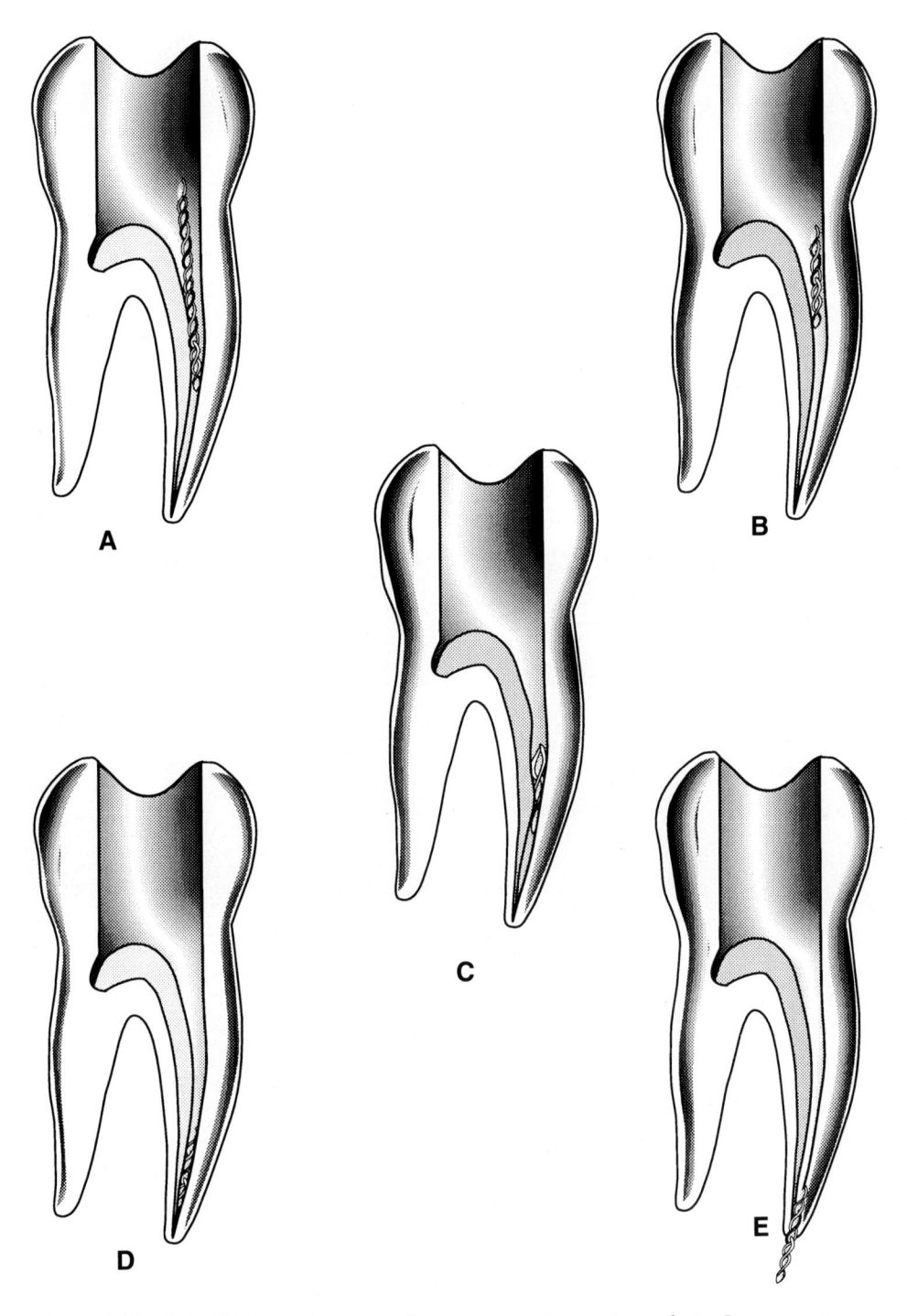

Figure 11-3 Classification of separated instruments in root canal. **A**, Instrument protruding in the pulp chamber. **B**, Instrument separated in the gingival third. **C**, Instrument separated in the middle third. **D**, Instrument separated in the apical third. **E**, Instrument protruding through the apex.

REMOVAL OF SEPARATED INSTRUMENTS PROTRUDING IN THE PULP CHAMBER

When an instrument is separated and visible in the pulp chamber and there is adequate space, it can be removed with a fine pair of forceps or right-angle pliers (Fig. 11-2, C). It can also be dislodged with the air scaler. Place the tip of the scaler on the instrument, activate to maximum power and the instrument will vibrate loose (Fig. 11-4). It may be necessary to retrieve it with a pair of Stieglitz forceps, a pair of hemostats, or silver point retrievers (Fig. 11-2, C).

An alternative treatment is to cut part of the crown from occlusal to gingival with a fissure bur and expose the instrument so that it can easily be removed with forceps or pliers. The tooth is then restored (Fig. 11-5).

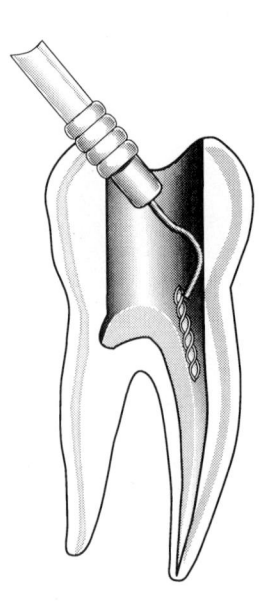

Figure 11-4 Activated ultrasound scaler touching broken instrument protruding in chamber.

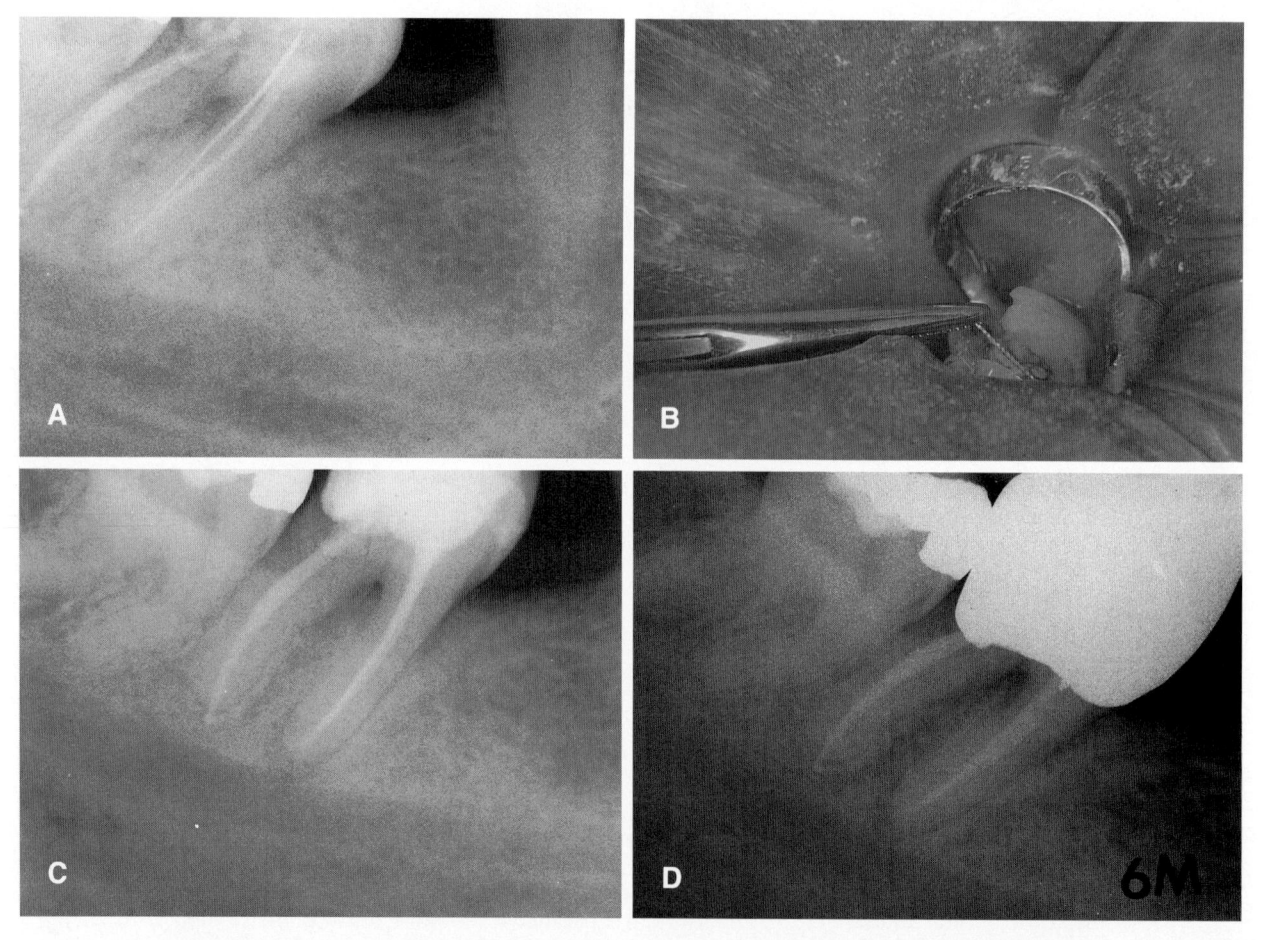

Figure 11-5 A, Separated file in the mesiobuccal canal and protruding in the pulp chamber of tooth No. 18. The patient had a dull ache in the tooth for 2 years and a slight radiolucent area is evident at the apex of the mesial root. **B,** Part of the buccal wall was removed with a fissure bur and the visible instrument was removed with straight hemostats. **C,** The canals are cleaned, shaped, and filled with gutta percha. **D,** The coronal portion of the tooth was restored with a crown and a 6 months check-up radiograph shows the radiolucent area to be reducing in size.

REMOVAL OF SEPARATED INSTRUMENTS FROM GINGIVAL, MIDDLE, OR APICAL THIRD AND NOT VISIBLE IN THE CROWN

When an instrument is separated in the gingival, middle, or apical third and not visible in the crown, it should be bypassed. Place some RC Prep (urea peroxide) in the canal with a small file or injection syringe and attempt to bypass it with a new No. 6, 8, or 10 K-type file. The files are carefully worked with ¼ to ½ turns back and forth motion. It may be a slow tedious process (Fig. 11-6). If a No. 15 is able to bypass it then a No. 15 ultrasound file is placed in the canal bypassing the separated instrument and the ultrasound is activated. Sound waves will travel down the file to the separated instrument and dislodge it and vibrate it toward the gingival direction. When the instrument is loose a small Hedstrom file may be

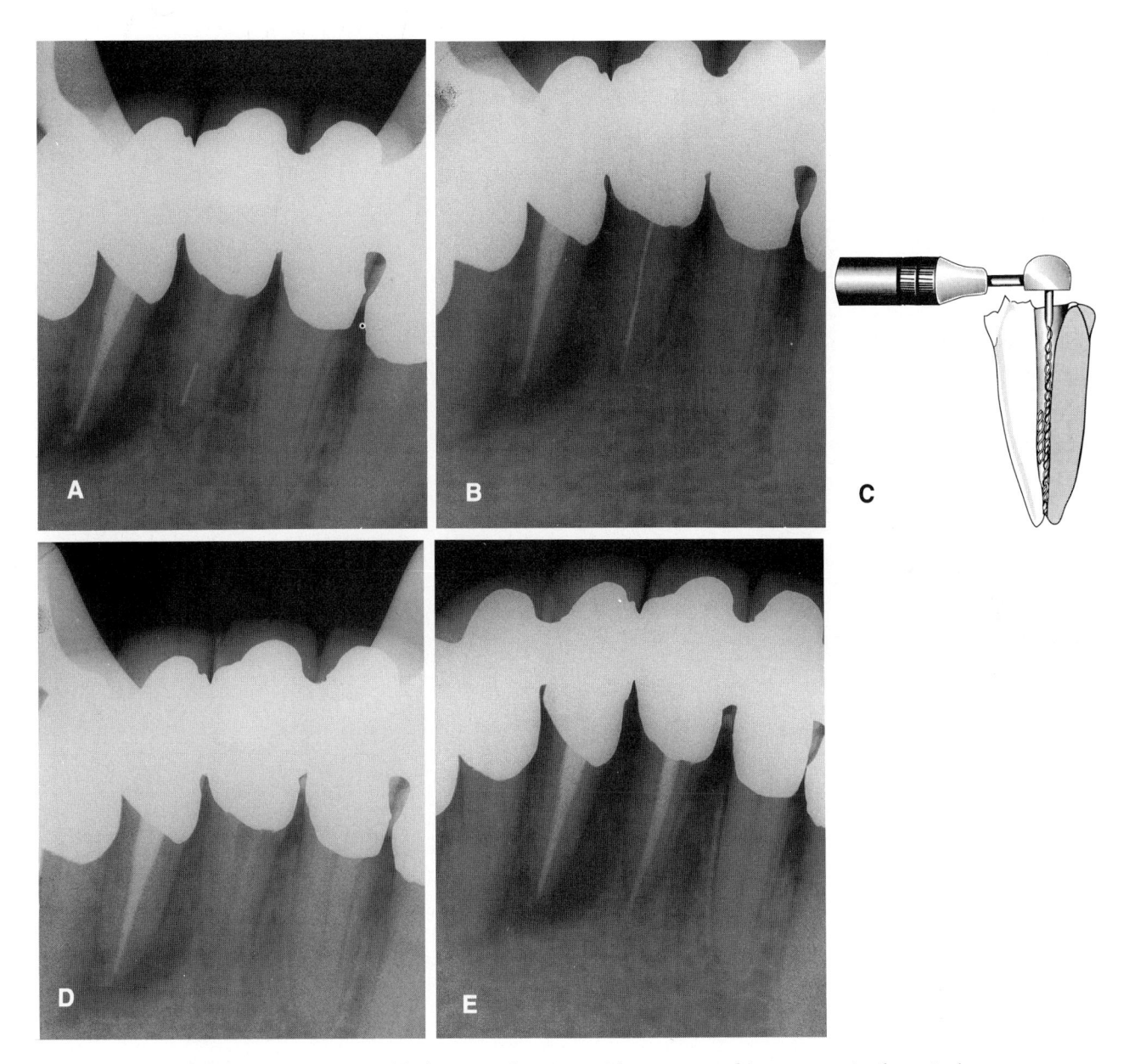

Figure 11-6 **A**, A mandibular central incisor with a separated instrument in the apical third. **B**, The instrument is bypassed by using a No. 8 file and then a No. 10 file. RC Prep (urea peroxide) is placed on the tip of the file and it is worked in $\frac{1}{4}$ to $\frac{1}{2}$ turns to bypass the separated instrument. A No. 15 file is shown bypassing the instrument. **C**, The No. 15 ultrasound file is placed in the canal bypassing the instrument and it is activated to maximum power until vibrated loose. If a hedstrom can be worked in the canal bypassing the instrument, the flutes of the instrument may engage the instrument and remove it. **D**, The instrument removed with ultrasound. **E**, Canal filled after cleaning and shaping. (Courtesy of Drs. Augusto and Mercedes Posada.)

worked down along side the instrument and it is rotated so the flutes of the file will engage it and it can be carefully removed (Fig. 11-7).

The operator must be careful not to perforate the root in an attempt to bypass the instrument. Careful use and probing with small files (No. 8 or No. 10) and the use of a lubricant RC Prep will aid in preventing perforations.

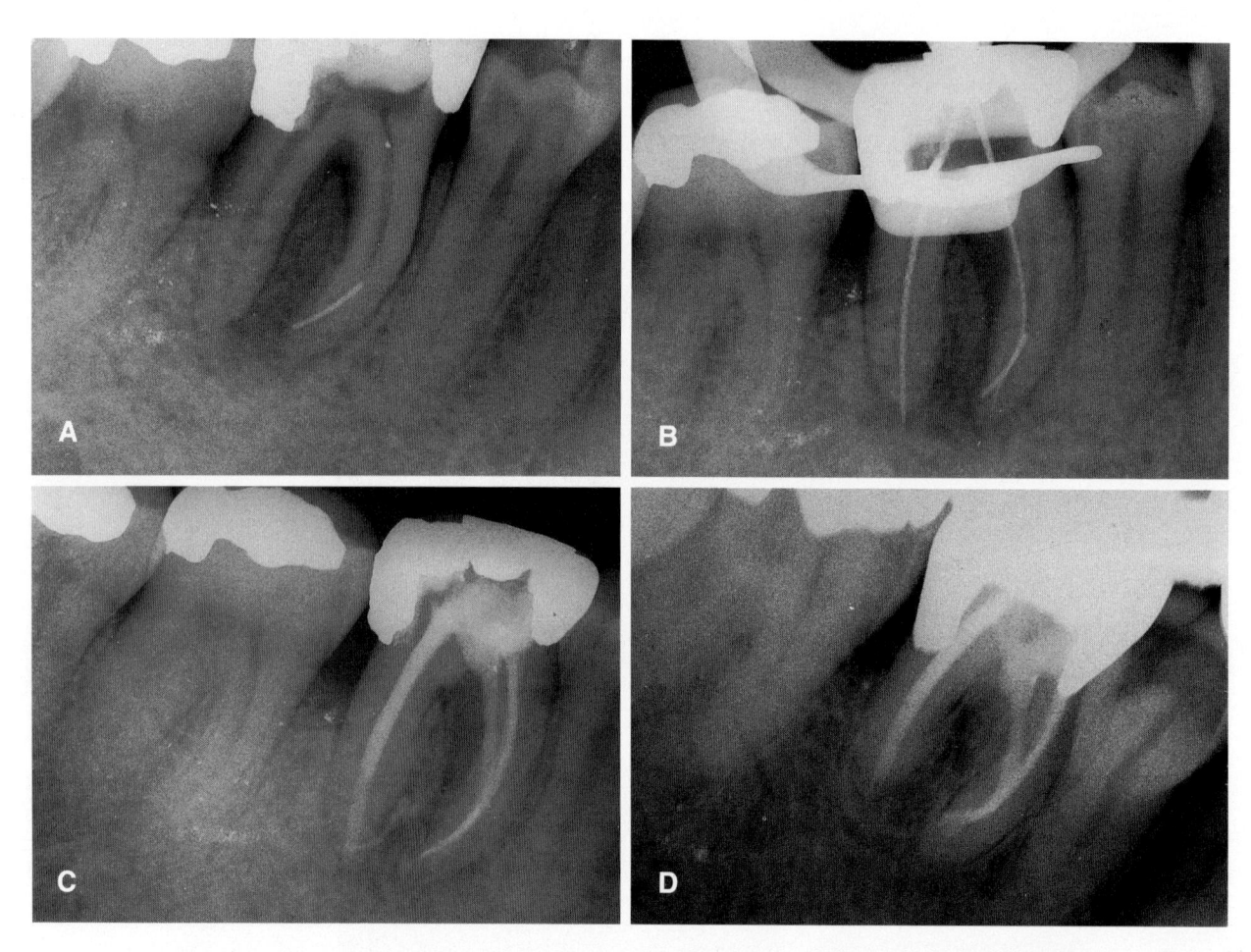

Figure 11-7 **A**, An instrument separated in the apical third of the mesial-buccal canal in mandibular first molar. **B**, The other canals were measured and the instrument was bypassed first using a No. 10 and No. 15 file with RC Prep. The instrument was removed by engaging it with a small No. 15 hedstrom file. **C**, The canals are cleaned, shaped, and filled. **D**, A 5-year postoperative radiograph showing complete healing.

WHEN AN INSTRUMENT IS SEPARATED AND UNABLE TO BE RETRIEVED

When an instrument is separated and unable to be retrieved, the canal is instrumented to that point. If the instrument is able to be bypassed and unable to be retrieved it is left in the canal. Once the instrument is bypassed and wedged against a wall, the same path of insertion is used each time so as not to dislodge it. Passive instrumentation with the instrument that bypasses it is essential (i.e., do not go to a higher instrument until the working instrument files loosely). When the canal is cleaned it is coated with sealer and injected with Firm set or Regular set Ultrafil. The viscosity of the Ultrafil allows it to flow around the instrument and seal the canal (Fig. 11-8).

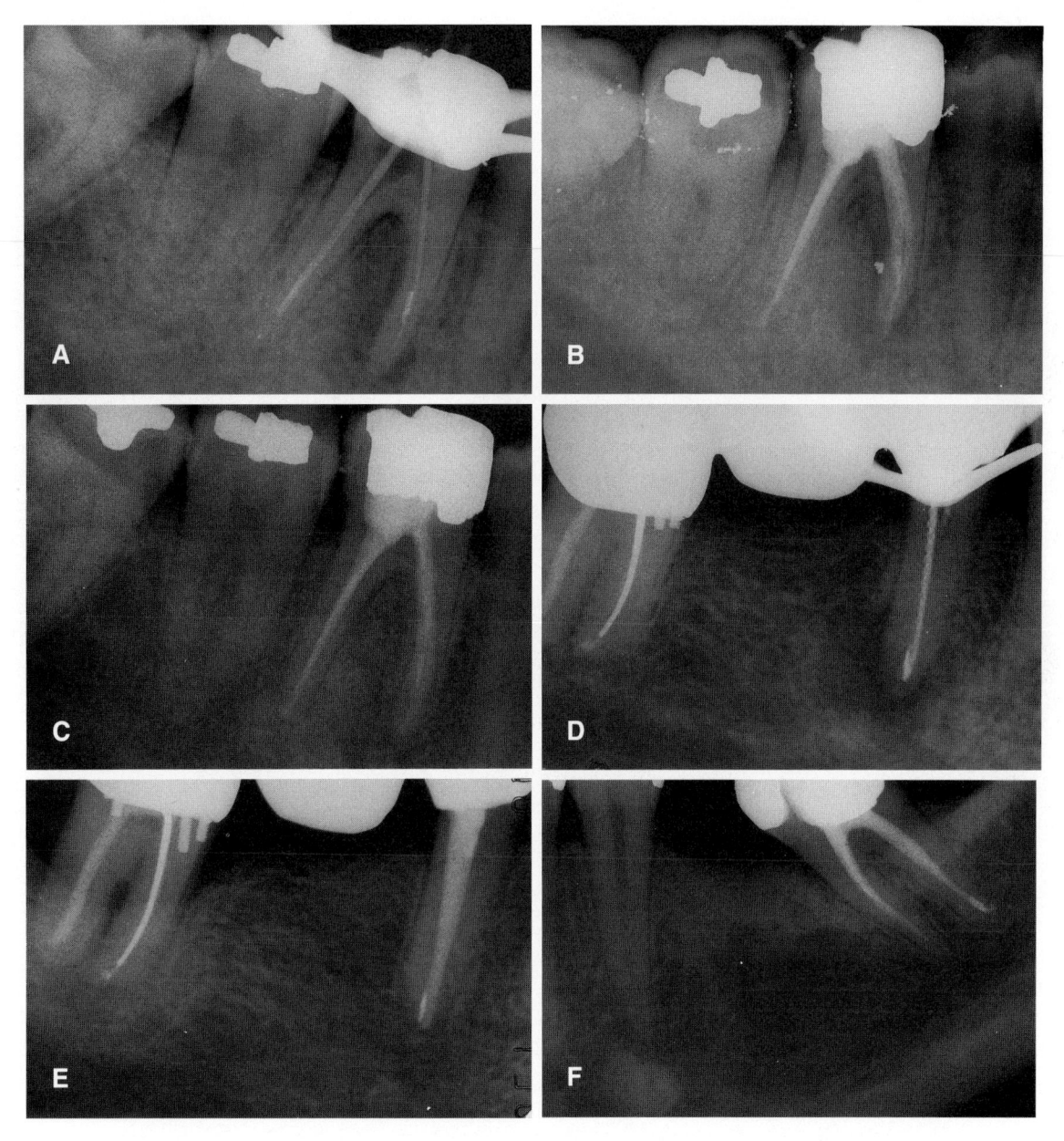

Figure 11-8 **A**, An instrument separated in the middle third of the mesial-lingual root of tooth No. 19. The instrument was bypassed and cones fitted. **B**, Canals filled with lateral condensation around the separated instrument. **C**, A 2-year check-up radiograph showing complete healing and the instrument bypassed with gutta percha. **D**, A No. 40 hedstrom file is shown bypassing the instrument. **E**, A 2-year postoperative radiograph shows complete healing and the gutta percha filling the canal beyond the instrument with Ultrafil. **F**, A mandibular molar with a separated instrument in the apical third of the distal root filled with Regular set Ultrafil. Note the gutta percha that flowed passed the instrument.

204 PRACTICAL ENDODONTICS

SEPARATED INSTRUMENTS BEYOND THE FORAMEN

Separated instruments beyond the foramen usually require surgery. However, if the canal is sealed, the tooth is painless, and there is no pathosis, it may be left in the canal without surgery. Postoperative pain usually dictates the modality (Fig. 11-9).

Dr. Roig Greene developed a unique method to retrieve separated instruments by taking an injection needle and looping a steel wire through it and then passing it over the separated instrument. The ends of the wire are twisted tightly around the instrument with a pair of hemostats and removed from the canal (Fig. 11-10).

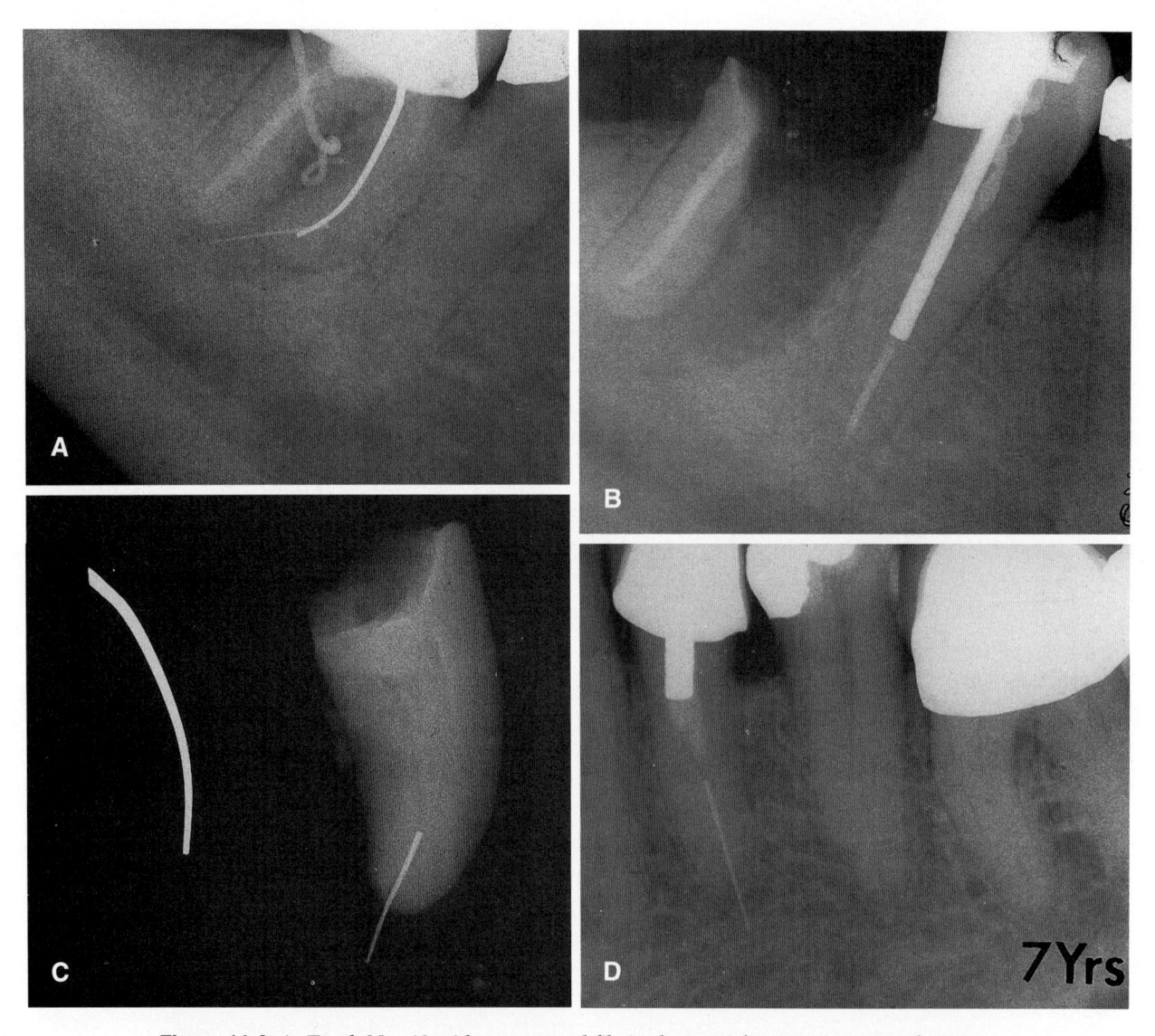

Figure 11-9 **A**, Tooth No. 19 with a separated file in the mesial root approximately 3 mm beyond the foramen and a silver cone in the canal. The patient had chronic pain for 1 ½ years. A gutta percha tracer was placed in the furca where suppuration was active. **B**, The tooth was hemisected in lieu of proximity to the mandibular canal and the furcal involvement. **C**, A sagittal view of the root with the extruded instrument and silver cone. The patient became asymptomatic following surgery. (Courtesy of Andrew M. Michanowicz.) **D**, A 7-year postoperative radiograph of separated instrument beyond the apical foramen in a mandibular bicuspid.

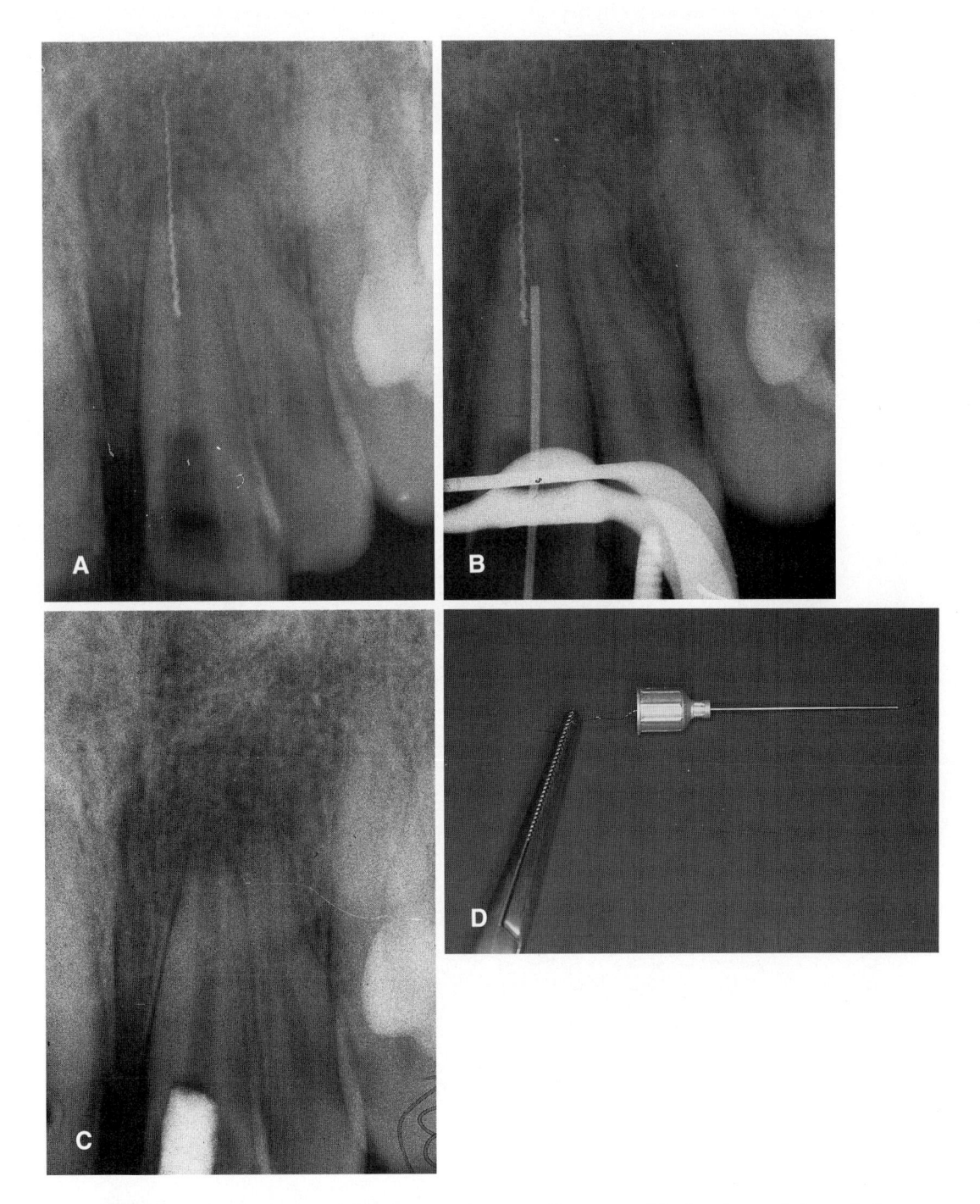

Figure 11-10 **A**, A separated instrument in a maxillary central incisor beyond the apical foramen. **B**, A radiograph of the needle and wire loop placed into the canal with the loop placed over the instrument. The other end of the wire is twisted and tightened, then withdrawn out of the canal. **C**, Instrument removed. **D**, The wire is inserted through an injection needle and one end held with hemostats.

REMOVAL OF SEPARATED BURS

A separated bur in the canal is removed by bypassing the bur with a hedstrom file dipped in RC Prep. It is engaged with the flutes of the hedstrom file and withdrawn. The file can also be left in place and the ultrasound scaler activated against the file to vibrate the bur out of the canal. The Roto Pro Scalers (see Fig. 11-16, *C*) can also be used to remove the separated bur and instruments such as Gates Glidden drills (Fig. 11-11, *A*, *B*, and *C*).

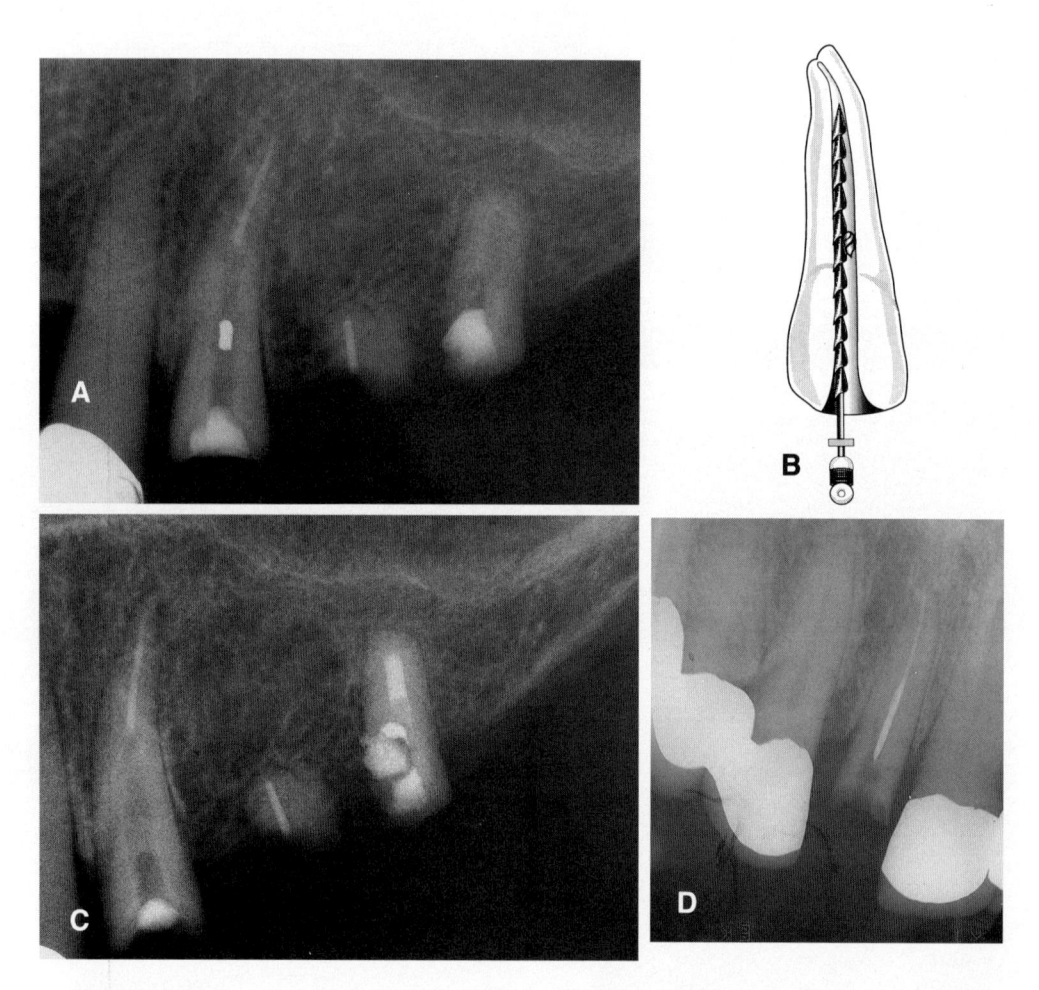

Figure 11-11 **A**, A separated pear-shaped bur in the middle third of the root canal of tooth No. 6. **B**, Bur bypassed with a hedstrom file. **C**, Bur removed. **D**, Separated Gates Glidden drill.

Continued.

Chapter 11 ♦ Nonsurgical Retreatment 207

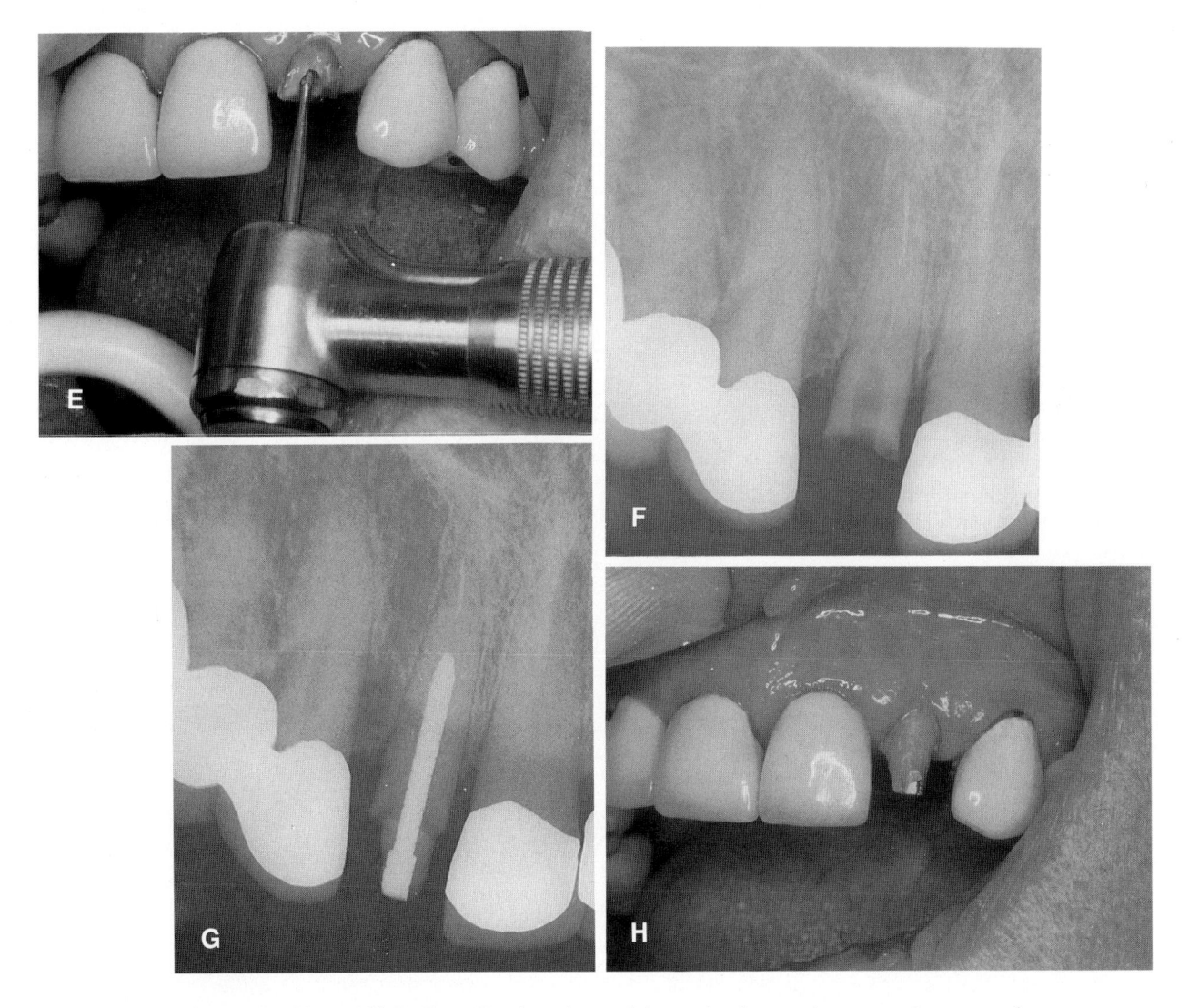

Figure 11-11, *cont'd* **E,** Roto Pro bur is used in a circular motion around separated Gates Glidden drill. **F,** Instrument removed. **G,** New post. **H,** Core placed. (Courtesy of Dr. Robert D. Westerman.)

208 PRACTICAL ENDODONTICS

REMOVAL OF POSTS

Determine the position, size, and type (tapered, passive, active, or parallel) of post and, if possible, the cementing media for the post. Active posts are much more difficult to remove than passive posts because active posts are threaded and twisted into the canal and they must be reversed and twisted to deactivate them. To date, there is no solvent for post cementing media such as oxyphosphate or carboxylate cements. There is a debonder X-7 for cured cyanoacrylates (Durelon) that may help to soften it, however it does not dissolve it. The bonding media for the posts must be physically separated from the dentin.

Instruments

- Hemostats (Fig. 11-12, *B*)
- Roto Pro Burs (see Fig. 11-16, *C*)
- Ultrasound scaler (see Fig. 11-2, *B*)
- Sonic Air Scaler (Fig. 11-12, *A*)
- Clev-dent pliers (Fig. 11-12, *A*)
- Right-angle pliers
- Eggler post pullers (Fig. 11-12, *B*)
- Stewart double-ended explorer (Fig. 11-12, *A*)

Posts may have to be removed from teeth in which the crown is intact or in teeth in which the crown and/or post has fractured. It is much easier to remove a post when the crown is removed since the operator can visibly see the type of post, core material, and the amount of remaining tooth structure. At times it may not be prudent to remove the crown. Whether the crown is removed or occlusal access is made into the crown, the cement and/or the bonding material must be detached from the post. Occlusal access is made with a fissure bur while being careful not to cut additional tooth structure or the post. As you approach the gingival and/or the post and the chamber floor, chip away the cement with a Stewart explorer and/or Sonic air scaler or ultrasound. This prevents perforation with a bur (Fig. 11-13).

When the post is exposed, place the ultrasound scaler on the post and activate. Move the scaler in a circular motion around the post. It may take several minutes to several hours. When the bond is broken, deactivate the post by twisting and remove with forceps or curved pliers (Fig. 11-14). When a post fractures and the root canal does not have to be retreated then only the post is removed and the length of the post space is increased (Fig. 11-15).

Posts can also be removed with use of the "Ellman" Roto Pro Tips. A Roto tip is used with light pressure moved from side to side around the post until it is vibrated loose (Fig. 11-16, 11-17, and 11-18).

Parallel posts and tapered posts may also be removed with the use of an Eggler post puller (Fig. 11-12, B). This type of post extractor can only be used when several millimeters of post can be grasped in

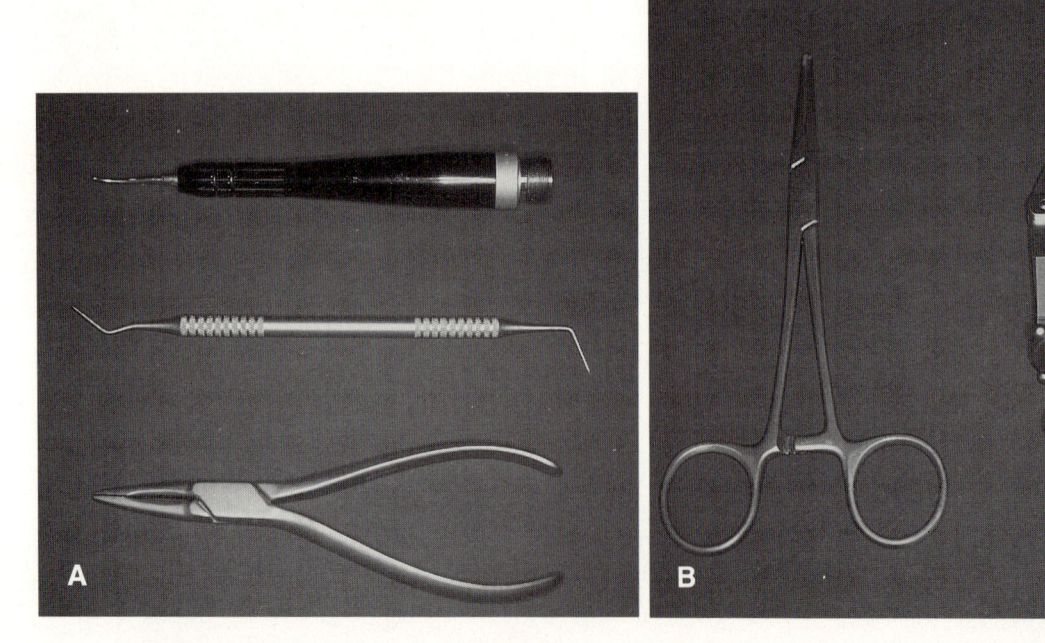

Figure 11-12 Armamentarium necessary to remove posts. **A,** Sonic air scaler, Stewart double-ended explorer, and Clev-dent pliers. **B,** Eggler post puller and straight hemostats.

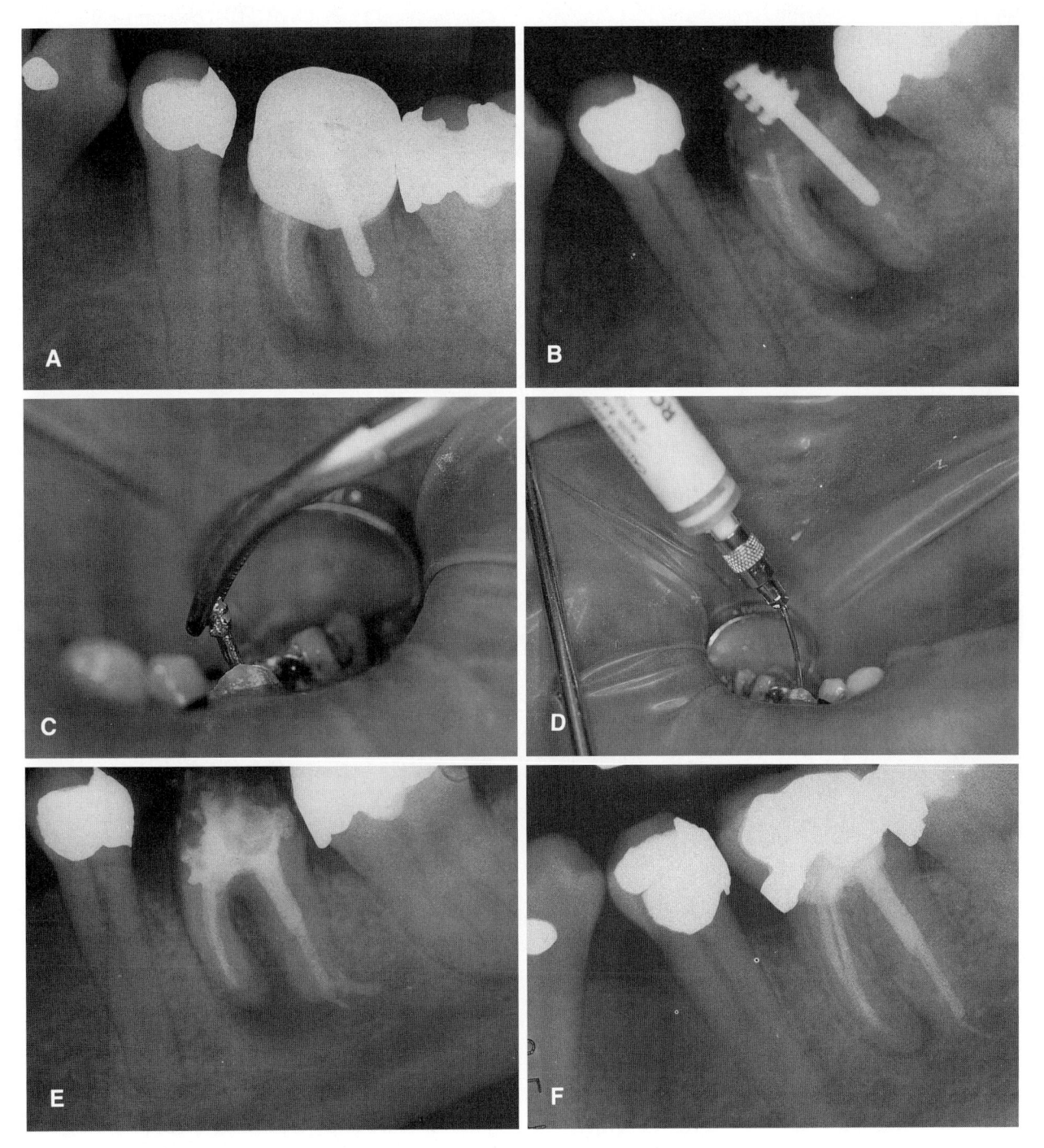

Figure 11-13 A, A mandibular molar with an ill-fitting root canal and a chronic apical periodontitis circumscribing both roots. There is a parallel post in distal canal. Retreatment is indicated as well as a new crown. **B**, The crown was removed and core was chipped away with a Stewart explorer and the ultrasound scaler. **C**, The post was removed with curved hemostats after it was vibrated loose with the ultrasound scaler. **D**, The canals were enlarged and cleaned, and calcium hydroxide (Root-Cal) was placed in the chamber and carried into the canal with absorbent points. **E**, The tooth was refilled. **F**, A 2-year radiograph showing healing.

the crown and there is adequate room for the post puller. The core is cut laterally to the gingival margin to expose the post and shoulder. The extractor is attached to the post by turning a knob and the force is applied to the gingival portion of the tooth after the post is engaged (Fig. 11-19).

At times a post is fractured below the gingival and wedged tightly in the canal and does not lend itself to ultrasound or post pullers. There are several options. It can be drilled out of the canal with a Beaver bur. The process is slow and the risk of perforation is present.

The endo extractor kit that uses a trepan bur may also be used (Fig. 11-20, A). The hollow bur that fits over the post is selected and a channel is made around the post. A hollow tube filled with cyanoacrylate is placed over the post and allowed to set and bond to the post. Force can now be applied to the tube to withdraw it from the canal (Fig. 11-20, B). The Gonon post extractor kit (R. Chige Inc., Valley Stream, NY), which uses a trephine and extractor pliers, can also be used to remove gingival fractured posts (Fig. 11-21).

Text continued on p. 218.

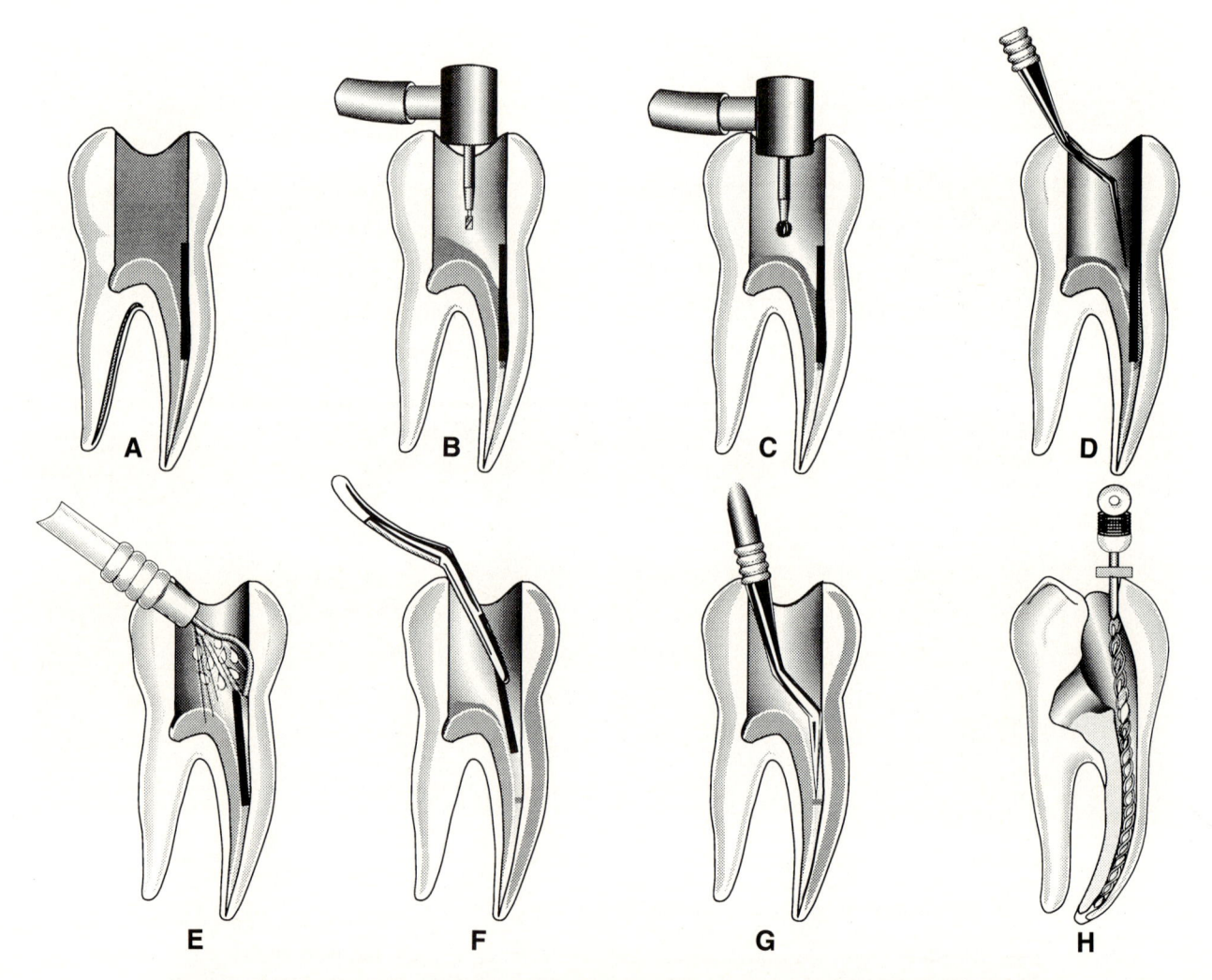

Figure 11-14 A, The core is exposed. B, The post is exposed with a fissure bur. C, The post is further exposed with dull round bur. D, The cement around the post on the gingival floor and in the canal is removed with the Stewart explorer. E, The post is vibrated loose with ultrasound scaler or sonic air scaler. F, Post removed with hemostats. G, The cement at base of post is removed with the Stewart double-ended explorer to expose the root filling. H, The canal is measured for length and retreated.

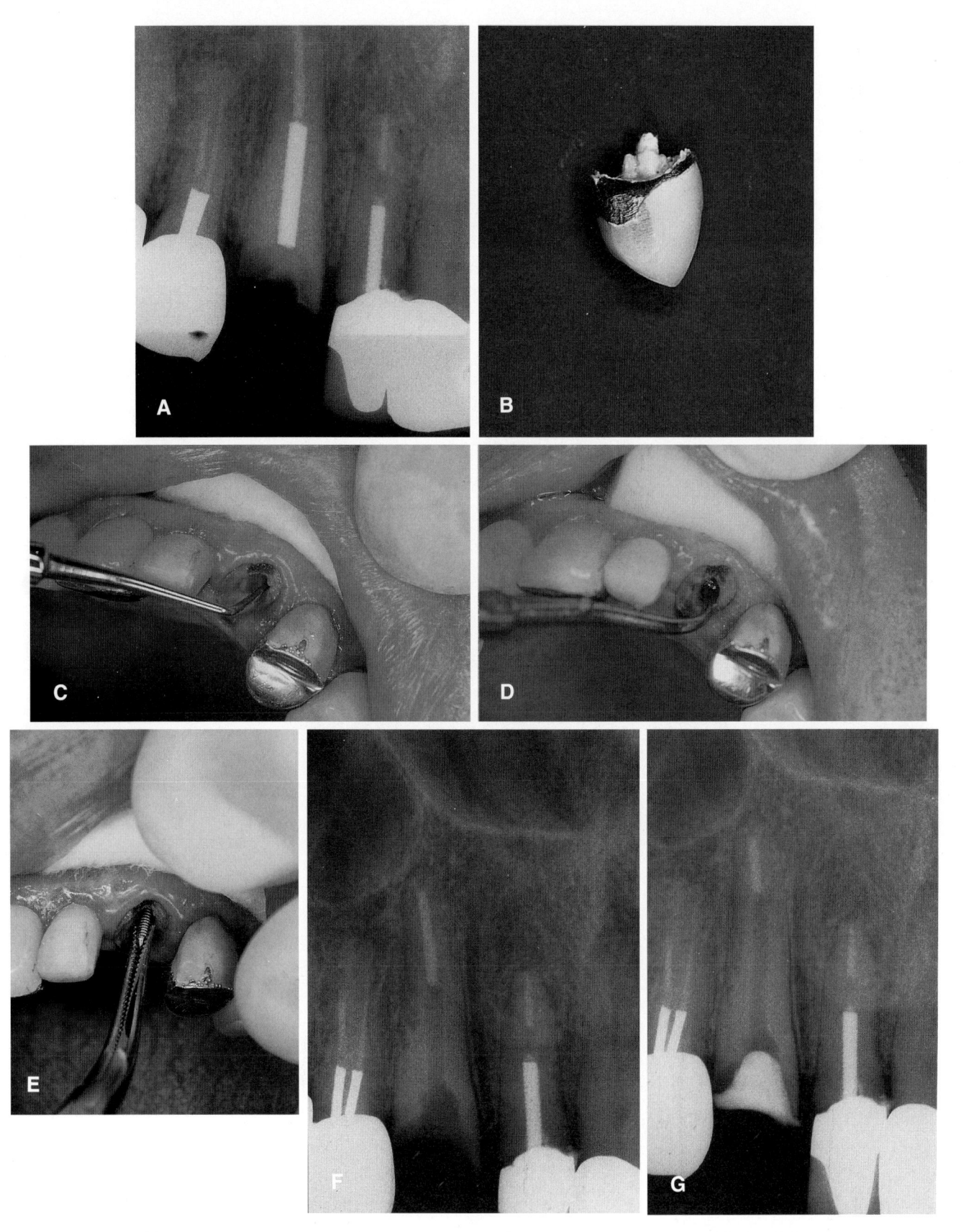

Figure 11-15 **A**, A maxillary cuspid with post fractured into the canal. **B**, Photo of the broken crown and post. **C**, The cement around the post is removed with a Stewart explorer. **D**, The ultrasound scaler is placed on the post and activated. It is moved around the post in a circular motion. **E**, The loosened post is removed with hemostats. **F**, Post removed from canal. **G,** Post length increased.

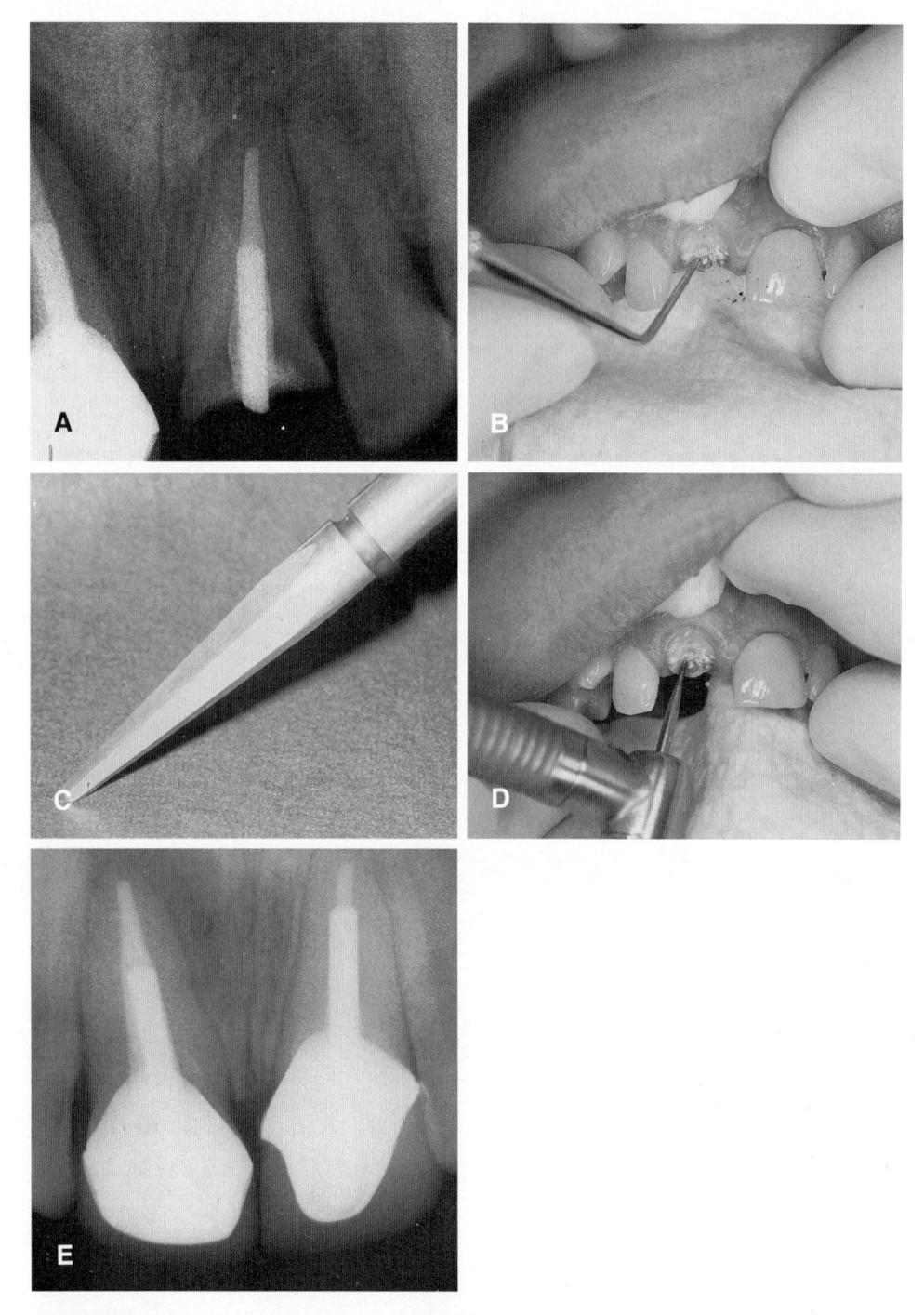

Figure 11-16 **A**, A crown and post fractured in maxillary central incisor. **B**, The cement surrounding the post is chipped away with a double-ended explorer. **C**, The Roto Pro tip showing the pointed end and flattened sides. **D**, The Roto Pro tip is inserted between the dentin and post and moved back and forth in a circular motion. **E**, One-year recall with new post and core. (Courtesy of Dr. Robert D. Westerman.)

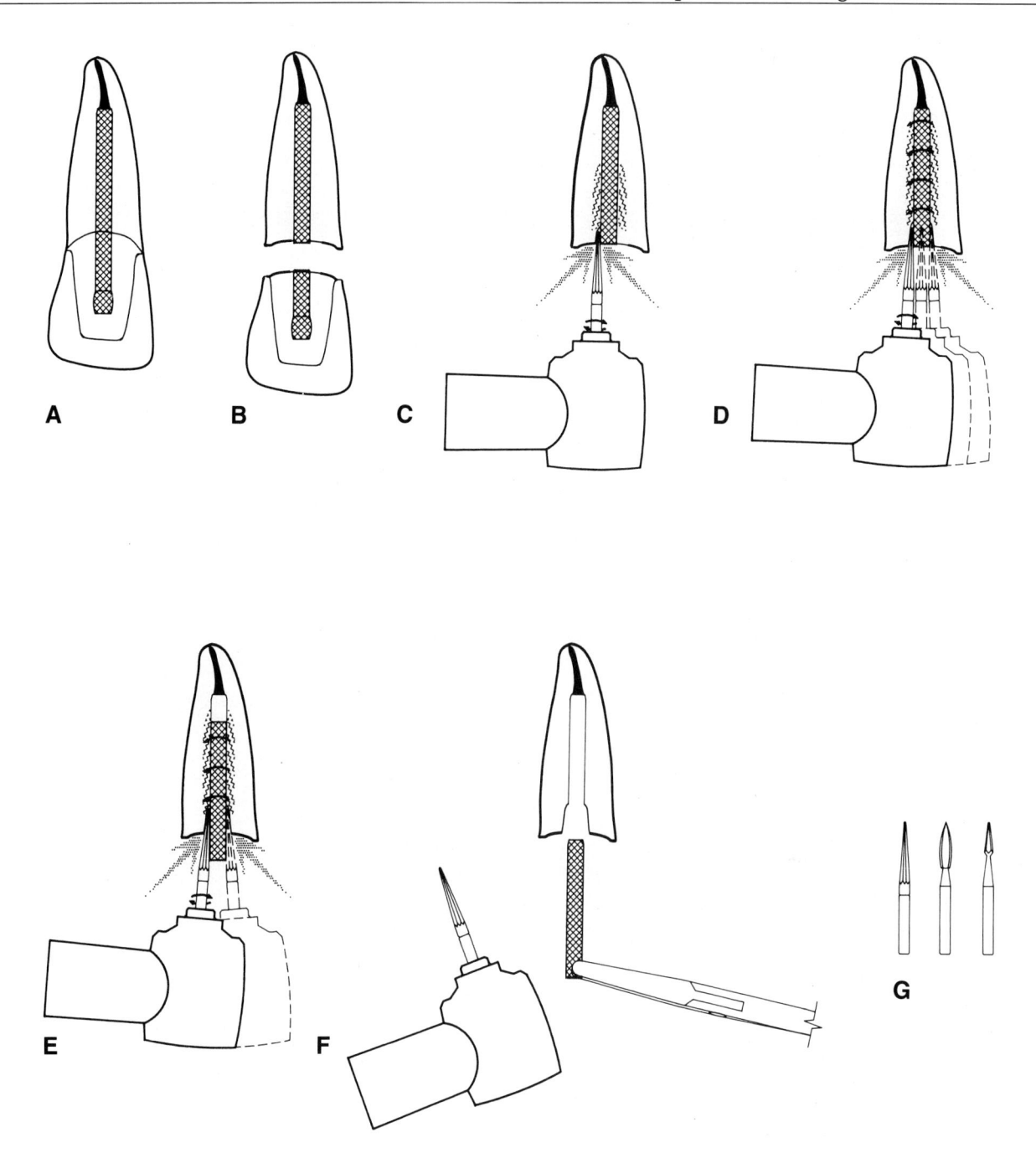

Figure 11-17 A, A parallel post cemented in a central incisor with a crown. **B,** A gingival fracture of the post within the crown. **C,** A tip is selected that can be inserted between the post and the dentin. The handpiece with the tip and water spray is moved circumferentialy around post using very light pressure. If the post is snug against the dentin with a thin layer of cement it may be necessary to remove a small amount of dentin with a bur to allow access to the post. **D,** When the slightest rotation is observed, an attempt is made to vibrate the post in the opposite direction as the tip is moved from side to side. **E,** The circumferential side to side movement is repeated until the post becomes loose. **F,** The post is removed with hemostats or Stieglitz forceps. **G,** The Roto Pro burs are six sided, noncutting, and tapered. They rotate and vibrate at 20,000 cycles per second pulverizing the cement that traps the post. (Courtesy of Dr. Robert D. Westerman.)

214 PRACTICAL ENDODONTICS

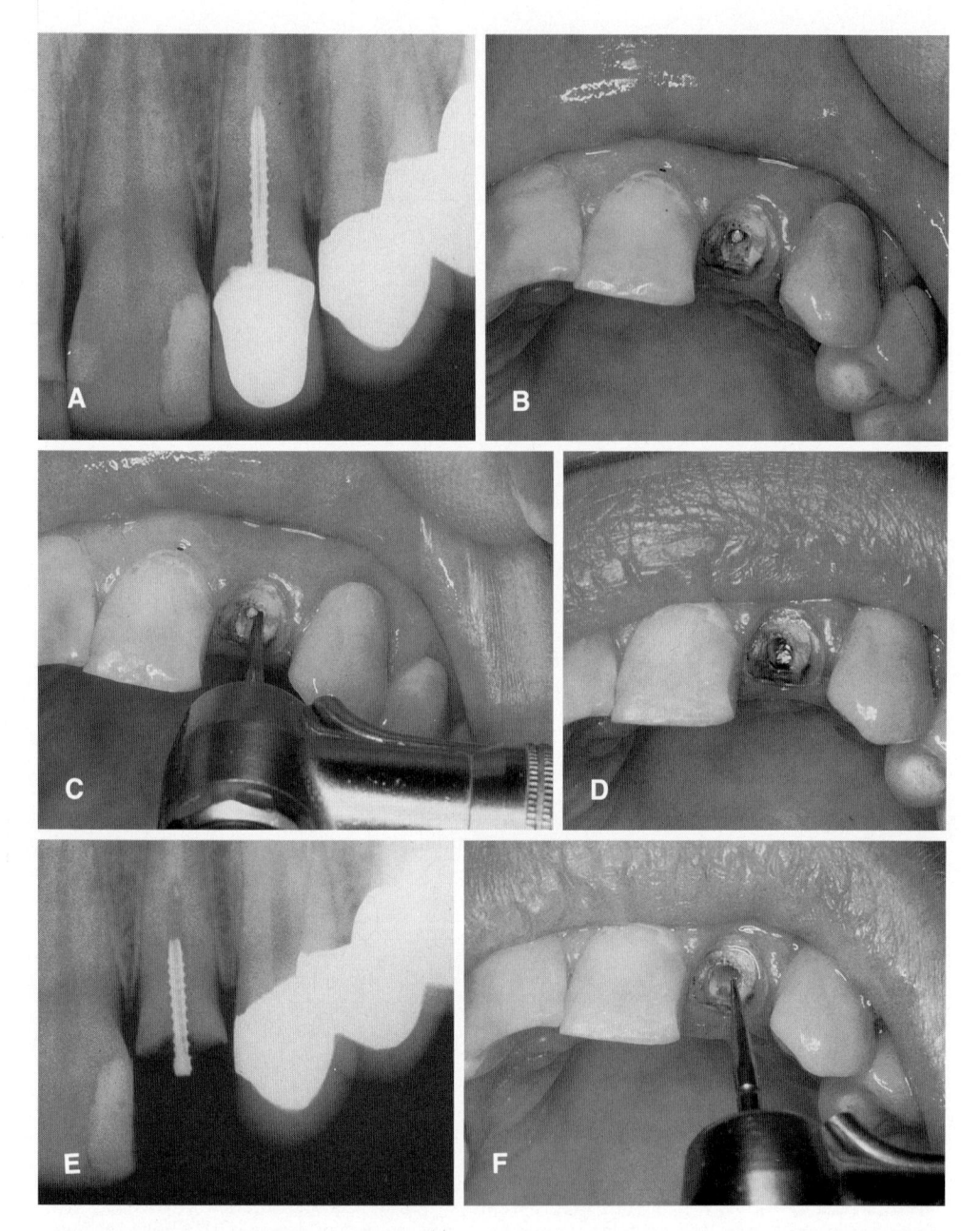

Figure 11-18 **A**, Maxillary lateral incisor with a loose fitting crown and flexi post. **B**, Crown removed. **C**, Roto Pro tip inserted between separated post and dentin. **D**, Post loosened. **E**, Dislodged post. **F**, Post vibrated out of canal. (Courtesy of Dr. Robert D. Westerman.)

Chapter 11 ♦ Nonsurgical Retreatment 215

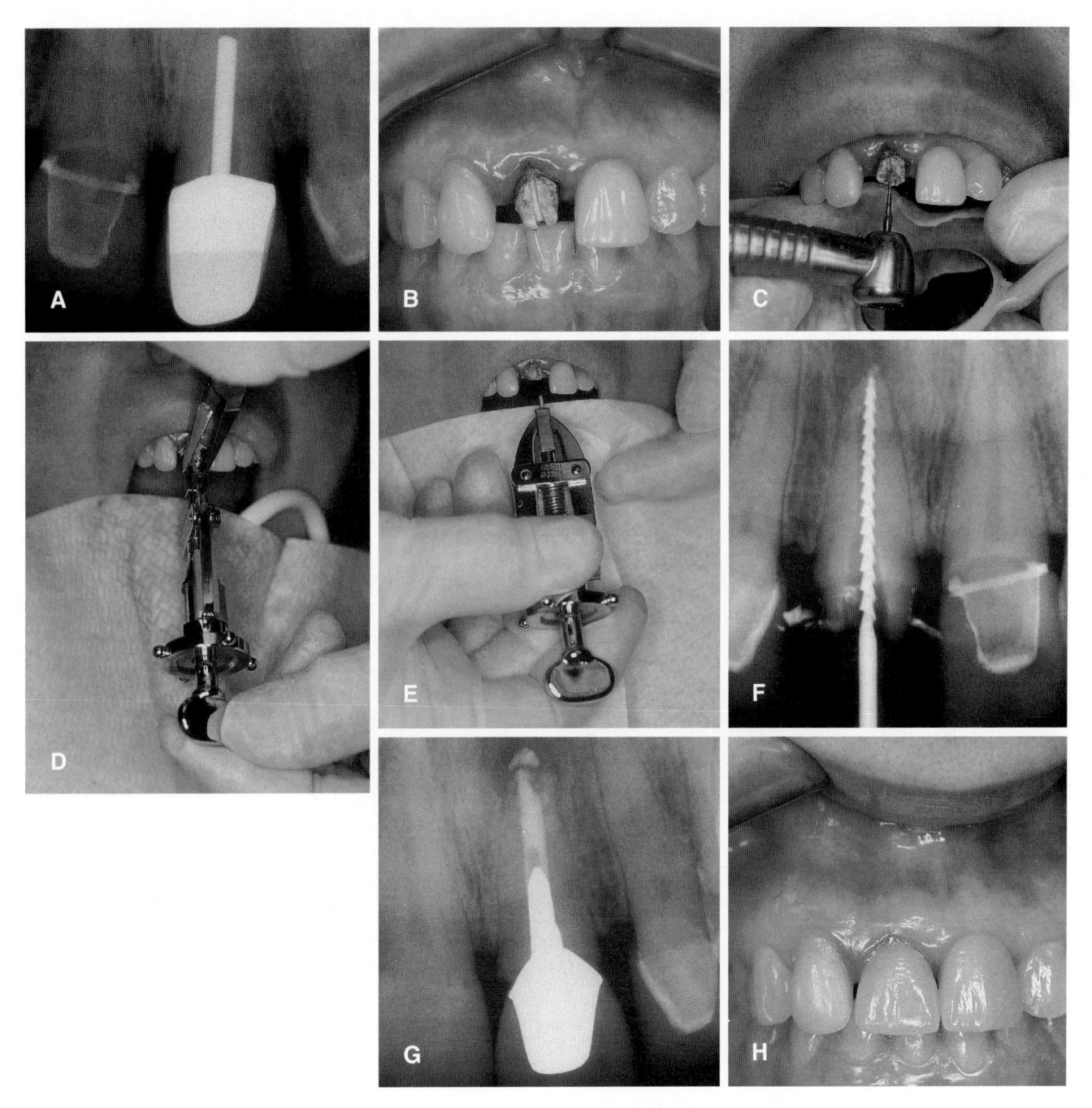

Figure 11-19 **A** and **B**, Maxillary central incisor with a post, crown, and incomplete root canal. **C**, Crown removed and the core is cut out. **D**, The Eggler post extractor is attached to the post and pressure is applied by turning the knob. Since the shoulders were small, the feet of the extractor were held together with Cleve-dent pliers to prevent slipping. **E**, The removed post is attached to the extractor. **F**, The tooth is measured, cleaned, and shaped with hedstrom files. **G**, Canal refilled, new post, and crown. **H**, Photo of new crown.

216 PRACTICAL ENDODONTICS

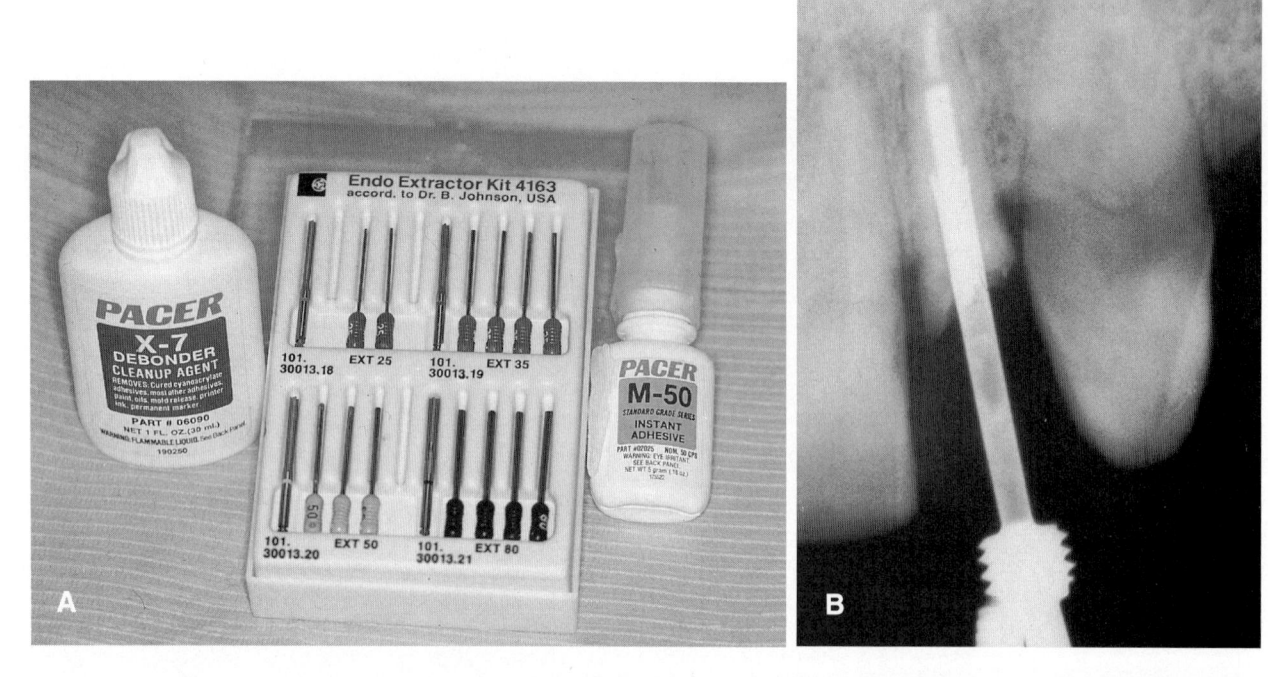

Figure 11-20 **A**, The extractor kit. **B**, The tube cemented to the post.

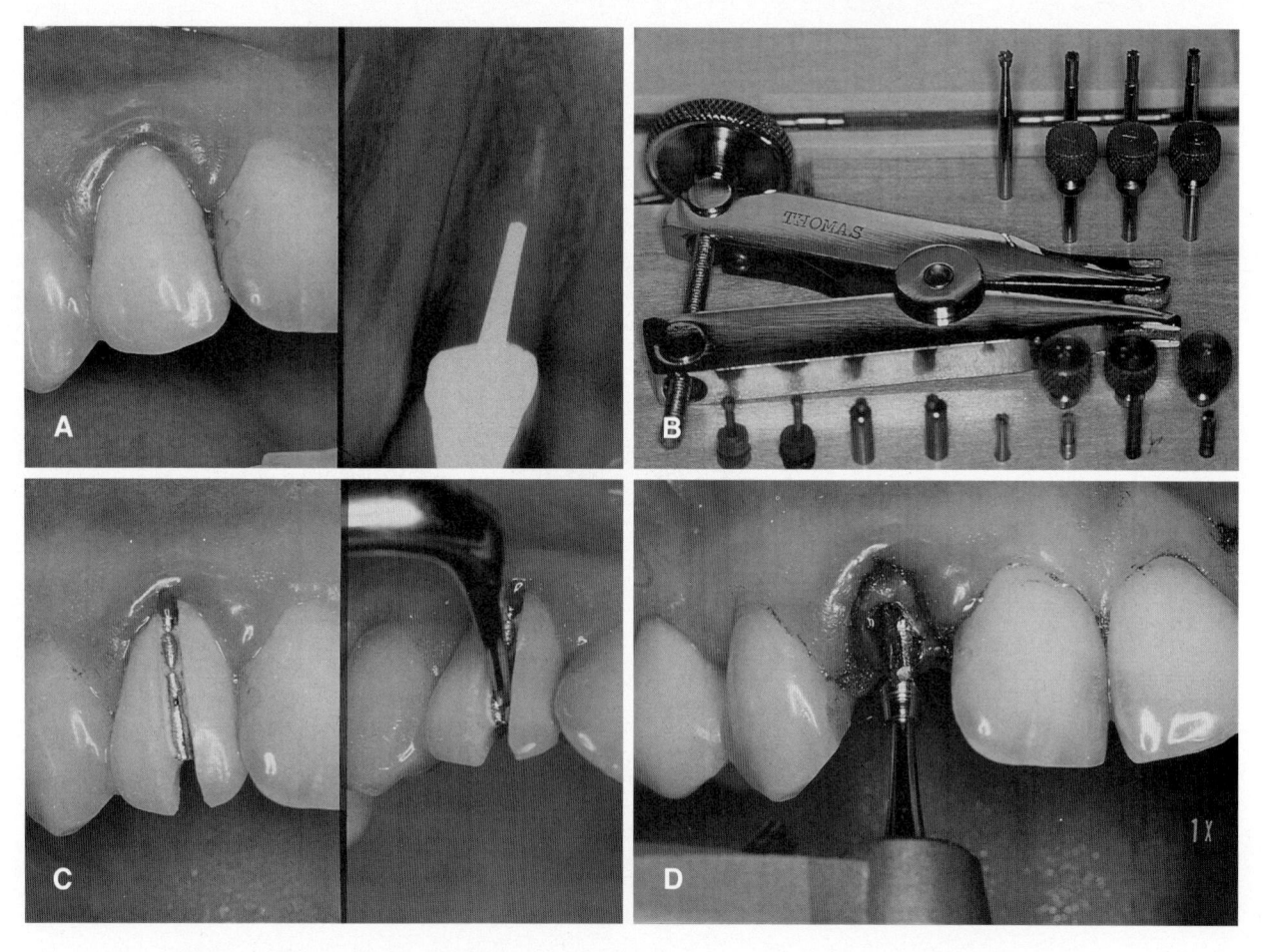

Figure 11-21 **A**, Poor endo treatment. **B**, Gonon post system. **C**, Crown sectioned and separated. **D**, Use of the trephine.

Continued.

Chapter 11 ♦ Nonsurgical Retreatment 217

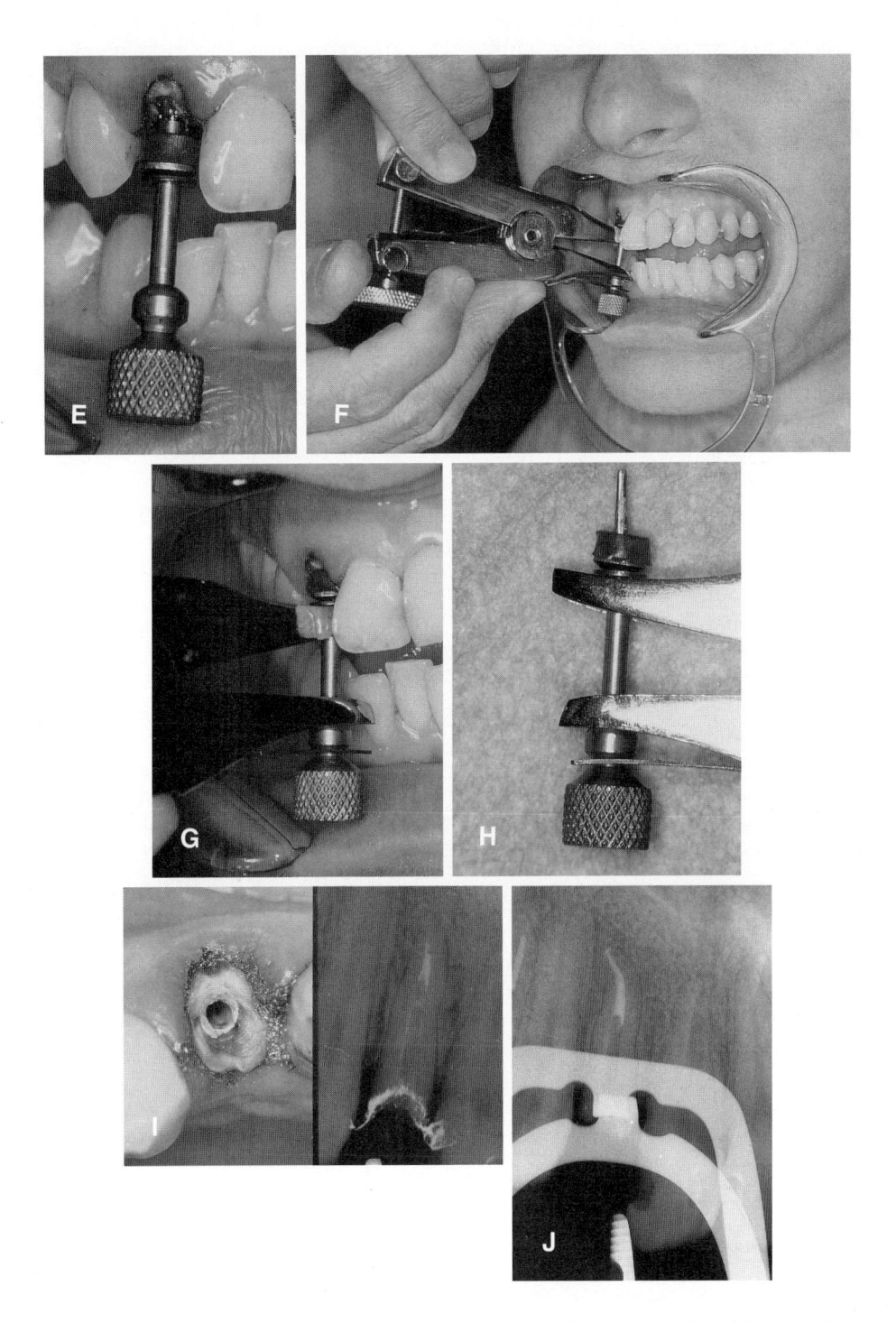

Figure 11-21, *cont'd* **E**, Threading the post. **F**, Positioning of the beaks of Ganon pliers. **G**, Extracting pliers on the threaded mandrel. **H**, The post removed. **I**, The empty canal. **J**, Endodontic retreatment completed. (Courtesy of Pierre Machtou, DCD, DSO, Paris.)

REMOVAL OF SILVER CONES

Silver cones sealed in the canal with several millimeters of the cone in the pulp chamber are removed by making a slightly larger access cavity and carefully exposing the silver cones with a No. 2 round bur or fissure bur. The operator must be extremely cautious not to cut off the silver cones. The gutta percha in the chamber can be softened with a warm instrument or chloroform and removed with a double-ended explorer or small spoon excavator. The loose cones can be grasped with silver cone pliers and removed (Fig. 11-22). Those that are cut off at the gingival or below are much more difficult to remove. Amalgam or cement on the gingival floor makes the task even more difficult. The amalgam must be drilled away with a bur and the cement must be drilled and chipped away carefully so as not to cut off the protruding silver cone. Use a fissure bur to make access and then proceed to a No. 2 or No. 4 round bur when the silver cone is identified. Remove the restorative material in the crown without touching the silver cone (Fig. 11-23). The ultrasound scaler can be used to chip away the restorative material surrounding the cone. A bur is more likely to cut the silver cone and should be used with utmost care. Remove the gutta percha (if present) that may be packed around the silver cone with chloroform and reamers (No. 15, 20, and 25). When loose, remove the silver cone with silver cone forceps. Once the silver cone is removed, the canal is irrigated with sodium hypochlorite and working length is established. Files are now used to cleanse the dentin walls.

Do not attempt to remove the silver cone if resistance is met when engaging with silver cone pliers or forceps. Silver is ductile and may stretch; part of it will separate and remain in the canal, which makes it more difficult to retrieve. Loosen the silver cone with files or ultrasound and determine if the cone is loose before tugging at it again. Several techniques may be used to remove silver cones:

1. An ultrasound scaler is placed against it and activated to vibrate it loose (Fig. 11-24).
2. A No. 15 K-file is used to bypass it partially or completely. The instrument is left in place and activated with an ultrasound scaler. The sound waves are transmitted to the silver cone and will vibrate it loose and out of the canal (Fig. 11-25).
3. A hedstrom file is used to partially bypass it and twisted so the sharp flutes of the hedstrom bite into the silver cone and allow it to be removed (Fig. 11-26).
4. A forked silver cone remover (Caufield) instrument may aid in removing it when part of it becomes visible in the crown and it is loose. The neck of the fork is placed against the silver cone and lifted out of the canal (Fig. 11-27).
5. Silver cones may also be removed by using the Roig Greene technique as previously described for a separated instrument (Fig. 11-10).
6. In straight canals the silver cone can be reamed out by passing it with a small reamer and increasing the reamer size incrementally. Since silver is softer than dentin it can be reamed out of the canal.
7. The silver cone is first bypassed with a No. 15 K-file. A No. 15 ultrasound file is placed along side the silver cone and activated. The ultrasound loosens the cement bond and vibrates the silver cone loose (Fig. 11-28).

The endo extractor kit can also be used when the silver cones are separated inside the canal (Fig. 11-20, A). It is the least desirable because tooth structure must be sacrificed. A trepan bur that fits over the silver cone is used to make a channel around the cone. A snug hollow tube is placed over the cone with a drop of cyanoacrylate cement and allowed to bond. The tube and silver cone is then removed out of the canal (Fig. 11-29).

Text continued on p. 225.

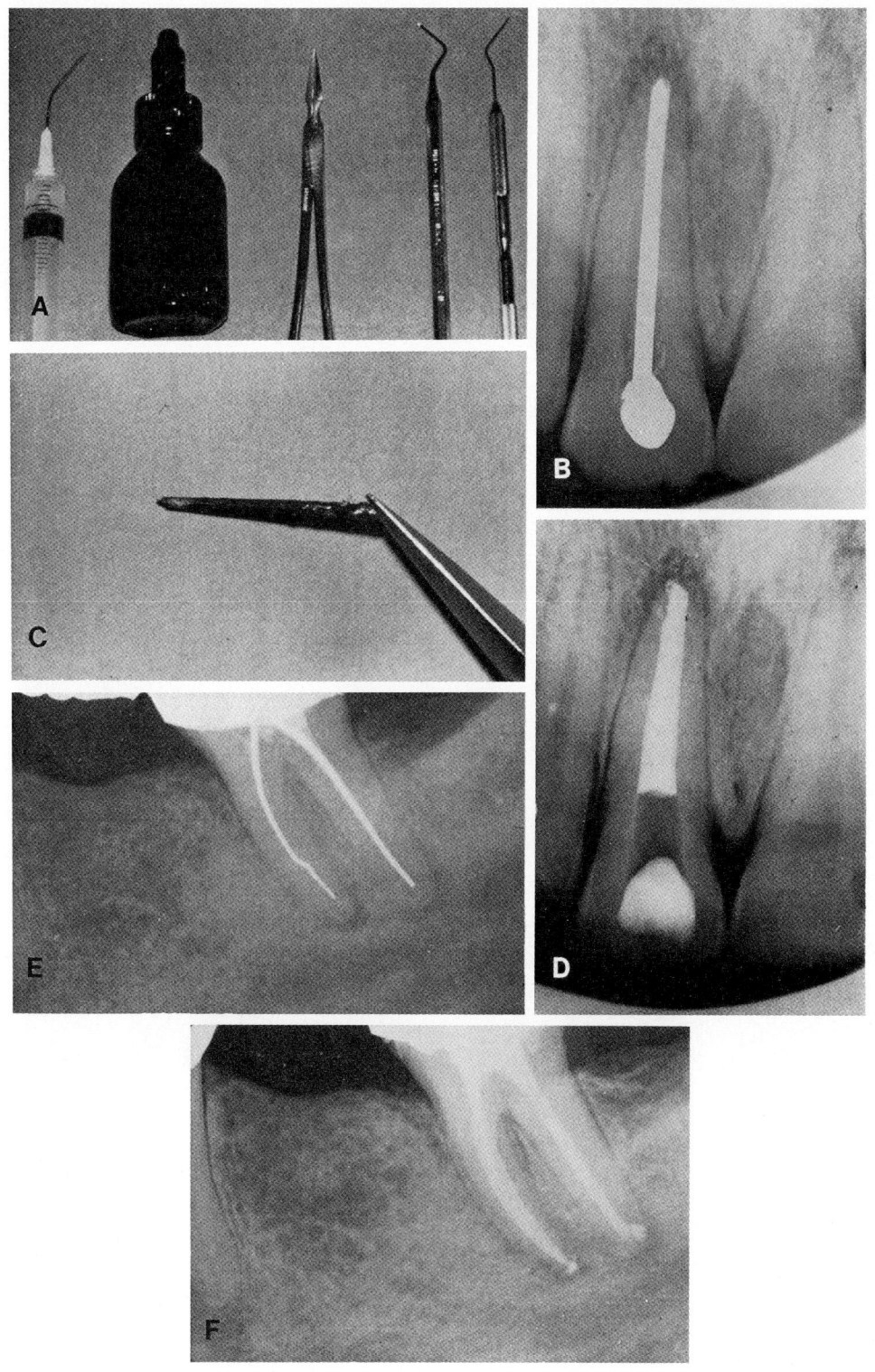

Figure 11-22 **A**, Armamentarium used in retrieving silver points from root canals. From *left* to *right:* syringe filled with chloroform used as a dissolvent to soften the cement around the silver point, chloroform bottle, Stieglitz forcep used to remove the silver point, spoon excavator used to lift up the silver point when the Stieglitz forcep cannot fit into the canal, DG-16 explorer used to chip away the cement around the silver point and act as a wedge between the dentinal wall and the silver point. **B**, Maxillary right central incisor filled with a silver point. Notice space between the silver point and the lateral walls of the canal. The patient presented with an acute periapical abscess. **C**, Silver point removed with the Stieglitz forcep. Notice the corrosion of the silver point. **D**, Postoperative radiograph immediately after the root canal was filled. The root canal was cleansed, reshaped, and filled in a two-visit procedure. **E**, Mandibular molar after being treated inadequately with silver point technique. **F**, Postoperative radiograph after retreating this same case with gutta percha.

220 PRACTICAL ENDODONTICS

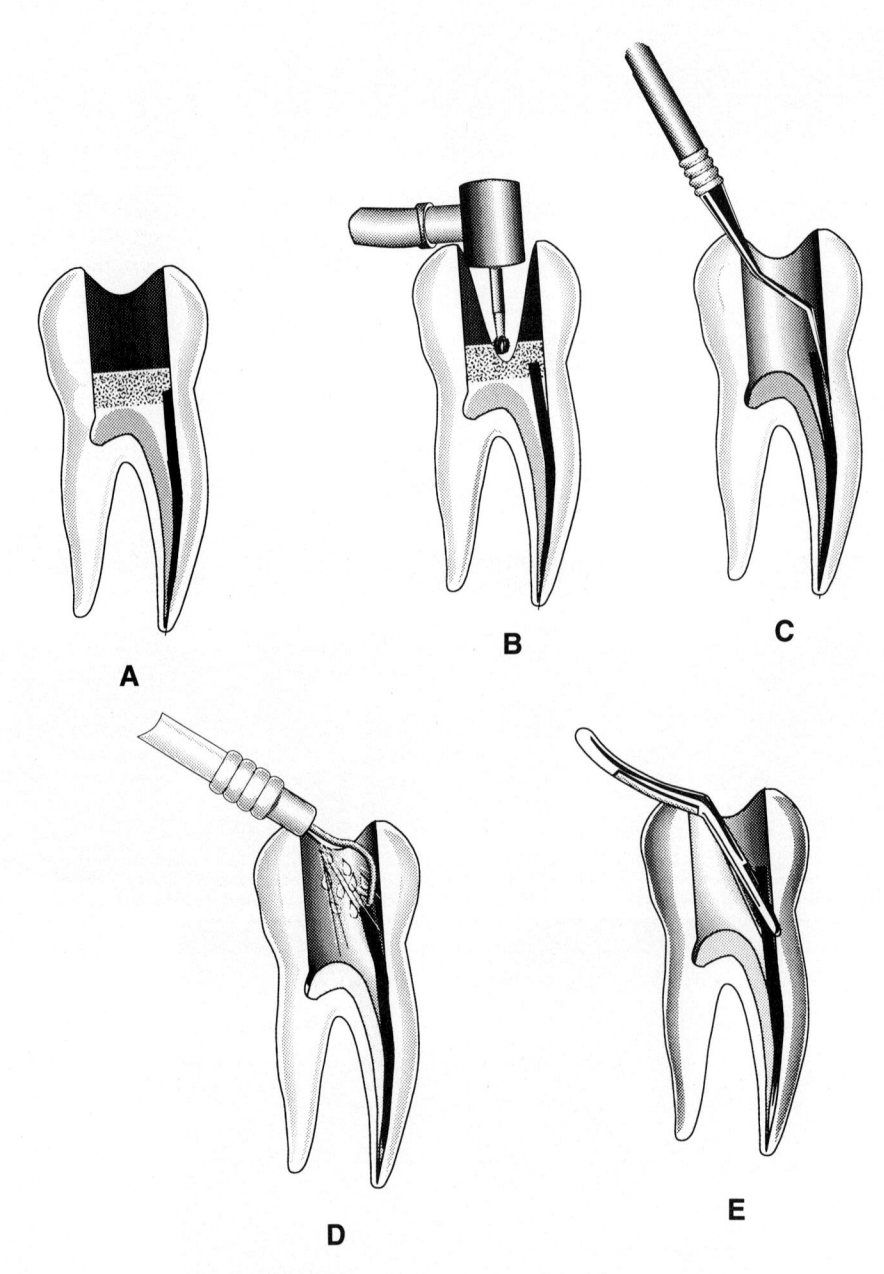

Figure 11-23 **A,** Silver cone sealed in canal. **B,** The cement core is carefully removed with a round or fissure bur until the silver cone is visible. **C,** The remaining cement close to the silver cone is chipped away with a Stewart double-ended explorer. **D,** The silver cone is vibrated loose with the ultrasound scaler. **E,** The loose silver cone is removed with silver cone pliers.

Chapter 11 ♦ Nonsurgical Retreatment 221

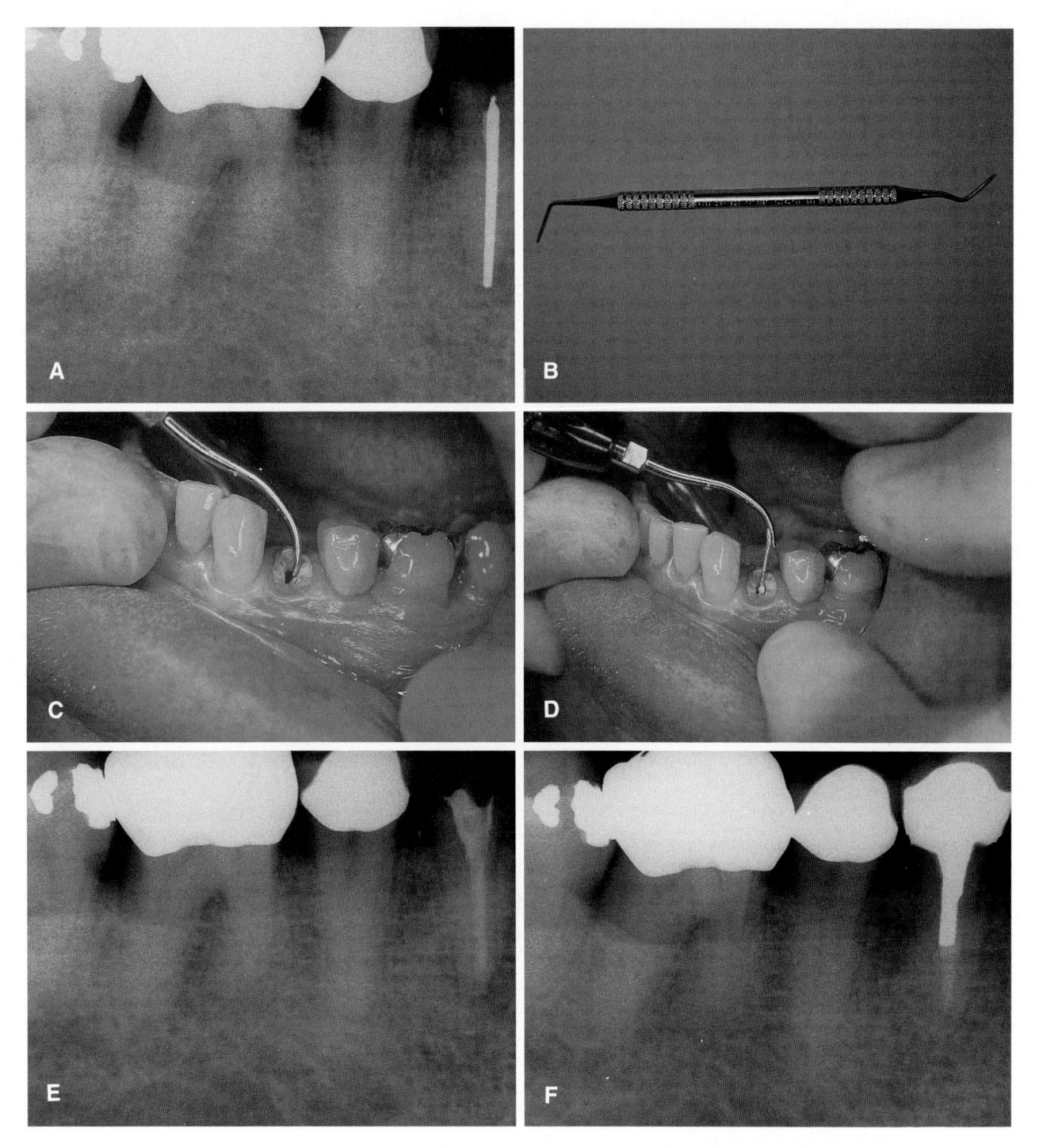

Figure 11-24 **A**, Tooth No. 21 showing crown fracture with a silver cone below the gingival margin. **B**, A Stewart double-ended explorer is used to pick away the cement around the silver cone. **C**, The ultrasound scaler is placed against the silver cone and activated to maximum power. The scaler will remove any remaining cement and loosen the silver cone. **D**, The silver cone is vibrated out of the canal. **E**, A radiograph showing the root canal completed. **F**, Two-year radiograph showing post, core, and crown.

222 PRACTICAL ENDODONTICS

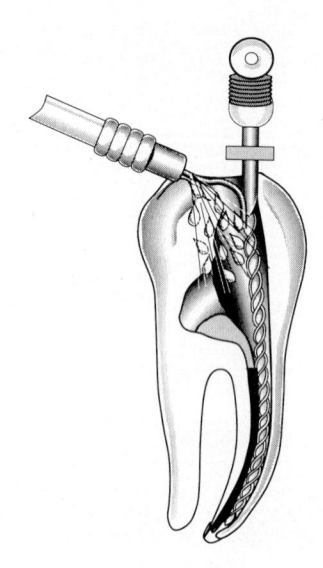

Figure 11-25 The ultrasound scaler touching the instrument that bypassed the silver cone.

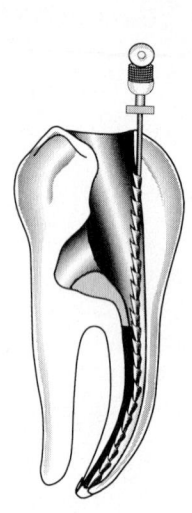

Figure 11-26 Hedstrom file bypassing and engaging a silver cone in a molar.

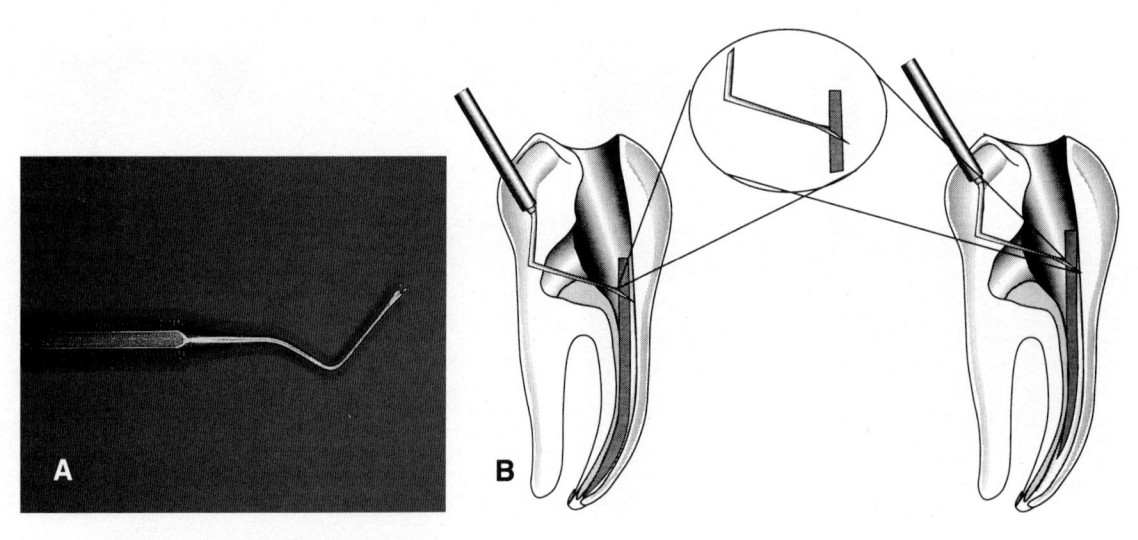

Figure 11-27 A, The Caufield silver point retriever. B, The silver cone is taken out of the canal with the Caufield instrument.

Chapter 11 ♦ Nonsurgical Retreatment 223

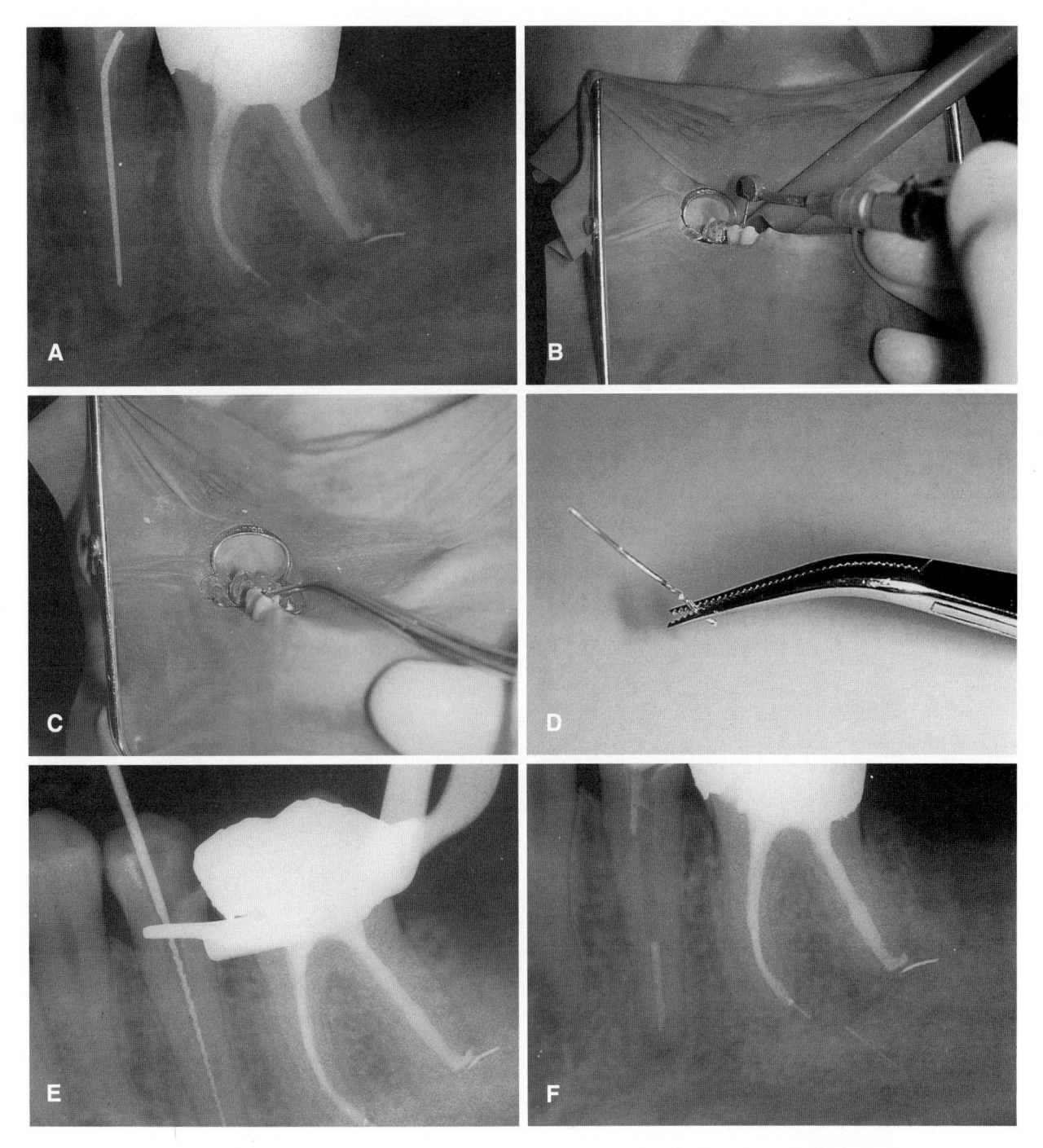

Figure 11-28 **A**, A fractured crown with a silver cone in tooth. **B**, A No. 15 ultrasound file being activated to maximum power against the silver cone. **C**, The loosened silver cone is removed with silver point pliers. **D**, The silver cone was darkened from oxidation. **E**, Instrument in the canal to established working length. **F**, The tooth was filled and prepared for a post. Note the separated instrument and silver cone beyond the foramen and in the medullary bone with no apparent pathosis or symptoms.

224 PRACTICAL ENDODONTICS

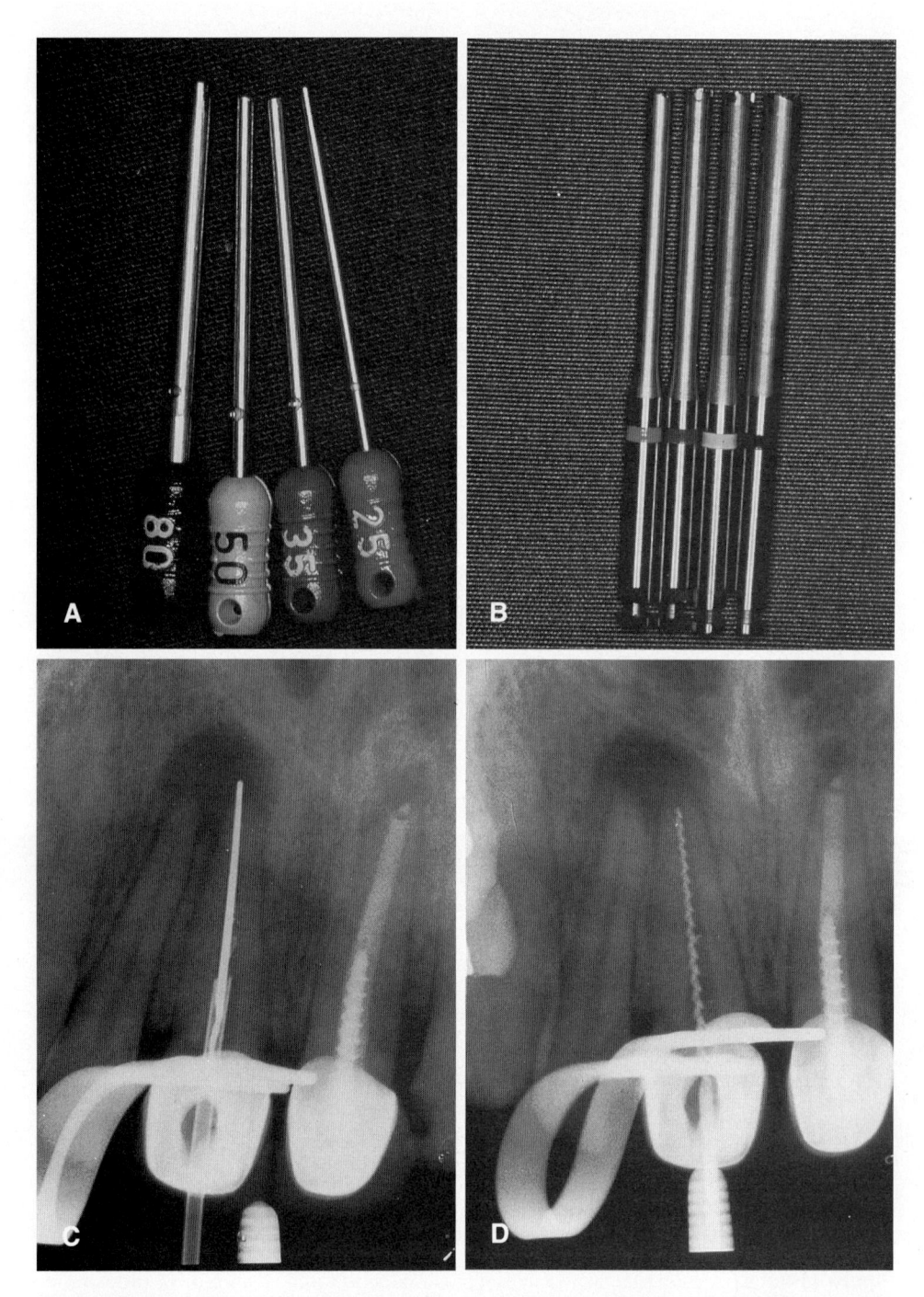

Figure 11-29 Endo Extractor Tubes. **A**, The Endo Extractor Tubes #25-#80. **B**, A trepan bur is selected that will fit over the silver cone and room is made for the extractor. **C**, A radiograph of the extractor tube seated over the silver cone. **D**, Radiograph showing silver cone removed and a file in place for working length.

REMOVAL OF GUTTA PERCHA

Gutta percha fillings are removed with a solvent such as chloroform (Fig. 11-30, A). The tissue is protected with petrolatum such as Velvachol (a water-miscible vehicle) (Fig. 11-30, B and C). A tight-fitting rubber dam is placed and the gutta percha is exposed (Fig. 11-30, D). It is best to use the same access into the pulp chamber whenever possible. Chloroform is carried into the chamber with treatment pliers or a 2-cc syringe using a 23-gauge needle (Fig. 11-30, E). A smaller gauge needle is used to confine the chloroform to the pulp chamber. A double-ended explorer is worked in and out to help soften and penetrate the gutta percha. A No. 25 reamer is used to penetrate the canal with back and forth reaming motion. The No. 25 reamer is used because it has some resistance and is less likely to bend. The reamer is removed and the softened gutta percha is wiped off and the instrument is reinserted (Fig. 11-30, F). The apical third is approached with a No. 25 reamer, then a No. 15 reamer is carried to the apex (Fig. 11-30, G). Once the apex is reached with a No. 15 the canal is cleansed with subsequently larger reamers. The sequential sizing of reamers prevents perforations. If the canal is somewhat large a broach can be used to aid in removing the gutta percha.

When the gutta percha is removed, conventional cleansing, shaping, and filling is completed (Fig. 11-30, H).

PASTES AND CEMENTS

There are no known solvents for pastes used in the root canal such as ZOE. They must be hand reamed out of the canal. It is best to use a No. 25 reamer because it is not too rigid and will bend rather than perforate. It is a slow and tedious process. Chloroform at times seems to help, but presently there is no solvent. The use of a double-ended explorer is useful in picking out the cement. The picking and reaming action are helpful.

Cements such as oxyphosphate and carboxylate are rarely used as root canal fillings. There are no known solvents to remove them. An ultrasound scaler will aid in removing the cements from the crown (Fig. 11-2).

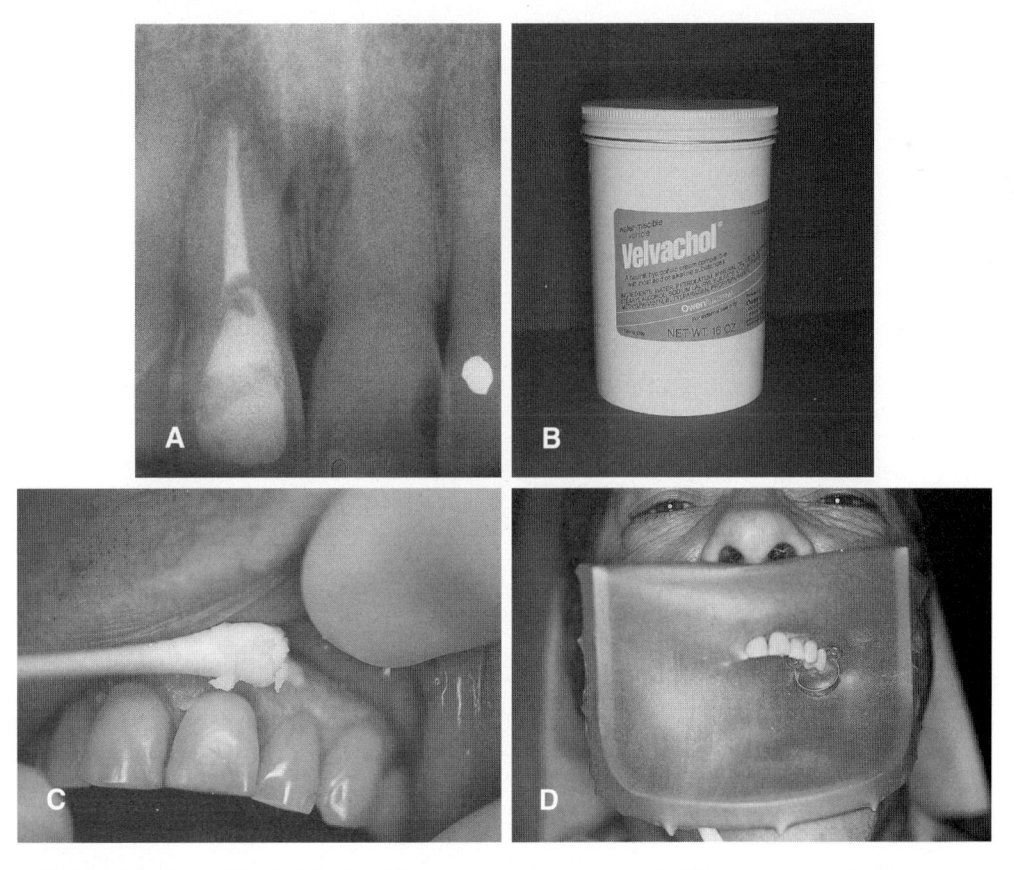

Figure 11-30 **A**, Tooth No. 9 with gutta percha root canal filling and an apical periodontitis. **B**, Velvachol. **C**, Velvachol is placed on gingival tissue with cotton swab. **D**, A rubber dam placed.

Continued.

226 PRACTICAL ENDODONTICS

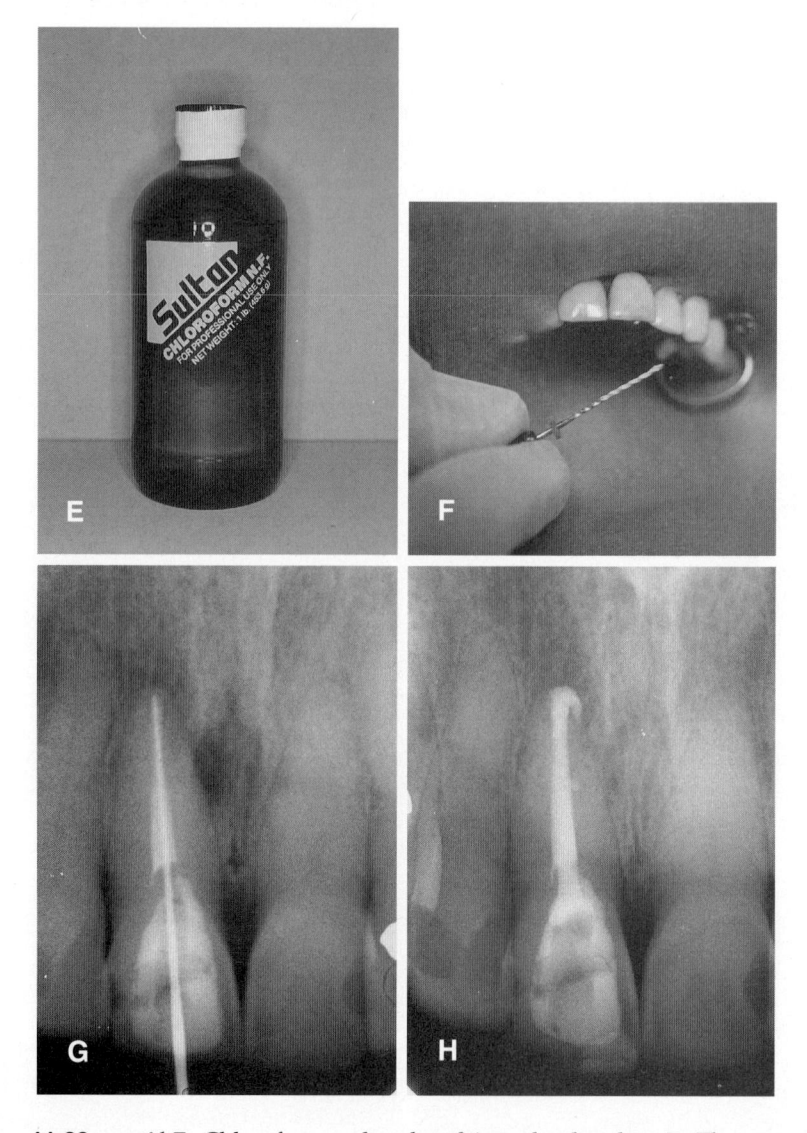

Figure 11-30, *cont'd* **E**, Chloroform to be placed in pulp chamber. **F**, The reamer with gutta percha. **G**, Working length is established with No. 15 reamer placed in canal and radiograph taken. **H**, Tooth is refilled.

12

Surgical Endodontics

Most endodontic procedures can be treated without surgery, however there are some cases in which surgical intervention is indicated and prudent. This chapter will deal with the surgical approach and outline in detail a technique for both anterior and posterior surgery. This chapter will also include incision and drainage, trephination, marsupialization, apicoectomy of anterior and posterior teeth, apical seal (retrograde filling) hemisection, and root amputation.

INDICATIONS

1. Calcified canals with lesions.
2. Teeth with constant discomfort and persistent drainage.
3. Teeth with post and cores that cannot be treated nonsurgically.
4. Perforations and teeth that were ledged and unmanageable with conventional endodontic procedure.
5. Teeth with curved roots, i.e., S-shaped root apices not negotiable with conventional endodontics.
6. Incomplete apical formation that will not respond to apexification.
7. Root resorption—external resorption that altered the root canal, chamber, or apex.
8. Excess overfilling of the root canal apex with persistent exacerbation.
9. Root fractures associated with periapical lesions.

ARMAMENTARIUM

The surgical procedure requires a broad array of surgical instruments that includes the following (Figs. 12-1 and 12-2):

ALLIS TISSUE FORCEPS
BONE WAX
BONE FILES
CURETTES (various sizes)

DEMINERALIZED BONE
GELFOAM (oxymethylcellulose)

HEMOSTATS

NU GAUZE SPONGES (J & J)
SCALERS
SCALPEL No. 12

SOFT TISSUE CURETTES
SURGICAL RULER
SUTURE SCISSORS

BONE AWL
BONE BURS
BONE RONGUERS
CURVED EXPLORER
DISPOSABLE
 SUCTION TIPS
HANDPIECES
IRRIGATING
 SYRINGE
PERIOSTEAL
 ELEVATOR
SALINE SOLUTION
SCALPEL No. 15
SPECIMEN BOTTLE
 (formalin)
SUTURES
TISSUE RETRACTOR

Apicoectomy

Apicoectomy is the resection of the apex and the total curettement of the diseased tissue from the apical region of a non-vital tooth (Fig. 12-3).

228 PRACTICAL ENDODONTICS

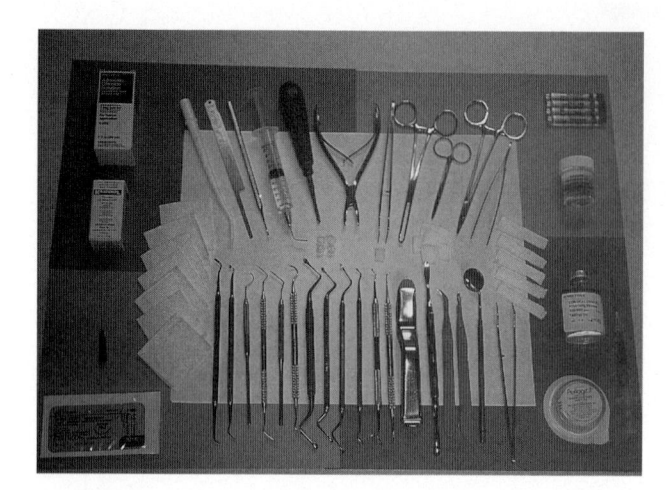

Figure 12-1 Standard tray set up for surgical endodontics.

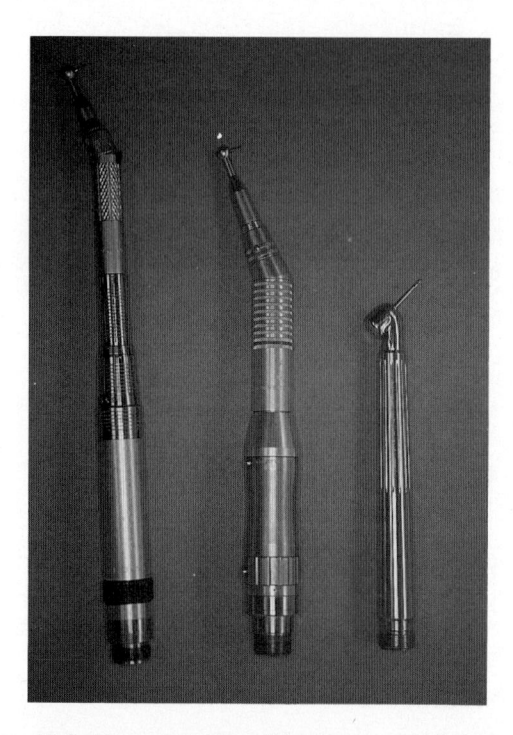

Figure 12-2 Micro mini-handpieces are used for apical seals, which provides access to the apex of the involved tooth (Courtesy of Moyco Union Broach, Inc., Emigsville, PA). The impact air 45 surgical handpiece is used with a surgical friction grip tapered fissure bur 1702 for making access to the apex (Courtesy of Innovations, Inc., Jefferson City, MO).

PROCEDURES

The area in which the apicoectomy is to be performed should be totally anesthetized.

Anesthesia

The maxillary teeth are infiltrated on the labial surface of the muccolabial fold with a 27-gauge needle with 1:50,000 lidocaine with epinephrine (Fig. 12-4, *A*). The epinephrine aids in controlling the hemorrhage in the surgical site. The lingual tissue is anesthetized by using the nasopalatine injection (Fig. 12-4, *B*).

Flap Design

The triangular flap is the most applicable surgical flap for the maxillary and mandibular teeth. However, the rectangular and extended semilunar flaps can also be used. The rectangular flap is used predominantly on teeth with long roots and/or large lesions (Fig. 12-5). Before using the scalpel it is best to gently outline the design on the soft tissue with the pointed end of the periosteal elevator (Fig. 12-5, *F*). The gingival margin fibers are first released around each tooth included in the flap, and a vertical incision is made to include at least one tooth mesially and distally of the involved tooth (Fig. 12-5, *G*). The incision should always be made on sound bone (Fig. 12-5, *H*). The incision is made with a Bard Parker No. 12 scalpel. The tissue is reflected with a periosteal elevator by gently releasing the tissue and including the periosteum by holding

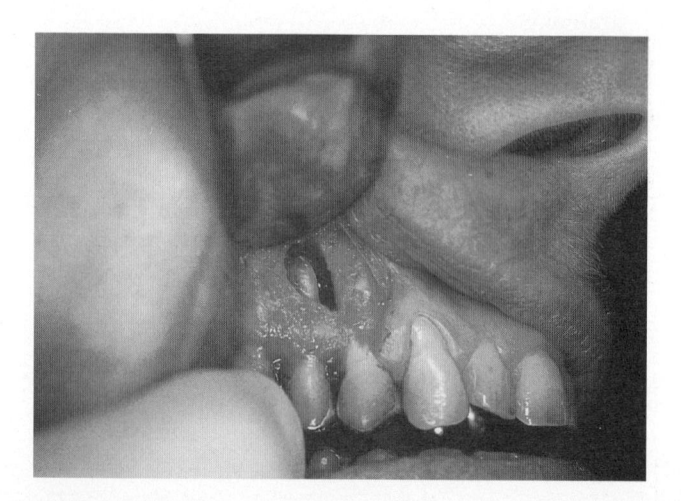

Figure 12-3 Apicoectomy root resected and beveled at a 45-degree angle.

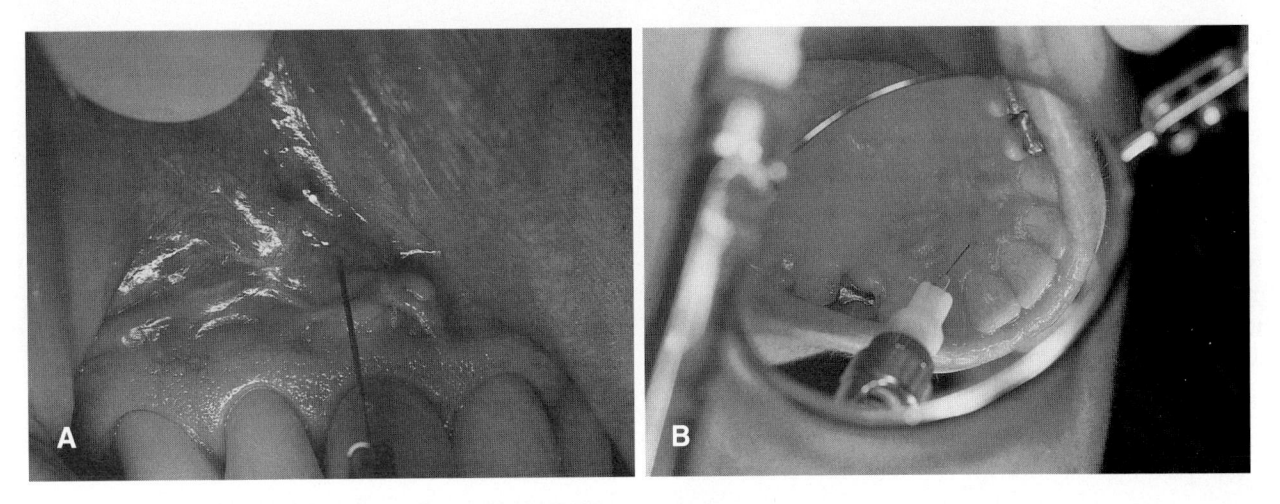

Figure 12-4 **A,** Infiltration anesthesia. **B,** Nasopalatine injection.

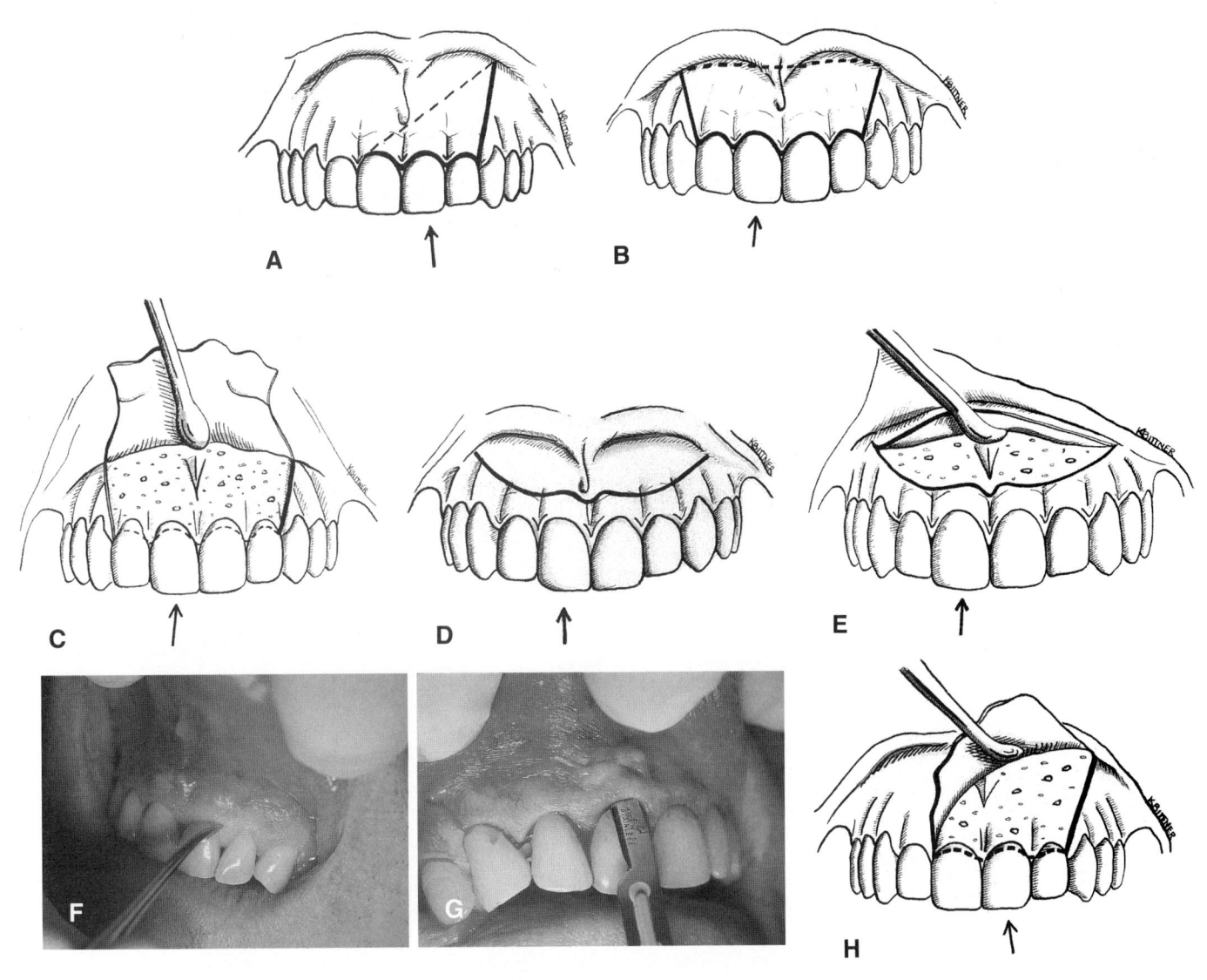

Figure 12-5 **A,** Outline of triangular flap. **B,** Outline of rectangular flap. **C,** Flap reflected exposing the labial plate to the gingival. **D,** The extended semilunar flap is made several millimeters above the gingival margin of the teeth. This flap preserves the integrity of the margins when crowns are present. **E,** The flap is utilized when the surgery is confined to the apical area. **F,** Scribing incision with periosteal elevator. **G,** The gingival margins are released around each tooth involved in the surgical flap. **H,** The incision rests on sound bone.

230 PRACTICAL ENDODONTICS

the elevator tightly against the bone and pushing it apically (Fig. 12-6). The flap is retracted with a Minnesota retractor (Fig. 12-7). The surgical ruler is placed on the labial plate of bone at the length of the root (Fig. 12-8, *A*). When the labial plate is intact the surgical tack is used to locate the apex (Fig. 12-8, *B*). The surgical tack is placed in the cancellous bone and a radiograph is taken. A surgical bone bur (Bur-L-1) is used to remove bone around the apex of the root (Fig. 12-9). Constant flow of saline is used so the bone is not overheated. Enough bone should be removed to expose the margin of the bony defect. When a lesion is present it is detached from the bony defect by using a sharp curette, releasing it from the entire cavity (Fig. 12-10). During the curettement the lesion is grasped with Allis tissue forceps

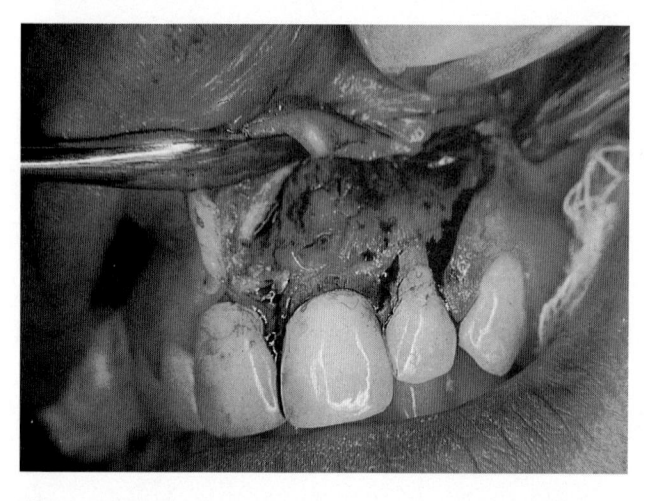

Figure 12-6 The tissue is reflected with a periosteal elevator.

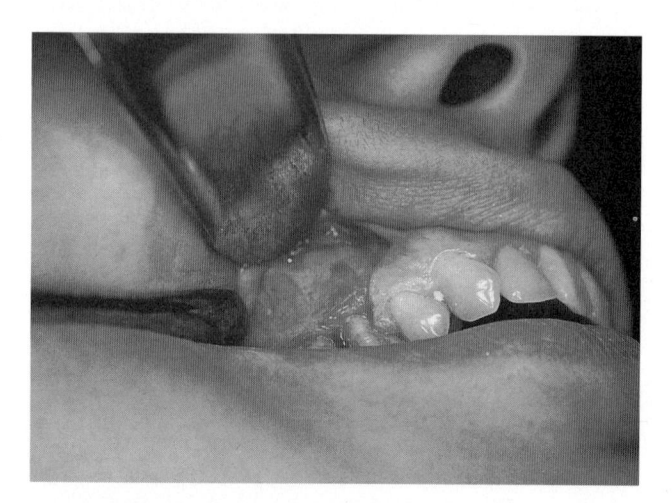

Figure 12-7 The flap is retracted.

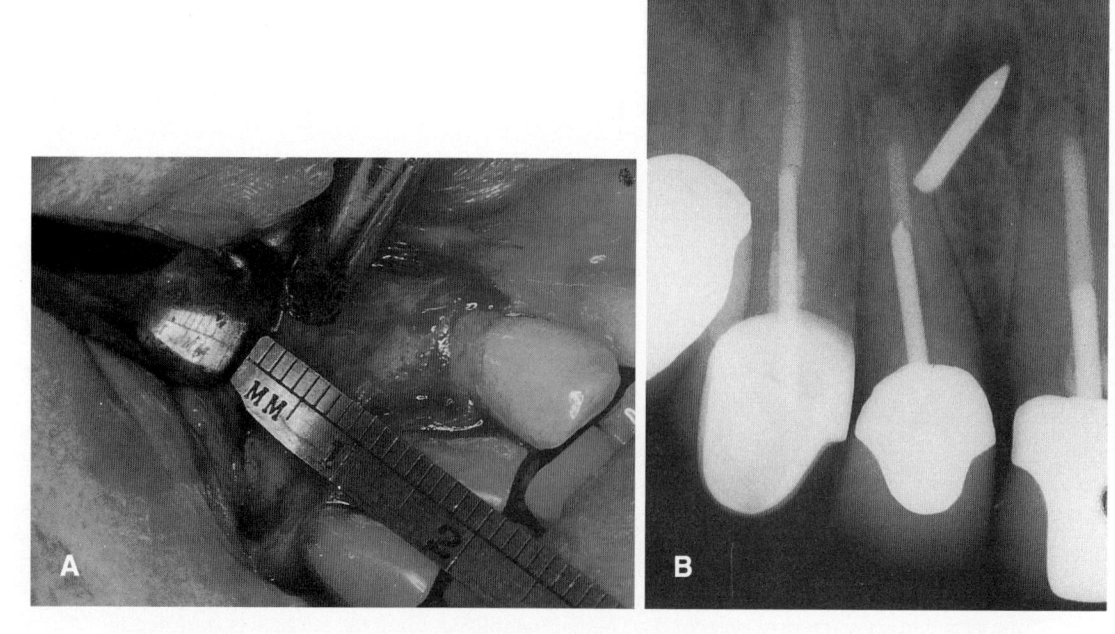

Figure 12-8 A, The surgical ruler measuring length of tooth. **B,** Radiograph of surgical tack locating apex.

(Fig. 12-11, *A*); this helps to prevent the lesion from fragmenting during the procedure. An effort should be made to remove the entire lesion (Fig. 12-11, *B*). The specimen should be placed in a specimen bottle of formalin and sent for histopathological analysis (Fig. 12-12). A radiograph is taken of the completed procedure before suturing. The area is irrigated with saline. Gelfoam (oxymethylcellulose) is placed in the cavity to aid in clot formation. The flap is gently repositioned and held firmly with finger pressure for a few seconds (Fig. 12-13, *A*). Sutures (either silk or vicryl) are placed from loose to fixed tissue beginning at a site near the mucobuccal fold (Fig. 12-13, *A*, *B*, and *C*).

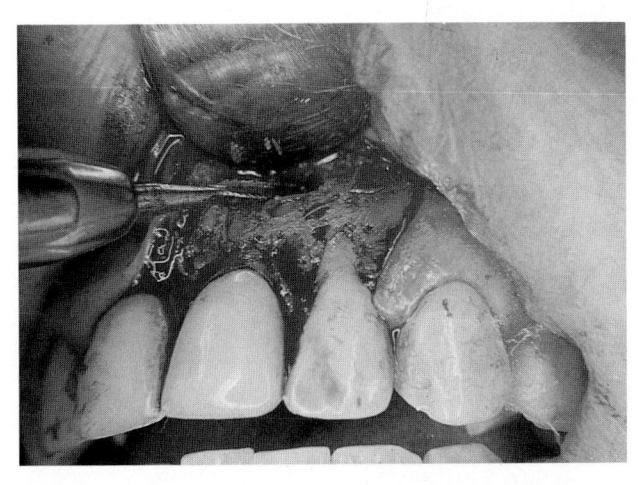

Figure 12-9 Tapered fissure bur No. 1702 is exposing the apex.

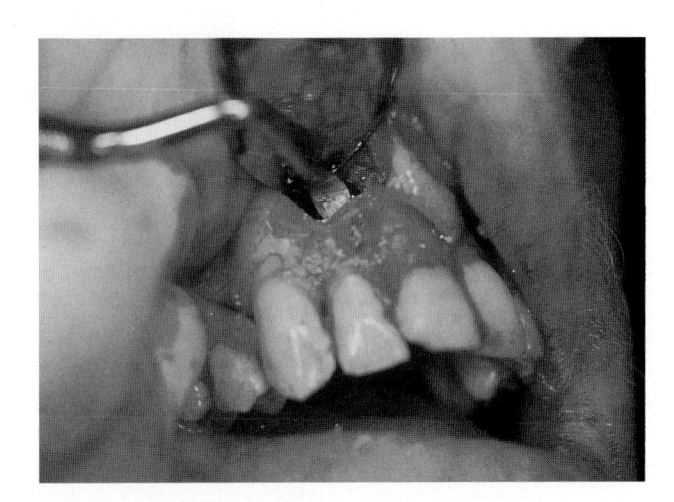

Figure 12-10 Detaching lesion with sharp curette.

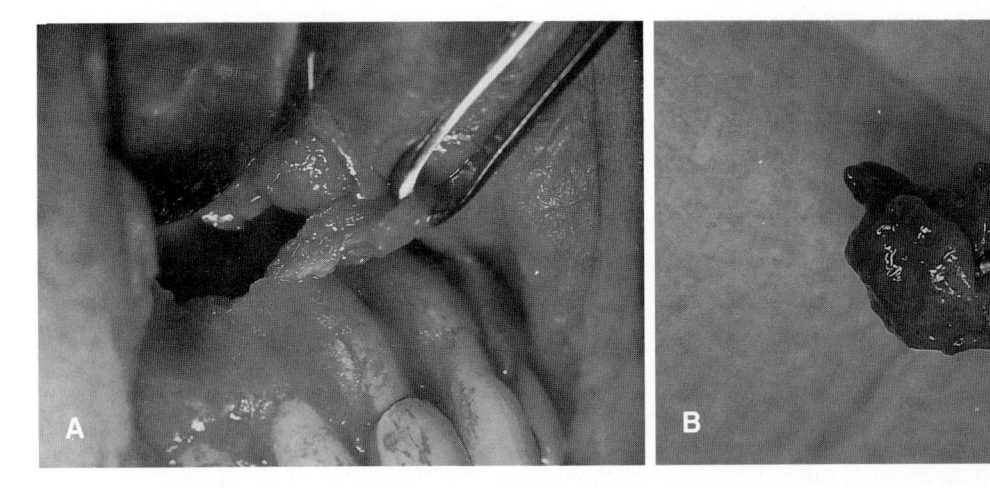

Figure 12-11 A, The lesion is grasped with Allis forceps. **B,** Lesion removed intact.

232 PRACTICAL ENDODONTICS

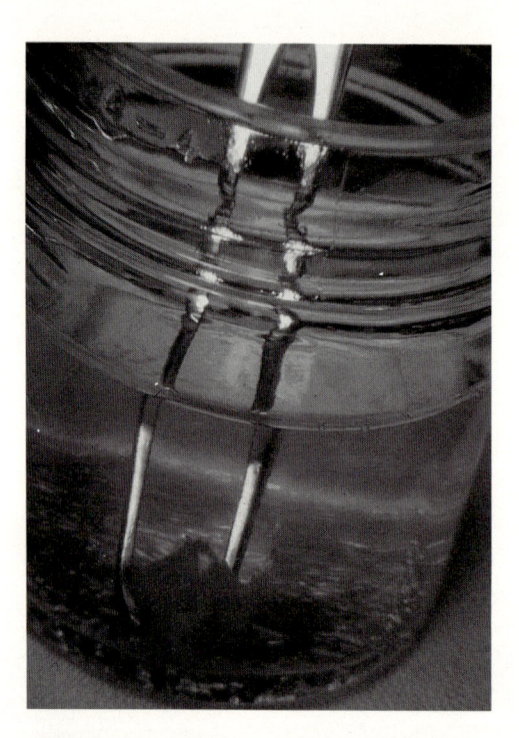

Figure 12-12 The specimen placed in formalin.

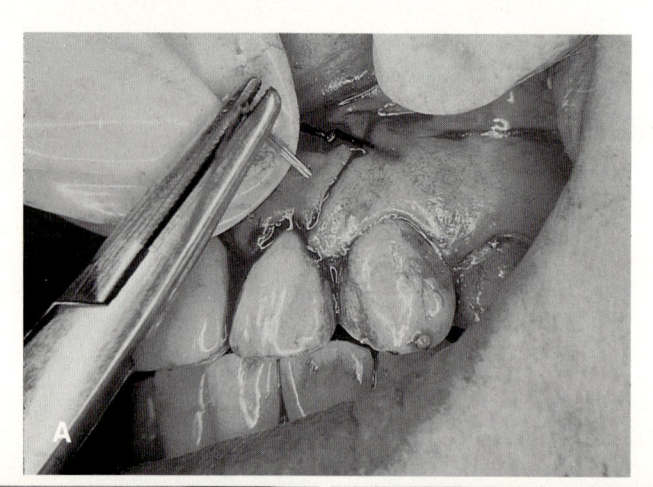

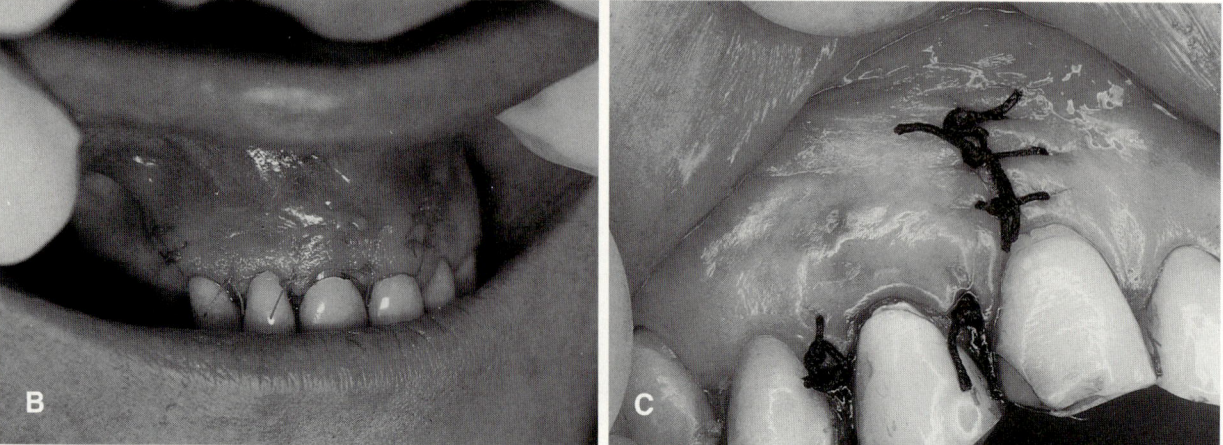

Figure 12-13 A, Tissue is sutured from loose to fixed tissue with 3-0 suture. B, 3-0 vicryl sutures. C, 3-0 silk sutures.

Maxillary Posterior Teeth

The area is infiltrated in the mucobuccal fold with 1:50,000 lidocaine and the palatine nerve is anesthetized. A triangular flap is used to expose the roots (Fig. 12-14). The flap is made on sound bone one tooth anterior of the involved tooth.

Mandibular Teeth

The inferior alveolar nerve is anesthetized with 1:100,000 lidocaine. When excess hemorrhage or discomfort are present supplemental anesthesia may be necessary. Following a vertical incision and release of the margin fibers (Fig. 12-15, *A* and *B*), the buccal and lingual surfaces of the surgical site are infiltrated with 1:50,000 lidocaine to aid in vasoconstriction (Fig. 12-15, *C*). A triangular flap is used to expose the roots. The labial plate of bone is removed, exposing the entire lesion and root apices (Fig. 12-15, *D*). The lesion is curetted and excised. The roots are resected and beveled on 45-degree angles (Fig. 12-15, *E*). The cavity is irrigated with saline; gelfoam is placed in the cavity (Fig. 12-15, *F*), and the incision is sutured (Fig. 12-15, *G*). The sutures are removed in 5 to 7 days (Fig. 12-15, *H* and *I*).

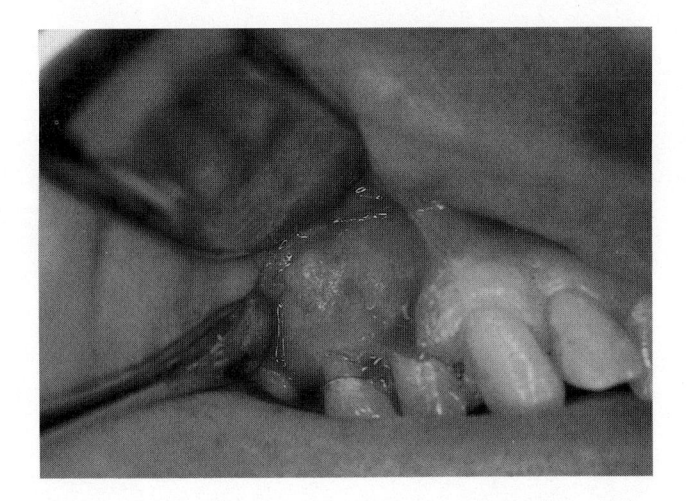

Figure 12-14 A triangular flap for maxillary second bicuspid exposing the eroded buccal plate and large lesion.

234   PRACTICAL ENDODONTICS

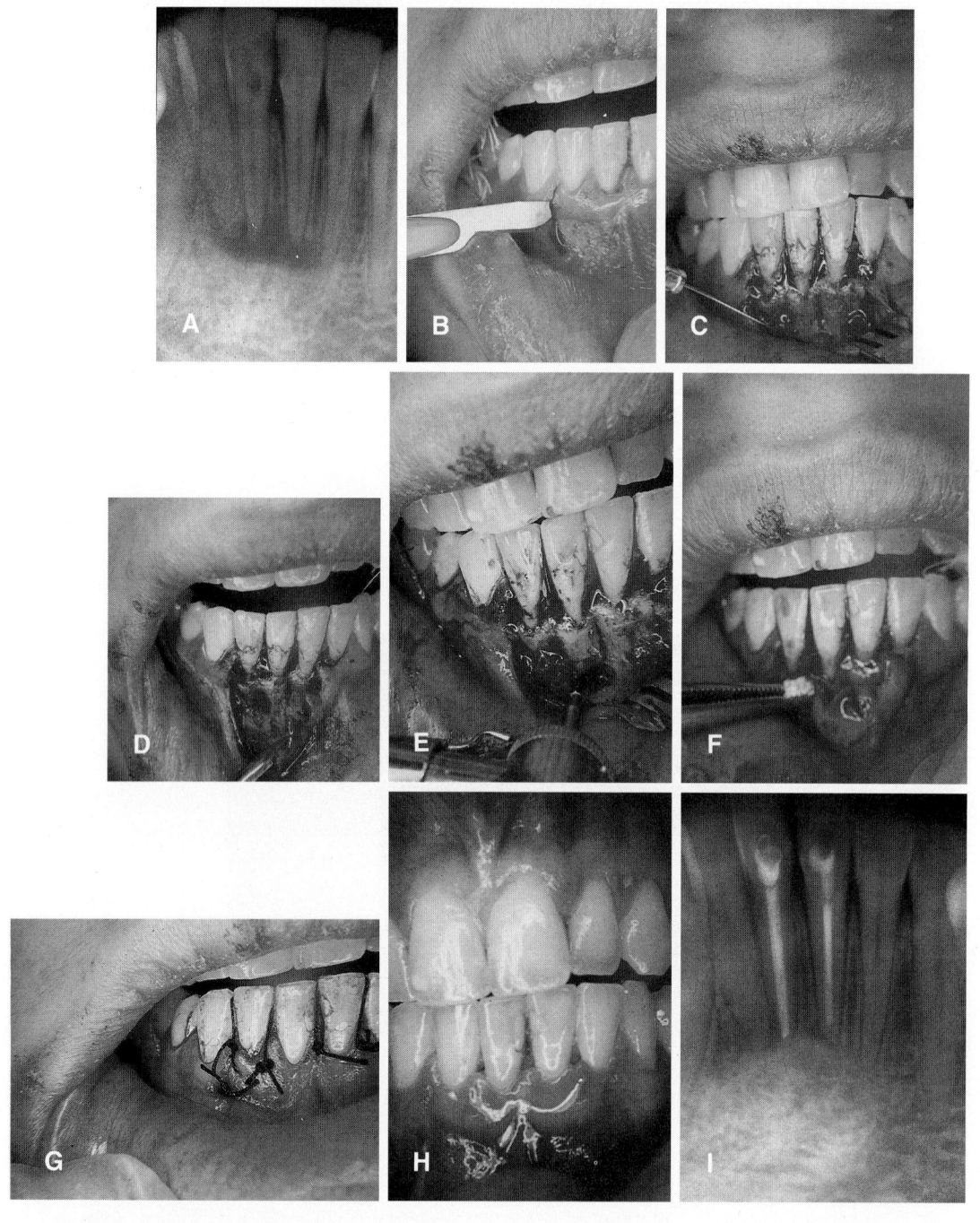

Figure 12-15 **A**, Diagnostic radiograph of No. 24 and No. 25. **B**, Vertical incision. **C**, Supplemental anesthesia. **D**, Triangular flap showing eroded labial plate with lesion. **E**, Roots are beveled with tapered fissure bur. **F**, Placing gelfoam. **G**, 3.0 silk sutures are placed interproximal and in vertical incision. **H**, Seven days postoperative healing. **I**, Three years postoperative radiograph.

Apical Seal

The root end is exposed and beveled at a 45-degree angle with a fissure bur. The canal is prepared with a ½ round bur using a mini-surgical handpiece 2 to 3 mm in depth (Fig. 12-16, *A*). The base of the preparation is undercut with a 33½ inverted cone bur using mini-surgical handpiece (Fig. 12-16, *B*). The preparation is irrigated with saline and dried with Nu gauze. Nu gauze strips are packed in the cavity to prevent excess filling material from flowing into the surgical cavity (Fig. 12-16, *C*). A small amount of root canal sealer is carried into the cavity preparation with a bent reamer or a double-ended explorer (Fig. 12-16, *D*). The preparation is injected with Firm set or Endoset Ultrafil as the apical seal (Fig. 12-16, *E*). After 20 to 30 seconds the gutta percha is condensed with a plugger (Fig. 12-16, *F*). A radiograph is taken before suturing (Fig. 12-16, *G*).

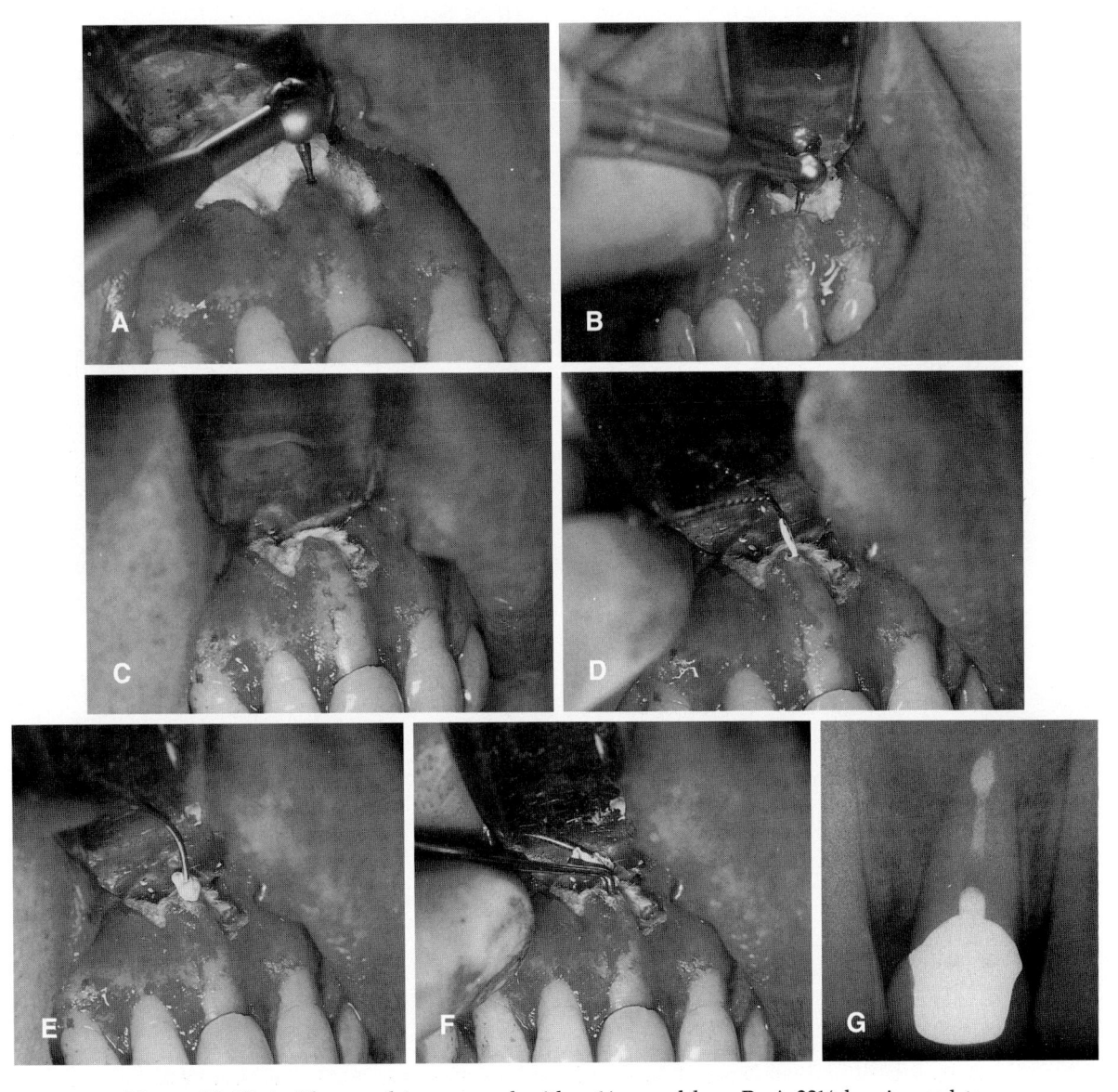

Figure 12-16 **A**, The canal is prepared with a ½ round bur. **B**, A 33½ bur is used to undercut the preparation. **C**, Cavity is packed with nu gauze. **D**, Sealer is carried into preparation with reamer bent at a right angle. **E**, Endoset Ultrafil (green cannule) is injected into the preparation. **F**, The gutta percha is compacted with a plugger. **G**, A radiograph of apical seal.

Hemisection

The radiograph is examined to determine that fusion of the roots is not present (Fig. 12-17, *A*). Endodontic treatment is completed on the root to be retained. The chamber and root to be resected is condensed with amalgam (12-17, *B*). The area is anesthetized and the coronal segment of the tooth is sectioned with a fissure bur. The bur is placed in the bifurcation and moved in the buccal and lingual direction until the entire crown is severed. The bur is then moved in the apical direction to sever the furca. When the crown and furca are severed a periosteal elevator is used to release the periodontal attachment and luxate the root. Extraction forceps are used to grasp and luxate the section to be removed. A radiograph is taken to determine all of the overhanging furca is removed (Fig. 12-17, *C*). The buccal and lingual plates are compressed with finger pressure. Sutures are not usually required. Tooth is restored with a crown (Fig. 12-17, *D*).

Crown Sectioning

Crown sectioning is indicated when the furca is perforated (Fig. 12-18, *A*). It is completed in a similar manner to the hemisection except the roots are retained. Post preparations are completed before sectioning the tooth. The crown and furca are sectioned with a No. 558 tapered fissure bur. The fissure bur is placed on the occlusal surface and extended apically to the furca in a buccal and lingual direction until both roots are separated. The sharp edges of the furca are removed. The roots are individually prepared with posts, cores, and crowns (Fig. 12-18, *B*).

Root Sectioning

Root sectioning is indicated when one or more roots are totally circumscribed with bone loss, external root resorption, vertical fracture of the root, and perforations of the cervical, middle third of the root (12-19, *A* and *B*). Root sectioning is accomplished by sectioning

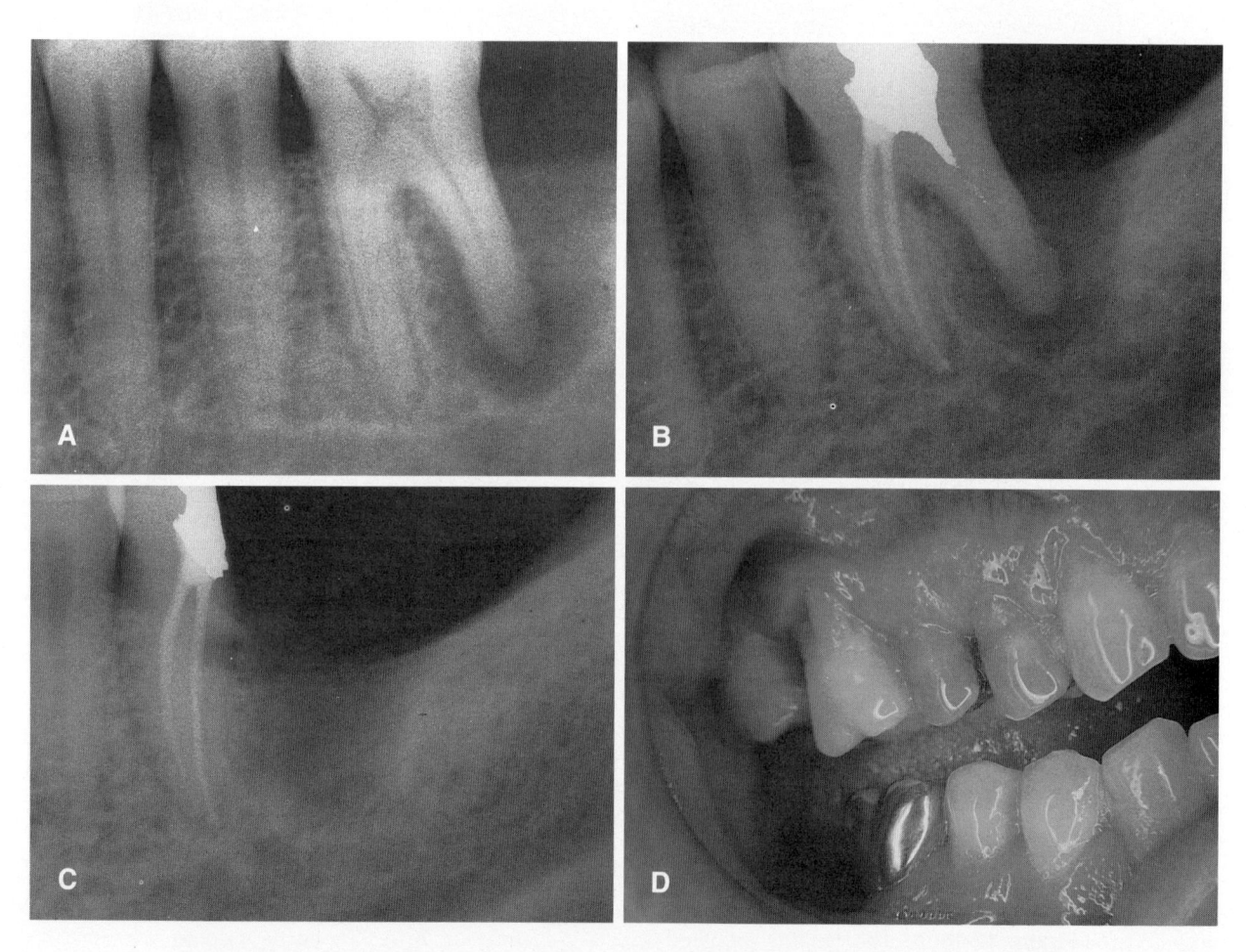

Figure 12-17 **A**, A large periapical lesion circumscribes the distal root and roots are not fused together. **B**, Mesial root filled with gutta percha and distal root and chamber are filled with amalgam. **C**, Radiograph of completed hemisection. **D**, Crown in place. (Courtesy of Dr. S. Rand Werrin.)

the root to the furca. The gingival portion of the root is enlarged with a No. 2 or No. 3 Gates Glidden drill. The root to be sectioned should be filled with amalgam or glass ionomer. The root is then sectioned with a fissure bur to the furca leaving the furca intact (Fig 12-19, C and D). The crown is recontoured with a diamond bur to reduce the occlusal-gingival stresses on the remaining root or roots.

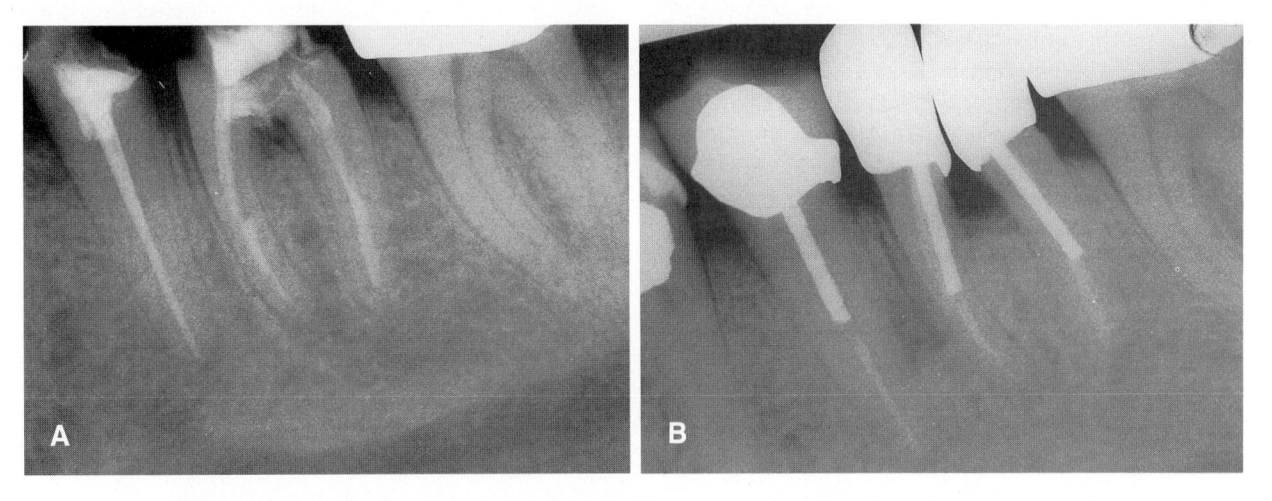

Figure 12-18 **A**, Perforation of the furca. **B**, Posts were placed and two separate crowns made. (Courtesy of Dr. S. Rand Werrin.)

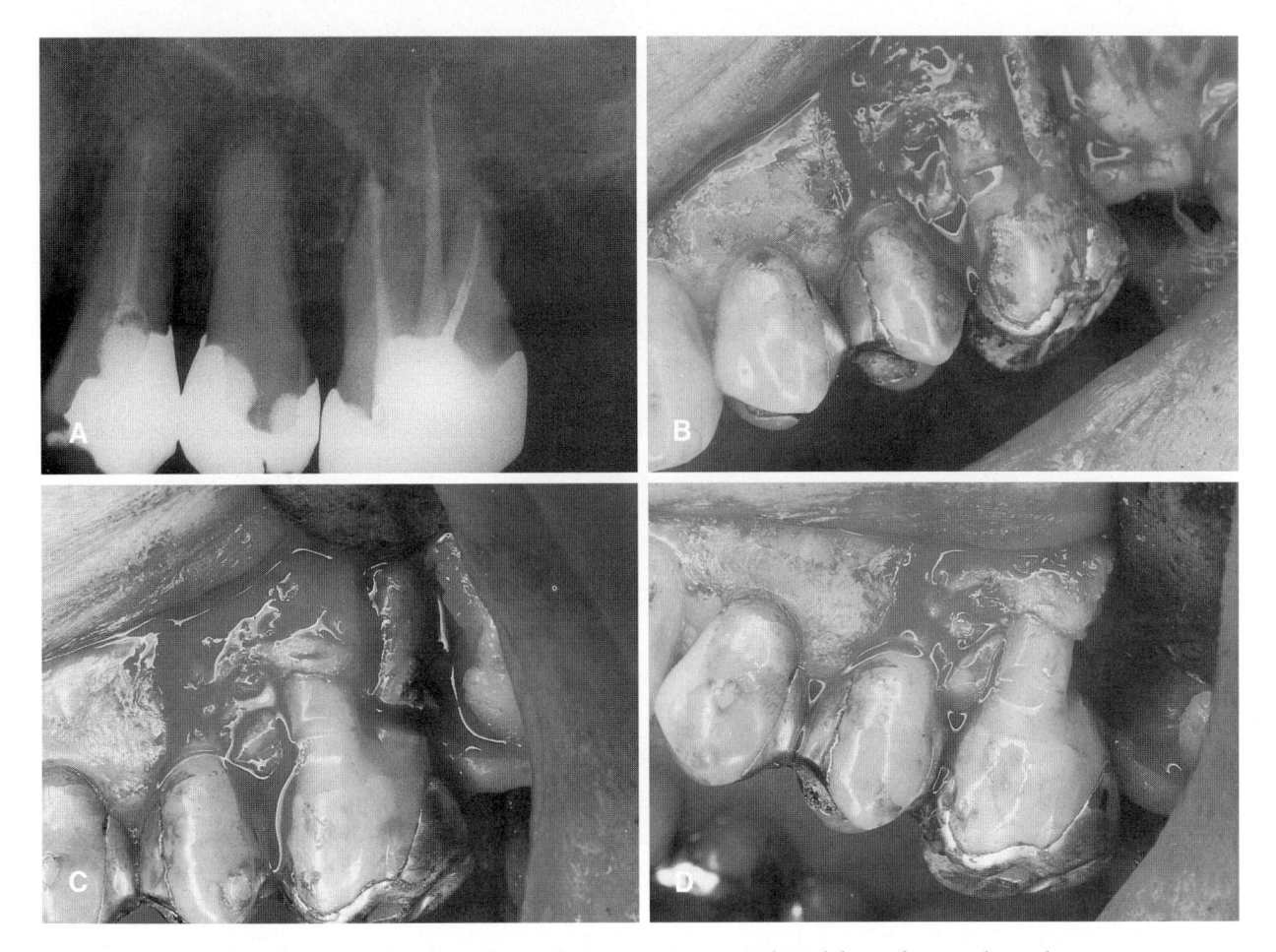

Figure 12-19 A, Distobuccal root has excessive periodontal bone loss and amalgam placed in distobuccal root. **B**, Distobuccal root completely denuded. **C**, Distobuccal is sectioned. **D**, The furca was beveled with a tapered diamond.

Incision and Drainage

Incision and drainage is required when an acute exacerbation occurs with localized swelling (Fig. 12-20, A and B). An acute exacerbation may occur after treating a tooth (non-vital) or during the final stages of an alveolar abscess. The patient is clinically in distress from lack of sleep and pain. The patient may also be emotionally fatigued. The tooth should first be opened to determine if intracanal drainage is possible. The area should be incised when intracanal drainage is minimal, the pain is not relieved, and the tissue is soft and fluctuant.

The mandibular teeth can be anesthetized with an inferior alveolar block. When localized swelling is present in the maxilla, the area is anesthetized by injecting a few drops of 1:100,000 lidocaine distal and mesial to the affected area. Direct injection into the fluctuant area is contraindicated so as not to force the infection deeper. A Bard Parker No. 11 scalpel is used to incise the area (Fig. 12-20, C). The incision of approximately 5 mm is made at the softest pointed part of the swelling. The scalpel is inserted into the area and the incision is made as the scalpel is withdrawn (Fig. 12-20, D-F). With slight finger pressure the suppuration is expelled. A pair of treatment pliers or hemostats is inserted into the incision and opened to ensure complete access and drainage (Fig. 12-20, G). With treatment pliers a rubber dam T-drain is placed in the incision. Grasping the T portion of the drain and placing it in the incision allows it to open and drain. No sutures are usually necessary and the drain is kept in position 5 to 7 days (Fig. 12-20, H). The patient is placed on an antibiotic for 7 to 10 days. Relief is usually immediate. If the drain fits loosely it may be necessary to suture the drain in position.

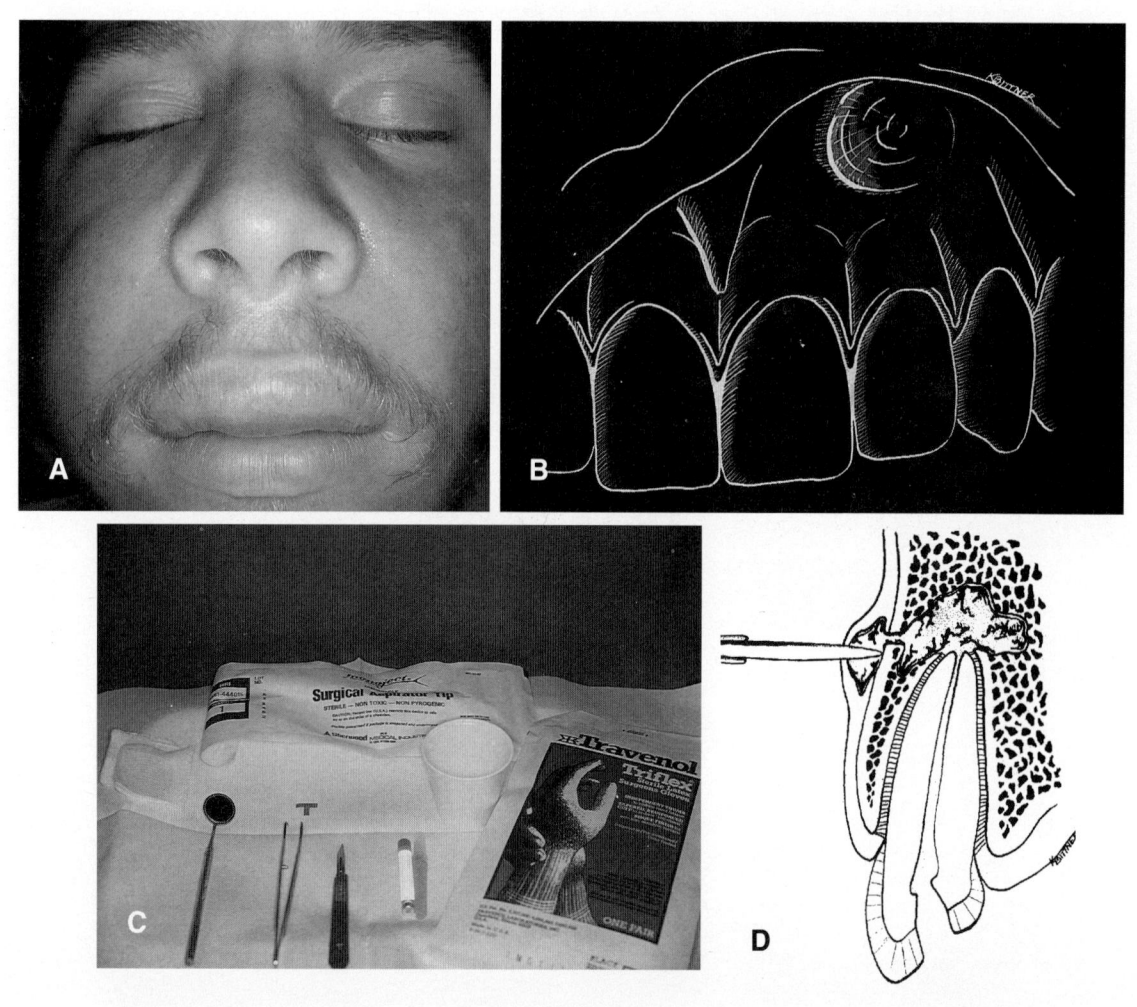

Figure 12-20 **A**, Acute facial swelling. **B**, Most fluctuant point. **C**, An incision and drain set-up. The incision tray usually includes No. 11 scalpel, saline, surgical aspirator tip, surgical gloves, treatment pliers, 2 x 2 gauze and rubber dam T-drain. **D** and **E**, The incision is made into the most fluctuant point.

Continued.

Chapter 12 ♦ Surgical Endodontics 239

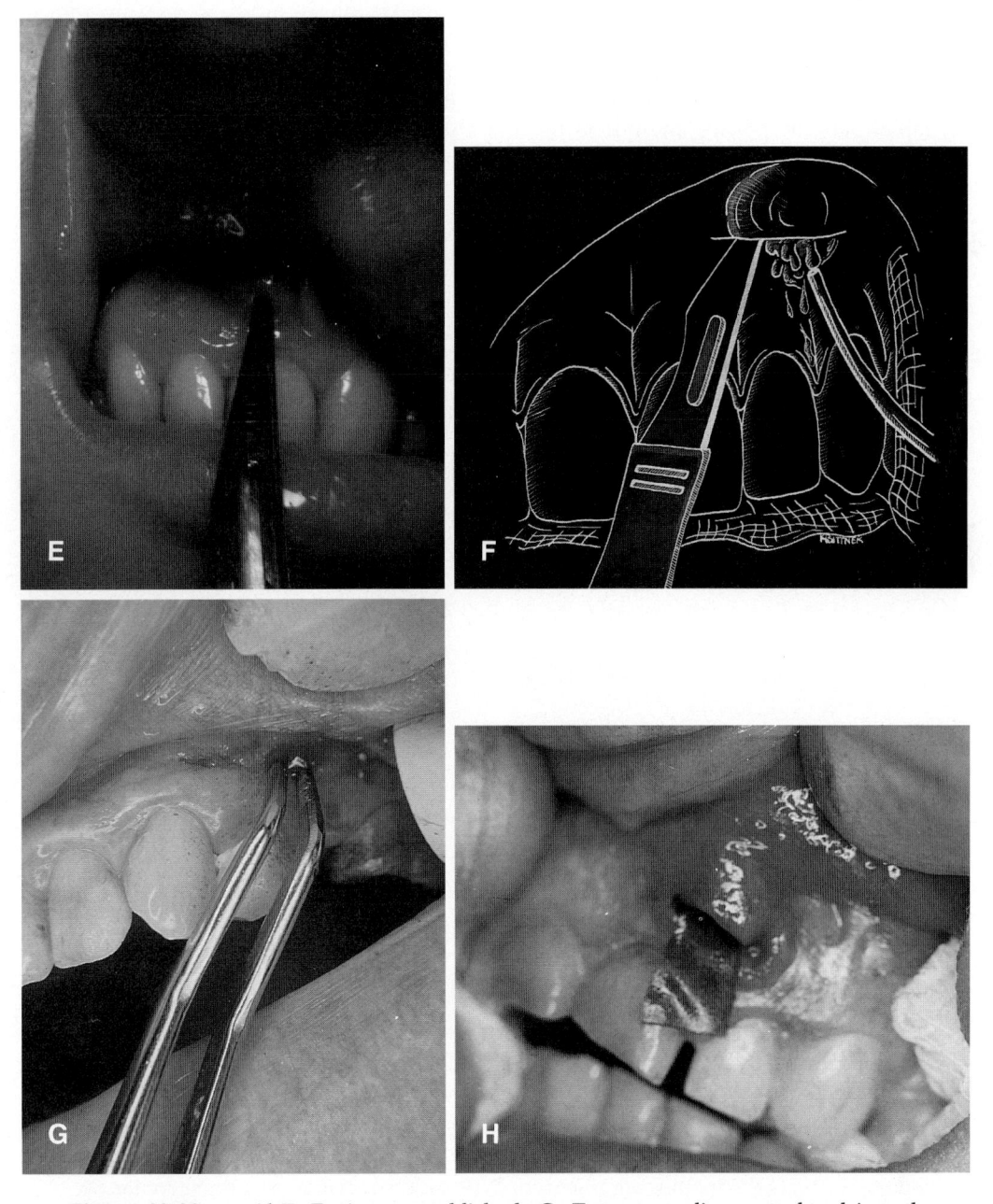

Figure 12-20, *cont'd* **F,** Drainage established. **G,** Treatment pliers are placed into the incision to ensure complete access for drainage. **H,** The T-drain is placed in incision.

Trephination

Trephination is used when the patient is experiencing severe pain and intracanal drainage is not accomplished. An artificial fistula is made in the labial or buccal plate of bone at the root apex. On mandibular posterior teeth it is made in the bifurcation.

The tooth is anesthetized and the apex of the tooth is located by measuring with a surgical ruler (Fig. 12-21, A and B). If the root length is not known it can be determined by measuring the radiograph. A surgical tack is inserted into the buccal or labial plate by rotating back and forth in the area of the apex (Fig. 12-21, C). A radiograph is taken to confirm the position. The fistulator is placed in the desired area and held firmly against the tissue. The fistulating bur is used in a slow contra angle and an opening is made in the buccal or labial plate by placing the bur in the eye of the fistulator (Fig. 12-21, D). The operator will feel the bur drop into the alveolar space.

Marsupialization

Marsupialization is indicated when a radiolucent area is so large that surgical removal jeopardizes the vitality of the adjacent teeth (Fig. 12-22, A). Marsupialization of a large cavity is best accomplished by placing a polyethylene tube into the lesion and reducing the internal pressure so that it no longer increases in size. The area is anesthetized and a small 3 to 4 mm incision is made with a No. 15 scalpel (Fig. 12-22, B). The labial plate is soft and penetrated with the pointed end of the periosteal elevator by rotating it back and forth. The cavity is aspirated with a 20-gauge needle in a 5-cc syringe to remove the cavity fluid (Fig. 12-22, C). Polyethylene tubing with a lip on both ends is inserted and sutured so that the lip of the tube is lying flat on the labial surface and extends to the lingual wall of the cavity (Fig. 12-22, D and E). The suture is removed in 5 days and the patient is placed on a prescription of antibiotics for 7 to 10 days

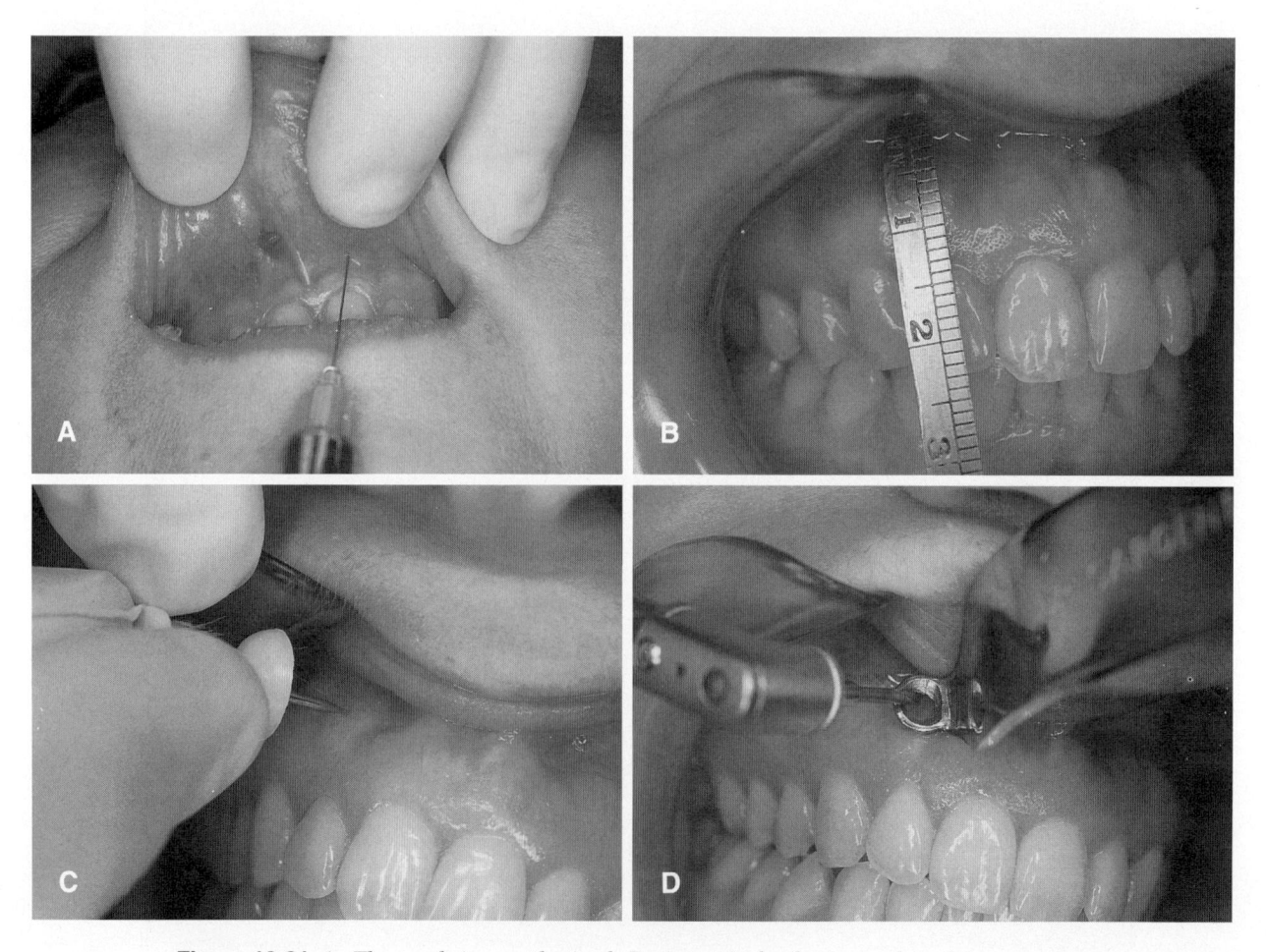

Figure 12-21 A, The tooth is anesthetized. B, A surgical ruler is used to determine the length of the root. C, Surgical tack is placed in the labial plate at the root length. D, The labial plate is perforated with the trephination bur.

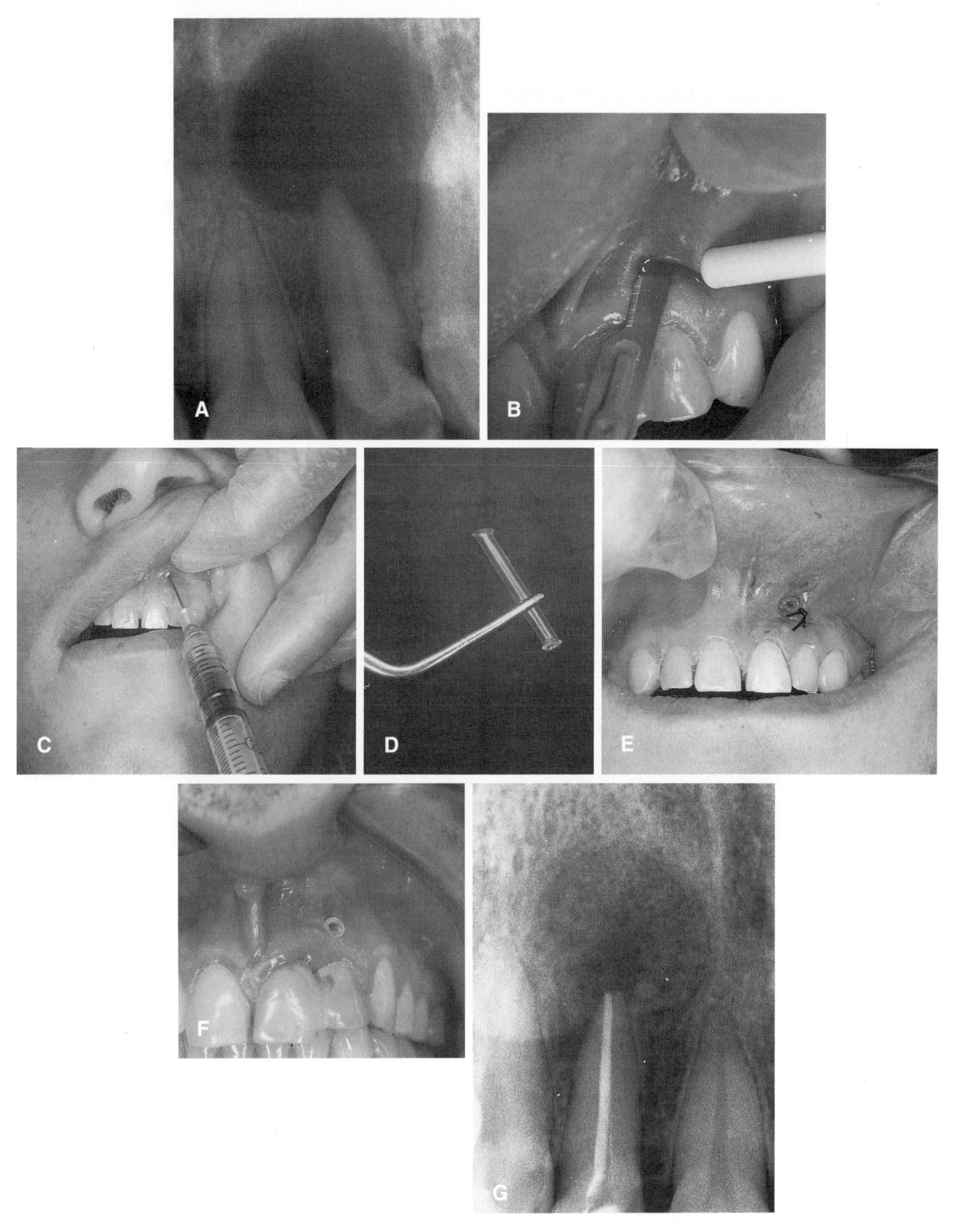

Figure 12-22 **A**, A large radiolucent lesion 1.25 x 1.75 cm. Calcium hydroxide was placed in the canal. **B**, A small incision is made with No. 15 scalpel. **C**, The fluid is aspirated from the lesion with a 20-gauge needle and a 5-cc syringe. **D**, A polyethylene tube with inner diameter .047 inch and an outer diameter .067 inch. Both ends have a lip so tube is not displaced inwardly or outwardly. The lips are made by passing the tubing quickly through an open flame. **E**, The tube is held in place with a single suture. **F**, The suture is removed in 5 days. **G**, One-year radiograph showing repair without surgery.

(Fig. 12-22, *F*). Root canal therapy is completed after suture is removed. The patient is recalled at 3, 6, and 9 month intervals to determine the amount of healing. When healing is adequate so the vitality of the adjacent teeth are no longer in jeopardy, surgery is completed. It is possible for the area to reduce in size and heal completely so surgery may not be necessary (Fig. 12-22, *G*).

POSTOPERATIVE INSTRUCTIONS FOR THE PATIENT

1. Do not raise the lip to look at the sutures.
2. Place an ice pack on the outside of the face, 20 minutes out of every 1 ½ hours for the first 24 hours.
3. Beginning with the second day, place ½ teaspoon of table salt in a glass of warm water and rinse 3 times daily.
4. Do not chew any hard foods with the tooth for 1 week.
5. A rather soft diet is suggested for the first 4 days.
6. Do not brush in the area of the surgery for 1 week, however, brush the remaining teeth as usual.
7. Take the medication as prescribed by the doctor.
8. Should an emergency occur as a result of the surgery or medication, please call the office. The telephone answers 24 hours daily.

13

Traumatic Injuries

Injuries to teeth occur in a significant number and they occur at unscheduled times, which adds another degree of difficulty. The initial diagnosis and treatment is important for early recovery and to help in preventing and intercepting future problems Before treatment a thorough clinical and radiographic examination should be made.

EXAMINATION

The examination should include the accident history of how the accident happened, type of injury, where the injury occurred, was there a prior injury, and if any previous treatment had been initiated.

The clinical examination should consist of:
1. Radiographs
2. Soft tissue examination
3. Hard tissue examination

RADIOGRAPHS

Radiographs should be taken at several angles to detect root fractures, labial or lingual plate fractures, socket perforations, and foreign bodies. If a radiograph is taken at the same plane of the fracture it may not be visible. The tube should be shifted horizontally but kept in the same vertical plane and another radiograph taken (Fig. 13-1).

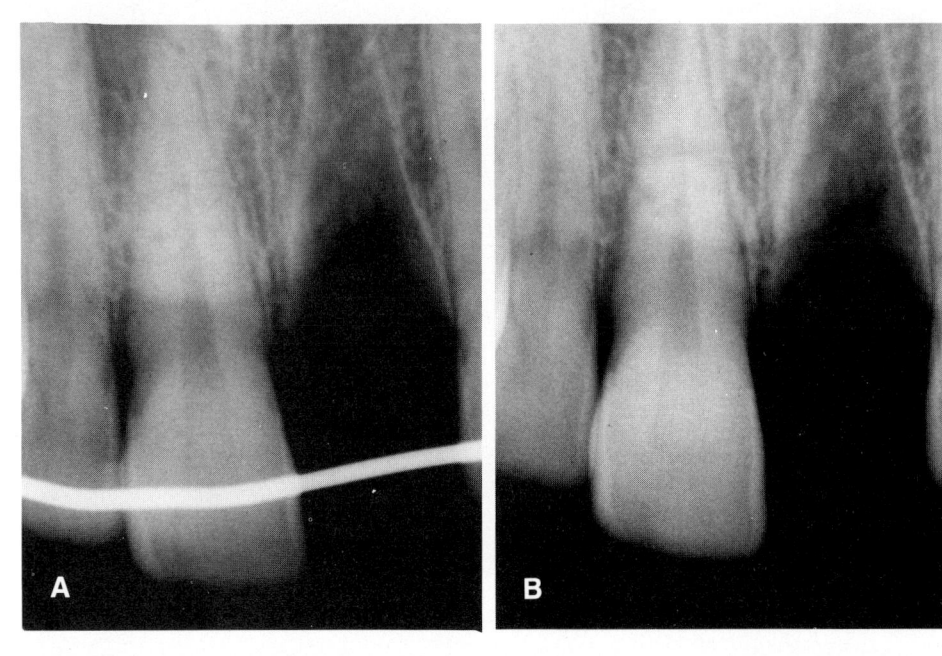

Figure 13-1 **A,** Radiograph of root fracture of tooth No. 9 not apparently evident in the apical third. **B,** The radiograph was taken with a different horizontal angulation and the root fracture is now apparent.

SOFT TISSUE

The soft tissue should be examined for lacerations, contusions and bruises, foreign bodies, and displaced fragments of teeth or bone (Fig. 13-2).

HARD TISSUE

The teeth should be examined for vitality (thermal and electric), color, mobility, percussion sensitivity, displacement (intruded or extruded), rotated, malalignment, occlusion, avulsion, root development, enamel cracks and crazings (with transillumination), and coronal and root fractures (Fig. 13-3).

VITALITY OF TEETH

Teeth may test non-vital to both (thermal and electric) after an injury and may continue for several months. It is possible for a tooth to test vital to the electric pulp tester and negative to thermal testing. The vascular and neural bed may be torn, bruised, or crushed and the (non-vital) reading may be temporary. If the tooth tests non-vital it should be examined at 4 to 5 week intervals and retested for vitality. It is possible to wait as long as 4 months following an injury for vitality to return (Fig. 13-4). If the tooth becomes symptomatic and if discoloration progresses the pulp should be removed and root canal completed.

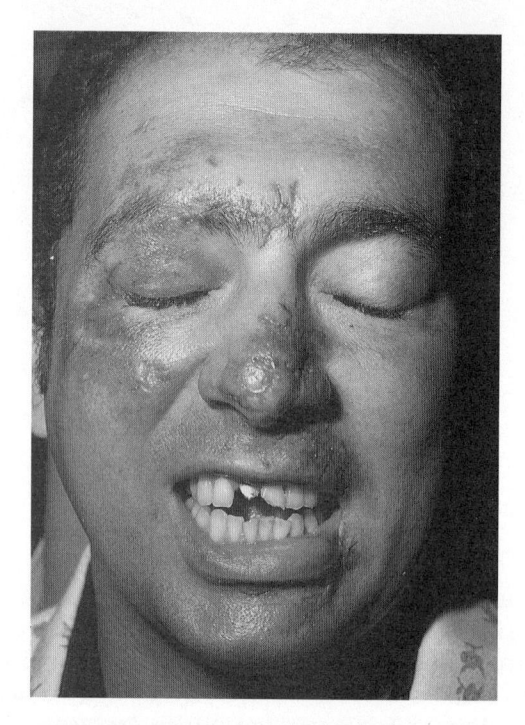

Figure 13-2 Lacerations of lip, contusions of chin and face, and crown fractures of both maxillary central incisors. The soft tissue should be examined for foreign bodies, such as tooth fragments and debris. Dycal was placed over the exposed pulp until the soft tissue was manageable.

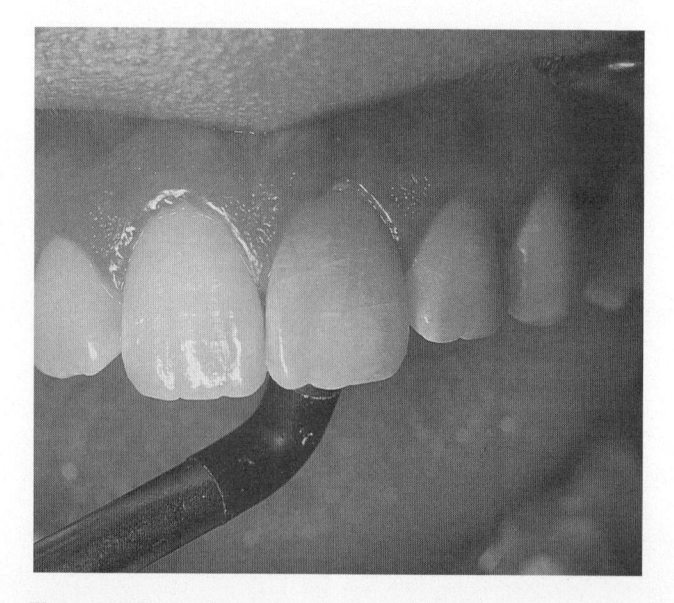

Figure 13-3 Cracks and crazings are easily seen with transillumination.

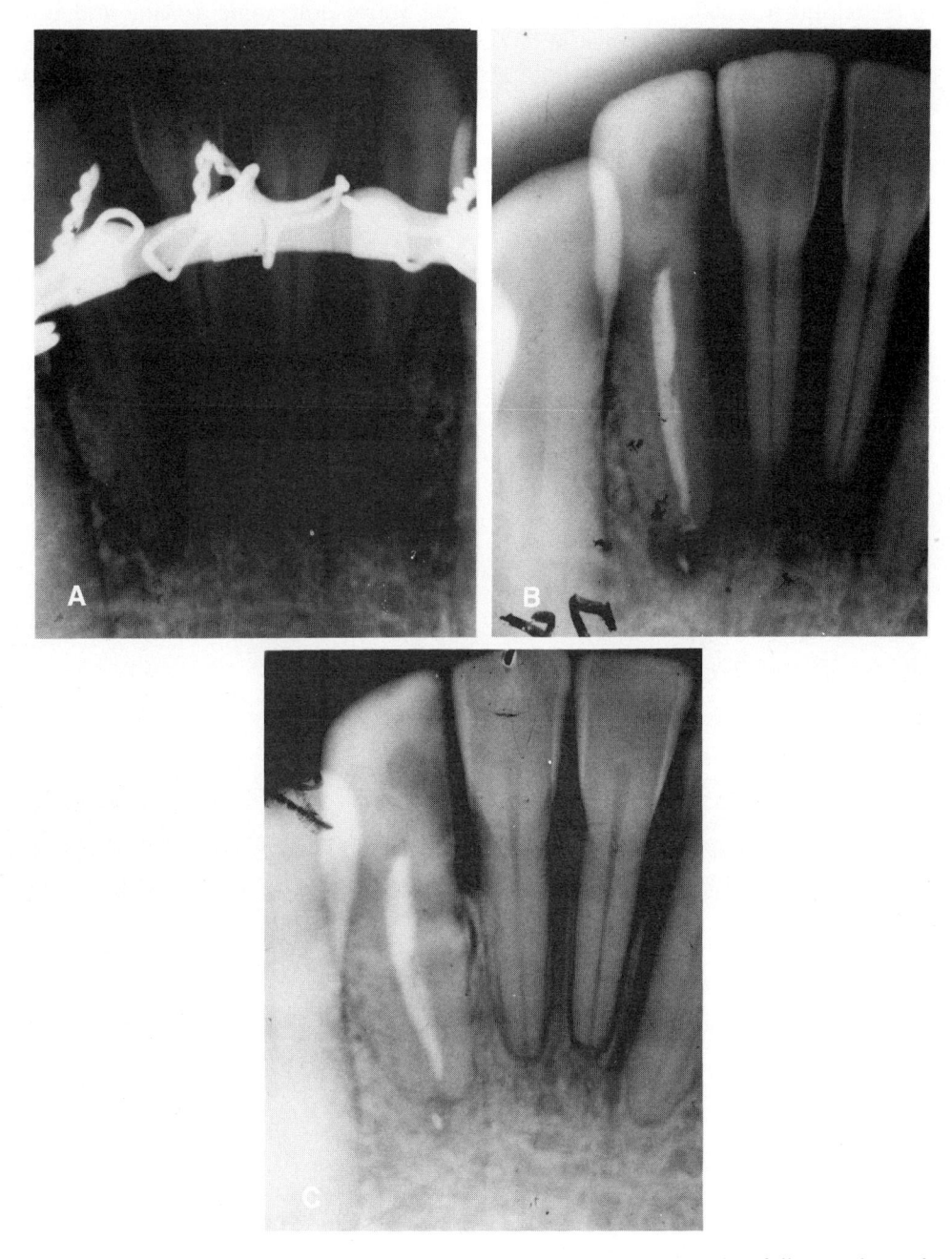

Figure 13-4 A, A full arch bracket placed on teeth No. 22, 23, 24, and 25 following lingual displacement. Note radiolucent area at the apices and periodontal thickening. Teeth No. 22, 23, and 24 tested negative to ice and vitalometer and No. 25 tested positive. **B,** A 4-month recall shows almost complete resolution of the radiolucent areas and only a slight periodontal thickening of both central incisors, which now tested vital to ice and vitalometer, however a root canal was completed on tooth No. 22, which became nonvital. **C,** A radiograph 2½ year posttreatment shows normal lamina dura at the apex of the four mandibular incisors. Teeth No. 23, 24, and 25 tested positive to both ice and the vitalometer.

DISCOLORATION

Discoloration is not a positive indicator of loss of vitality, although it is helpful in making a diagnosis. Teeth may become discolored temporarily because of internal hemorrhage of the pulp and may regain both vitality and color. If the color is pink or red it is more likely to remain vital. A pink to red color will occur following extravasation of the red blood cells and is indicative of a pulpal ischematic infarct. Infarcted, discolored pulp in the chamber may be walled off and the apical pulp remains vital and usually begins to calcify. A pulpectomy should be performed to prevent calcification of the canal that is unmanageable without surgery (Fig. 13-5). A blue or gray discoloration may be an early sign of degeneration and permanent loss of vitality. Early removal of such pulp helps control discoloration and prevents further calcification.

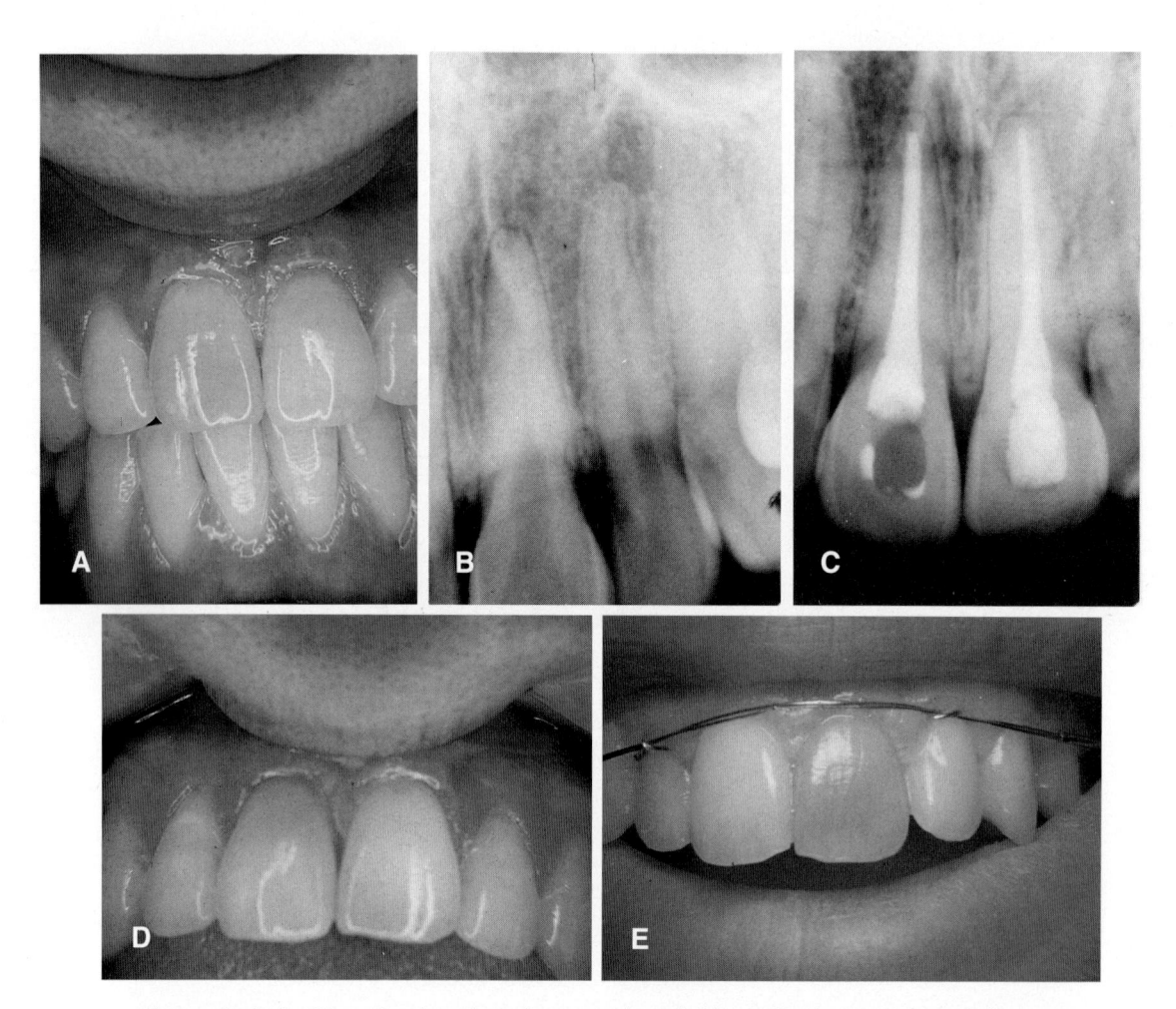

Figure 13-5 **A,** Gray discoloration of crown of tooth No. 8. **B,** A narrowing of the root canal of No. 8 above gingival third and an apparent ischemic infarction in crown, 1 year following a traumatic injury. Note how wide the pulp chamber is in the coronal third. **C,** Interceptive endodontics was initiated and root canal completed. **D,** The tooth was whitened considerable with a walking bleach of 30% peroxide and sodium perborate for 2 treatments 1 week apart. **E,** A gray discoloration of No. 9. Three months posttrauma the tooth tested non-vital and was becoming progressively darker. Rapid and continuous discoloration is an indication for endodontic therapy.

SIMPLE ENAMEL FRACTURES

Cracks and crazings of enamel are evident under transillumination and require no specific treatment (Fig. 13-3). Small enamel surface fractures may be treated by smoothing the edges with a disc (enameloplasty). Larger noticeable enamel fractures may be repaired with acid etch restorations (Fig. 13-6).

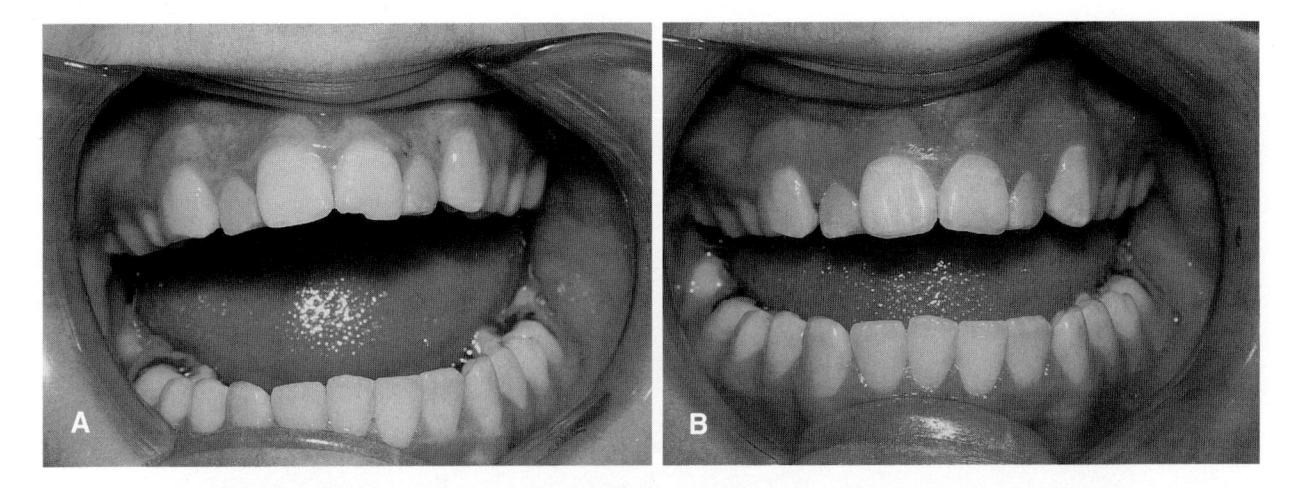

Figure 13-6 Photo of enameloplasty of No. 9. **A,** A very small segment of the mesial incisal edge was fractured. **B,** The mesial incisal edge of No. 9 was made smooth with a fine disk. (Courtesy of Dr. Jack Perchersky.)

FRACTURES OF ENAMEL AND DENTIN WITH NO PULP EXPOSURE

When both enamel and dentin are fractured, the dentin (which is highly organic) must be protected. The tubules may serve as a pathway for organisms and toxic material to the pulp. Calcium hydroxide offers the best protection to the pulp. Place a layer of Dycal over the dentin, acid etch the enamel, and place a composite restoration to restore the tooth (Fig. 13-7).

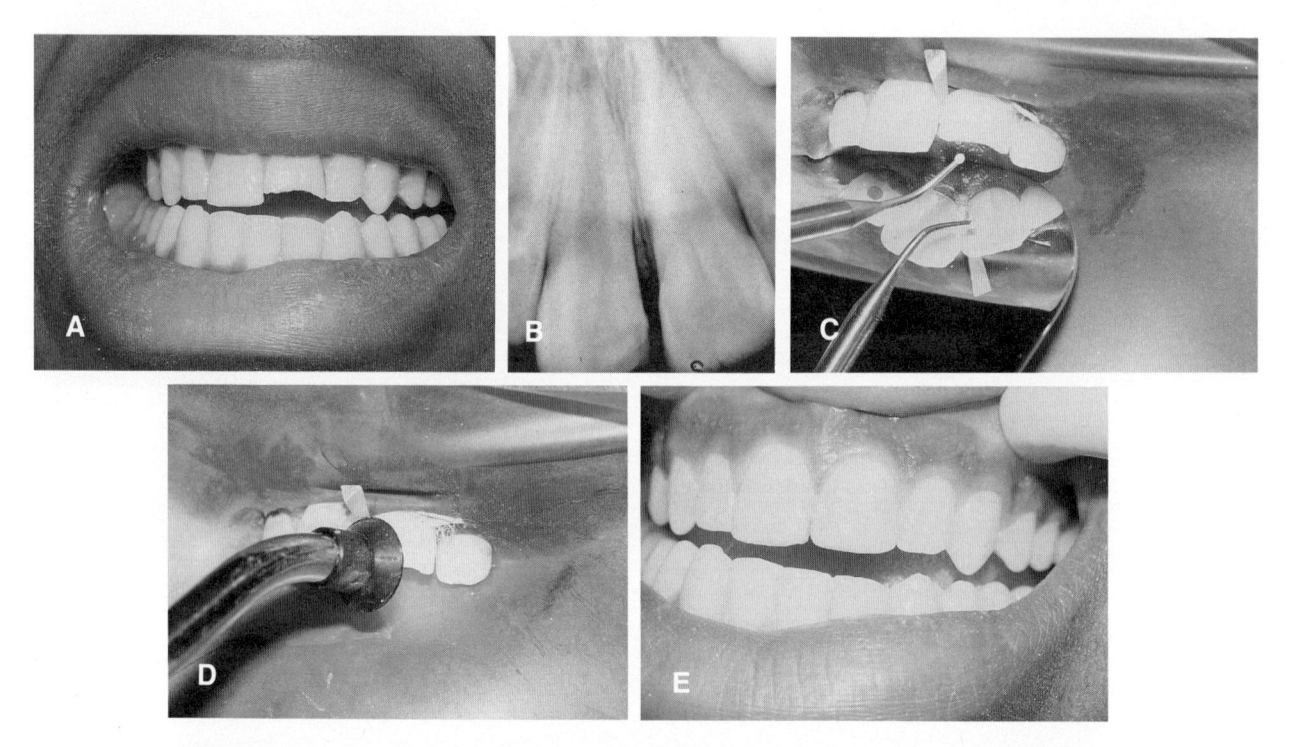

Figure 13-7 Acid etch repair of No. 9 with calcium hydroxide (Dycal) placed on dentin. **A,** Fracture of incisal third of tooth No. 9. **B,** Radiograph of fracture of enamel and dentin incisal third with no pulp exposure. **C,** CaOH (Dycal) is placed over dentin with a small, round-tipped applicator. **D,** The tooth is acid etched and light cured. **E,** Completed polished restoration. (Courtesy of Dr. Jack Perchersky.)

CROWN FRACTURE WITH PULP EXPOSURE (INCOMPLETE ROOT)

A crown fracture with a pulp exposure and an incompletely formed root requires a pulpotomy. Local anesthesia is given, the tooth is isolated, and the roof of the pulp chamber is removed with sterile No. 4 or No. 6 round bur or a very sharp spoon excavator. A pulpotomy is performed with a sterile, large, round bur or diamond, using a water coolant and intermittent light pressure. The hemorrhage is wiped out of the chamber with a cotton pellet and a clot is allowed to form (several minutes). Calcium hydroxide (Root-Cal or Calysept) is injected over the pulp stump and covered with a ZOE temporary cement. The tooth should be examined in 3 months, then every 6 months until root formation is completed. When the root is developed the dressing is removed and endodontic treatment is completed (Fig. 13-8). The root canal many times is not evident in the apical portion of the root and the root canal should be instrumented and filled to the point of calcification.

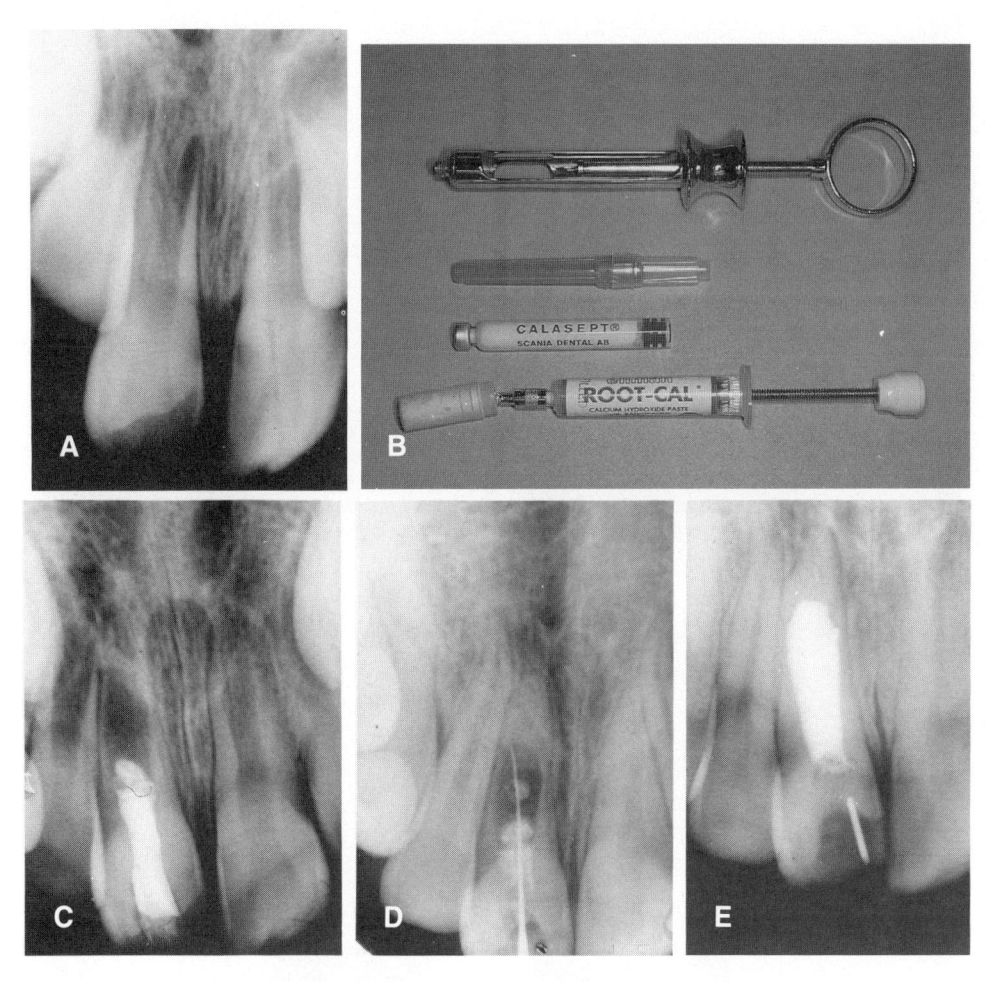

Figure 13-8 **A,** A radiograph of tooth No. 9 with fractured incisal one third, a pulp exposure, and incompletely formed root on an 8-year-old child. **B,** Following the pulpotomy calcium hydroxide (Root-Cal) was injected over the pulp stump and covered with a temporary seal of ZOE. Calasept (CaoH) or U.S.P. calcium hydroxide mixed with sterile water to a dry paste can also be used. **C,** A 10-month radiograph showing pulpotomy complete. Slight root formation is evident. **D,** A 4-year postpulpotomy radiograph shows complete root formation with no evidence of a canal in the apical third. The root length was obtained with a file placed in the canal and probed for a possible opening. **E,** An 8-year post operative radiograph shows the root canal filled to the level of calcification and the lamina dura is intact.

CROWN FRACTURE WITH PULP EXPOSURE AND ROOT FULLY FORMED

A pulpectomy is performed in teeth where the crown is fractured, the pulp is exposed, and the root is fully formed. The root canal may be completed in the same appointment if time permits and the canal is prepared for a post (Fig. 13-9).

CROWN FRACTURE SUBGINGIVALLY

If tooth is fractured below the alveolar crest, a root canal is performed, a post is placed, and the tooth is extruded orthodontically. It should take about 3 months and held into position for another 3 months to prevent re-intrusion (Fig. 13-10).

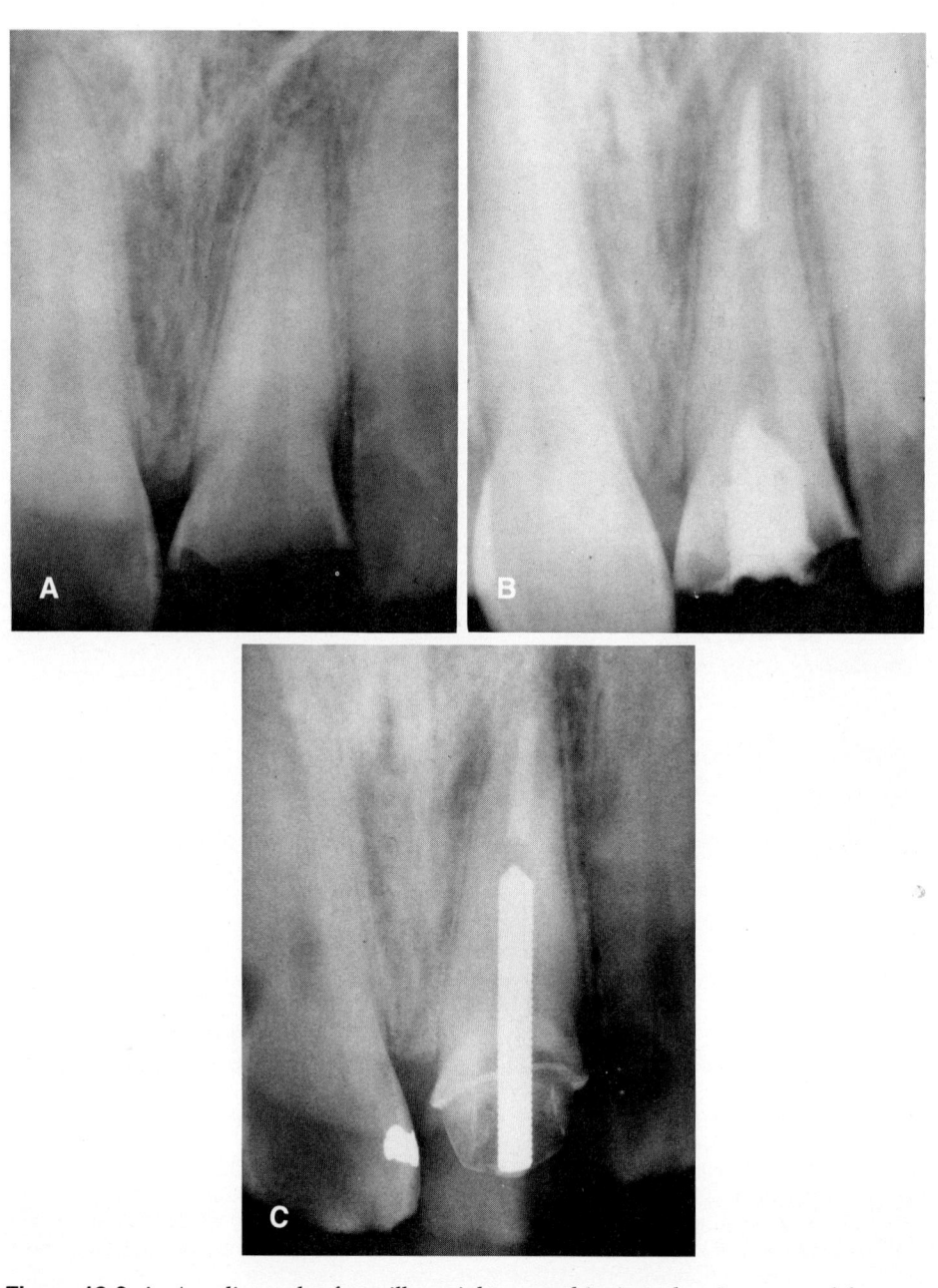

Figure 13-9 **A,** A radiograph of maxillary right central incisor showing coronal fracture to the gingival third with pulp exposure and root fully formed. **B,** Root canal is completed at same appointment and prepared for a post. **C,** Radiograph of post and core.

Chapter 13 ♦ Traumatic Injuries 251

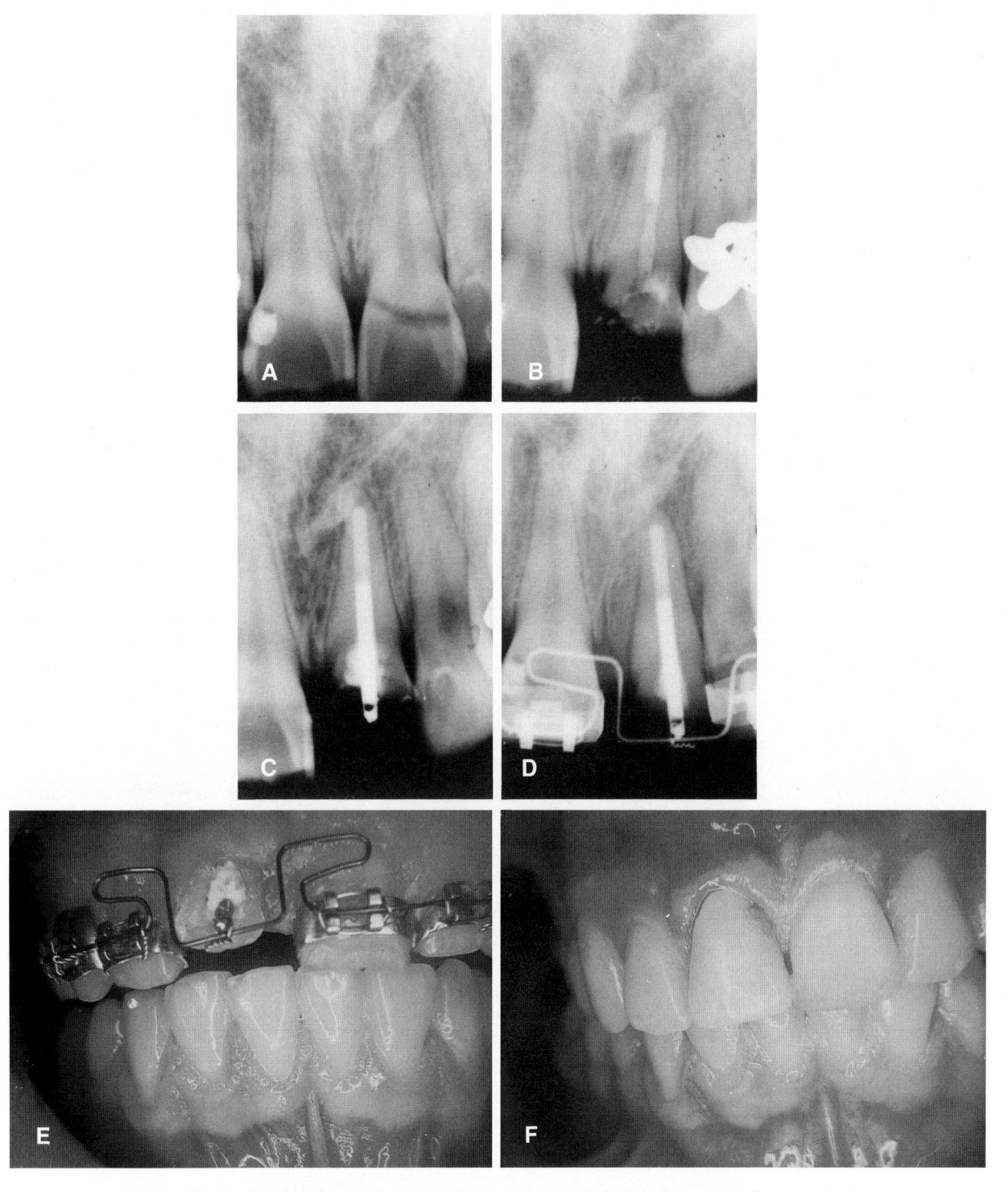

Figure 13-10 **A,** A radiograph of maxillary right central with the crown fractured subgingivally and pulp exposed. **B,** A radiograph of tooth No. 8 root canal completed in one appointment and prepared for a post. **C,** Post sealed in canal with very thin oxyphosphate cement and a hole made in post with an inverted cone bur (33½) for wire placement. **D,** A radiograph of the orthodontic appliance in place to extrude tooth. **E,** Three months following extrusion with orthodontic appliance. The adjacent teeth are used as anchor teeth and should include at least two teeth on either side. **F,** Temporary crown is splinted to the incisal edge for an additional 60 to 90 days to prevent reintrusion.

TRAUMATIZED IMMATURE NON-VITAL TEETH

When an immature tooth is non-vital an apexification procedure is performed. The canal is cleaned with blunted hedstrom files, irrigated with sodium hypochlorite, and dried with paper points. A creamy mixture of calcium hydroxide and sterile water or CMCP (camphorated paramonochlorophenol) is mixed on a glass slab into a thick dry paste, carried into the canal (with an amalgam plugger), and condensed to the apex with a large No. 9 or No. 10 plugger. A small amount is first placed into the canal and packed into the apical area with a prefitted plugger. Root-Cal or Calysept can also be injected into the canal. The tooth is examined in 3 months and then at 6-month intervals until apexification is complete, which may take 1½ to 2 years. The dressing does not need to be changed unless it has been absorbed or the filling has percolated. If Hertwig's sheath remains vital, continued root formation results and the root increases in length. If it has been destroyed by necrosis or aging, apexogenesis occurs and a cementum bridge forms across the apical end of the root. Following either, the root canal is completed (Fig. 13-11).

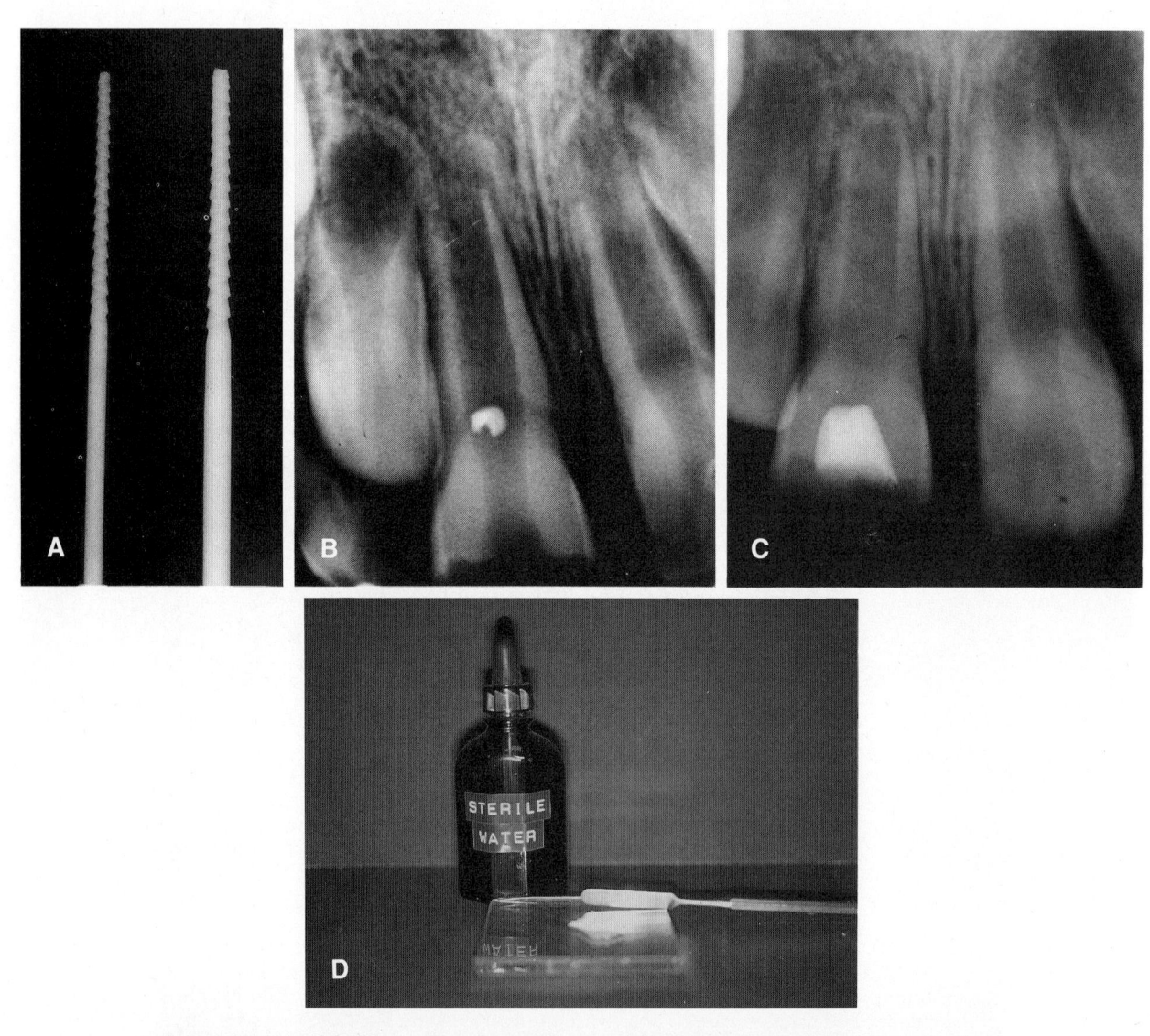

Figure 13-11 **A,** Hedstrom files shown blunted with a stone to keep the sharp tip from penetrating apical tissue. **B,** Radiograph of non-vital, immature, fractured maxillary left central incisor. **C,** A 4-month check-up of calcium hydroxide without barium sulfate placed in canal. Slight apexification is evident. **D,** The calcium hydroxide was mixed with sterile water on a sterilized slab.

Continued.

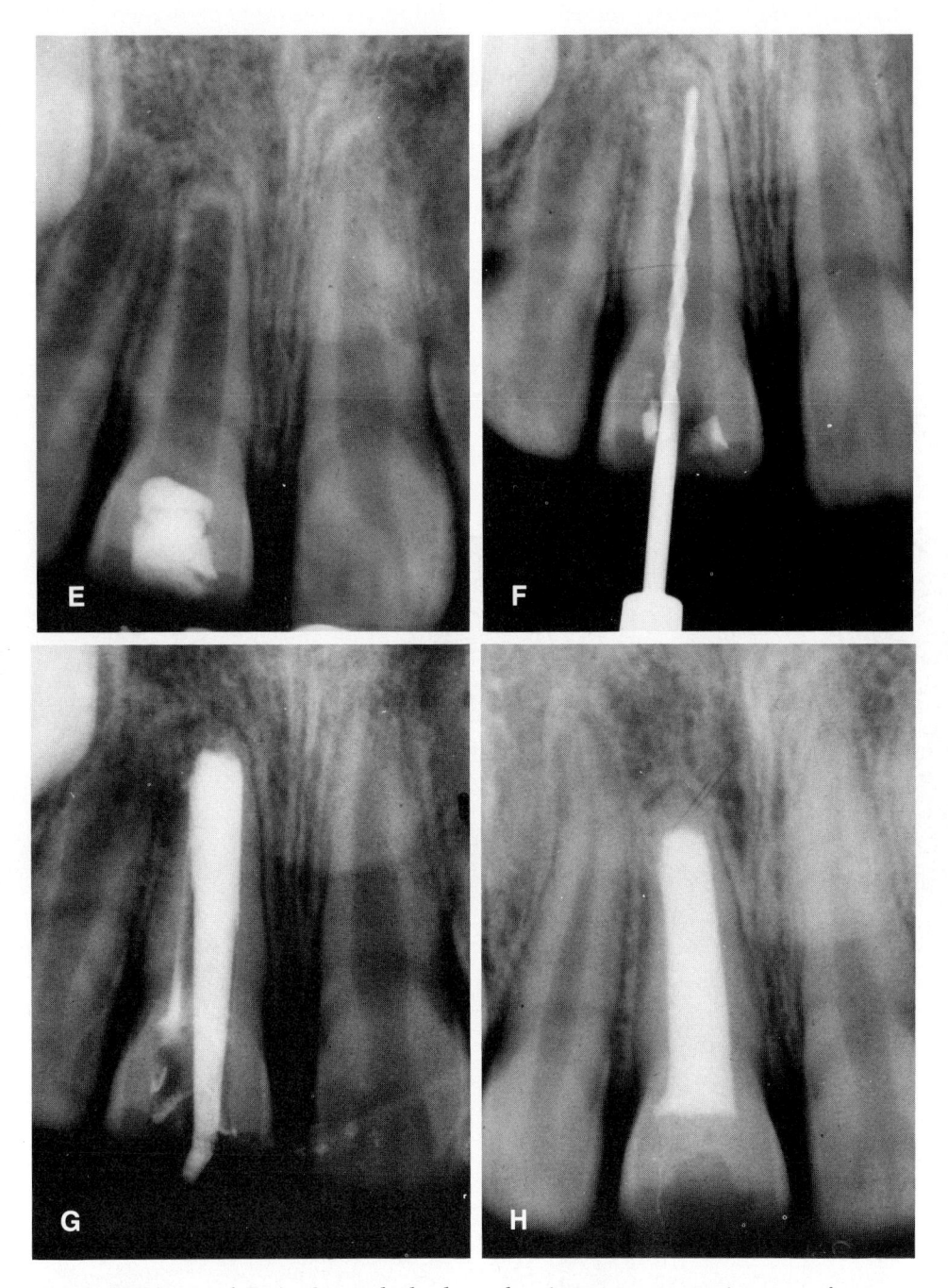

Figure 13-11, *cont'd* **E,** An 8-month check-up showing cementogenesis or cap of cementum at apex. **F,** Test file placed in canal to determine working length and test integrity of cemental cap for voids. **G,** An Inverted master cone placed in position for a tight fit at apex and the canal is filled. **H,** A 6-year postoperative examination showing root canal completed and lamina dura intact and adjacent teeth erupted.

LUXATED TEETH (LOOSENED, MALPOSITIONED)

Loosened teeth should be repositioned under local anesthesia and splinted for 6 weeks. When hemorrhage or gingival lacerations are present the repositioned teeth are splinted with an acrylic band. The acrylic is placed incisal to the contact point so as not to impinge on the interproximal tissue, which may cause blunting and recession (Fig. 13-12). The splint usually lasts 3 to 5 days, at which time hemorrhage is stopped and a more permanent splint is used, such as brackets or direct bonding with or without the use of a wire, bar, or nylon cord. This type of splint offers excellent stabilization for multiple loosened teeth (Fig. 13-13).

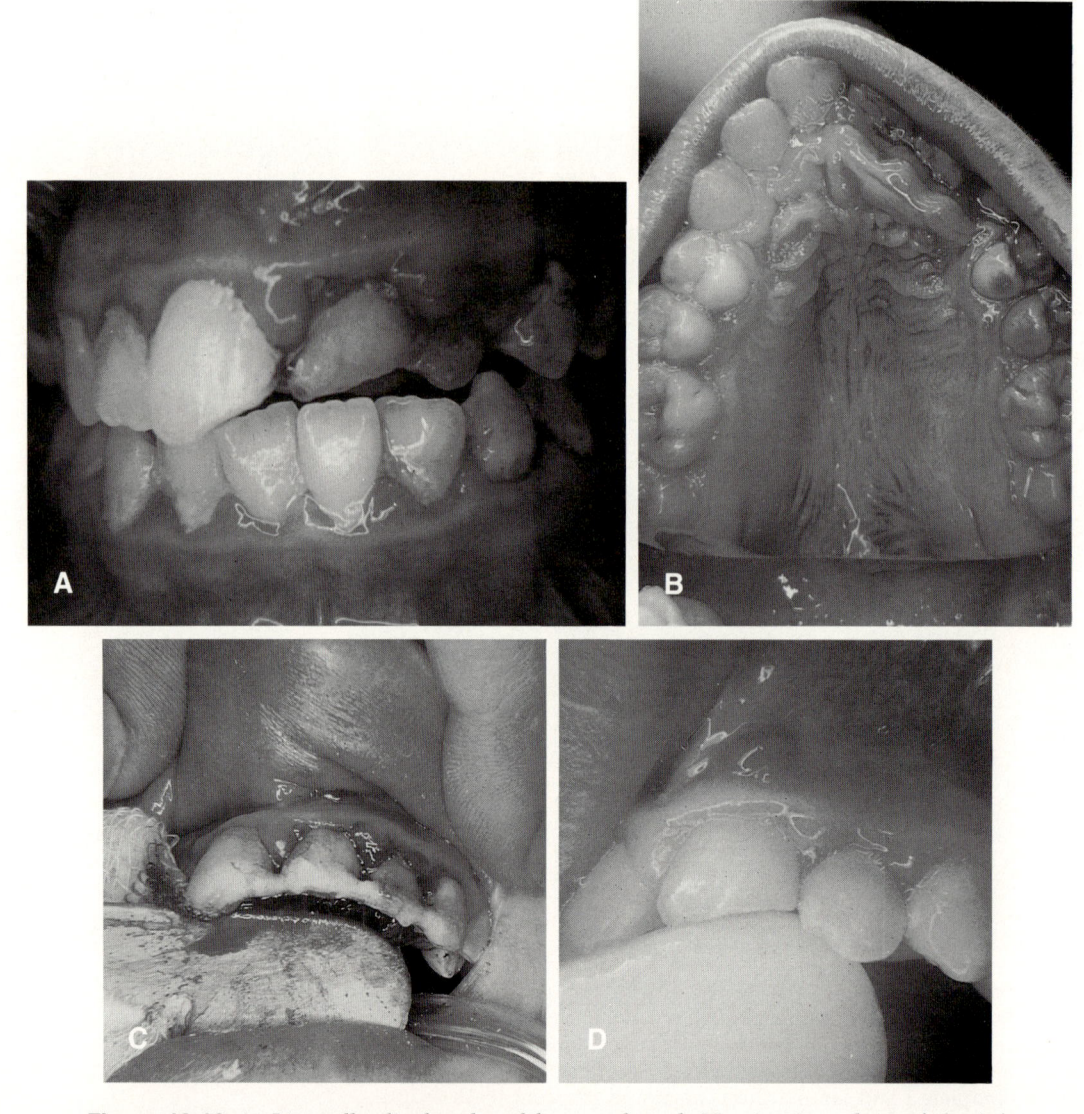

Figure 13-12 A, Lingually displaced and loosened teeth No. 9, 10, and 11 of the left pre-maxilla. Note extensive hemorrhage. **B,** A palatal view showing collapse of premaxilla. **C,** Teeth repositioned with finger pressure and a tongue depressor to obtain desired curvature and incisal edge alignment. An acrylic splint was placed incisal to contact point. **D,** A 7-day postoperative repair of soft tissue without hemorrhage. The teeth are now ready for a more secure splint such as brackets or bonding.

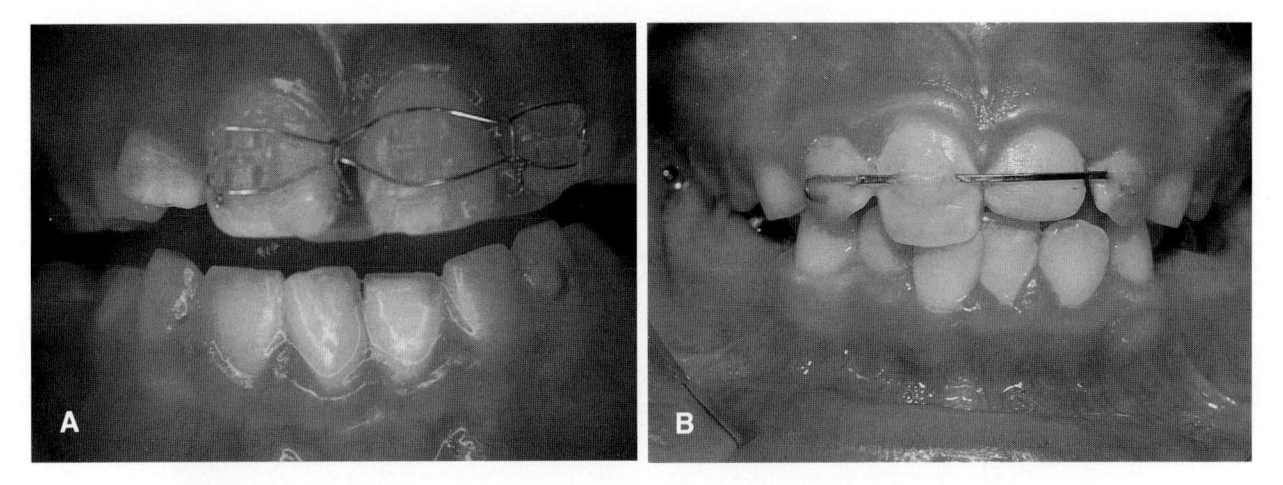

Figure 13-13 A, Anterior teeth ligated with brackets bonded to teeth. **B,** An orthodontic bar is placed over the luxated maxillary central incisor and bonded to the adjacent teeth.

EXTRUDED AND INTRUDED TEETH

Extruded teeth are repositioned under local anesthetic as soon as possible and the labial and lingual plates should be compressed slightly with finger pressure for several minutes. Teeth that are intruded extensively should be repositioned orthodontically and extruded into position over a period of several months. The use of forceps to surgically reposition increases the chances of resorption (Fig. 13-14). Following repositioning, teeth should be maintained with a splint for an additional 3 months to prevent redrifting.

Teeth that are intruded in the eruptive state and are in good vertical alignment can be left to reerupt. A normal eruption pattern usually occurs and the resorption factor is minimized.

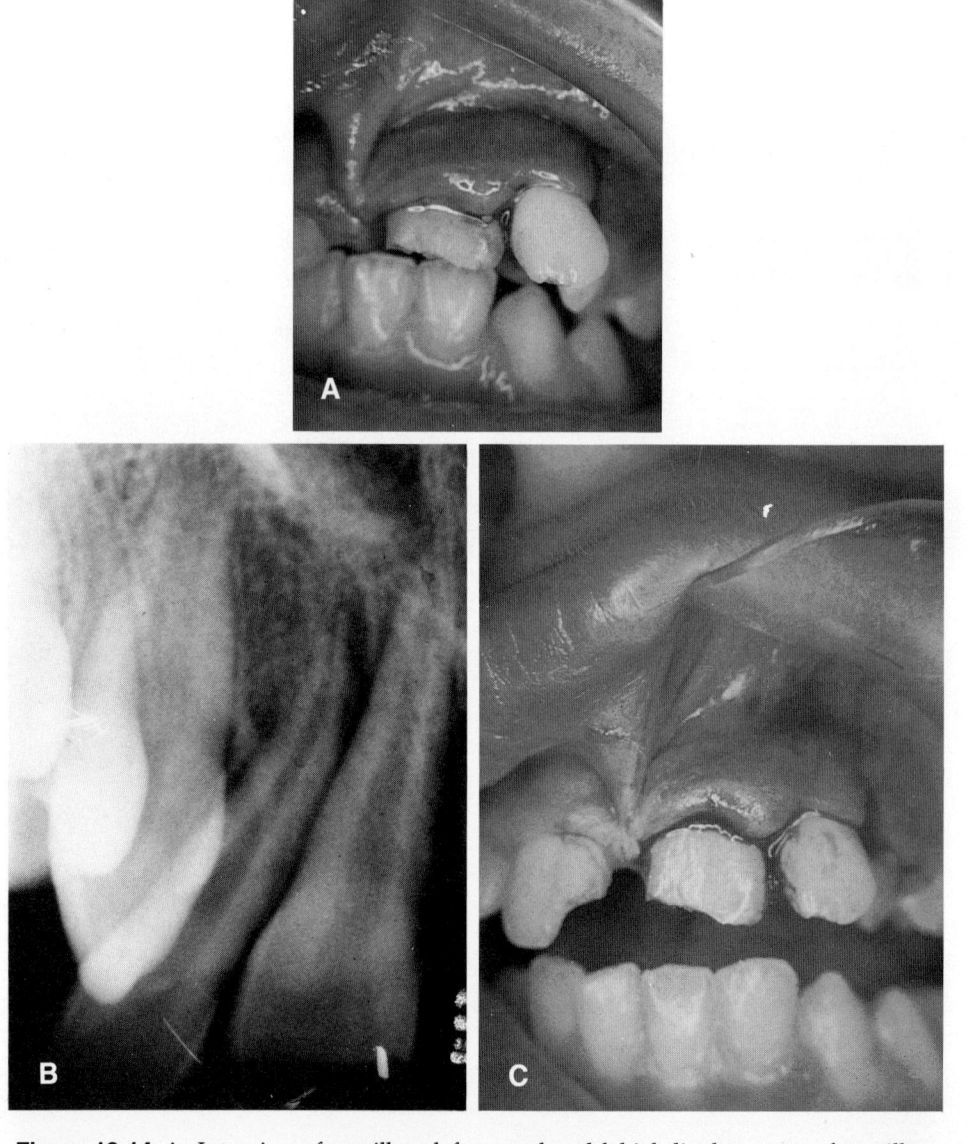

Figure 13-14 **A,** Intrusion of maxillary left central and labial displacement of maxillary left lateral incisor. **B,** Radiograph of teeth showing apex of No. 9 forced through socket and No. 10 extruded out of socket. **C,** Partial realignment with finger pressure under local anesthetic.

Continued.

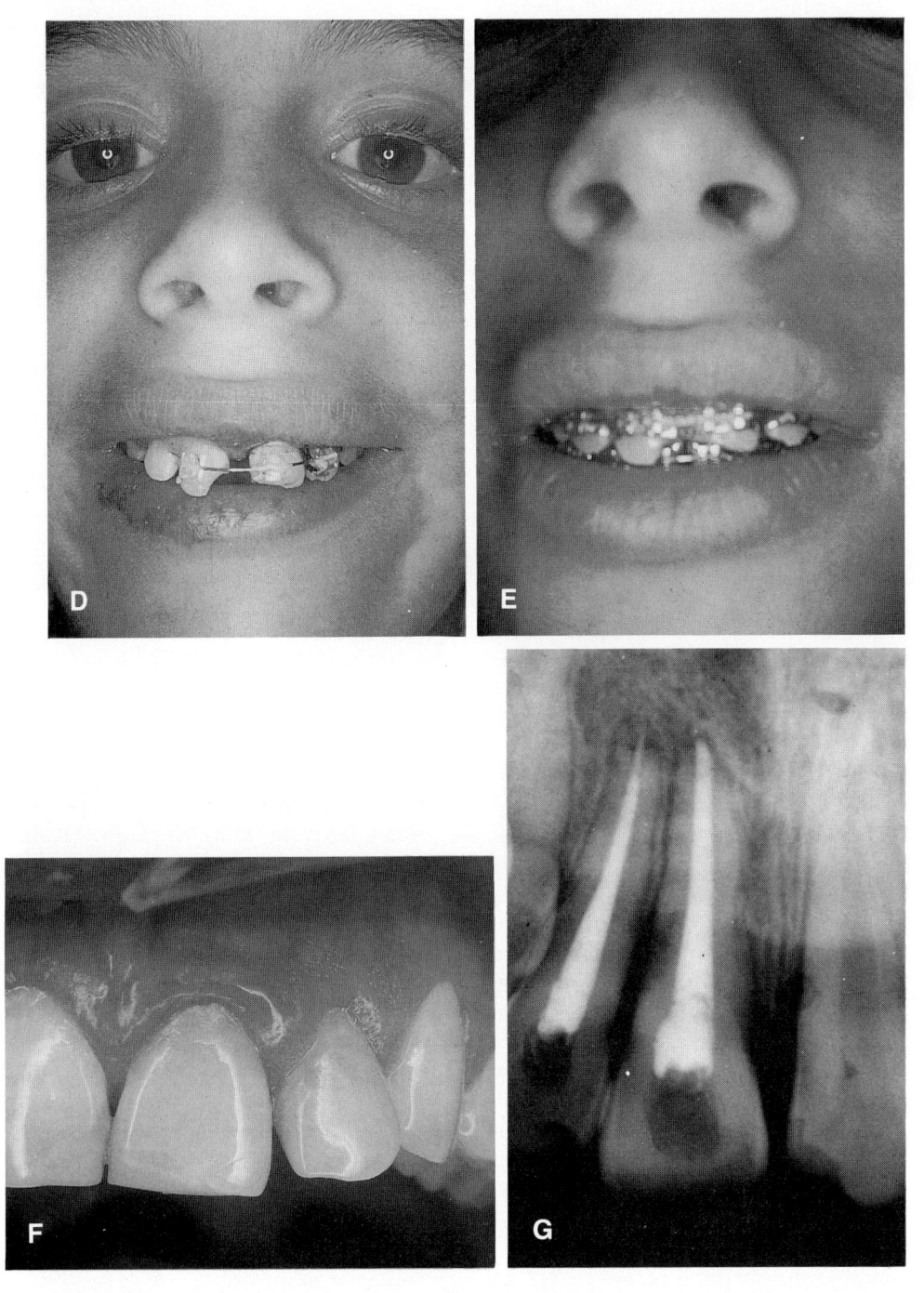

Figure 13-14, *cont'd* **D,** Teeth partially repositioned and ligated with passive arch wire and brackets. **E,** Five days later orthodontic brackets were placed to extrude No. 9 and align remaining teeth. **F,** A 10-year examination showing teeth in alignment. **G,** A 10-year radiograph showing endodontic treatment completed on both teeth following placement of CaOH for 6 weeks and lamina dura is intact. There is slight replacement resorption on mesial of tooth No. 9 and distal of tooth No. 10.

AVULSED TEETH

The majority of reimplanted teeth resorb (Fig. 13-15), however replantation is a viable alternative to immediate loss and reduces the psychological shock. The resorption may take several months or many years. Avulsion usually occurs when the energy of the injury is displaced over the crown, soft tissue, and root. Avulsed teeth should be replanted and repositioned as soon as possible (preferably at the scene of the accident), and then the patient taken to the dentist. The longer the tooth remains out of the socket and the more the tooth is manipulated, the greater the chance of resorption. The tooth can be stored in saline, milk, or patient's saliva because they have a similar osmotic balance with the periodontal and pulp tissues. If it is necessary to cleanse the root, it can be flushed with saline. When a clot is present in the socket it should be curetted and removed from the socket before replantation to minimize ankylosis.

STABILIZATION

The tooth is repositioned and ligated for a period of 1 to 3 weeks with passive splinting; a loop of .020 wire, orthodontic brackets, or a passive bar acid etched to the teeth can be used to passively stabilize the tooth or teeth (Fig. 13-16).

The patient is placed on a prescription of antibiotics, penicillin, or erythromycin prophylactically for 1 week and a tetanus shot is given when indicated. After 1 week the pulp tissue is removed, the canal is debrided, and a dressing of calcium hydroxide is placed. Root-cal or Calasept (Fig. 13-8,B) may be injected into the canal or a mixture of Calcium Hydroxide U.S.P. and sterile water are sealed in the canal (Fig. 13-11,C) until the splint must be removed. Before removing the splint, the root canal is completed. The calcium hydroxide dressing may slow, arrest, and prevent resorption.

The types of resorption that may occur are inflammatory resorption and replacement resorption. Inflammatory resorption is usually associated with necrotic and inflammatory tissue in the pulp canal. As the cementum is resorbed it is replaced by inflammatory tissue. Replacement resorption occurs when the resorbed cementum is replaced by bone and ankylosis occurs (Fig. 13-17). It can be partial, isolated, or complete. There is no apparent treatment for replacement resorption.

The teeth should be observed every 6 months for several years to detect possible resorption and ankylosis. Ankylosis is determined by tapping the tooth lightly with a blunted metal instrument. An ankylosed tooth has a sharp resonating sound that vibrates from the tooth through the skull. In a normal tooth the sound and percussion is absorbed by the periodontal ligament and has a dull sound. Radiographically there is a loss of periodontal ligament and the tooth is attached directly to bone (Fig. 13-17). If ankylosis occurs in preadolescent patients in which the premaxilla is still growing, the tooth should be extracted. Because the premaxilla grows downward and outward the ankylosed tooth remains high on the ridge and produces an unsightly defect (Fig. 13-18).

Several types of splints may be used to stabilize avulsed and luxated teeth. One tooth on either side of the involved tooth is usually sufficient. The splint should be placed passively and not impinge on the interproximal tissue (Fig. 13-19). Types of splints include the following:

a. An acrylic band over several teeth.
b. Direct bonding to the teeth.
c. Bonding at least one tooth on either side of the involved tooth with a passive bar.
d. Brackets placed on the labial of the teeth on either side of the involved tooth ligated with .020 wire or a passive bar.
e. A single loop with interproximal tie.

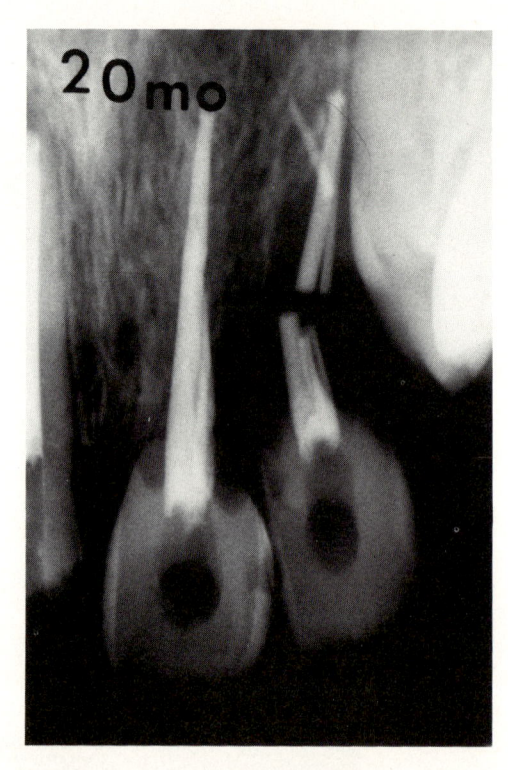

Figure 13-15 A 20-month postreplantation radiograph of teeth No. 7 and 8 showing both roots resorbed.

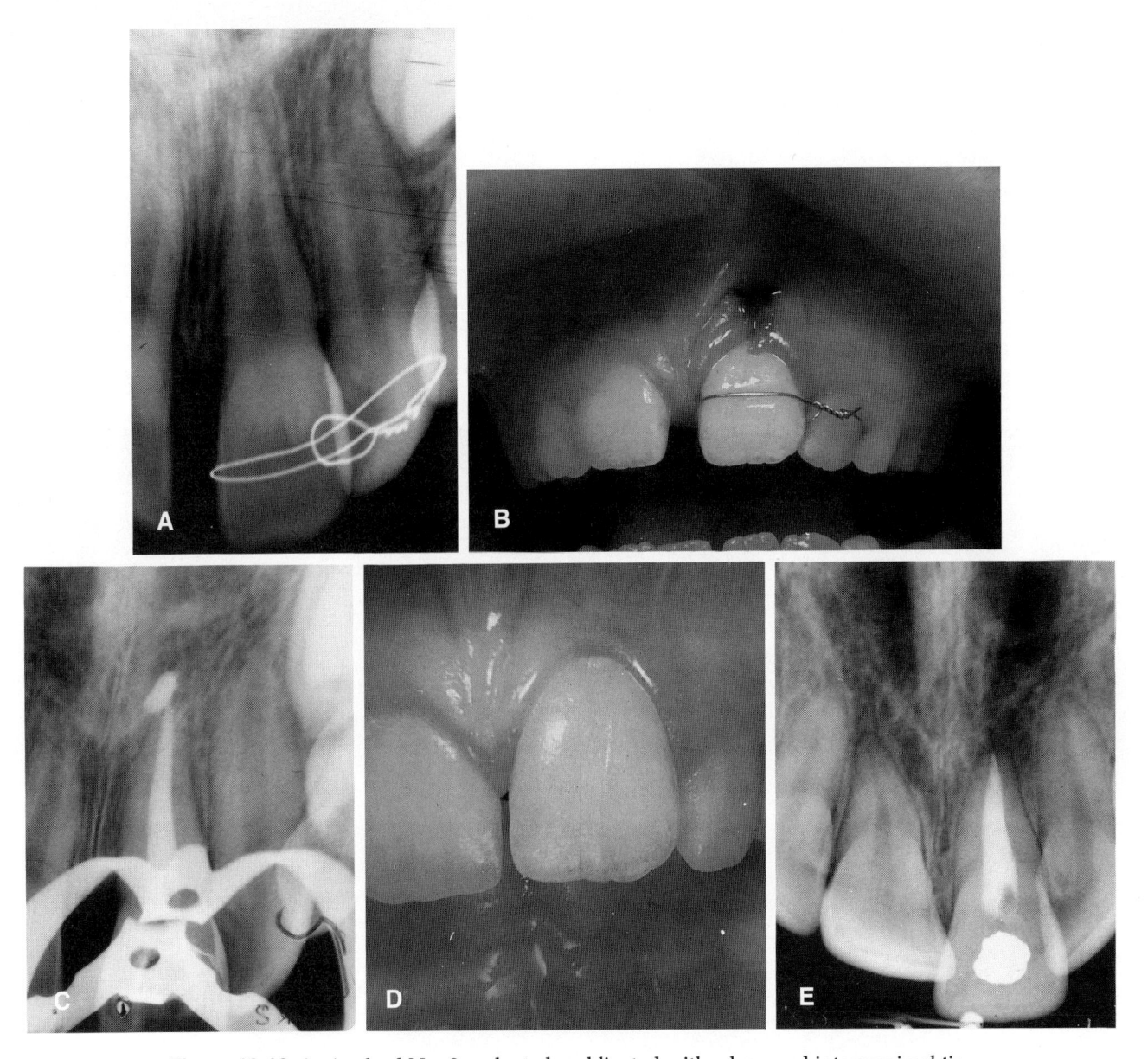

Figure 13-16 **A,** Avulsed No. 9 replanted and ligated with a loop and interproximal tie. **B,** Laceration of the gingival tissue and ligation above contact point not impinging on papilla. **C,** Root canal completed after 6 weeks of calcium hydroxide being placed in the canal. **D,** A 2-year examination shows slight ankylosis of clinical crown. **NOTE:** Gingival margin of No. 9 is slightly higher than No. 8. **E,** A postoperative 25-year radiograph showing periodontal space.

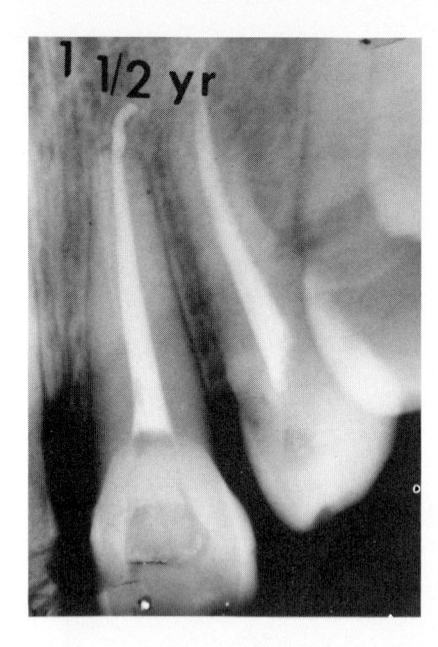

Figure 13-17 A 1½ year postreplantation radiograph of tooth No. 7. Root resorption with ankylosis is evident on the entire root and there is loss of the periodontal space.

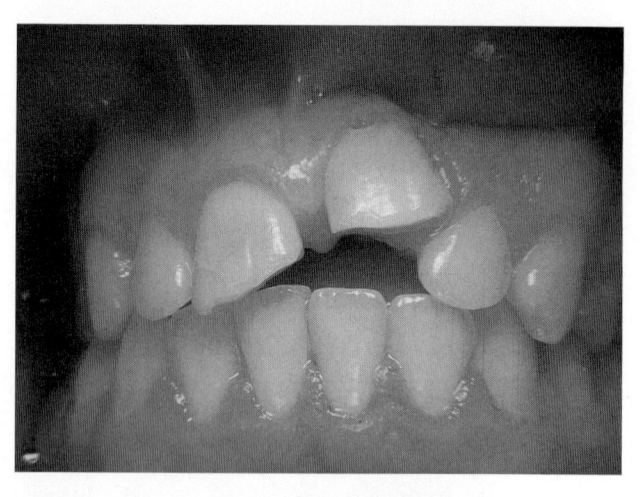

Figure 13-18 Tooth No. 9 ankylosed and remaining typically high on the ridge. The tooth was extracted.

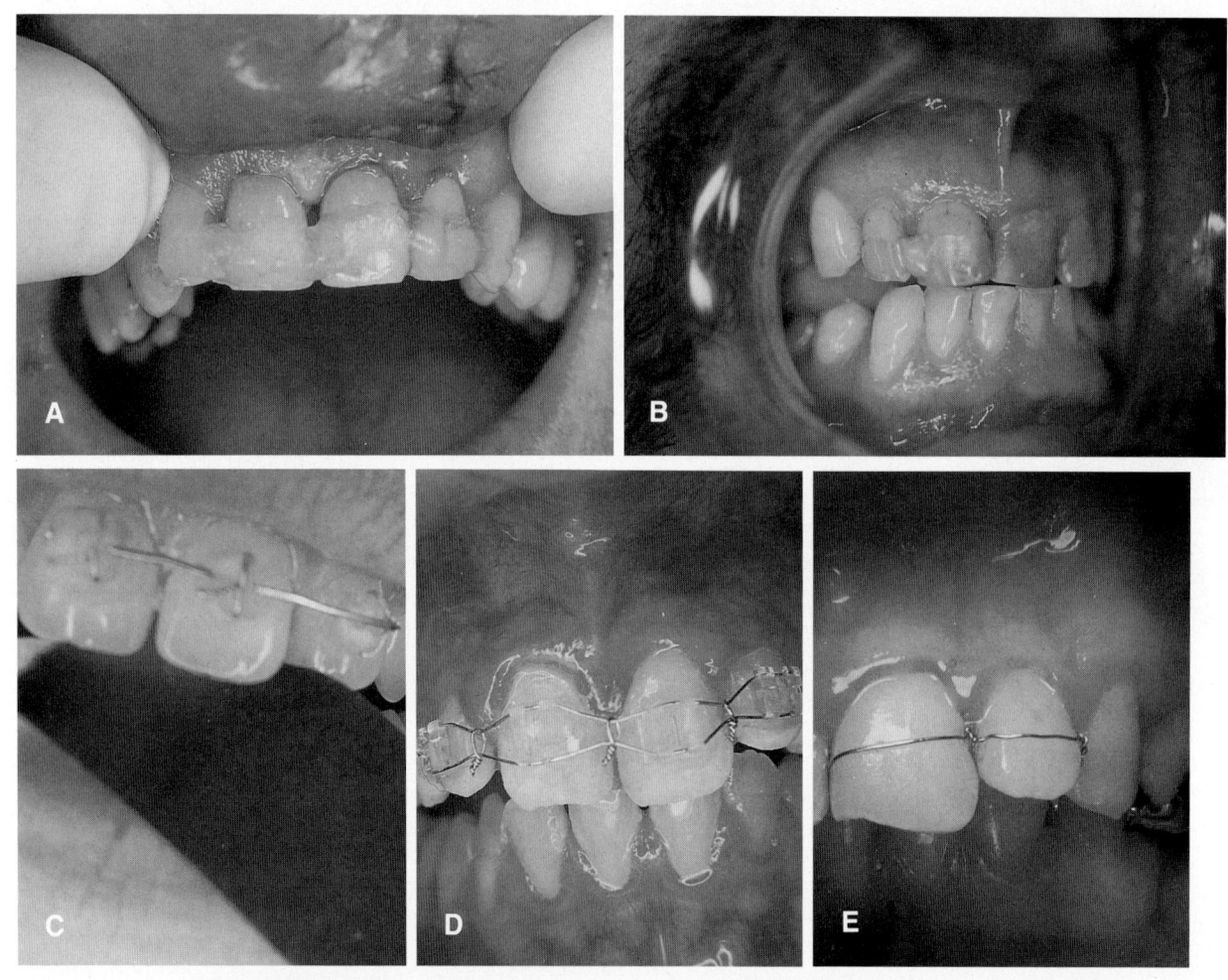

Figure 13-19 A, An acrylic band placed over labial surface. The acrylic is kept away from the interdental papilla so as not to cause recession. **B,** Direct bonding over several teeth. The bond could be strengthened with wire or nylon cord. **C,** Brackets bonded to the teeth with a passive wire and checked for occlusion. **D,** Bonded brackets and ligated with .020 wire with interproximal ties. **E,** A single loop of .020 arch wire with interproximal ties. The wire is kept away from the gingival papilla and above the contact point.

NON-VITAL TEETH—TREATED OR UNTREATED AND PARTIALLY ERUPTED

Non-vital teeth, treated or untreated and not fully erupted, erupt as any other teeth. Eruption of teeth is not dependent on the vitality of the pulp. Should partially erupted teeth become non-vital and lingual access is not feasible, treatment is delayed until the tooth erupts. If swelling and pain occur, antibiotic therapy and analgesics should be initiated (Fig. 13-20).

ROOT FRACTURES

Root fractures may be vertical or horizontal. The horizontal fracture may also be comminuted (Fig. 13-21).

Vertical

The prognosis for vertical root fractures is generally poor. When the fracture is separated and communication exists with sulcus and saliva, the tooth may be

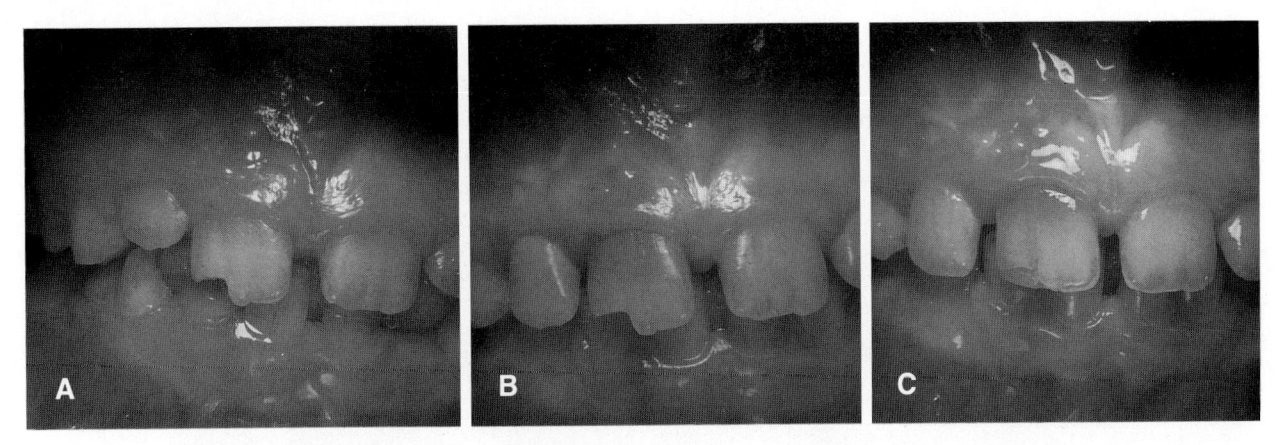

Figure 13-20 **A,** Partially erupted non-vital tooth No. 8. **B,** No. 8 at 8 months showing continued eruption. **C,** Twelve months post trauma showing eruption of crown and tooth is now ready for endodontic therapy.

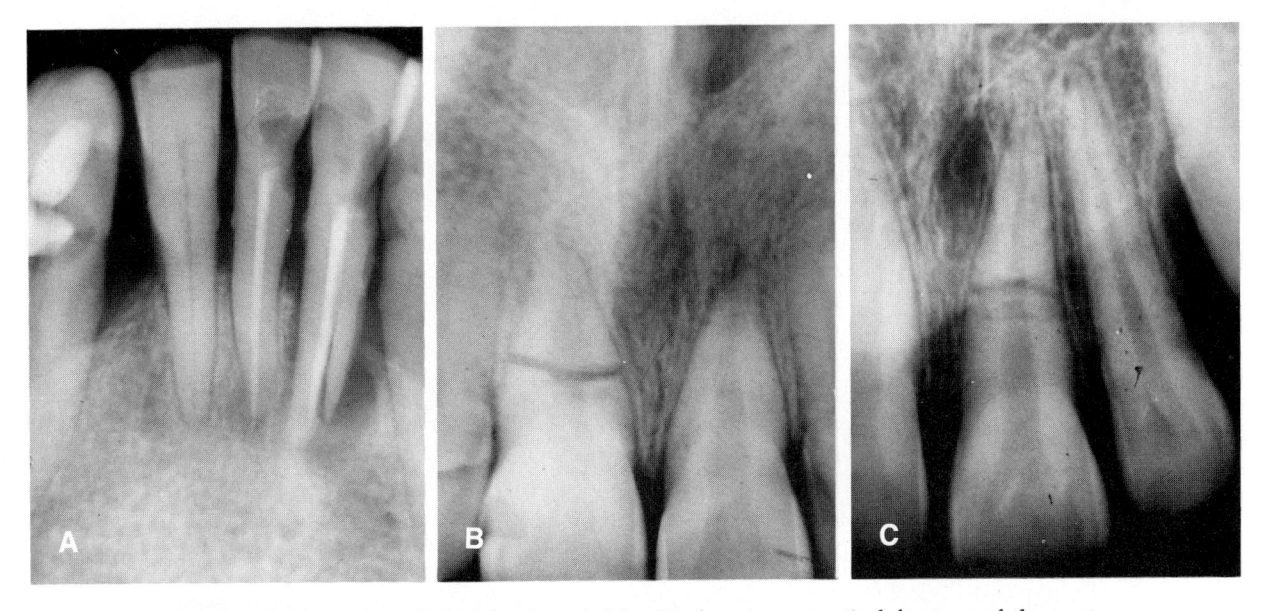

Figure 13-21 **A,** A radiograph of tooth No. 25 showing a vertical fracture of the root following excessive lateral condensation. **B,** Radiograph of No. 9 showing horizontal fracture in apical third following blow from a punch to the face. **C,** Radiograph of tooth No. 8 showing comminuted fracture in middle third.

considered hopeless (Fig. 13-22). The almost pathognomonic symptoms known as the *Cracked Tooth Syndrome* of a vertical fracture are pain to biting and no specific cause for the discomfort is able to be determined.

CRACKED TOOTH SYNDROME ♦ A vertical fracture should be suspected when:
- A halo lesion encircles the entire root.
- Crestal widening of the periodontal ligament.
- Isolated periodontal pocket.
- History of a very sharp pain when biting something hard (Fig. 13-23).
- Pain during insertion of a post or seating of an inlay.
- Inconsistent occurrences during routine treatment.
- Unexplainable failure of root canal.
- Pain to biting in certain planes.
- Persistent drainage or bleeding or pain elicited in unusual areas in the root canal.
- A history of repeated loosening and dislodging of a post and core.
- A very wide diameter post.
- Preendodontic and postendodontic pain (Fig. 13-22).

Most vertical fractures occur in posterior teeth; however, they can also occur in anterior teeth. They usually occur in teeth in which the cusps have been undermined from decay and extensive restoration, leaving weak enamel surfaces. The placement of a coronal restoration to reduce occlusal stresses such as an onlay or crown helps reduce occurrence of vertical fractures.

Vertical fractures may develop under unusual masticatory stresses (Fig. 13-23). They may also occur during unusual heavy lateral and vertical condensation of gutta percha (Fig. 13-22) and during the placement of posts, especially those that are tapered and very large (Fig. 13-22).

Transillumination, dye staining with methylene blue, and having the patient bite in specific occlusal planes to elicit pain are excellent diagnostic aids in detecting a vertical fracture. When the patient describes the symptoms of pain when biting in certain planes and all the tests are negative and no definitive

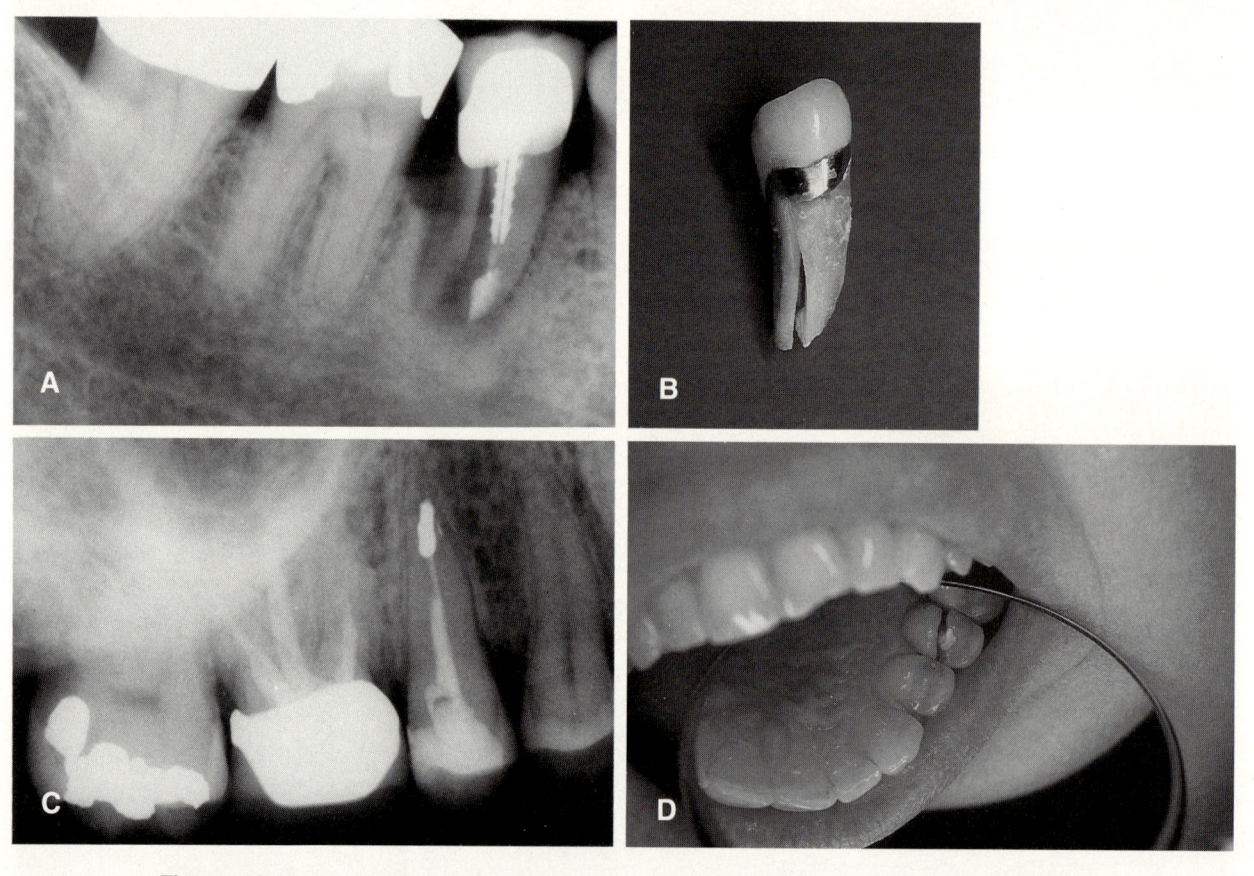

Figure 13-22 **A,** A radiograph of tooth No. 20 showing extensive widening of root fracture and a radiolucent area extending to the crestal bone. A Flexi post is in the canal. **B,** Lingual view of fracture showing widening in apical third. **C,** A radiograph of fracture of clinical crown that became apparent after patient bit on hard crust of bread and experienced a sudden sharp thrust of pain. **D,** The fracture extended through the lingual and buccal. The tooth was extracted.

tests are conclusive, it usually indicates a microscopic vertical fracture. The tooth should be crowned for protection from further fracture and the prognosis is good. Such fractures are usually not detectable with a radiograph (Fig. 13-23).

TREATMENT ♦ When a vertical fracture is evident, the tooth should immediately be protected from separation by placing a band or crown around the tooth and the root canal completed and taken out of occlusion. The pulp chamber walls are cleaned of all sealer with alcohol, and a core paste (Den-Mat) is used to bond the fractured segments together. The core paste is injected into the entire chamber. The paste will bond to the dentin, form a tight union, and seal out moisture. The tooth is then crowned (Figs. 13-24 and 13-25). The Den-Mat core paste has shown unusual clinical success for teeth with vertical fractures that were once considered hopeless.

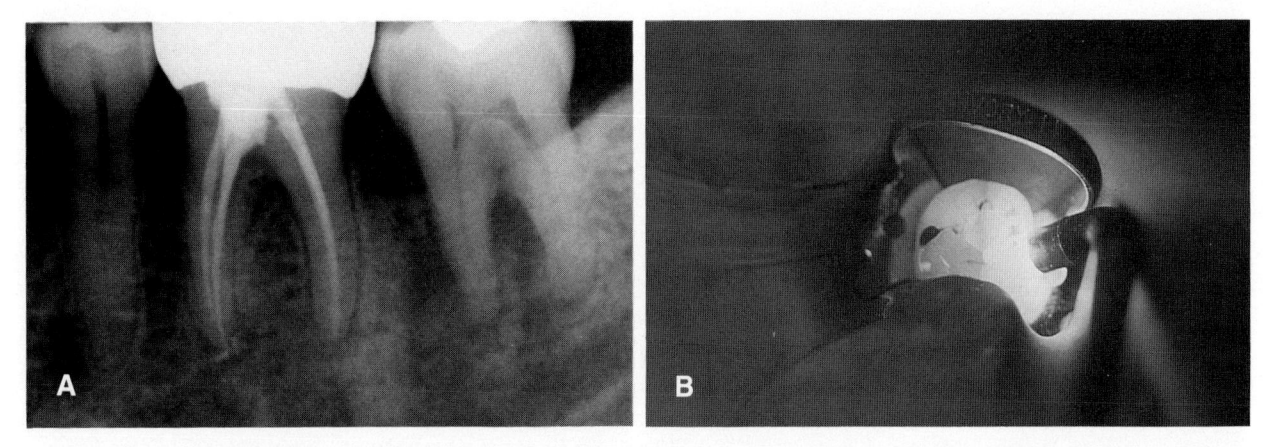

Figure 13-23 Vertical fracture of tooth without root canal caused by biting a cherry pit. **A,** Radiograph of tooth No. 31 showing a large radiolucent lesion circumscribing the mesial root and a very small occlusal restoration. Tooth was very tender to biting. **B,** Transillumination of tooth shows vertical fracture from mesial to distal marginal ridge. The tooth was extracted.

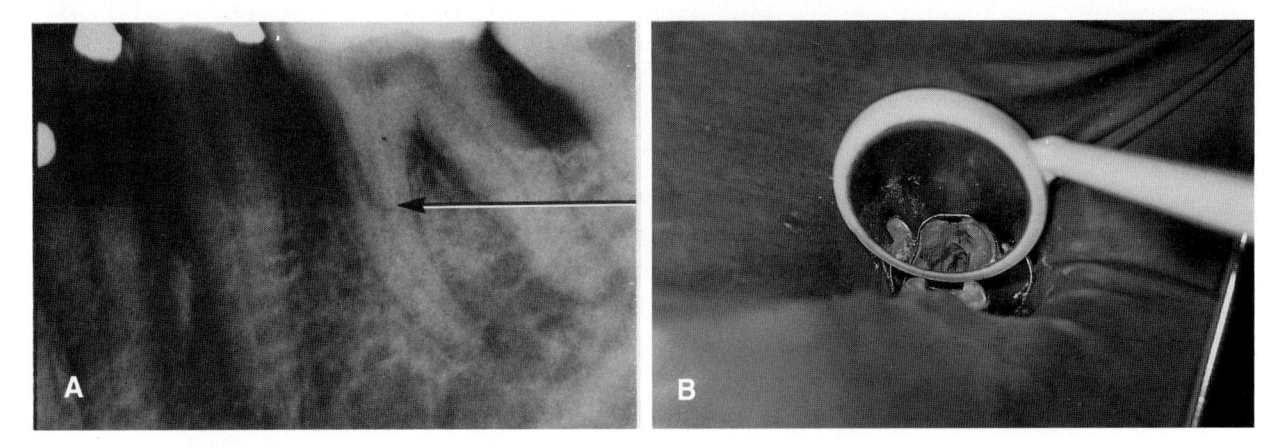

Figure 13-24 Vertical fracture — repair with Den-Mat Core Paste. **A,** A radiograph of tooth No. 30 with a large occlusal restoration. Patient recalls biting on an olive pit and experiencing sharp pain apparently 1 year prior. A diagonal fracture was evident on the mesial root on the radiograph and extended through the furca to the distal marginal ridge. Patient was having pain when biting. **B,** The occlusion was reduced, a copper band was placed, and the restoration removed. A clinical fracture was evident on the distal wall and extending to the gingival floor.

Continued.

264 PRACTICAL ENDODONTICS

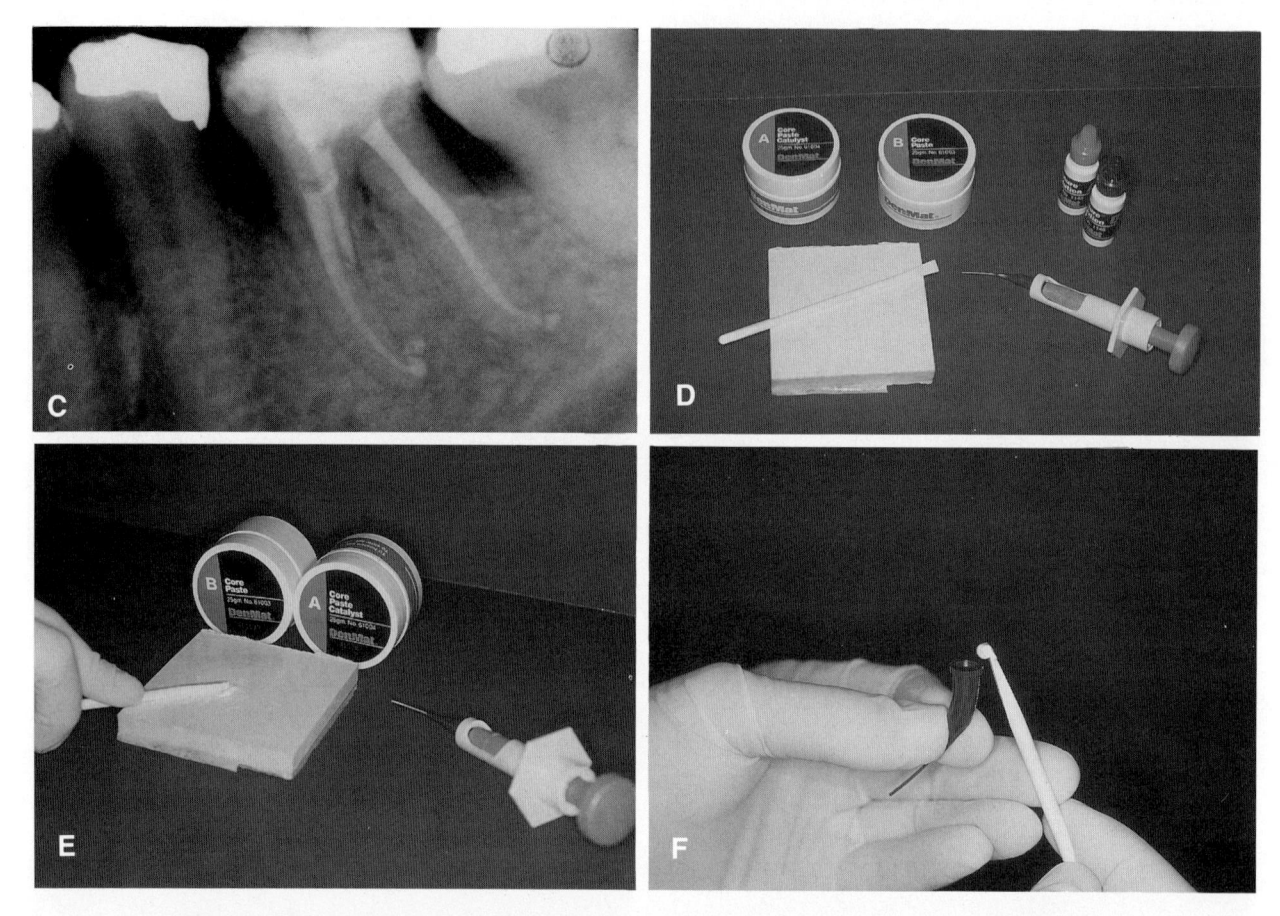

Figure 13-24, *cont'd* **C,** A radiograph of the completed root canal. The pulp chamber was cleaned with a cotton pellet moistened in alcohol and the dentin walls were prepared with bonding agent (Tenure). The entire pulp chamber was injected with Den-Mat core paste, and the tooth crowned. **D,** The Den-Mat kit consists of the core paste, catalyst, bonding agent, and syringe. **E,** Equal amounts of core paste and catalyst are mixed. **F,** The mixture is placed in the injection cartridge.

Continued.

Chapter 13 ♦ Traumatic Injuries   265

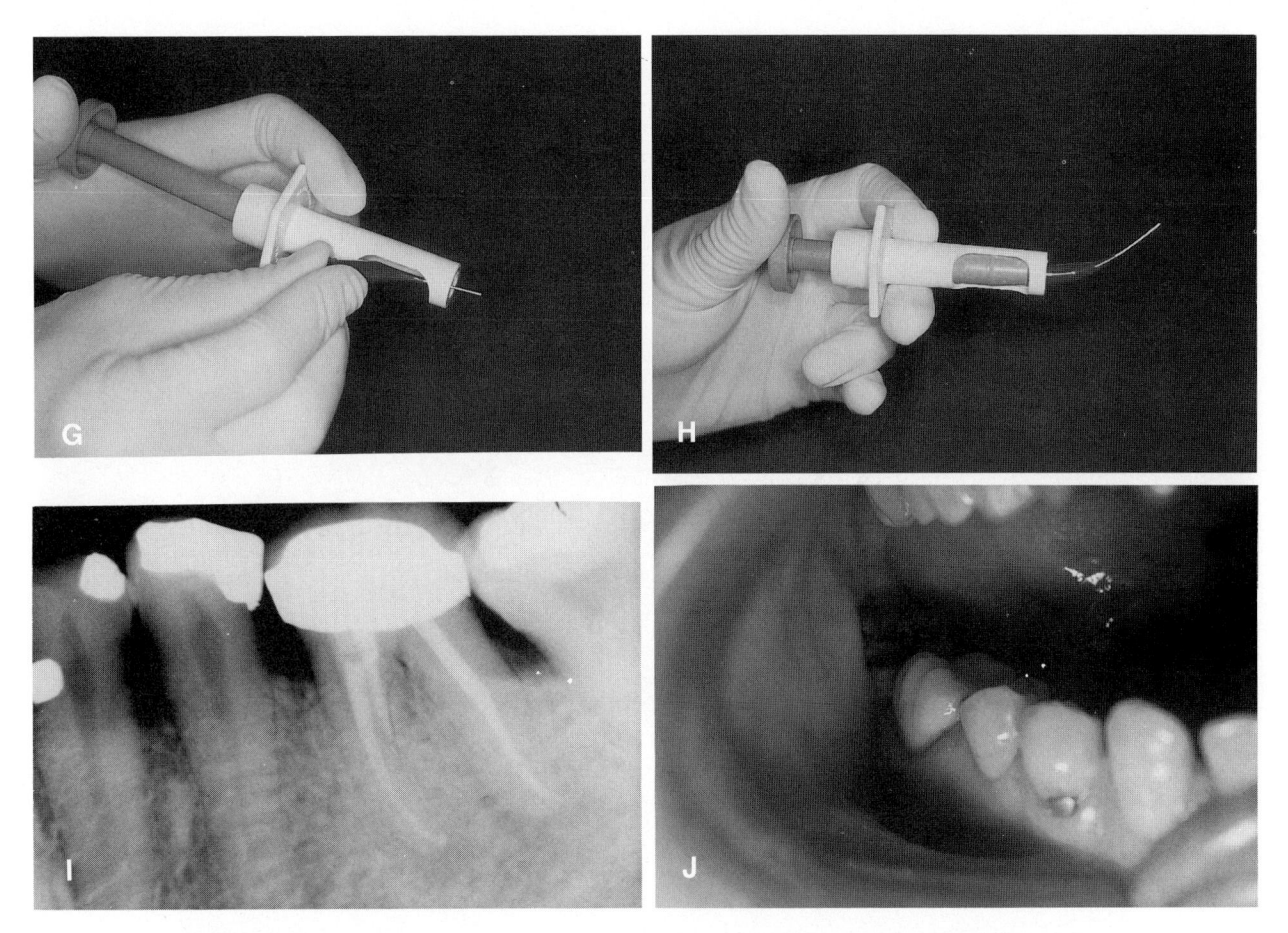

Figure 13-24, *cont'd* **G,** placed in the syringe. **H,** A small amount is extruded to determine flow and carried to the tooth. **I,** A 1½ year postoperative radiograph showing a normal lamina dura. **J,** A photo of the crown in place.

266   PRACTICAL ENDODONTICS

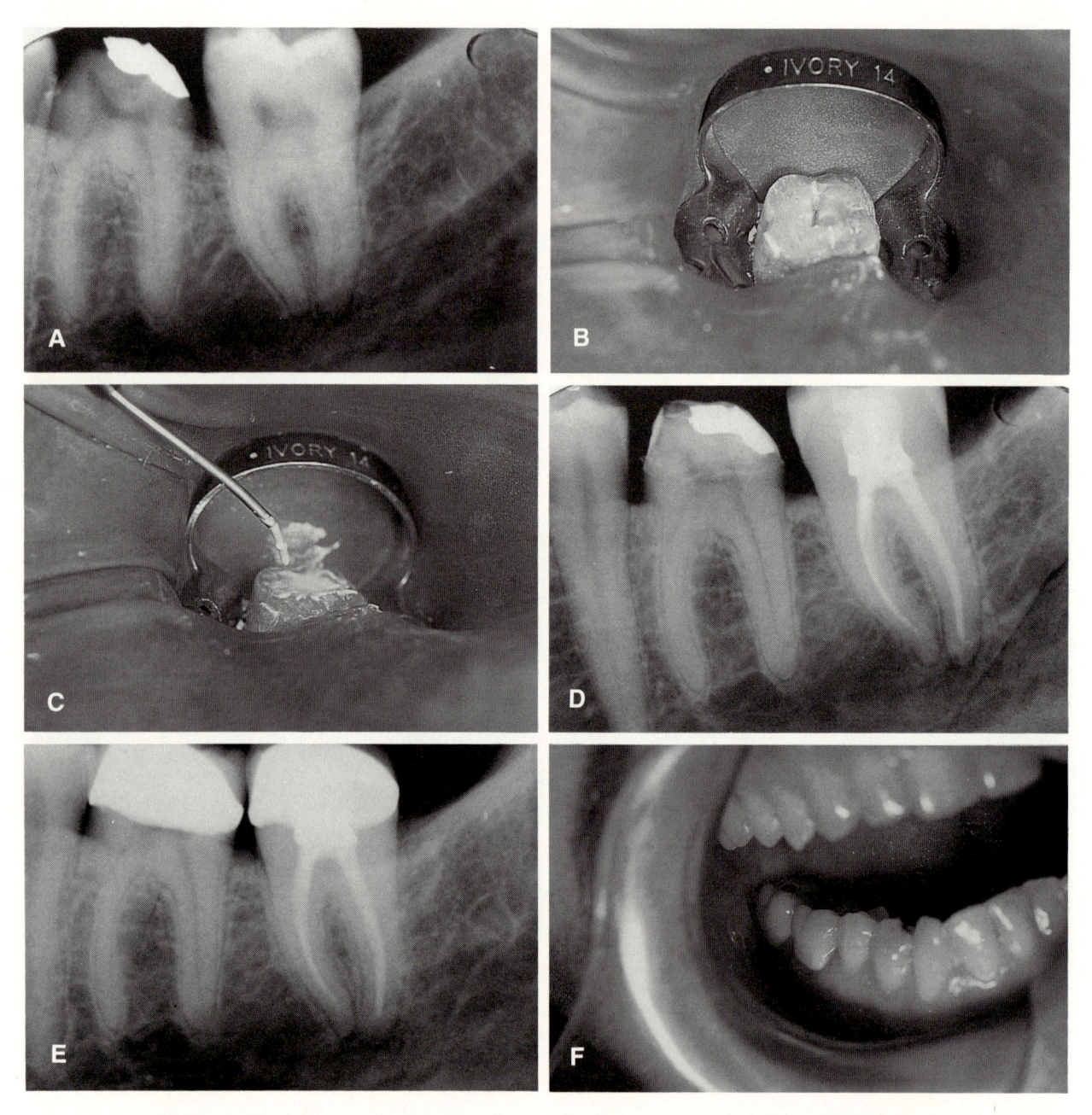

Figure 13-25 A, A radiograph of tooth No. 31. A fracture is not evident. There is no restoration in the tooth, however the patient had pain when biting and referred pain to the ear. **B,** A photo of clinical fracture on the distal marginal ridge that extended to the floor of the pulp chamber. A tight rubber dam clamp was placed to hold the fracture together and the root canal was completed in one appointment. **C,** Den-Mat core paste is shown injected into the chamber. **D,** A radiograph of completed root canal and core paste in the chamber. **E,** A 6-month postoperative radiograph showing a normal lamina dura. **F,** Crown in place.

Horizontal

Horizontal root fractures are usually caused by a severe blow in which the energy is dissipated over the entire crown. They may occur at the gingival, middle, or apical third and may be diagonal or comminuted (Fig. 13-21, B and C). Several radiographs from different horizontal angulation may have to be taken to detect the fracture (see Fig. 13-1, A and B) The fracture is treated like a long bone fracture and is reduced with finger pressure under local anesthetic and ligated passively to its original position for a period of 6 weeks (Fig. 13-26). When multiple teeth are fractured the brackets are extended to the adjacent teeth on either side of those fractured.

Horizontal root fractures usually repair with cementum or a combination of bone, cementum, and dentin. The pulp, periodontal ligament, and surrounding bone all respond to repair the fracture. In most instances the pulp remains vital, however it is not essential for repair of the fracture and splinting is usually the only treatment necessary. There are five types of repair of fractures that may take place.

1. A union of both segments with a continuous periodontal ligament (Fig. 13-27).
2. A separation of the coronal segment from the apical segment and each has its own periodontal ligament (Fig. 13-28).
3. Repair of a non-vital segment to a vital segment in which endodontic treatment is completed on

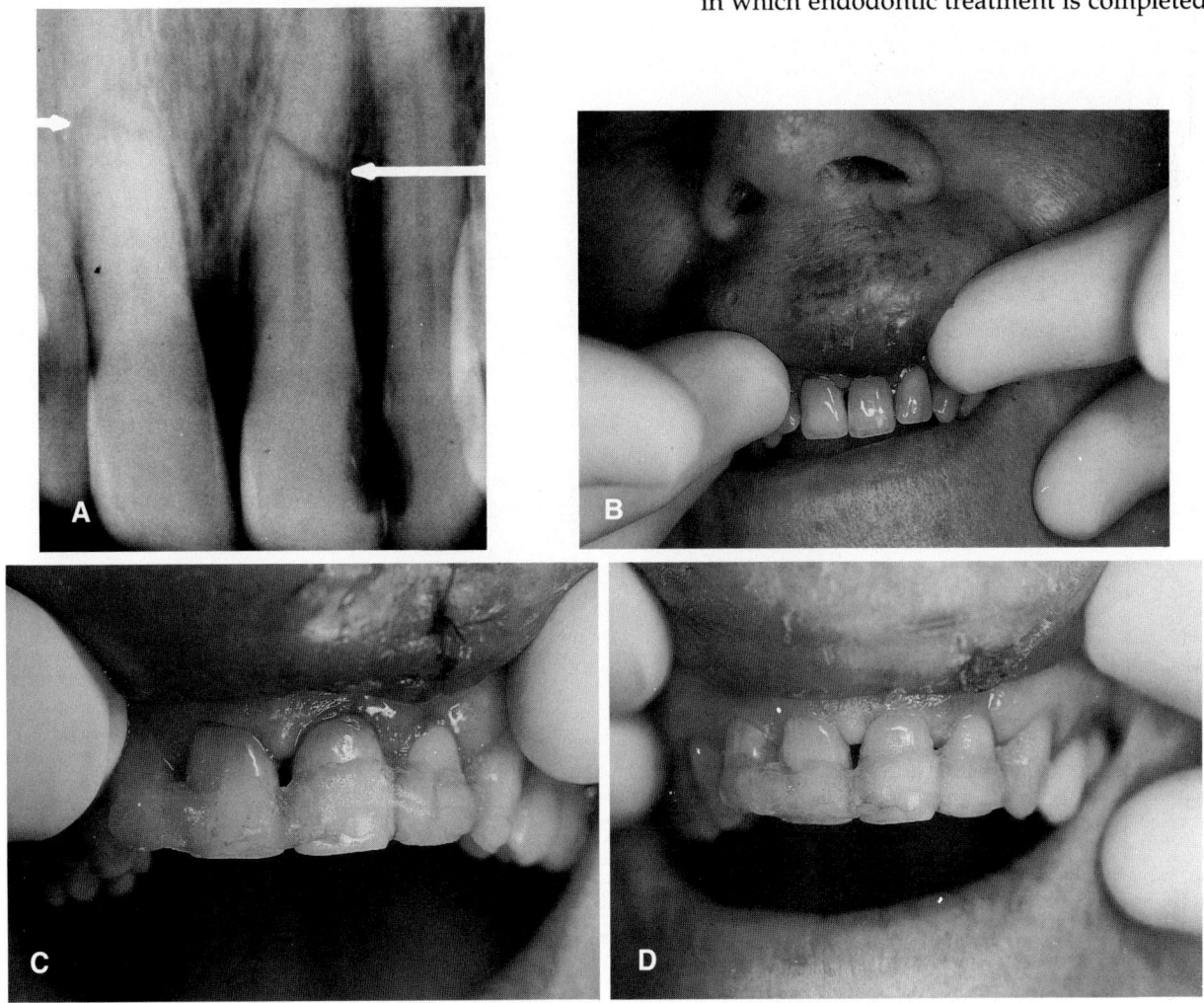

Figure 13-26 **A**, A radiograph of horizontal fracture of both No. 8 and 9 in the apical middle third of the roots. **B**, Degree of displacement and extrusion of teeth, contusion, and laceration of soft tissue and lip. The soft tissue was examined for debris. **C**, The lip was sutured and the teeth repositioned with finger pressure under local anesthetic. A temporary acrylic splint was placed to stabilize the teeth. Note acrylic is not placed on gingival papilla and kept above contact point. **D**, A photo 5 days posttrauma showing repair of soft tissue and no hemorrhage.

Continued.

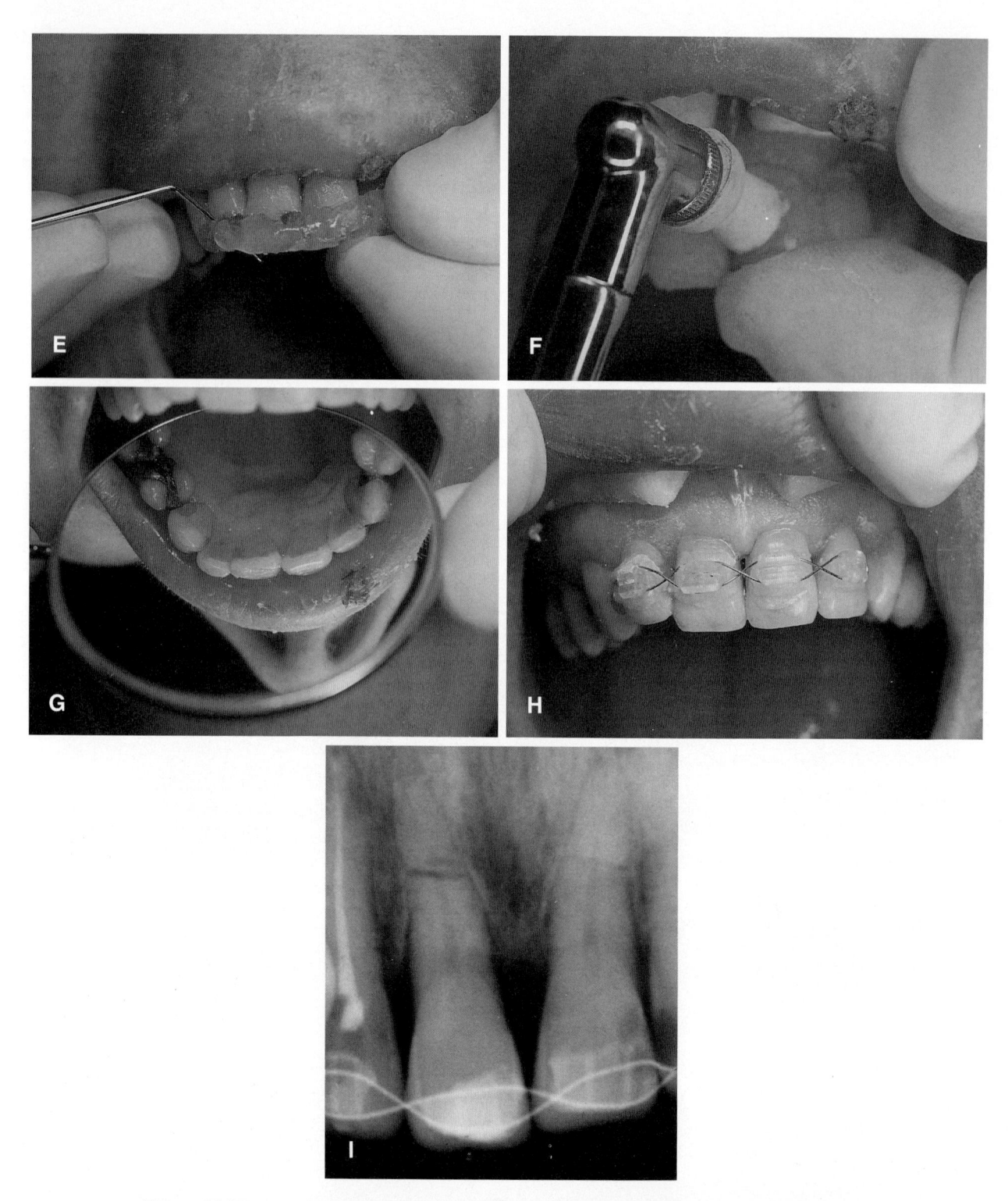

Figure 13-26, *cont'd* **E,** The temporary splint is removed with a double-ended explorer. **F,** The teeth are pumiced lightly and prepared for brackets. The teeth should be supported with finger pressure. **G,** Lingual view of teeth repositioned before placing brackets to determine incisal edge alignment. **H,** Brackets placed and .020 wire loop was placed and tightened on one end. The suture was removed. **I,** Radiograph of repositioned teeth after placing brackets for 6 weeks. The teeth responded vital to testing.

the coronal segment that had become inflamed or non-vital (Fig. 13-29).
4. Repair of two non-vital segments. Repair may occur when a fracture occurs on an endodontically treated tooth (Fig. 13-30).
5. Repair of minute (1 to 2 mm) horizontal apical root fractures. The teeth usually remain vital, remodeling of the apex occurs, and no specific treatment is usually necessary (Fig. 13-31).

Horizontal fractures occurring 2-3 mm in the apical third require no treatment. The fracture usually repairs and resorption of the apical fragment occurs over an extended period (Fig. 13-31).

If the splint is removed in 6 weeks and the tooth is still mobile, it is resplinted for another 6 weeks. The splint may have been loosened or the tooth may have been in traumatic occlusion. If the tooth is kept in constant motion, cementogenesis will not occur and a fibrous union will persist and the tooth will remain mobile.

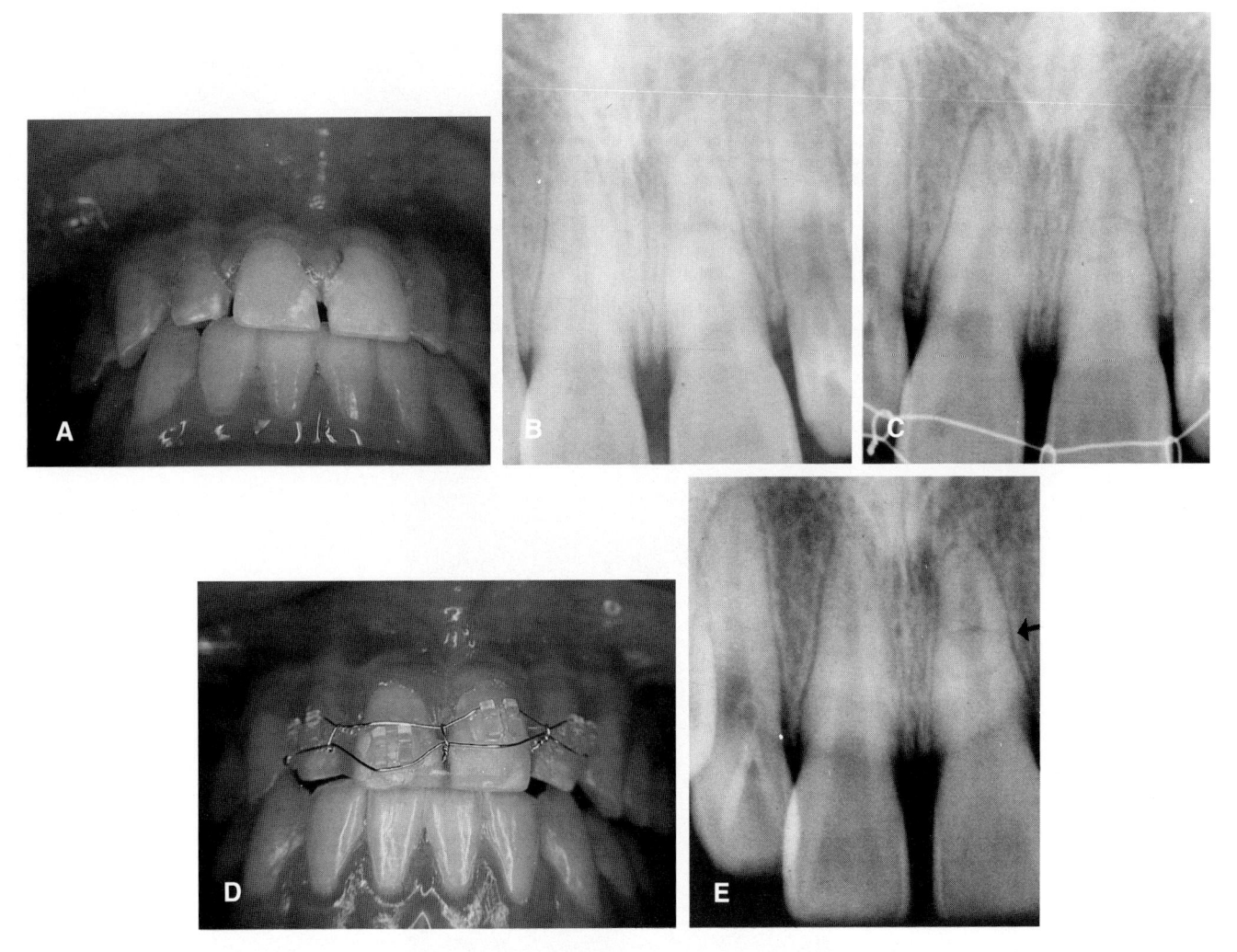

Figure 13-27 A, Labial displacement of tooth No. 8 and edematous and inflamed interdental papilla. Tooth was mobile and tender to touch. **B,** A radiograph showing comminuted horizontal fracture in the apical third of tooth No. 8. The tooth tested vital to ice and vitalometer. **C,** Radiograph of the fracture reduced and brackets placed. The fracture was reduced under local anesthesia with finger pressure and held in position while tightening the wire. **D,** A 5-day postoperative examination of splint with brackets and .020 arch wire loop with interproximal ties. The tissue was no longer inflamed. **E,** A 1-year postoperative radiograph showing lamina dura intact. Tooth responds normal to vitality testing.

270   PRACTICAL ENDODONTICS

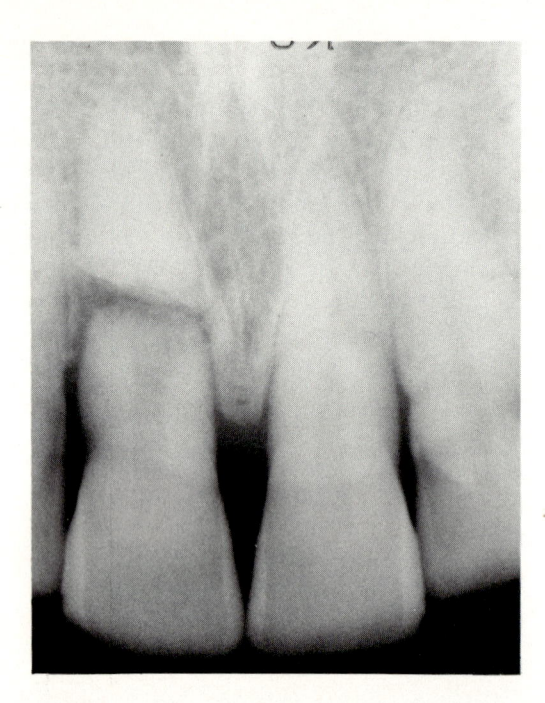

Figure 13-28 A 20-year radiograph of healing showing separation of the coronal and apical fractured segments. Each segment has a periodontal ligament. The tooth responds vital.

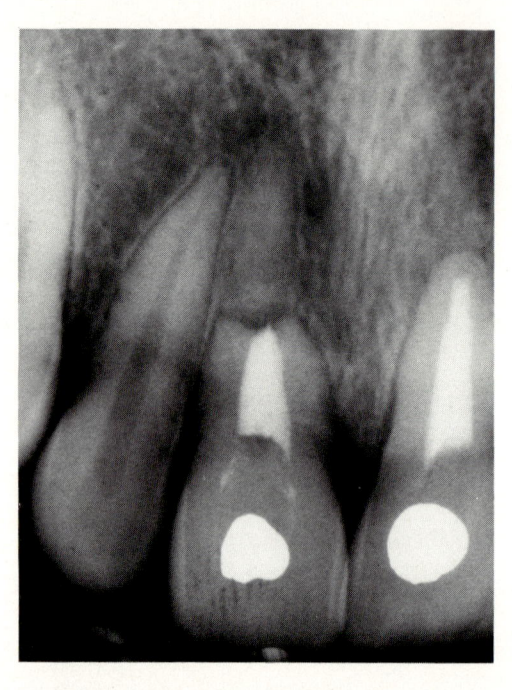

Figure 13-29 A 10-year radiograph showing repair of non-vital coronal segment to the vital apical segment. The tooth became symptomatic and the root canal was completed on the coronal segment and lamina dura remained intact on the apical segment.

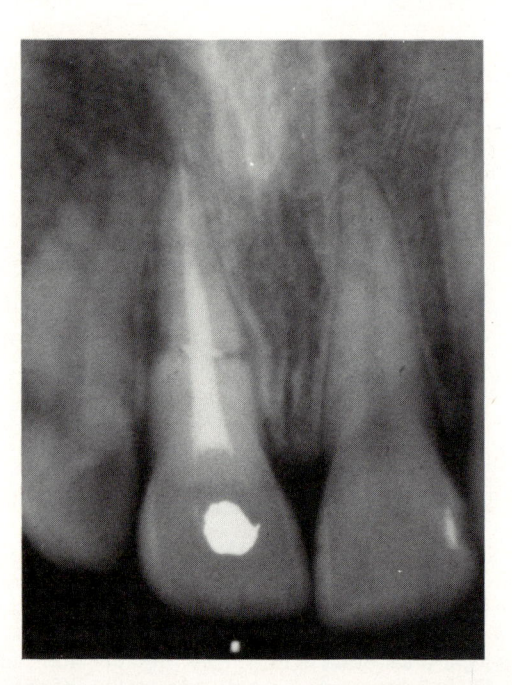

Figure 13-30 An 8-year posttrauma radiograph of tooth No. 9 showing repair of the non-vital coronal and apical segments. The fracture occurred on tooth No. 9 with a previously treated root canal. The root canal was retreated and the tooth was splinted.

Chapter 13 ♦ Traumatic Injuries   271

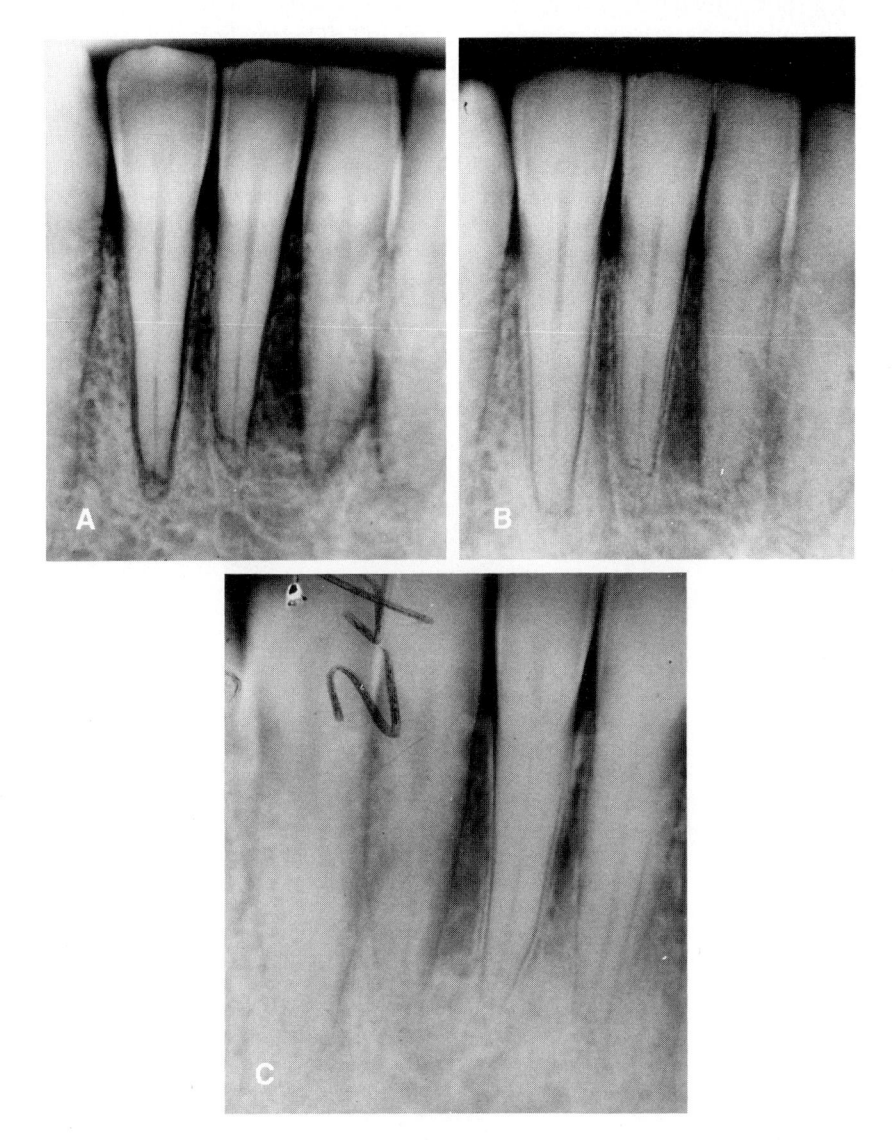

Figure 13-31 **A,** A minute horizontal fracture occurring in lower 2 mm of apex of No. 25 and 26. The periodontal ligament is widened, the teeth test vital, no mobility is present, and no splinting was necessary. **B,** A 14-year postoperative radiograph shows resorption and remodeling of the minute fractured segments. **C,** A 25-year postoperative radiograph shows normal lamina dura with narrowing of the pulp canals. All of the teeth respond vital.

POSTOPERATIVE EXAMINATION AND MONITORING

Following an injury, discoloration, resorption, calcification, ankylosis, necrosis, and other disorders may occur. Some of these problems can be prevented and controlled with interceptive endodontics (i.e., removal of the pulp). It is not unusual to examine a traumatized, fractured, or avulsed tooth and observe the adjacent tooth to become non-vital and calcify over an extended period. This occurs because the force of the injury causes fracture, displacement, or avulsion and the remaining energy of the trauma is absorbed by the adjacent teeth and soft tissue; the adjacent teeth and tissue may initially show no apparent signs of distress. Damage may not become obvious until months or years later (Fig. 13-32).

Calcification is indicated by the radiograph, reduction of vitality, and yellowish discoloration of the crown. When calcification is evident a decision should be made early enough to remove the pulp while it is still visible in the crown. If the pulp recedes above the chamber and calcification extends into the root, much of the tooth structure may be lost in an attempt to locate the canal and a labial root perforation becomes a possibility.

The teeth should be examined every 6 months for 2 years and then once annually thereafter. The examination should consist of radiographs, color examination, mobility, vitality testing (both thermal and electric), and transillumination.

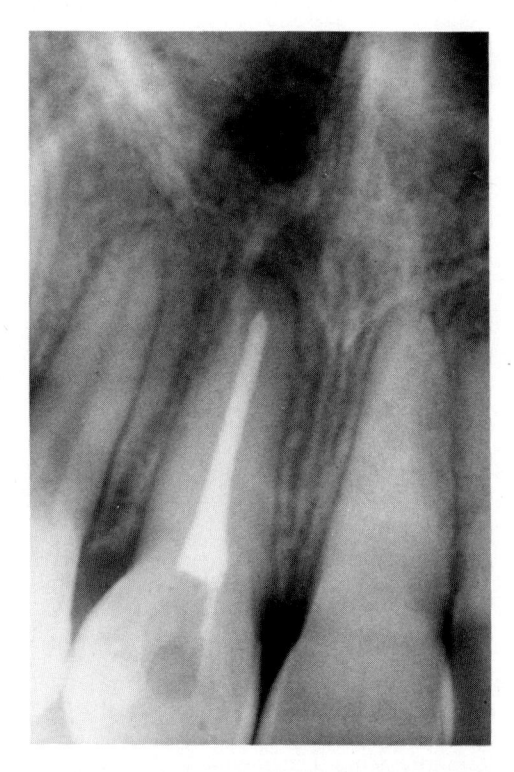

Figure 13-32 A radiograph of tooth No. 9 showing apparent calcification of the pulp canal 7 years after a traumatic injury.

Index

A
Absorbent paper points, 89
Access openings
 of mandibular anterior teeth, 119, 120
 of mandibular bicuspids, 122, 123
 of mandibular molars, 126, 127
 of maxillary anterior teeth, 114, 117, 118
 of maxillary bicuspids, 120, 121
 of maxillary molars, 124, 125
 in routine endodontic therapy, 114–127
Acid etching technique, splinting technique using, 14
Ad Post, 172
Alcoholism, limitations on endodontic therapy because of, 21, 23
Amphetamine, limitations on endodontic therapy because of, 21, 23
Anatomical landmarks, differential diagnosis of, from endodontic lesions, 36–39
Anatomical variations, 95–104
Anesthesia
 mandibular injection of, in routine endodontic therapy, 110, 111
 maxillary injection of, in routine endodontic therapy, 109–110
 in routine endodontic therapy, 109–111
 in surgical endodontics, 228, 229
Anesthetic test in diagnosis of endodontic problems, 26, 33
Antibiotics, prophylactic, limitations on endodontic therapy because of, 21, 23
Antidepressant drugs, limitations on endodontic therapy because of, 21, 23
Antidiabetic agents, oral, limitations on endodontic therapy because of, 21, 23
Antihypertensive drugs, limitations on endodontic therapy because of, 21, 23
Antiseptic handwash, dental office infection control program and, 66, 71
Antiseptic mouthrinse, dental office infection control program and, 66, 71
Apex, endodontic radiography and, 41
Apexification, 6, 7

APH, 179
Apical foramen, endodontic radiography and, 41, 45, 46
Apical seal in surgical endodontics, 235
Apicoectomy in surgical endodontics, 227, 228
Arch wire, splinting technique using orthodontic bands and, 13
Armamentarium, endodontic; *see* Endodontic instruments
Articulating paper in diagnosis of endodontic problems, 32
Aspirin, limitations on endodontic therapy because of, 21, 23
Autoclave, steam, sterilization and, 63, 65
Autoclave pack, 81
Avulsed tooth
 in traumatic injuries, 258, 259
 treatment of, 7, 12

B
Bacterial endocarditis, prevention of, 21, 24
Barbed broach, 85, 86
Barbiturates, limitations on endodontic therapy because of, 21, 23
BCH Post, 172
Beta Post, 172
Bicuspids
 mandibular, access openings of, 122, 123
 maxillary, access openings of, 118, 121
Biological chemical color indicator for monitoring steam and ethylene oxide sterilization, 75, 78
Bisecting angle radiographic technique, 105
Bite test in diagnosis of endodontic problems, 26, 33, 34–35, 36
Bleach, household, as surface disinfectant, 66
Bleaching, 7
 non-vital, 7, 14
 vital, 7, 15
BOR; *see* Buccal object rule
Broach, barbed, 85, 86
Broken root canal instruments as endodontic complication, 188–192
Buccal object rule (BOR), 53–55, 131
Burs, separated, removal of, 206–207

273

Index

C

Calcified canal as endodontic complication, 188, 189
Calcium hydroxide (Calysept; Root-Cal), 133, 137, 209, 249, 252, 258
Camphorated paramonochlorophenol (CMCP), 252
Canal
    calcified, as endodontic complication, 188, 189
    inadequate length control of, postoperative discomfort caused by, 185, 186
    preparation of, for low temperature thermoplasticized gutta percha, 143–144
Canal walls, preparation of, in restoration of endodontically treated tooth, 173–174
Cannules for low temperature thermoplasticized gutta percha, 142, 143
Carboxylate, removal of, 225
Caries, endodontics and, 1
Cast Gold, 175
Cast post and core technique in restoration of endodontically treated tooth, 181
Caulfield silver point retriever, 218, 222
Cavity, toilet of, in routine endodontic therapy, 132
CDJ; *see* Cementodentinal junction
Cement
    placement of, in restoration of endodontically treated tooth, 174, 175
    removal of, 225
Cementodentinal junction (CDJ), endodontic radiography and, 41, 46
Chemical vapor, sterilization and, 63, 65
Chloroform, removal of gutta percha with, 225
Chloropercha
    lateral condensation with, 164, 167
    vertical condensation with, 164–167
Cingulum, enamel defect above, 100
Clamps in routine endodontic therapy, 82, 83, 112, 113
Cleansing
    incomplete, postoperative discomfort caused by, 185, 186
    and shaping in routine endodontic therapy, 132–133, 134–135
Cleve-dent pliers, 208
Clinical observations in diagnosis of endodontic problems, 25–26
Clinical tests in diagnosis of endodontic problems, 26–36
    diagnostic armamentarium for, 28–32
CMCP; *see* Camphorated paramonochlorophenol
CNS stimulants, limitations on endodontic therapy because of, 21, 23
Cold thermal test in diagnosis of endodontic problems, 26, 28, 29
Complications, endodontic; *see* Endodontic complications
Composite Resins, 176
Comprehensive medical history, dental office infection control program and, 66, 67
Condensation
    lateral, with chloropercha, 164, 167
    vertical; *see* Vertical condensation
Condensing osteitis, endodontic radiography and, 51
Cones, silver, removal of, 218–224
Convenience form in routine endodontic therapy, 132
Convulsive disorders, limitations on endodontic therapy because of, 21, 23
Core
    additional, retention of, in restoration of endodontically treated tooth, 181
    placement of, in restoration of endodontically treated tooth, 178–179, 180
    selection of, in restoration of endodontically treated tooth, 175–176
Core Paste, 176

Coreforms, 179
Cracked tooth syndrome
    diagnosis of, 26, 33, 34–35, 36
    in traumatic injuries, 262, 263
Crawford hemostat, 56–57
Crown, separated instruments in gingival, middle, or apical third and not visible in, removal of, 201–202
Crown fracture
    with pulp exposure in
        and root fully formed, in traumatic injuries, 250
        in traumatic injuries, 249
    subgingivally, in traumatic injuries, 250, 251
Crown sectioning in surgical endodontics, 236, 237
Crown-root ratio in detection of extra root canals, 95, 101
Customized gutta percha point, 169–170

D

Den-Mat, 263
Dens in dente, 98–99
Dens Invaginatus, 98–99
Dental history
    dental office infection control program and, 66, 67
    in diagnosis of endodontic problems, 21–24
Dental office infection control program, minimum, sterilization and, 66–75, 76–77, 78, 79, 80
Dentin
    exposure of, endodontics and, 1
    fractures of, with no exposure of pulp, in traumatic injuries, 248
Dentin protection, 6
Devastated tooth, treatment of, in restoration of endodontically treated tooth, 183, 184
Diabinese, limitations on endodontic therapy because of, 21, 23
Diagnosis of endodontic problems, 21–39
    anesthetic test in, 26, 33
    articulating paper in, 32
    bite test in, 26, 33, 34–35, 36
    clinical observations in, 25–26
    clinical tests in, 26–36
        diagnostic armamentarium for, 28–32
    dental history in, 21–24
    diagnostic tests in, 26, 27, 28, 29, 30, 31, 32
    differential, of anatomical landmarks and pathological lesions from endodontic lesions, 36–39
    difficult, selective tests for, 33–36
    electric pulp test in, 26, 28
    gutta percha point tracing with radiograph in, 26, 33, 38
    medical history in, 21, 22, 23, 24
    mobility in, 26, 30, 31
    occlusal evaluation in, 26, 32
    palpation in, 26, 30, 31
    percussion in, 26, 30
    periodontal evaluation in, 26, 30, 31
    periodontal probe in, 30, 31
    radiography in; *see* Radiography, endodontic
    referred pain and, 39
    of root fracture, 26, 36, 37
    selective tests for difficult diagnostic situations in, 26, 28, 33, 34–35, 36, 38
    staining in, 26, 33, 34–35, 36
    subjective symptoms in, 25
    test cavity preparation in, 26, 33
    tests for cracked tooth syndrome in, 26, 33, 34–35, 36
    thermal test in
        cold, 26, 28, 29
        hot, 26, 30

Index

Diagnosis of endodontic problems—cont'd
  transillumination in, 26, 33, 34-35, 36
Diagnostic tests in diagnosis of endodontic problems, 26, 27, 28, 29, 30, 31, 32
Discoloration of teeth in traumatic injuries, 246
Discomfort, postoperative, as endodontic complication, 185, 186
Disinfectants, surface, sterilization and, 66
Disposable face mask, dental office infection control program and, 66, 72
Disposable gloves, dental office infection control program and, 66, 72, 80
Dowel
  placement of, in restoration of endodontically treated tooth, 175
  selection of, in restoration of endodontically treated tooth, 173
Drainage, incision and, in surgical endodontics, 238-239
Drill, Gates Glidden, 87, 206-207
Drug treatment plan, sample, for use during endodontic therapy, 187
Durelon, 208

E
Eggler post pullers, 208
Electric pulp test in diagnosis of endodontic problems, 26, 28
Elliptication as endodontic complication, 196
Emergencies, endodontic, 185-195
Enamel defect above cingulum, 100
Enamel fracture
  with no exposure of pulp in traumatic injuries, 248
  simple, in traumatic injuries, 247
Endo extractor kit, 210, 216, 218
Endo Extractor Tubes, 218, 224
Endocarditis, bacterial, prevention of, 21, 24
Endodontic armamentarium; see Endodontic instruments
Endodontic complications, 185-195
  broken root canal instruments as, 188-192
  calcified canal as, 188, 189
  postoperative discomfort as, 185, 186
Endodontic emergencies, 185-195
Endodontic implant, 7, 10
Endodontic instruments, 75-93
  enlarging, 75
  exploring, 75
  extirpating, 75
  filling, 75
  intracanal, 75, 85
  for obturation of root canal, 75-93
  for removal of posts, 208-217
  in retrieving silver points from root canals, 218, 219
  root canal, broken, as endodontic complication, 188-192
  separated; see Separated instruments
  sterilization procedures for, 63-75, 76-77, 78, 79, 80
  in surgical endodontics, 227, 228
  tray, 75, 80
Endodontic lesions, differential diagnosis of anatomical landmarks and pathological lesions from, 36-39
Endodontic radiography; see Radiography, endodontic
Endodontic surgery, 6, 8, 9
Endodontic therapy, 6-16
  basic concepts of, 17-20
  routine, 105-140
    access openings in, 114-127
    anesthesia in, 109-111
      "injection of last resort" in, 110, 111
      mandibular injection of, 110, 111
      maxillary injection of, 109-110

cleansing and shaping in, 132-133, 134-135
convenience form in, 132
extension in, 132
intracanal medication in, 133-137, 138, 139-140
length determination in, 130, 131
preaccess distances in, 114, 116
pretreatment in, 107-108
principles of root canal preparation in, 132
resistance form in, 132
retention form in, 132
rubber dam in, 112, 113
toilet of cavity in, 132
x-ray technique in, 105-107
sample drug treatment plan for use during, 187
scope of, 1-16
surgical; see Surgical endodontics
Endodontically treated tooth, restoration of; see Restoration of endodontically treated tooth
Endo-Ray, 57
Enlarging instruments, 75
Explorer, Stewart double-ended, 208, 209
Exploring instruments, 75
Extension in routine endodontic therapy, 132
External resorption, endodontics and, 2, 4, 5
Extirpating instruments, 75
Extruded teeth in traumatic injuries, 256-257
Eyewear, protective, dental office infection control program and, 66, 72

F
Face mask, disposable, dental office infection control program and, 66, 72
Filling instruments, 75
Fistula, intraoral, 26, 33, 38
Flap design in surgical endodontics, 228-231, 232
FluoroCore, 176
Foramen, separated instruments beyond, 204, 205
Foramina, transportation of, postoperative discomfort caused by, 185, 186
Fracture(s)
  crown; see Crown fracture
  of enamel and dentin with no pulp exposure in traumatic injuries, 248
  root; see Root fractures
  simple enamel, in traumatic injuries, 247
Funneling, canal preparation and, 143

G
Gates Glidden drill, 87, 206-207
Glass bead sterilizer, 75, 77
Gloves, disposable, dental office infection control program and, 66, 72, 80
Glutaraldehyde as surface disinfectant, 66
Gonadal effects of radiography, 61
Gonon post extractor kit, 210, 216-217
Gonon post system, 210, 216-217
Gout, limitations on endodontic therapy because of, 21, 23
Gowns, protective, dental office infection control program and, 66, 72
Gutta percha
  removal of, 225-226
    in restoration of endodontically treated tooth, 173
  warm, vertical condensation with, 160-163
Gutta percha points, 90-92
  customized, 169-170

H

Handpieces, sterilizable, dental office infection control program and, 66, 74
Handwash, antiseptic, dental office infection control program and, 66, 71
Hard tissue, examination of, in traumatic injuries, 244
Head injuries, limitations on endodontic therapy because of, 21, 23
Hedstrom file, 85, 87
Hemisection in surgical endodontics, 236
Hemisectomy, 6, 9
Hemostat, 208
    Crawford, 56–57
Hepatitis B, sterilization procedures and, 63, 75, 80
Hepatitis B vaccine, dental office infection control program and, 66
Herculite, 179
High Copper Spherical Amalgam, 175
History
    dental, in diagnosis of endodontic problems, 21–24
    medical, in diagnosis of endodontic problems, 21–24
HIV; see Human immune deficiency virus
Horizontal root fractures in traumatic injuries, 267–269, 270, 271
Hot thermal test in diagnosis of endodontic problems, 26, 30
Household bleach as surface disinfectant, 66
Human immune deficiency virus (HIV), sterilization procedures and, 63, 75, 80
Hyperthyroidism, limitations on endodontic therapy because of, 21, 23

I

Immature non-vital teeth, traumatized, in traumatic injuries, 252–253
Implant, endodontic, 7, 10
Incision and drainage in surgical endodontics, 238–239
Incisor
    mandibular, extra root canals in, 95–100
    maxillary central, extra root canals in, 101
    maxillary lateral, developmental anomalies of, 98, 99, 100
Incomplete cleansing and shaping, postoperative discomfort caused by, 185, 186
Incomplete root in traumatic injuries, 249
Incremental filling, canal preparation and, 143
Infection control program, dental office, minimum, sterilization and, 66–75, 76–77, 78, 79, 80
"Injection of last resort" anesthesia in routine endodontic therapy, 110, 111
Injuries, traumatic; see Traumatic injuries
Instruments; see Endodontic instruments
Intentional replantation, 7, 12
Internal resorption, endodontics and, 2, 3
Intracanal instruments, 75, 85
Intracanal medication in routine endodontic therapy, 88, 133–137, 138, 139–140
Intraoral fistula tracing, 26, 33, 38
Intruded teeth in traumatic injuries, 256–257
Invaginated teeth, classification of, 96
Iodophors as surface disinfectants, 66
Irrigating solutions, 84–85
Ivory No. 2 clamp in routine endodontic therapy, 83, 112, 113
Ivory No. 5 clamp in routine endodontic therapy, 83, 112, 113
Ivory No. 9 clamp in routine endodontic therapy, 82, 112

K

Ketec Silver, 176, 178
K-file, 85, 87

L

Lamina dura, endodontic radiography and, 46
Lateral condensation
    with chloropercha, 164, 167
    modified, obturation using, 133, 138
Ledge formation as endodontic complication, 192, 193
Legal considerations, endodontic radiography and, 61
Length
    tooth
        determination of, 130, 131
        versus working length, 130
    working, 104
Length-of-tooth radiograph in detection of extra root canals, 95
Liver damage, limitations on endodontic therapy because of, 21, 23
Loosened teeth in traumatic injuries, 254, 255
Low temperature thermoplasticized gutta percha (Ultrafil), 141–158
    adjunct hand instrument armamentarium for, 143
    advantages of, 141
    canal preparation for, 143–144
    cannules for, 142, 143
    Endoset, 143, 150, 151, 152, 153–154
    Firm set, 143, 144–145, 148, 153–154, 157
    injecting techniques for, 143
    injection and lateral condensation of, 153
    injection and master cone, 148–149
    injection and vertical compaction of, 150, 151, 152
    Regular set, 143, 144–145, 148, 153, 157
    syringe preparation for, 144
    technique for injection of entire canal with, 144–145
    Trifecta technique of, 141, 153–154
    types of, 143
Luxated teeth in traumatic injuries, 254, 255

M

Malpositioned teeth in traumatic injuries, 254, 255
Mandibular arch
    anatomic landmarks of, 41, 42
    endodontic radiography and, 41, 42, 53, 55
Mandibular bicuspids, access openings of, 122, 123
Mandibular incisors, extra root canals in, 95–100
Mandibular injection of anesthesia in routine endodontic therapy, 110, 111
Mandibular molars
    access openings of, 126, 127
    extra root canals in, 101
    variation of orifices in, 128
Mandibular teeth, surgical endodontics for, 233, 234
MAO inhibitors, limitations on endodontic therapy because of, 21, 23
Marsupialization in surgical endodontics, 240–242
Maxillary arch
    anatomic landmarks of, 41, 43–44
    endodontic radiography and, 41, 43–44, 53, 54
Maxillary bicuspids, access openings of, 120, 121
Maxillary central incisors, extra root canals in, 101
Maxillary injection of anesthesia in routine endodontic therapy, 109–110
Maxillary lateral incisor, developmental anomalies of, 98, 99, 100
Maxillary molars
    access openings of, 124, 125
    extra root canals in, 95–97
    variation of orifices in, 129
Maxillary posterior teeth, surgical endodontics for, 233
Maxillary premolars, extra root canals in, 101

Medical history
  comprehensive, dental office infection control program and, 66, 67
  in diagnosis of endodontic problems, 21, 22, 23, 24
Medically compromised patient, endodontic therapy and, 21, 23
Medication, intracanal, in routine endodontic therapy, 88, 133–137, 138, 139–140
Microcopy Fix-Off, 59, 60
Minimum dental office infection control program, sterilization and, 66–75, 76–77, 78, 79, 80
Miricle Mix, 176
Mobility in diagnosis of endodontic problems, 26, 30, 31
Molars
  mandibular
    access openings of, 126, 127
    extra root canals in, 101
    variation of orifices in, 128
  maxillary
    access openings of, 124, 125
    extra root canals in, 95–97
    variation of orifices in, 129
Mouthrinse, antiseptic, dental office infection control program and, 66, 71

N

Nonsurgical retreatment, 7, 16, 197–226
  removal of
    gutta percha in, 225–226
    pastes and cements in, 225
    posts in, 208–217
    separated burs in, 206–207
    silver cones in, 218–224
  separated instruments in, 198, 199
    beyond foramen, 204, 205
    removal of
      from gingival, middle, or apical third and not visible in crown, 201–202
      protruding in pulp chamber, 200
    when instrument is separated and unable to be retrieved, 203
Non-vital bleaching, 7, 14
Non-vital teeth
  traumatized immature, in traumatic injuries, 252–253
  treated or untreated and partially erupted, in traumatic injuries, 261

O

Obturation of root canal, 17, 19
  instruments for, 75–93
  using modified lateral condensation technique, 133, 138
Occlusal evaluation in diagnosis of endodontic problems, 26, 32
Occupational Safety and Health Agency (OSHA), 63, 68
Operator protection, endodontic radiography and, 61
Oral antidiabetic agents, limitations on endodontic therapy because of, 21, 23
Orthodontic bands and arch wire, splinting technique using, 13
OSHA; see Occupational Safety and Health Agency
Overmedication, postoperative discomfort caused by, 185, 186
Oxyphosphate, removal of, 225

P

Pain, referred, in diagnosis of endodontic problems, 39
Palatal groove defect, 100
Palpation in diagnosis of endodontic problems, 26, 30, 31
Panavia, 174
Paper points, absorbent, 89
Paralleling radiographic technique, 106
ParaPost, 172
Pastes, removal of, 225
Pathological lesions, differential diagnosis of, from endodontic lesions, 36–39
Peeso, selection of, in restoration of endodontically treated tooth, 173
Percussion in diagnosis of endodontic problems, 26, 30
Perforation as endodontic complication, 193–194, 195
Periapical and lateral pathology, endodontics and, 2, 5
Periapical lesion, persistent, as postoperative failure, 196
Periapical radiographic techniques, comparison of, 105, 106
Periapical surgery, 6, 8, 9
Periodontal evaluation in diagnosis of endodontic problems, 26, 30, 31
Periodontal pathology, endodontics and, 1–6
Periodontal probe in diagnosis of endodontic problems, 30, 31
Periodontal-endodontic lesions, endodontics and, 2, 6
Persistent periapical lesion as postoperative failure, 196
Phenoformin, limitations on endodontic therapy because of, 21, 23
Phenol combinations, synthetic, as surface disinfectants, 66
Phenol water sprays as surface disinfectants, 66
Phenol-alcohol sprays as surface disinfectants, 66
Phenylphenoe as surface disinfectant, 66
Pliers, Cleve-dent, 208
Posterior teeth, maxillary, surgical endodontics for, 233
Postexposure evaluation and follow-up, dental office infection control program and, 66
Postoperative discomfort as endodontic complication, 185, 186
Postoperative failures, 196
Postoperative instructions in surgical endodontics, 242
Posts
  removal of, 208–217
  in restoration of endodontically treated tooth, 171
  selection of, guidelines for, in restoration of endodontically treated tooth, 171–172
  size of, in restoration of endodontically treated tooth, 171, 172
Preaccess distances in routine endodontic therapy, 114, 116
Premolars, maxillary, extra root canals in, 101
Pretreatment in routine endodontic therapy, 107–108
Prophylactic antibiotics, limitations on endodontic therapy because of, 21, 23
Protective eyewear, dental office infection control program and, 66, 72
Protective gowns, dental office infection control program and, 66, 72
Pulp
  exposure of
    crown fracture with, in traumatic injuries, 249
    and root fully formed, crown fracture with, in traumatic injuries, 250
  no exposure of, fractures of enamel and dentin with, in traumatic injuries, 248
Pulp calcification, endodontics and, 2
Pulp capping, 6
Pulp chamber, separated instruments protruding in, removal of, 200
Pulp exposure, endodontics and, 1
Pulpal degeneration, endodontic radiography and, 48
Pulpal pathology, endodontics and, 1–6
Pulpectomy and root canal therapy, 6, 7
Pulpotomy, 6, 7

R

Radiography, endodontic, 26, 32, 41–62
  gonadal effects of, 61
  helpful hints in, 48–52

Radiography, endodontic—cont'd
  incorrect film placement in, 57
  legal considerations in, 61
  length-of-tooth, in detection of extra root canals, 95
  in location of extra root canals, 95, 101–104
  normal anatomic landmarks in, 41–47
  operator protection and, 61
  processing, 59–60
  safety of, 61
  somatic effects of, 61
  technique of
    helpful hints in, 56–59
    in routine endodontic therapy, 105–107
  terminology in, 41–47
  in traumatic injuries, 243
Radisectomy, 6, 9
RC Prep, 84–85
Reamer, 85, 87
Referred pain in diagnosis of endodontic problems, 39
Regulated waste disposal, dental office infection control program and, 66, 74
Reinforced Glass Ionomer, 176
Replantation, intentional, 7, 12
Reserpine, limitations on endodontic therapy because of, 21, 23
Resheathing devices, dental office infection control program and, 66, 73
Resistance form in routine endodontic therapy, 132
Restoration of endodontically treated tooth, 171–184
  additional core retention in, 181
  cast post and core technique in, 181–182
  cement in, 174
  cement placement in, 175
  combination of materials in, 179, 180
  core selection in, 175–176
  dowel placement in, 175
  dowel selection in, 173
  gutta percha removal in, 173
  initial preparation of, 173–178
  Peeso selection in, 173
  placement of core in, 178–179
  post selection guidelines in, 171–172, 173
  post size in, 171, 172
  posts in, 171
  preparation of canal walls in, 173–174
  restorative components in, 171, 172
  technique of, 173–178
  treatment of devastated tooth in, 183, 184
Restorative components in restoration of endodontically treated tooth, 171, 172
Restorative failure as postoperative failure, 196
Retention form in routine endodontic therapy, 132
Retreatment, nonsurgical; see Nonsurgical retreatment
Right-angle pliers, 208
Rinn Mini-Ray duplicator, 58, 59
Rinn Snap-A-Ray, 57
Rinn XCP, 56–57
Root(s)
  fully formed, crown fracture with pulp exposure and, in traumatic injuries, 250
  incomplete, in traumatic injuries, 249
Root amputation, 6, 9
Root canal(s)
  extra
    clues in locating, 101–104
    crown-root ratio in detection of, 95, 101
    length-of-tooth radiograph in detection of, 95
    often missed
      in mandibular incisors, 95–100
      in maxillary molars, 95–97
  obturation of; see Obturation of root canal
Root canal preparation, principles of, in routine endodontic therapy, 132
Root fractures
  diagnosis of, 26, 36, 37
  horizontal, in traumatic injuries, 267–269, 270, 271
  in traumatic injuries, 261–269, 270, 271
  vertical, in traumatic injuries, 261–265, 266
Root outline, endodontic radiography and, 48
Root sectioning in surgical endodontics, 236–237
Root-Cal; see Calcium hydroxide
Roto Pro Burs, 208, 212
Roto Pro Scalers, 206, 207, 208, 212
Routine endodontic therapy; see Endodontic therapy, routine
Rubber dam
  dental office infection control program and, 66, 73
  in routine endodontic therapy, 112, 113
Rubber dam set-up, 81

S

Safety, endodontic radiography and, 61
Scaler
  Roto Pro, 206, 207, 208, 212
  Sonic Air, 208
  ultrasound, 198, 208, 209, 218, 222
Sealing agents, 93
Separated burs, removal of, 206–207
Separated instruments, 198, 199
  beyond foramen, 204, 205
  removal of
    from gingival, middle, or apical third and not visible in crown, 201–202
    protruding in pulp chamber, 200
  unable to be retrieved, 203
Shaping
  and cleansing in routine endodontic therapy, 132–133, 134–135
  incomplete, postoperative discomfort caused by, 185, 186
Sharps containers, dental office infection control program and, 66, 73
Silver cones, removal of, 218–224
Sinus tract, endodontic radiography and, 50
Snap-A-Ray, 57
Soft tissue, examination of, in traumatic injuries, 244
Somatic effects of radiography, 61
Sonic Air Scaler, 208
Splinting technique
  using acid etching technique, 13
  using orthodontic bands and arch wire, 13
  using wire ligature splint, 12
Spray
  phenol water as surface disinfectants, 66
  phenol-alcohol, as surface disinfectant, 66
Spray-wipe-spray technique as surface disinfectant, 66, 75, 79
S.S. White No. 211 clamp in routine endodontic therapy, 82, 112
Stabilization of teeth in traumatic injuries, 258, 259, 260
Staining in diagnosis of endodontic problems, 26, 33, 34–35, 36
Steam autoclave, sterilization and, 63, 65
Sterilizable handpieces, dental office infection control program and, 66, 74
Sterilization, 63–75, 76–77, 78, 79, 80
  biological chemical color indicator for monitoring, 75, 78

glass bead, 75, 77
of intracanal instruments, 75
minimum dental office infection control program in, 66–75, 76–77, 78, 79, 80
spray-wipe-spray method of, 66, 75, 79
surface disinfectants in, 66
for tray procedures, 75, 80
Stewart double-ended explorer, 208, 209
Stimulants, CNS, limitations on endodontic therapy because of, 21, 23
Subjective symptoms in diagnosis of endodontic problems, 25
Successfil, 141, 153–154
Sulfonamides, limitations on endodontic therapy because of, 21, 23
Surface disinfectants, sterilization and, 66
Surgical endodontics, 227–242
anesthesia for, 228, 229
apical seal in, 235
apicoectomy in, 227, 228
armamentarium for, 227, 228
crown sectioning in, 236, 237
flap design in, 228–231, 232
hemisection in, 236
incision and drainage in, 238–239
indications for, 227
for mandibular teeth, 233, 234
marsupialization in, 240–242
for maxillary posterior teeth, 233
postoperative instructions for, 242
procedure in, 228–242
root sectioning in, 236–237
trephination in, 240
Synthetic phenol combinations as surface disinfectants, 66

T
Teeth
anatomical variations in, 95–104
avulsed
in traumatic injuries, 258, 259
treatment of, 7, 12
discoloration of, in traumatic injuries, 246
endodontically treated, restoration of; see Restoration of endodontically treated tooth
extruded, in traumatic injuries, 256–257
intruded, in traumatic injuries, 256–257
invaginated, classification of, 96
length of, versus working length, 104, 130, 131
loosened, in traumatic injuries, 254, 255
luxated, in traumatic injuries, 254, 255
malpositioned, in traumatic injuries, 254, 255
mandibular, surgical endodontics for, 233, 234
mandibular anterior, access openings of, 119, 120
maxillary anterior, access openings of, 114, 117, 118
maxillary posterior, surgical endodontics for, 233
with most developmental anomalies, 98, 99, 100
non-vital; see Non-vital teeth
stabilization of, in traumatic injuries, 258, 259, 260
vitality of, in traumatic injuries, 244, 245
Telescoping, canal preparation and, 143
p-Tertiary amylphenol as surface disinfectant, 66
Test cavity preparation in diagnosis of endodontic problems, 26, 33
Tests
clinical
in diagnosis of endodontic problems, 26–36
diagnostic armamentarium for, 28–32

diagnostic, in diagnosis of endodontic problems, 26, 27, 28, 29, 30, 31, 32
selective, in diagnosis of endodontic problems, 26, 28, 33, 34–35, 36, 38
Tetracycline, limitations on endodontic therapy because of, 21, 23
Thermal test
cold, in diagnosis of endodontic problems, 26, 28, 29
hot, in diagnosis of endodontic problems, 26, 30
Toilet of cavity in routine endodontic therapy, 132
Touch 'N Heat instrument, 92, 162
Transillumination in diagnosis of endodontic problems, 26, 33, 34–35, 36
Transportation of foramina, postoperative discomfort caused by, 185, 186
Traumatic injuries, 243–272
avulsed teeth in, 258, 259
cracked tooth syndrome in, 262, 263
crown fracture subgingivally in, 250, 251
crown fracture with pulp exposure in, 249
and root fully formed in, 250
discoloration of teeth in, 246
examination of, 243
extruded teeth in, 256–257
fractures of enamel and dentin with no pulp exposure in, 248
hard tissue examination in, 244
horizontal root fractures in, 267–269, 270, 271
incomplete root in, 249
intruded teeth in, 256–257
loosened teeth in, 254, 255
luxated teeth in, 254, 255
malpositioned teeth in, 254, 255
non-vital teeth, treated or untreated and partially erupted, in, 261
postoperative examination and monitoring of, 272
radiographs of, 243
root fractures in, 261–269, 270, 271
simple enamel fractures in, 247
soft tissue examination in, 244
stabilization of teeth in, 258, 259, 260
traumatized immature non-vital teeth in, 252–253
vertical root fractures in, 261–265, 266
vitality of teeth in, 244, 245
Traumatized immature non-vital teeth in traumatic injuries, 252–253
Tray instruments, 75, 80
Trephination in surgical endodontics, 240
Tytin, 176

U
Ulcers, limitations on endodontic therapy because of, 21, 23
Ultrafil; see Low temperature thermoplasticized gutta percha
Ultrasonic cleaner, dental office infection control program and, 66, 75
Ultrasound scaler, 198, 208, 209, 218, 222
Universal precautions, dental office infection control program and, 66, 68–70

V
Vaccine, hepatitis B, dental office infection control program and, 66
Valient, 176
Vapor, chemical, sterilization and, 63, 65
Velvachol, 225
Versadowel, 172, 179
Vertical condensation
with chloropercha, 164–167

Vertical condensation—cont'd
  with warm gutta-percha, 160–163
Vertical root fractures in traumatic injuries, 261–265, 266
Vital bleaching, 7, 15
Vitality of teeth in traumatic injuries, 244, 245

W
Waste disposal, regulated, dental office infection control program and, 66, 74
Wire ligature splint, splinting technique using, 13

Working length versus tooth length, 104, 130, 131
Written exposure control plan, dental office infection control program and, 66, 68

X
XCP film holder, 106, 107
X-rays; *see* Radiography, endodontic

Z
ZOE, removal of, 225